T0252622

# Color Image Processing

## Methods and Applications

# IMAGE PROCESSING SERIES

Series Editor: Phillip A. Laplante, Pennsylvania State University

## *Published Titles*

**Adaptive Image Processing: A Computational Intelligence Perspective**
Stuart William Perry, Hau-San Wong, and Ling Guan

**Color Image Processing: Methods and Applications**
Rastislav Lukac and Konstantinos N. Plataniotis

**Image Acquisition and Processing with LabVIEW™**
Christopher G. Relf

**Image and Video Compression for Multimedia Engineering**
Yun Q. Shi and Huiyang Sun

**Multimedia Image and Video Processing**
Ling Guan, S.Y. Kung, and Jan Larsen

**Shape Analysis and Classification: Theory and Practice**
Luciano da Fontoura Costa and Roberto Marcondes Cesar Jr.

**Software Engineering for Image Processing Systems**
Phillip A. Laplante

# Color Image Processing

## Methods and Applications

### Edited by

## Rastislav Lukac
*University of Toronto*
*Toronto, Ontario, Canada*

## Konstantinos N. Plataniotis
*University of Toronto*
*Toronto, Ontario, Canada*

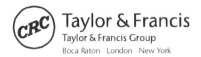 Taylor & Francis
Taylor & Francis Group
Boca Raton   London   New York

CRC is an imprint of the Taylor & Francis Group,
an informa business

CRC Press
Taylor & Francis Group
6000 Broken Sound Parkway NW, Suite 300
Boca Raton, FL 33487-2742

© 2007 by Taylor & Francis Group, LLC
CRC Press is an imprint of Taylor & Francis Group, an Informa business

No claim to original U.S. Government works
Printed in the United States of America on acid-free paper
10 9 8 7 6 5 4 3 2 1

International Standard Book Number-10: 0-8493-9774-X (Hardcover)
International Standard Book Number-13: 978-0-8493-9774-5 (Hardcover)

**Visit the Taylor & Francis Web site at**
**http://www.taylorandfrancis.com**

**and the CRC Press Web site at**
**http://www.crcpress.com**

*Color television! Bah, I won't believe it until I see it in black and white.*

—*Samuel Goldwyn, movie producer*

# *Dedication*

*To my dear parents, whose constant love and support*

*have made my achievements possible.*

*R. Lukac*

*To the loving memory of my father.*

*K.N. Plataniotis*

# *Preface*

Over the last two decades, we have witnessed an explosive growth in both the diversity of techniques and the range of applications of image processing. However, the area of color image processing is still sporadically covered, despite having become commonplace, with consumers choosing the convenience of color imaging over traditional grayscale imaging. With advances in image sensors, digital TV, image databases, and video and multimedia systems, and with the proliferation of color printers, color image displays, DVD devices, and especially digital cameras and image-enabled consumer electronics, color image processing appears to have become the main focus of the image-processing research community. Processing color images or, more generally, processing multichannel images, such as satellite images, color filter array images, microarray images, and color video sequences, is a nontrivial extension of the classical grayscale processing. Indeed, the vectorial nature of multichannel images suggests a different approach — that of vector algebra and vector fields — should be utilized in approaching this research problem. Recently, there have been many color image processing and analysis solutions, and many interesting results have been reported concerning filtering, enhancement, restoration, edge detection, analysis, compression, preservation, manipulation, and evaluation of color images. The surge of emerging applications, such as single-sensor imaging, color-based multimedia, digital rights management, art, and biomedical applications, indicates that the demand for color imaging solutions will grow considerably in the next decade.

The purpose of this book is to fill the existing literature gap and comprehensively cover the system, processing and application aspects of digital color imaging. Due to the rapid developments in specialized areas of color image processing, this book has the form of a contributed volume, in which well-known experts address specific research and application problems. It presents the state-of-the-art as well as the most recent trends in color image processing and applications. It serves the needs of different readers at different levels. It can be used as a textbook in support of a graduate course in image processing or as a stand-alone reference for graduate students, researchers, and practitioners. For example, the researcher can use it as an up-to-date reference, because it offers a broad survey of the relevant literature. Finally, practicing engineers may find it useful in the design and the implementation of various image- and video-processing tasks.

In this book, recent advances in digital color imaging and multichannel image-processing methods are detailed, and emerging color image, video, multimedia, and biomedical processing applications are explored. The first few chapters focus on color fundamentals, targeting three critical areas: color management, gamut mapping, and color constancy. The remaining chapters explore color image processing approaches across a broad spectrum of emerging applications ranging from vector processing of color images, segmentation, resizing and compression, halftoning, secure imaging, feature detection and extraction, image retrieval, semantic processing, face detection, eye tracking, biomedical retina image analysis, real-time processing, digital camera image processing, spectral imaging, enhancement for plasma display panels, virtual restoration of artwork, image colorization, superresolution image reconstruction, video coding, video shot segmentation, and surveillance.

Discussed in Chapters 1 to 3 are the concepts and technology essential to ensure constant color appearance in different devices and media. This part of the book covers issues related to color management, color gamut mapping, and color constancy. Given the fact that each digital imaging device exhibits unique characteristics, its calibration and characterization using a *color management system* are of paramount importance to obtain predictable and accurate results when transferring the color data from one device to another. Similarly, each media has its own achievable color gamut. This suggests that some colors can often not be reproduced to precisely match the original, thus requiring *gamut mapping* solutions to overcome the problem. Because the color recorded by the eye or a camera is a function of the reflectances in the scene and the prevailing illumination, *color constancy* algorithms are used to remove color bias due to illumination and restore the true color information of the surfaces.

The intention in Chapters 4 through 7 is to cover the basics and overview recent advances in traditional color image processing tasks, such as filtering, segmentation, resizing, and halftoning. Due to the presence of noise in many image processing systems, noise filtering or estimation of the original image information from noisy data is often used to improve the perceptual quality of an image. Because edges convey essential information about a visual scene, edge detection allows imaging systems to better mimic human perception of the environment. Modern *color image filtering* solutions that rely on the trichromatic theory of color are suitable for both of the above tasks. *Image segmentation* refers to partitioning the image into different regions that are homogeneous with respect to some image features. It is a complex process involving components relative to the analysis of color, shape, motion, and texture of objects in the visual data. Image segmentation is usually the first task in the lengthy process of deriving meaningful understanding of the visual input. *Image resizing* is often needed for the display, storage, and transmission of images. Resizing operations are usually performed in the spatial domain. However, as most images are stored in com-pressed formats, it is more attractive to perform resizing in a transform domain, such as the discrete cosine transform domain used in most compression engines. In this way, the computational overhead associated with the decompression and compression operations on the compressed stream can be considerably reduced. *Digital halftoning* is the method of reducing the number of gray levels or colors in a digital image while maintaining the visual illusion that the image still has a continuous-tone representation. Halftoning is needed to render a color image on devices that cannot support many levels or colors e.g., digital printers and low-cost displays. To improve a halftone image's natural appearance, color halftoning relies heavily on the properties of the human visual system.

Introduced in Chapter 8 is *secure color imaging* using secret sharing concepts. Essential encryption of private images, such as scanned documents and personal digital photographs, and their distribution in multimedia networks and mobile public networks, can be ensured by employing secret sharing-based image encryption technologies. The images, originally available in a binary or halftone format, can be directly decrypted by the human visual system at the expense of reduced visual quality. Using the symmetry between encryption and decryption functions, secure imaging solutions can be used to restore both binarized and continuous-tone secret color images in their original quality.

Important issues in the areas of object recognition, image matching, indexing, and retrieval are addressed in Chapters 9 to 11. Many of the above tasks rely on the use of discriminatory and robust *color feature detection* to improve color saliency and determine structural elements, such as shadows, highlights, and object edges and corners. Extracted features can help when grouping the image into distinctive parts so as to associate them with individual chromatic attributes and mutual spatial relationships. The utilization of both color and spatial information in *image retrieval* ensures effective access to archives and repositories of digital images. *Semantic processing* of color images can potentially increase the usability and applicability of color image databases and repositories. Application areas, such as in surveillance and authentication, content filtering, transcoding, and human and computer interaction, can benefit directly from improvements of tools and methodologies in color image analysis.

Face and eye-related color image processing are covered in Chapters 12 to 14. Color cues have been proven to be extremely useful in *facial image analysis*. However, the problem with color cue is its sensitivity to illumination variations that can significantly reduce the performance of face detection and recognition algorithms. Thus, understanding the effect of illumination and quantifying its influence on facial image analysis tools have become emerging areas of research. As the pupil and the sclera are different in color from each other and from the surrounding skin, color can also be seen as a useful cue in *eye detection and tracking*. Robust eye trackers usually utilize the information from both visible and invisible color spectra and are used in various human-computer interaction applications, such as fatigue and drowsiness detection and eye typing. Apart from biometrics and tracking applications, color image processing can be helpful in biomedical applications, such as in *automated identification of diabetic retinal exudates*. Diagnostic analysis of retinal photographs by an automated computerized system can detect disease in its early stage and reduce the cost of examination by an ophthalmologist.

Addressed in Chapters 15 through 18 is the important issue of color image acquisition, real-time processing and displaying. *Real-time imaging systems* comprise a special class of systems that underpin important application domains, including industrial, medical, and national defense. Understanding the hardware support is often fundamental to the analysis of real-time performance of a color imaging system. However, software, programming language, and implementation issues are also essential elements of a real-time imaging system, as algorithms must be implemented in some programming languages and hardware devices interface with the rest of the system using software components. A typical example of a real-time color imaging system is a digital camera. In the most popular camera configuration, the true color visual scene is captured using a color filter array-based single-image sensor, and the acquired data must be preprocessed, processed, and postprocessed to produce the captured color image in its desired quality and resolution. Thus, *single-sensor camera image processing* typically involves real-time interpolation solutions to complete demosaicking, enhancement, and zooming tasks. Real-time performance is also of paramount importance in *spectral imaging* for various industrial, agricultural, and environmental applications. Extending three color components up to hundreds or more spectral channels in different spectral bands requires dedicated sensors in particular spectral ranges and specialized image-processing solutions to enhance and display the spectral image data. Most display technologies have to efficiently render the image data in the highest visual quality. For instance, *plasma display panels* use image enhancement to faithfully reproduce dark areas, reduce dynamic false contours, and ensure color fidelity.

Other applications of color image enhancement are dealt with in Chapters 19 to 21. Recent advances in electronic imaging have allowed for *virtual restoration of artwork* using digital image processing and restoration techniques. The usefulness of this particular kind of restoration consists of the possibility to use it as a guide to the actual restoration of the artwork or to produce a digitally restored version of the artwork, as it was originally. *Image and video colorization* adds the desired color to a monochrome image or movie in a fully automated manner or based on a few scribbles supplied by the user. By transferring the geometry of the given luminance image to the three-dimensional space of color data, the color is inpainted, constrained both by the monochrome image geometry and the provided color samples. Apart from the above applications, *superresolution color image reconstruction* aims to reduce the cost of optical devices and overcome the resolution limitations of image sensors by producing a high-resolution image from a sequence of low-resolution images. Because each video frame or color channel may bring unique information to the reconstruction process, the use of multiple low-resolution frames or channels provides the opportunity to generate the desired output in higher quality.

Finally, various issues in color video processing are discussed in Chapters 22 through 24. *Coding of image sequences* is essential in providing bandwidth efficiency without sacrificing video quality. Reducing the bit rate needed for the representation of a video sequence enables the transmission of the stream over a communication channel or its storage in an optical medium. To obtain the desired coding performance, efficient video coding algorithms usually rely on motion estimation and geometrical models of the object in the visual scene. Because the temporal nature of video is responsible for its semantic richness, temporal video segmentation using *shot boundary detection* algorithms is often a necessary first step in many video-processing tasks. The process segments the video into a sequence of scenes, which are subsequently segmented into a sequence of shots. Each shot can be represented by a key-frame. Indexing the above units allows for efficient video browsing and retrieval. Apart from traditional video and multimedia applications, the processing of color image sequences constitutes the basis for the development of *automatic video systems for surveillance applications*. For instance, the use of color information assists operators in classifying and understanding complex scenes, detecting changes and objects on the scene, focusing attention on objects of interest and tracking objects of interest.

The bibliographic links included in the various chapters of the book provide a good basis for further exploration of the topics covered in this edited volume. This volume includes numerous examples and illustrations of color image processing results, as well as tables summarizing the results of quantitative analysis studies. Complementary material including full-color electronic versions of results reported in this volume are available online at http://colorimageprocessing.org.

We would like to thank the contributors for their effort, valuable time, and motivation to enhance the profession by providing material for a fairly wide audience, while still offering their individual research insights and opinions. We are very grateful for their enthusiastic support, timely response, and willingness to incorporate suggestions from us, from other contributing authors, and from a number of colleagues in the field who served as reviewers. Particular thanks are due to the reviewers, whose input helped to improve the quality of the contributions. Finally, a word of appreciation goes to CRC Press for giving us the opportunity to edit a book on color image processing. In particular, we would like to thank Dr. Phillip A. Laplante for his encouragement, Nora Konopka for initiating this project, Jim McGovern for handling the copy editing and final production, and Helena Redshaw for her support and assistance at all times.

**Rastislav Lukac and Konstantinos N. Plataniotis**
University of Toronto, Toronto, Ontario, Canada
lukacr@ieee.org, kostas@dsp.utoronto.ca

# The Editors

**Rastislav Lukac** (www.colorimageprocessing.com) received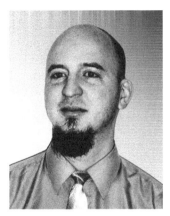
the M.S. (Ing.) and Ph.D. degrees in telecommunications from
the Technical University of Kosice, Slovak Republic, in 1998
and 2001, respectively. From February 2001 to August 2002, he
was an assistant professor with the Department of Electronics
and Multimedia Communications at the Technical University
of Kosice. From August 2002 to July 2003, he was a researcher
with the Slovak Image Processing Center in Dobsina, Slovak
Republic. From January 2003 to March 2003, he was a postdoctoral fellow with the Artificial Intelligence and Information Analysis Laboratory, Aristotle University of Thessaloniki,
Greece. Since May 2003, he has been a postdoctoral fellow
with the Edward S. Rogers Sr. Department of Electrical and
Computer Engineering, University of Toronto, Toronto, Canada. He is a contributor to four
books, and he has published over 200 papers in the areas of digital camera image processing,
color image and video processing, multimedia security, and microarray image processing.

Dr. Lukac is a member of the Institute of Electrical and Electronics Engineers (IEEE),
The European Association for Signal, Speech and Image Processing (EURASIP), and IEEE
Circuits and Systems, IEEE Consumer Electronics, and IEEE Signal Processing societies.
He is a guest coeditor of the *Real-Time Imaging*, Special Issue on Multi-Dimensional Image
Processing, and of the *Computer Vision and Image Understanding*, Special Issue on Color Image
Processing for Computer Vision and Image Understanding. He is an associate editor for the
*Journal of Real-Time Image Processing*. He serves as a technical reviewer for various scientific
journals, and he participates as a member of numerous international conference committees.
In 2003, he was the recipient of the North Atlantic Treaty Organization/National Sciences
and Engineering Research Council of Canada (NATO/NSERC) Science Award.

**Konstantinos N. Plataniotis** (www.dsp.utoronto.ca/~kostas)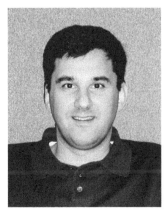
received the B. Engineering degree in computer engineering
from the Department of Computer Engineering and Informatics, University of Patras, Patras, Greece, in 1988 and the M.S.
and Ph.D. degrees in electrical engineering from the Florida
Institute of Technology (Florida Tech), Melbourne, Florida, in
1992 and 1994, respectively. From August 1997 to June 1999,
he was an assistant professor with the School of Computer
Science at Ryerson University. He is currently an associate
professor at the Edward S. Rogers Sr. Department of Electrical
and Computer Engineering where he researches and teaches
image processing, adaptive systems, and multimedia signal
processing. He coauthored, with A.N. Venetsanopoulos, a

book entitled *Color Image Processing & Applications* (Springer Verlag, May 2000), he is a contributor to seven books, and he has published more than 300 papers in refereed journals and conference proceedings in the areas of multimedia signal processing, image processing, adaptive systems, communications systems, and stochastic estimation.

Dr. Plataniotis is a senior member of the Institute of Electrical and Electronics Engineers (IEEE), an associate editor for the *IEEE Transactions on Neural Networks*, and a past member of the IEEE Technical Committee on Neural Networks for Signal Processing. He was the Technical Co-Chair of the Canadian Conference on Electrical and Computer Engineering (CCECE) 2001, and CCECE 2004. He is the Technical Program Chair of the 2006 IEEE International Conference in Multimedia and Expo (ICME 2006), the Vice-Chair for the 2006 IEEE Intelligent Transportation Systems Conference (ITSC 2006), and the Image Processing Area Editor for the IEEE Signal Processing Society e-letter. He is the 2005 IEEE Canada Outstanding Engineering Educator Award recipient and the corecipient of the 2006 IEEE Transactions on Neural Networks Outstanding Paper Award.

# Contributors

**Abhay Sharma**   Ryerson University, Toronto, Ontario, Canada

**Hiroaki Kotera**   Chiba University, Chiba, Japan

**Ryoichi Saito**   Chiba University, Chiba, Japan

**Graham D. Finlayson**   University of East Anglia, Norwich, United Kingdom

**Bogdan Smolka**   Silesian University of Technology, Gliwice, Poland

**Anastasios N. Venetsanopoulos**   University of Toronto, Toronto, Ontario, Canada

**Henryk Palus**   Silesian University of Technology, Gliwice, Poland

**Jayanta Mukherjee**   Indian Institute of Technology, Kharagpur, India

**Sanjit K. Mitra**   University of California, Santa Barbara, California, USA

**Vishal Monga**   Xerox Innovation Group, El Segundo, California, USA

**Niranjan Damera-Venkata**   Hewlett-Packard Labs, Palo Alto, California, USA

**Brian L. Evans**   The University of Texas, Austin, Texas, USA

**Rastislav Lukac**   University of Toronto, Toronto, Ontario, Canada

**Konstantinos N. Plataniotis**   University of Toronto, Toronto, Ontario, Canada

**Theo Gevers**   University of Amsterdam, Amsterdam, The Netherlands

**Joost van de Weijer**   INRIA, Grenoble, France

**Harro Stokman**   University of Amsterdam, Amsterdam, The Netherlands

**Stefano Berretti**   Università degli Studi di Firenze, Firenze, Italy

**Alberto Del Bimbo**   Università degli Studi di Firenze, Firenze, Italy

**Stamatia Dasiopoulou**   Aristotle University of Thessaloniki, Thessaloniki, Greece

**Evaggelos Spyrou**   National Technical University of Athens, Zografou, Greece

**Yiannis Kompatsiaris**   Informatics and Telematics Institute, Thessaloniki, Greece

**Yannis Avrithis**   National Technical University of Athens, Zografou, Greece

**Michael G. Strintzis**   Informatics and Telematics Institute, Thessaloniki, Greece

**Birgitta Martinkauppi**   University of Joensuu, Joensuu, Finland

**Abdenour Hadid**   University of Oulu, Oulu, Finland

**Matti Pietikäinen**   University of Oulu, Oulu, Finland

**Dan Witzner Hansen**   IT University of Copenhagen, Copenhagen, Denmark

**Alireza Osareh**   Chamran University of Ahvaz, Ahvaz, Iran

**Phillip A. Laplante**   Penn State University, Malvern, Pennsylvania, USA

**Pamela Vercellone-Smith**   Penn State University, Malvern, Pennsylvania, USA

**Matthias F. Carlsohn**   Engineering and Consultancy Dr. Carlsohn, Bremen, Germany

**Bjoern H. Menze**   University of Heidelberg, Heidelberg, Germany

**B. Michael Kelm**   University of Heidelberg, Heidelberg, Germany

**Fred A. Hamprecht**   University of Heidelberg, Heidelberg, Germany

**Andreas Kercek**   Carinthian Tech Research AG, Villach/St. Magdalen, Austria

**Raimund Leitner**   Carinthian Tech Research AG, Villach/St. Magdalen, Austria

**Gerrit Polder**   Wageningen University, Wageningen, The Netherlands

**Choon-Woo Kim**   Inha University, Incheon, Korea

**Yu-Hoon Kim**   Inha University, Incheon, Korea

**Hwa-Seok Seong**   Samsung Electronics Co., Gyeonggi-Do, Korea

**Alessia De Rosa**   University of Florence, Firenze, Italy

**Alessandro Piva**   University of Florence, Firenze, Italy

**Vito Cappellini**   University of Florence, Firenze, Italy

**Liron Yatziv**   Siemens Corporate Research, Princeton, New Jersey, USA

**Guillermo Sapiro**   University of Minnesota, Minneapolis, Minnesota, USA

**Hu He**   State University of New York at Buffalo, Buffalo, New York, USA

**Lisimachos P. Kondi**   State University of New York at Buffalo, Buffalo, New York, USA

**Savvas Argyropoulos**   Aristotle University of Thessaloniki, Thessaloniki, Greece

**Nikolaos V. Boulgouris**   King's College London, London, United Kingdom

**Nikolaos Thomos**   Informatics and Telematics Institute, Thessaloniki, Greece

**Costas Cotsaces**   University of Thessaloniki, Thessaloniki, Greece

**Zuzana Cernekova**   University of Thessaloniki, Thessaloniki, Greece

**Nikos Nikolaidis**   University of Thessaloniki, Thessaloniki, Greece

**Ioannis Pitas**   University of Thessaloniki, Thessaloniki, Greece

**Stefano Piva**   University of Genoa, Genoa, Italy

**Carlo S. Regazzoni**   University of Genoa, Genoa, Italy

**Marcella Spirito**   University of Genoa, Genoa, Italy

# Contents

# 1

## ICC Color Management: Architecture and Implementation

**Abhay Sharma**

## CONTENTS

## 1.1 Introduction

Color imaging devices such as scanners, cameras, and printers have always exhibited some variability or "personal characteristics." To achieve high-quality and accurate color, it is necessary to have a framework that accommodates these characteristics. There are two ways of making allowances for device characteristics. The old way is called closed-loop color, and the new way is known as open-loop color, that is, color management. Until the 1970s and 1980s, digital color was controlled using closed-loop systems in which all devices were designed and installed by one vendor. As the conditions for a closed-loop system (skilled personnel and a fixed workflow) disintegrated, something had to be done to get consistent, accurate color. The answer is an open-loop environment, also known as a color management system, such as that specified by the International Color Consortium (ICC). Open- and closed-loop color control systems are described in detail in Section 1.2.

The ICC color management system is based on various CIE (Commission Internationale de l'Eclairage) color measurement systems. CIE color measurement systems meet all technical requirements of a color specification system and provide the underpinning framework for color management today. In Section 1.3, we look at the specification of color using CIE XYZ, CIE LAB, and CIE Yxy.

The implementation of an ICC workflow requires an understanding of and adherence to the ICC specification. The current version of the specification is *Specification ICC.1:2004-10 (Profile version 4.2.0.0) Image technology colour management — Architecture, profile format, and data structure*. This is a technical document that describes the structure and format of ICC profiles including the profile header and tags. The document is designed for those who need to implement the specification in hardware and software. In Section 1.4, we describe salient aspects of the specification as applicable to practical implementation of an ICC system.

A color management process can be described as consisting of three "C"s: calibration, characterization, and conversion (Section 1.5). Calibration involves establishing a fixed, repeatable condition for a device. Calibration involves establishing some known starting condition and some means of returning the device to that state. After a device has been calibrated, its characteristic response is studied in a process known as characterization. In color management, characterization refers to the process of making a profile. During the profile generation process, the behavior of the device is studied by sending a reasonable sampling of color patches (a test chart) to the device and recording the device's colorimetric response. A mathematical relationship is then derived between the device values and corresponding CIE LAB data. This transform information is stored in (ICC standardized) single and multidimensional lookup tables. These lookup tables constitute the main component of an ICC profile. An explanation for lookup tables is presented in Section 1.5.3. Section 1.5.3 examines lookup tables in real profiles, thus clearly illustrating the whole basis for ICC color management.

The third *C* of color management is conversion, a process in which images are converted from one color space to another. Typically, for a scanner-to-printer scenario this may mean converting an image from scanner RGB (red, green, blue) via the scanner profile into LAB and then into appropriate CMYK (cyan, magenta, yellow, and black) via a printer profile, so that the image can be printed. The conversion process relies on application software (e.g., Adobe® Photoshop), system-level software (e.g., Apple® ColorSync), and a color management module (CMM). The three *C*s are hierarchical, which means that each process is dependent on the preceding step. Thus, characterization is only valid for a given calibration condition. The system must be stable, that is, the device must be consistent and not drift from its original calibration. If the calibration changes (e.g., if the response of the device changes), then the characterization must be redetermined. If the characterization is inaccurate this detrimentally affects the results of the conversion.

Creating products for an ICC-based workflow utilizes skills in software engineering, color science, and color engineering. This chapter serves as an introduction to some of the terminology, concepts, and vagaries that face software engineers and scientists as they seek to implement an ICC color managed system.

## 1.2 The Need for Color Management

Why do we need color management? Why do we have a problem with matching and controlling colors in digital imaging? Why can we not just scan a picture, look at it on the screen, and print it out and have the color match throughout? A fundamental issue with color imaging is that each device behaves differently. There are differences between two Hewlett-Packard (HP) scanners of the same make and model and even bigger differences between an HP and a Umax scanner. All digital imaging devices exhibit a unique characteristic, if device characteristics are left unchecked, this can lead to unpredictable and inaccurate results.

To illustrate the concept of device characteristics, consider the example of a scanner. An image from a scanner will generally be an RGB image in which each pixel in the image is specified by three numbers corresponding to red, green, and blue. If we use different scanners to scan the same sample, we get slightly different results. Figure 1.1 shows an experiment that was conducted with three scanners in the author's workplace. A simple red patch was scanned on HP, Heidelberg, and Umax scanners. The RGB pixel response of the HP scanner was 177, 15, 38; the Heidelberg scanner produced 170, 22, 24; and the Umax scanner produced 168, 27, 20. It is true that all results are indeed red, with most information in the red channel, but the results are slightly different, with each scanner creating a unique interpretation of identical scanned material.

Differences due to device characteristics are equally obvious when we print an image. CMYK values are instructions for a device and represent the amount of each colorant that is required to create a given color. Suppose we create a simple block image and fill it with some CMYK pixel values. Another test was conducted in the author's workplace, the simulated results of which are shown in Figure 1.2. The CMYK image was sent to three printers, each

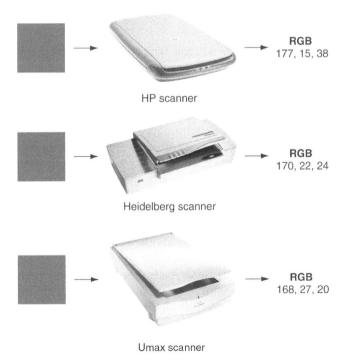

HP scanner

Heidelberg scanner

Umax scanner

**FIGURE 1.1**
Imaging devices exhibit unique characteristics. In an experiment, the same original when scanned on different scanners produced different RGB scan values.

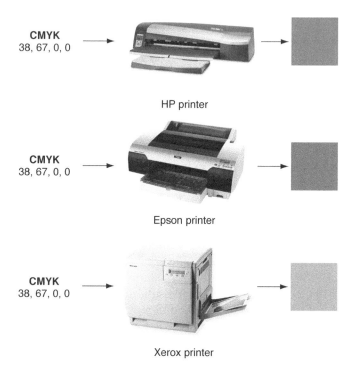

**FIGURE 1.2**
An image was created with CMYK values of 38, 67, 0, 0 and printed on HP, Epson, and Xerox printers. We see that the same digital file created very different results on each printer.

device received identical CMYK instructions, which instructed the printer to drop varying amounts of cyan, magenta, yellow, and black colorant on the paper. However, individual printers have different printing technologies, different inks, and different paper, and the colorants themselves may differ in color. Therefore, even if the instructions are meticulously obeyed by each printer, because the characteristics of each printing system are different, the printed results can be (and often are) dramatically different.

We see that at the scanner stage, the same color gets translated into different pixel values, due to camera or scanner characteristics. There are variations due to monitor characteristics that affect the displayed image. And, as clearly demonstrated by the printer example, every printer in an imaging chain has a unique (different) response to a given set of device instructions.

A common requirement of a color management system is to replicate the color produced by one device on a second system. To replicate the color produced by the HP printer on the Epson printer, for example, a color management system would alter the pixel value instructions destined for the Epson printer such that the instructions would be different but the printed color would be the same. Color management systems seek to quantify the color characteristics of a device and use this to alter the pixel values that must be sent to a device to achieve the desired color.

### 1.2.1  Closed-Loop Color Control

To achieve a desired color, it is necessary to alter the pixel values in a systematic way that is dependent on the characteristics of the destination device. There are two ways of making allowances for device characteristics. The old way is called closed-loop color, and the new way is known as open-loop color (e.g., a color management system such as that specified by the ICC).

Affordable devices for color imaging are a recent development that have come about because cheaper computer systems have brought the technology within the reach of the mass market. Until the 1970s and 1980s, digital color was the preserve of high-end systems such as those marketed by Crosfield Electronics, Hell, or Dainippon Screen. The same manufacturer would sell a color imaging suite that included the monitor, software, scanner, output, and so on. These were closed-loop systems in which all devices were designed and installed by one vendor. In this closely controlled situation, it was relatively easy to obtain the color we wanted. However, two important conditions had to be met: skilled personnel and a fixed workflow.

Closed-loop color was able to achieve high-quality results. In fact, closed-loop systems are still used in many color workflows today. However, there are many instances in which the demands of the modern imaging industry make closed-loop color appear very expensive, inflexible, proprietary, and personnel dependent.

## 1.2.2 Open-Loop Color Management

For many years, closed-loop color worked very well. The operator learned the device characteristics and then compensated for the devices' behavior by manually altering the image pixel values. Why is it not possible to simply extend that way of working to today's imaging environment? As shown in Figure 1.3, in modern workflows, images come from a number of places, are viewed on different displays, and are printed on different printer technologies. The closed-loop system of trying to compensate for the behavior of each device on

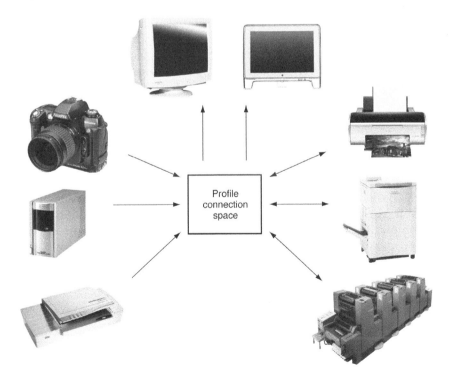

**FIGURE 1.3**

An open-loop color managed system uses a central connection space to connect many devices. Images arriving from a scanner can be sent to a monitor for viewing or a printer for printing.

a device-by-device basis is impractical and when used in modern workflows would lead to a large number of connections.

As the conditions for a closed-loop system (skilled personnel and a fixed workflow) disintegrated, something had to be done to get consistent, accurate color. The answer is an open-loop environment, also known as a color management system, such as that specified by the ICC. An ICC color management system provides an elegant solution to the issue of color control. Instead of connecting every device to every other device, a color management system connects all devices into and out of a central connecting space or "hub" (Figure 1.3). The official name for the central hub is the profile connection space (PCS). Computer files called ICC profiles are used to bring an image "into" or send an image "out of" the PCS. Thus, we need a scanner profile for a scanner, a monitor profile for a monitor, and a printer profile for a printer. An ICC profile encapsulates the characteristics of an imaging device and provides an automated compensation mechanism such that the correct (intended) color can be communicated and reproduced on any device in the imaging chain.

It is possible to calculate the number of connections required in the open- versus closed-loop systems. If you are trying to connect a group of devices $a$ to another group of devices $b$, in the closed-loop way of working, this requires $a \times b$ relationships, whereas for an open-loop system, these devices can be connected with a much smaller number of $a + b$ relationships.

### 1.2.2.1  *Device-Dependent and Device-Independent Color Specification*

Color specification, in this context, falls into two main categories — device-dependent and device-independent color. RGB and CMYK are instructions for a device and are necessarily in units that the device can understand and use. From the experiment described earlier, it is clear that the RGB values from a scanner are not a universal truth but are in fact very dependent on which scanner was used to scan the original. We also described an experiment in which the same CMYK pixel values were sent to different printers. You will recall that the same CMYK pixel values created a different color on each printer. In a device-dependent color specification, RGB or CMYK, for example, pixel values are merely instructions for a device, and the color that is produced will depend on the device being used.

CIE stands for Commission Internationale de l'Eclairage, which translates to International Commission on Illumination. CIE systems are standardized and dependable systems, so when a color is specified by one of these systems, it means the same thing to any user anywhere. One of the most useful CIE systems is CIE 1976 L*, a*, b*, with the official abbreviation of CIELAB. For clarity and brevity in this chapter, CIELAB is further shortened to LAB. The central color space (PCS) is encoded in LAB. LAB is dealt with in more detail in Section 1.3. CIE-based systems use a measuring instrument to sample a color and produce a numeric result. The measuring instrument does not need to know about the printer that produced a sample, it just measures the printed color patch. Therefore, we can say that CIE systems are independent of the underlying processes of any particular printer, scanner, or monitor system that produced the color. Unlike RGB and CMYK, a CIE color specification is not in a format that a device can understand or implement; more accurately, it can be thought of as a description or specification of a color. CIE color specification systems are scientifically proven, well-established methods of color measurement and form the backbone of nearly every color management process today.

### 1.2.2.2  *Profile Connection Space*

Let us return to our original problem. Why can we not take an image from a scanner, send it to a printer, and get the colors we want? The problem lies in specifying the color we want. For a scanner, an ICC profile is used to relate device-dependent RGB values to

LAB values. Thus, a profile contains data to convert between the RGB value each scanner produces and the LAB number for a color. Without the profile, we would be presented with a set of different RGB numbers with no way of knowing what color they are supposed to represent. In an ICC system, each scanner needs to have a different profile, and the profile must accompany the image from that scanner, thus allowing the device-dependent RGB values to be correctly interpreted. When you print an image, the process is reversed. That is, we specify a color in terms of LAB, and the printer profile establishes the necessary CMYK instructions specific to that printer to produce that color. In summary, the solution provided by ICC color management is to use a central common color scale and to relate device-specific scales to this central scale using profiles [1], [2].

Now that we have established the necessary vocabulary, we are in a position to provide a technical explanation for a color management system. A color management system uses software, hardware, and set procedures to control color across different media [3], [4]. In technical terms, an ICC color management system can be defined as a system that uses input and output profiles to convert device-dependent image data into and out of a central, device-independent PCS. Data in the PCS can be defined in terms of CIE LAB or CIE XYZ. Device characterization information is stored in profiles such that an input profile provides a mapping between input RGB data and the PCS, and an output profile provides a mapping between the PCS and output RGB/CMYK values.

## 1.3   CIE Color Measurement

In order to understand color measurement and color management it is necessary to consider human color vision. There are three things that affect the way a color is perceived by humans. First, there are the characteristics of the illumination. Second, there is the object. Third, there is the interpretation of this information in the eye/brain system of the human observer. CIE metrics incorporate these three quantities, making them correlate well with human perception.

### 1.3.1   CIE Color Matching Functions

Let us look in more detail at what constitutes the CIE color systems [5], [6]. There are three things that affect the way a color is perceived — the characteristics of the illumination, the object, and the interpretation of this information in the eye/brain system of the human observer. The light source is specified by data for the spectral energy distribution of a CIE illuminant and is readily available from a variety of literature sources [7]. The measured transmission or reflection spectrum describes the sample. Finally, it is necessary to quantify the human response. To contend with the issue of all observers seeing color slightly differently, the CIE has developed the concept of the "standard observer." The standard observer is assumed to represent the average of the human population having normal color vision [6]. The CIE specified three primary colors and conducted experiments to work out how much of each of the primaries are needed to match colors in the spectrum. The CIE transformed the original primaries into new primaries and in 1931 published the results as graphs called the color-matching functions (Figure 1.4). The color-matching functions are designated $\bar{x}, \bar{y}, \bar{z}$, (pronounced "xbar, ybar, zbar").

The CIE makes a significant contribution to the whole area of color measurement by providing data for the characteristics of an average human observer via the color-matching

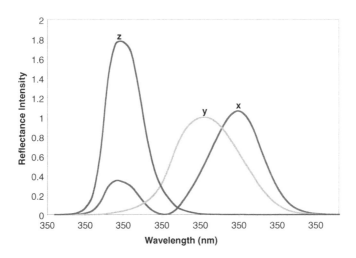

**FIGURE 1.4**
The CIE color-matching functions are assumed to represent the color-matching results of the average of the human population having normal color vision.

functions. Once we have the color-matching functions, then the measurement of color is derived from purely physical data (easily measured spectrophotometric data) and is based entirely on instrumental measurement.

### 1.3.2 CIE XYZ

In CIE systems, the starting point for all color specification is CIE XYZ. XYZ are known as tristimulus values, and it is customary to show them in capital letters to distinguish them from other similar notations. To arrive at X, Y, and Z values, we multiply together the three spectral data sets representing the light source $l(\lambda_i)$, the sample $r(\lambda_i)$, and the color-matching functions, $\bar{x}(\lambda_i)$, $\bar{y}(\lambda_i)$, or $\bar{z}(\lambda_i)$:

$$X = k \sum_{i=0}^{N-1} \bar{x}(\lambda_i) \, l(\lambda_i) \, r(\lambda_i)$$

$$Y = k \sum_{i=0}^{N-1} \bar{y}(\lambda_i) \, l(\lambda_i) \, r(\lambda_i)$$

$$Z = k \sum_{i=0}^{N-1} \bar{z}(\lambda_i) \, l(\lambda_i) \, r(\lambda_i) \tag{1.1}$$

where $(\lambda_i)_{i=0}^{N-1}$ are uniformly spaced wavelengths covering the visible region of the spectrum. The summation is specified at 1 nm intervals over the range of visible wavelengths, but for practical purposes, the summation may be approximated by coarser wavelength intervals of $\Delta\lambda = 5$ or 10 nm. Equation 1.1 is subject to a normalization process. CIE XYZ tristimulus values are fundamental measures of color and are directly used in a number of color management operations, especially, for example, in monitor profiles, where there is a relationship between input pixel values and tristimulus values. CIE XYZ does not give an immediately obvious representation of color, and for many user-level implementations, XYZ values can be transformed into other representations described in the following sections.

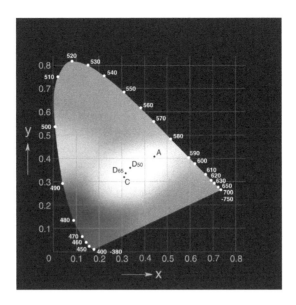

**FIGURE 1.5 (See color insert.)**
On the 1931 CIE *x*, *y* chromaticity diagram, the locus is labeled with the wavelength of the dominant hue. (Courtesy of X-Rite Incorporated.)

### 1.3.3 CIE *x*, *y* Chromaticity Diagram

The first system to consider is the CIE 1931 chromaticity diagram. In this system, a color is represented by its *x*, *y* coordinates and is plotted on a horseshoe-shaped diagram, an example of which is shown in Figure 1.5. This diagram is called the *x*, *y* chromaticity diagram, and *x*, *y* are known as chromaticity coordinates. It is possible to make a small calculation based on the XYZ value of a sample to obtain *x*, *y* which can then be plotted on this diagram to show the position of a color in this color space. From XYZ values, we can calculate *x*, *y* chromaticity coordinates using the following simple equations:

$$x = \frac{X}{(X+Y+Z)} \qquad\qquad y = \frac{Y}{(X+Y+Z)} \tag{1.2}$$

here *x*, *y* are the chromaticity coordinates, and *X*, *Y*, and *Z* are tristimulus values. By convention, the lowercase *x*, *y* is reserved for the chromaticity coordinates, and uppercase (capital) XYZ for the predecessor tristimulus values.

### 1.3.4 CIE LAB

Color scientists continue to develop new color spaces and variations of the XYZ color space with the goal of providing better correlation with the human perception of color. In the previous section, we saw how XYZ can be used as the basis for; in this section, we see how XYZ can be used as the basis for LAB, which is an improvement over the system.

The LAB diagram is a three-dimensional color diagram, a slice of which is shown in Figure 1.6. The color of a sample is specified by its "position" in this three-dimensional volume, expressed in LAB coordinates. The LAB system separates the color information into lightness ($L^*$) and color information ($a^*$, $b^*$) on a red/green ($a^*$) and yellow/blue ($b^*$) axis. The lightness of a color changes as a function of $L^*$, with $L^*$ of 0 representing black and $L^*$ of 100 representing white. As the position of a color moves from the central region toward the edge of the sphere, its saturation (or chroma) increases. As we go around the

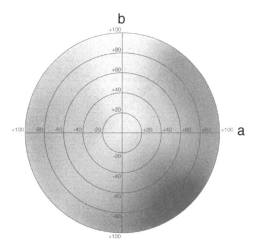

**FIGURE 1.6  (See color insert.)**
A slice through the CIE 1976 CIE L\*a\*b\* diagram shows colors arranged on a red/green ($a^*$) and yellow/blue ($b^*$) axis.

sphere, the hue angle (or dominant wavelength) changes. Thus, we see that all the attributes of color are clearly defined in the LAB system.

XYZ is used to derive LAB as follows:

$$L^* = 116 \left(\frac{Y}{Y_n}\right)^{1/3} - 16$$

$$a^* = 500 \left[\left(\frac{X}{X_n}\right)^{1/3} - \left(\frac{Y}{Y_n}\right)^{1/3}\right]$$

$$b^* = 200 \left[\left(\frac{Y}{Y_n}\right)^{1/3} - \left(\frac{Z}{Z_n}\right)^{1/3}\right] \tag{1.3}$$

here, $X$, $Y$, and $Z$ are the tristimulus values of the sample, and $X_n$, $Y_n$, and $Z_n$ are the tristimulus values of the reference illuminant (light source). There is a further correction to this equation for very dark colors. Note how much more complicated the LAB Equation 1.3 is compared to the $x, y$ Equation 1.2. The additional computation helps make the LAB system more perceptually uniform. In particular, note how the LAB equation involves functions raised to the power of 1/3 (a cube root function). The cube root function is a nonlinear function, which means that it compresses some values more than others — exactly the sort of correction we need to see happen to the colors in the $x, y$ chromaticity diagram. This equation is responsible for the better spacing of colors in the LAB diagram, such as in the green region. The other aspect of the XYZ to LAB conversion worth noting is that the equation explicitly considers the viewing illuminant, shown in the equation as $X_n$, $Y_n$, and $Z_n$. The interpretation of this is that LAB expresses the color of a sample as viewed under a particular illuminant, so that if we wanted to predict the color of a sample under a different illuminant, we could change the values of $X_n$, $Y_n$, and $Z_n$ in the equation.

A very important tool in color management is the ability to specify the color difference between two samples by a single number. Delta E is a measure of color difference and is the Euclidian distance between two samples in LAB space. There are a number of proposed improvements to the Delta E calculation. The new versions of Delta E are still based on LAB; the only thing that has changed is the way in which the calculation is done [6]. The new versions of Delta E are intended to improve perceptual uniformity [8]. The four main versions of Delta E are $\Delta E_{ab}^*$, $\Delta E_{CMC}$, $\Delta E_{94}^*$, and $\Delta E_{00}^*$. The version that has been referred to so far is $\Delta E_{ab}^*$. We have mentioned that the human eye is less sensitive to changes in lightness and more sensitive to changes in chroma. The Color Measurement Committee (CMC) of the Society of Dyers and Colourists in England uses a variation of Delta E in their work on textiles and threads. Their modification is called $\Delta E_{CMC(l:c)}$, which improves the prediction for very dark colors and near-neutral colors by introducing two variables, lightness and chroma ($l$ and $c$), whose ratio can be varied to weight the relative importance of lightness to chroma. Because the eye will generally accept larger differences in lightness ($l$) than in chroma ($c$), a default ratio for ($l$:$c$) is 2:1. The $\Delta E_{CMC}^*$ standard was adapted and adopted to become the CIE 1994 color-difference equation, bearing the symbol $\Delta E_{94}^*$ and the abbreviation CIE94. In 2000, another variation of Delta E was proposed, called the CIEDE2000 (symbol $\Delta E_{00}^*$).

## 1.4 ICC Specification and Profile Structure

An ICC profile is a data file that represents the color characteristics of an imaging device. ICC profiles can be made for scanners, digital cameras, monitors, or printers. There are even nondevice profiles such as device link profiles, and color space profiles for special situations. The structure of a profile is standardized by the ICC and strictly regulated so that a wide range of software, from many different vendors and at different parts of the workflow (e.g., image editing, preview, processing, Internet preparation, and printing), can open a profile and act on its contents.

The ICC is a regulatory body that supervises color management protocols between software vendors, equipment manufacturers, and users. Today's color management is basically "ICC-color management." The eight founding members of the ICC are Adobe, Agfa, Apple, Kodak, Taligent, Microsoft, Sun, and Silicon Graphics. Today, the ICC is open to all companies who work in fields related to color management. Members must sign a membership agreement and pay the dues. Currently, the ICC has over 70 member companies. The main work of the ICC is done via working groups, each dedicated to looking at a specific issue. Currently, there are Architecture, Communications, Digital Motion Picture, Digital Photography, Graphic Arts, Profile Assessment, Proof Certification, Specification Editing, and Workflow working groups. The outcomes of the ICC deliberations are communicated to users and vendors via the ICC profile specification. This is a technical document that describes the structure and format of ICC profiles and the Profile Connection Space. The document is designed for those who need to implement the specification in hardware and software. The specification continues to change and evolve. The current version of the specification is always available from the ICC Web site (www.color.org). At the time of writing, the current version and name of the document are *Specification ICC.1:2004-10 (Profile version 4.2.0.0) Image technology colour management — Architecture, profile format, and data structure.*

### 1.4.1 Profile Header

In accordance with the ICC specification, profiles consist of two parts (Figure 1.7): a header and tags. The profile header provides the necessary information to allow a receiving system to properly parse and sort a profile. The header is populated by the program that makes the profile. The profile header is 128 bytes in length and contains 18 fields. Each field in the header has a fixed byte position (offset), field length, and content. Having a header with a fixed size and structure allows for performance enhancements in profile searching

```
                    Size:  54,500 bytes
            Preferred CMM:  Apple
       Specification Version:  2.2.0
                   Class:  Output
                   Space:  CMYK
                     PCS:  Lab
                 Created:  11/4/02 12:00:12 PM
                Platform:  Apple
                   Flags:  Normal Quality
       Device Manufacturer:  Apple
            Device Model:
          Device Attributes:  00000000 00000000
          Rendering Intent:  Perceptual
            PCS Illuminant:  0.96420, 1.00000, 0.82491
                 Creator:  Apple
            MD5 Signature:
```

**FIGURE 1.7**
An ICC profile header contains 18 fields and tells us what type of profile it is, such as scanner, monitor, or printer.

and sorting. There are instances, in color space and abstract profiles for example, where some of these fields are not relevant and may be set to zero. Throughout the ICC architecture, in general, if a function is not needed, it may be set to zero. This process encourages inter-operability as it ensures that the profile has all required components and is in compliance with the specification.

Let us look at some of the important parts of the profile header. The value in the *Size* field will be the exact size obtained by combining the profile header, the tag table, and all the tagged element data. One of the first fields in the header is the *Preferred CMM*. CMM stands for color management module; it is the color engine that does the color conversions for an image on a pixel-by-pixel basis. When an image and profiles are sent to the CMM, the role of the CMM is to convert each pixel in the image from one color space encoding to another using the information in the profiles. CMMs are available from various vendors, including Adobe, Kodak, Heidelberg, and Apple. The CMM field in a profile header specifies the default CMM to be used. In many instances, software applications will offer a user-level menu that will override the CMM entry in the profile header. There may be a difference in the results obtained using different CMMs, but the intention is for all CMMs to behave in the same way. The *Specification Version* field corresponds to the version number of the ICC specification. Older profiles have version numbers of 2.0, and newer profiles should be 4.0. The version number is only changed when it is necessary that the CMM be upgraded in order to correctly use a profile.

One of the most significant parts of the header is the *Class* field. The profile or device Class tells us what type of profile it is, such as scanner, monitor, printer, and so on. There are seven profile Classes: display (mntr), input (scnr), output (prtr), device link (link), color space (spac), abstract (abst), and named color (nmcl). The reason the Class entry is important is that it indicates what sorts of tags to expect in the body of the profile. Most processing software will look first at the Class field. The *Space* and *PCS* fields indicate which color spaces the profile can convert between. Space refers to the device color space, and PCS refers to the Profile Connection Space. The device color Space will be either RGB or CMYK, and the PCS will be either CIE XYZ or CIE LAB. Profiles generally have the ability to convert data in both directions; that is, from PCS to device color Space and vice versa. The direction used to process the data is determined automatically, depending on the order in which the profiles are selected and presented to the CMM.

The profile header contains a *Flags* field. The Flags field is often neglected but can be very important. Part of the Flags field is reserved for use by the ICC and is used to specify issues such as whether the profile is embedded in an image or is a stand-alone profile. A color management system vendor, such as ColorSync, can use the remainder of the field. ColorSync uses the vendor's part of the Flags field for a quality setting. The quality setting controls the quality of the color-matching (conversion) process in relation to the time required to perform the match. There are three quality settings: normal (0), draft (1), and best (2). The procedure ColorSync uses to process image data is dependent on the quality setting. When you start a color-matching session, ColorSync sends the image and the required profiles to the CMM. The Apple CMM extracts the lookup tables it needs from the profiles and produces a new, single lookup table, in a process called lookup table concatenation. Using a single lookup table instead of separate lookup tables is a common technique in color imaging that speeds up conversion for runtime applications. The size of the new lookup table can be chosen so as to balance memory requirements, accuracy, and speed of color processing — the quality Flag directs how this is done. In current implementations, the normal and draft settings do similar things. When these quality settings are used, the Apple CMM is directed to make a new lookup table from the profiles sent to the CMM. In best-quality setting, however, the Apple CMM retains the original lookup tables from the profiles and does not create a new lookup table.

The *PCS Illuminant* is the reference light source. In the profile header, the light source would normally be D50, which has XYZ values of 0.9642, 1.000, and 0.8249. The illuminant is included as a changeable item as the ICC has long-term plans to extend the PCS to include other white points. Note that the white point in the header is different from the material/device white point. The PCS illuminant (reference white point) is specified in the header, and the white point of a monitor or inkjet paper is specified as a separate media white point tag in the tag field.

## 1.4.2 Profile Tags

Each profile contains a number of data records, called "tags." Some of the tags, such as those containing color lookup tables, provide data used in color transformations. The tag table acts as a table of contents for the tags and provides an index into the tag element data in the profile. The header is a standardized part of a profile and contains a fixed number of items. The tags, however, vary, depending on the type of device the profile is for (monitor, printer, and so on) and which profiling package was used to make the profile. The intent of requiring certain tags with each type of profile is to provide a common base level of functionality. If a proprietary color management procedure is not present, then the required tags should have enough information to allow the default engine to perform the requested color transformation.

The ICC specifies a list of generic tag encodings. For example, the red, green, blue, white point, and black point colorant tristimulus values are stored as an *XYZ Type* tag; copyright and characterization data are tags of *textType*; red, green and blue tone response curves are encoded as *curveType* tags. As many tags share a common tag type, this encourages tag type reuse and allows profile parsers to reuse code.

The ICC specifies a list of required tags for each class of profile. Without the required tags, the profiles are not a valid ICC profile. Properly written software applications should check a profile and reject it if it does not contain the minimum requirements for a particular profile class. We now look at required tags in more detail.

### 1.4.2.1 Lookup Table Tags

One of the main required tags in a profile is the lookup table tag. The color lookup table tag may be in either the Version 2 format (Figure 1.8) or Version 4 format (Figure 1.9). The version numbers refer to versions of the ICC specification. Both Version 2 and Version 4 lookup table tags consist of multiple components that provide parameters for color transformations between device space and the PCS. The lookup table tag can contain color conversion matrices, one-dimensional lookup tables, and multidimensional lookup tables [9]. The lookup table tag is very versatile and can transform between many color spaces;

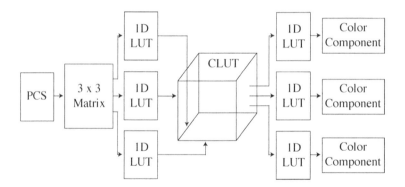

**FIGURE 1.8**
Version 2 ICC profiles have a number of components that can be used for color transformation.

for example, from scanner RGB to LAB, LAB to monitor RGB, LAB to CMYK, and CMYK to LAB. The number of channels at the input and the output of the lookup table will vary depending on the color space involved. It is not necessary for profile makers to use all elements in a lookup table tag, and in practice, they do not. If a vendor does not want to use part of a lookup table tag, the vendor can simply populate parts of the tag with null values (i.e., an identity response).

There are differences between Version 2 and Version 4 lookup table tags. The Version 2 data structure (Figure 1.8) has a matrix, a set of one-dimensional lookup tables, a multi-dimensional color lookup table (CLUT), and a final set of one-dimensional lookup tables. The Version 4 data structure (Figure 1.9) has a set of one-dimensional lookup tables, a matrix, another set of one-dimensional lookup tables, a multidimensional color lookup table (CLUT), and a final set of one-dimensional lookup tables. The lookup tables and associated structures are stored as an AToB or BToA tag in a profile. The interpretation of all the lookup tables is that AToB signifies a device-to-PCS lookup table, whereas the BToA tag is a PCS-to-device transform. Thus, an AToB lookup table is used to convert image data, for example, from RGB to LAB, while a BToA lookup table would be used to convert image data from LAB to RGB (or CMYK). Figure 1.9 shows the Version 4 "forward" (AToB) data structure, the Version 4 "inverse" (BToA) structure has the same blocks cascaded in the opposite order, improving composite transform accuracy when the forward and inverse transforms of a profile are combined.

Rendering intents are used to deal with differences between device gamuts and to deal with out of gamut colors. Four rendering intents (color rendering styles) are defined in the ICC specification (Table 1.1). Each rendering intent represents a different color

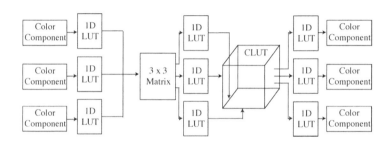

**FIGURE 1.9**
Version 4 ICC profiles can use a new lookup table data type that provides another set of one-dimensional lookup tables. An inverse form is also provided, in which the same blocks are cascaded in the opposite order.

**TABLE 1.1**

Rendering Intent and Lookup Table Designation

| Rendering Intent | Number | Tag Name | Tag Signature |
|---|---|---|---|
| Perceptual | 0 | AToB0/BToA0 | A2B0/B2A0 |
| Relative colorimetric | 1 | AToB1/BToA1 | A2B1/B2A1 |
| Saturation | 2 | AToB2/BToA2 | A2B2/B2A2 |
| Absolute colorimetric | 3 | — | — |

transformation pathway and is stored as a separate lookup table tag in an ICC profile. The perceptual intent operates on colorimetric values that are corrected in an as-needed fashion to account for any differences between devices, media, and viewing conditions. The perceptual intent is useful for general reproduction of pictorial images, and typically includes tone scale adjustments to map the dynamic range of one medium to that of another, and gamut mapping to deal with gamut mismatches. The color rendering of the perceptual intent is vendor specific, thus different vendors will populate the lookup tables with different transformations, even if working from the same input data. The colorimetric rendering intents operate directly on measured colorimetric values. When an exact color match is required for all in-gamut colors, the colorimetric rendering intent will define this. The saturation intent is used for images that contain objects such as charts or diagrams, and usually involves compromises such as trading off preservation of color accuracy in order to accentuate the vividness of pure colors. Table 1.1 shows no lookup table for the absolute colorimetric intent. Data for this lookup table is generated from data in the relative colorimetric lookup table.

## 1.4.3 Scanner Profile Tags

Now let us take a look at some of the required tags for each profile type. You will notice in the following tables that the first four tags are common to all profile types.

The scanner profile class can be used for devices such as scanners and digital cameras. It is typically used to convert RGB data into CIE LAB data. The minimum content of a scanner profile is outlined in Table 1.2. All profiles, including the scanner profile, must contain four tags: the Profile Description tag, Media White Point tag, Copyright tag, and Chromatic Adaptation tag. Conversion of RGB data to LAB data is done either by a matrix and tone reproduction curve tags or an AToB0 lookup table. Most vendors include both the matrix/tone curve tags and the lookup table. When data for more than one transformation

**TABLE 1.2**

Minimum Content of a Scanner Profile

| Tag | Tag Name | General Description |
|---|---|---|
| desc | Profile Description tag | Versions of the profile name for display in menus |
| wtpt | Media White Point tag | Media XYZ white point |
| cprt | Copyright tag | Profile copyright information |
| chad | Chromatic Adaptation tag | Method for converting a color from another illuminant to $D_{50}$ |
| rXYZ | Red Matrix Column tag | Matrix data for red column |
| gXYZ | Green Matrix Column tag | Matrix data for green column |
| bXYZ | Blue Matrix Column tag | Matrix data for blue column |
| rTRC | Red TRC tag | Red channel tone reproduction curve |
| gTRC | Green TRC tag | Green channel tone reproduction curve |
| bTRC | Blue TRC tag | Blue channel tone reproduction curve |
| A2B0 | AToB0 tag | Device-to-PCS lookup table |

method are included in the same profile, the CMM will always use the AToB0 lookup table, as this is a more accurate way of performing the conversion from RGB to LAB. In the situation where a profile is used as an input profile for a CMYK image, the matrix method does not suffice, and it is necessary to use the AToB0 lookup table form of the profile.

Occasionally, confusion arises due to changes in the ICC specification. In the early ICC specification, scanner profiles had only one lookup table, called the AToB0 tag. In the 1998 specification, the AToB1 and AToB2 tags for the scanner profile were mentioned but were undefined. In the current ICC specification (Version 4.2.0.0), all lookup tables are defined so that a scanner profile can contain the same set of lookup tables as all other profile types. Due to this historical background, there is potential for confusion with scanner profiles. Some applications can interpret the AToB0 tag in a scanner profile in the old sense, as simply the basic lookup table. However, in the new context, the AToB0 tag is a lookup table containing a specific rendering intent (the perceptual rendering intent) and is simply one of many lookup tables that can also include AToB1 (relative colorimetric) and AToB2 (saturation) lookup tables. It is important that profile-making programs, profile-using programs, and the CMM implement the new interpretation of these tags. An example of this problem occurs in Photoshop 6. Photoshop can use the Adobe CMM, called the Adobe Color Engine (ACE). In Photoshop 6, when the Image>Mode>Convert to Profile command is used, there is the option of selecting the rendering intent. When users select perceptual, relative colorimetric, or saturation intent, they expect to use the AToB0, AToB1, or AToB2 tag, respectively. However, the ACE CMM in Photoshop 6 always uses the AToB0 tag, irrespective of the user choice of rendering intent. This function has been corrected in Photoshop 7 onward. Another problem occurs when vendors do not use the rendering intent tags in accordance with the specification. A vendor may place colorimetric data (AToB1) in the perceptual (AToB0) tag or vice versa. It is interesting to note that the default behavior of GretagMacbeth ProfileMaker 5 is to make a scanner profile in which the colorimetric lookup table tag (AToB1) contains the contents of the perceptual lookup table (AToB0). To avoid any confusion, it is recommended that vendors populate lookup tables in complete accordance with the ICC specification and that Adobe® Photoshop be unambiguous in its use of rendering intents in all parts of the workflow.

### 1.4.4 Monitor Profile Tags

Monitor or display-class profiles can be used for cathode-ray tube (CRT) monitors or liquid crystal display (LCD) panels. The ICC specifies a list of required tags for this class of profile, as outlined in Table 1.3. Monitor profiles are required to have the same basic tags as do other

**TABLE 1.3**

Minimum Content of a Monitor Profile

| Tag | Tag Name | General Description |
| --- | --- | --- |
| desc | Profile Description tag | Versions of the profile name for display in menus |
| wtpt | Media White Point tag | Media XYZ white point |
| cprt | Copyright tag | Profile copyright information |
| chad | Chromatic Adaptation tag | Method for converting a color from another illuminant to $D_{50}$ |
| rXYZ | Red Matrix Column tag | Matrix data for red column |
| gXYZ | Green Matrix Column tag | Matrix data for green column |
| bXYZ | Blue Matrix Column tag | Matrix data for blue column |
| rTRC | Red TRC tag | Red channel tone reproduction curve |
| gTRC | Green TRC tag | Green channel tone reproduction curve |
| bTRC | Blue TRC tag | Blue channel tone reproduction curve |
| A2B0 | AToB0 tag | Device-to-PCS lookup table |
| B2A0 | BToA0 tag | PCS-to-device lookup table |

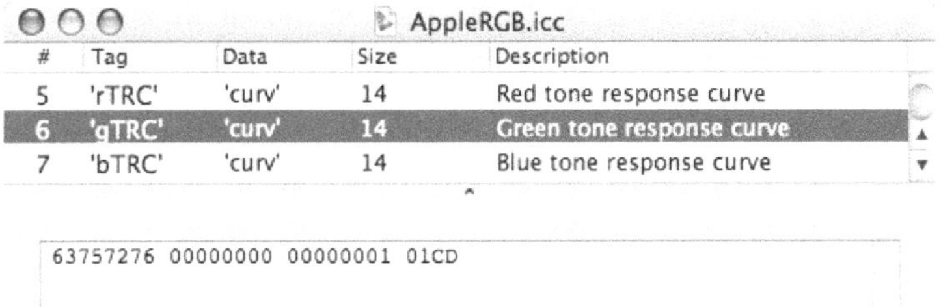

**FIGURE 1.10**
Apple ColorSync Utility can be used to view in detail the encoding of a TRC monitor tag as described in the text.

profile types. In addition to the basic tags, a monitor profile must have matrix and tone reproduction curve tags or lookup tables (AToB0 and BToA0).

As an example, let us look closer at one of the tags in a monitor profile. The lower part of Figure 1.10 shows the contents of the green response curve tag in a profile. (These details are obtained by using the alt-option key in Apple's ColorSync Utility.) This is a curveType tag. The tag signature is "curv," which is hex encoded in the first four bytes of the tag. For example, hex 63 = decimal 99 = ascii "c" and hex 75 = decimal 117 = ascii "u", and so forth. The next four bytes are reserved for future use and are set to 0. The next four bytes are a count value that specifies the number of entries to follow. If the count value is 0, then an identity response is assumed. If the count value is 1, then the value in the last part of the tag is interpreted as a gamma value. The data in the last part of the tag in this instance are stored as fixed unsigned two-byte/16-bit quantity that has eight fractional bits, so $01CD = 1 + \frac{205}{256} = 1.80$. In situations where the count value is greater than 1, the values that follow define a curve that embodies a sampled one-dimensional transfer function.

### 1.4.5  Printer Profile Tags

Printer profiles are used for output devices. They may be RGB devices (inkjet printers with a printer driver) or CMYK devices (inkjet printers with a Raster Image Processor (RIP) driver, laser printers, or printing presses), and they may have more color channels, depending on the process. In common with other profile types, the ICC specifies that a printer profile must contain four basic tags. A printer profile must also contain six lookup tables and a gamut tag as listed in Table 1.4. A printer profile contains tags for the perceptual, relative colorimetric, and saturation lookup tables. As described earlier, a profile does not contain a lookup table containing data for the absolute colorimetric rendering intent.

**TABLE 1.4**

Minimum Content of a Printer Profile

| Tag | Tag Name | General Description |
|---|---|---|
| desc | Profile Description tag | Versions of the profile name for display in menus |
| wtpt | Media White Point tag | Media XYZ white point |
| cprt | Copyright tag | Profile copyright information |
| chad | Chromatic Adaptation tag | Method for converting a color from another illuminant to $D_{50}$ |
| A2B0 | AToB0 tag | Device-to-PCS lookup table, perceptual intent |
| A2B1 | AToB1 tag | Device-to-PCS lookup table, relative colorimetric intent |
| A2B2 | AToB2 tag | Device-to-PCS lookup table, saturation intent |
| B2A0 | BToA0 tag | PCS-to-Device lookup table, perceptual intent |
| B2A1 | BToA1 tag | PCS-to-Device lookup table, relative colorimetric intent |
| B2A2 | BToA2 tag | PCS-to-Device lookup table, saturation intent |
| gamt | Gamut tag | Information on out-of-gamut colors |

The lookup tables in a printer profile are multidimensional, thus printer profiles can be quite large, with a file size of 2 to 3 MB. There is a way to make the file size smaller using the tag offset. The tag offset indicates the location of the tag's data. If you look closely at the tag offset in a profile, you will often see that some tags have identical offsets. In this way, the same data are reused for different tags. This technique is often used in profiles where a vendor must include a number of required tags to produce a valid ICC profile, but the vendor has not prepared special data for that tag content. Reusing tags can be done in all profile types and can be used to reduce file size. The structure of a printer profile lookup table tag is described in more detail in Section 1.5.3.

## 1.5   Device Calibration and Characterization

The practical implementation of color management can be described as consisting of three "C"s: calibration, characterization, and conversion. Calibration involves establishing a fixed, repeatable condition for a device. For a scanner, this may involve scanning a white plaque; for a monitor, this may mean adjusting the contrast and brightness controls; for a printer, this may involve software ink limiting and linearization and agreeing on a paper and ink combination. Anything that alters the color response of the system must be identified and "locked down." Calibration thus involves establishing some known starting condition and some means of returning the device to that state. It is important for subsequent processes that the device maintain a fixed color response.

After a device has been calibrated, its characteristic response is studied in a process known as characterization. In color management, characterization refers to the process of making a profile. During the profile generation process, the behavior of the device is studied by sending a reasonable sampling of color patches (a test chart) to the device and recording the device's response. A mathematical relationship is then derived between the device values and corresponding LAB data. This transform information is stored in single and multidimensional lookup tables. During characterization, the gamut of the device is implicitly quantified.

Conversion is a process in which images are converted from one color space to another using a CMM. We now consider the calibration and characterization procedures for scanner, monitor, and print processes.

### 1.5.1   Scanner Characterization

In an ICC system, the input profile provides a transformation between scanner RGB and device-independent CIE XYZ or CIE LAB. The process of generating and storing this transform is called characterization. To construct the transform, a scan is made of a standard characterization test chart such as the IT8.7/1 (transparency) or IT8.7/2 (reflection) target to obtain scanner RGB values (Figure 1.11). The test chart patches are also measured using an instrument such as a spectrophotometer to provide corresponding LAB colorimetry.

The characterization process seeks to determine the relationship between scanner RGB and corresponding LAB or XYZ values. A number of different ways to establish this transform relationship are described in the literature. It is possible to use data-fitting processes that can range from a simple linear matrix approximation to higher-order polynomial regression [10]. Due to the nonlinear relationship between dye density and tristimulus value, Charge-Coupled Device (CCD) flatbed scanners that are primarily designed to measure photographic densities are poorly characterized by a linear transformation [11]. The transform between scanner RGB and LAB is, therefore, most commonly computed using

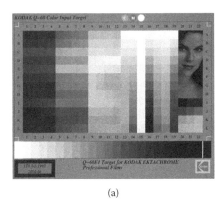 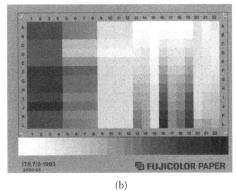

(a)                    (b)

**FIGURE 1.11 (See color insert.)**
(a) The IT8.7/1 is a transparency scanner target, and (b) the IT8.7/2 is for reflection prints.

polynomial regression. It may be necessary to use a higher-order polynomial least squares fit process to adequately characterize the scanner response [12]. The order of the polynomial needs to be carefully chosen so as to maximize colorimetric accuracy without introducing unwanted artifacts. To create a better fit to the data, polynomial regression analysis can be used in conjunction with some prelinearization [13], and often, it is found that mapping RGB to XYZ is preferable to mapping RGB to LAB.

It is often necessary to evaluate the accuracy of an input profile. To test an input profile, we first make an input profile in the normal way. To construct an input profile, a scan is made of the standard characterization test chart to obtain scanner RGB values. The reference file for the test chart containing corresponding XYZ/LAB values is obtained. The scan of the chart and the reference file are provided to a commercial profile-making package that computes the mapping transform between RGB and LAB, populates the lookup tables, and saves the result as an ICC input profile.

To compute a Delta E accuracy metric, the RGB values of the scanned chart image are processed through the input profile to arrive at processed LAB values. A program such as Adobe Photoshop can be used to do this. The processed LAB values are compared to reference LAB values. Ideally, the processed data should be numerically equivalent to the reference data. Due to fitting processes and interpolation errors, there is likely to be a difference between these two values. A Delta E difference can be calculated between the processed LAB data, and the reference LAB data, and this forms a metric for input profile quality. This simple result is a guide to the accuracy of the input profile and is a useful metric that can be used to assess the relative quality of input profiles from different sources for the same data set. A recent study compared accuracies of ICC device profiles made by different vendors [14].

### 1.5.2 Monitor Characterization

Characterization for a monitor is the process of describing the color characteristics of a monitor and creating a profile within which to store that data. The response of a monitor is generally characterized by a linear expression (the phosphor matrix) combined with a nonlinear expression (the $\gamma$ curve) [15], [16]. Thus, monitor profiles are simple profiles that contain primarily a matrix, a set of tone reproduction curves, and the device's white point. Monitor profiling often combines calibration and characterization into a single step. It is possible to calibrate a monitor (i.e., adjust the response of the monitor to some predetermined condition, for examples, a chosen white point and gamma). To calibrate a monitor,

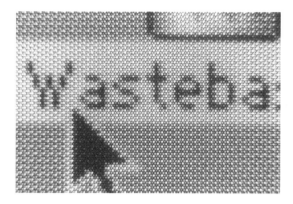

**FIGURE 1.12** (See color insert.)
CRT displays create color using red, green, and blue phosphor dots. The "color" of the monitor phosphors is measured in terms of XYZ. The phosphor dot pitch is 0.2 mm.

special lookup tables can be downloaded to the computer's video card to alter the response of the monitor. These lookup tables can change a monitor's white point and gamma. The monitor is then characterized by saving information regarding this new condition in a monitor profile. We can say that calibration is an active process during which we adjust the behavior of the monitor, and characterization is a passive process in which we simply record the characteristics of the device in its new current state.

CRT displays create images using phosphor dots that are electrically excited, causing them to glow and produce emissive light (Figure 1.12). The "color" of the phosphor dots can vary from monitor to monitor and manufacturer to manufacturer. In addition, aging effects can alter the phosphor emissivity. As all monitor phosphors are slightly different, characterization involves measuring the color of the phosphors and storing this information in a profile. To do this, the red, green, and blue phosphor groups are turned on by sending to the monitor RGB pixel values of (255, 0, 0), (0, 255, 0), and (0, 0, 255), respectively. The XYZ chromaticity values of the red, green, and blue phosphors are measured using an externally applied measuring instrument and are stored in the profile in the rXYZ, gXYZ, and bXYZ tags (Figure 1.13a). A white patch is created by displaying RGB pixel values (255, 255, 255), and the XYZ values of this patch are measured and stored in the white point (wtpt) tag (Figure 1.13b).

To determine the gamma of a display, we create a red ramp on the monitor consisting of RGB pixel values (0, 0, 0), (15, 0, 0) . . . (255, 0, 0). The luminance (Y) of these patches is measured. If we plot log normalized RGB versus log normalized Y, and fit a straight line to the data, then the slope of the line is defined as the gamma of the display. We repeat the process for the green and blue channels. After the gamma has been measured, it is stored in the TRC (tone reproduction curve) tag in the profile (Figure 1.13c). It is possible to have different gamma values for each of the red, green, and blue channels, and thus a monitor profile contains three tags: rTRC, gTRC, and bTRC. When an image is being sent to the display, the program finds out about the monitor condition from the content of the TRC tag and adjusts for the gamma value being used on that display. This is how images can look correct on different gamma systems (e.g., on Macintosh or Windows PC). It is less important to have a particular gamma value (1.8, 2.0, 2.2, etc.); it is more important that the gamma value of your monitor is accurately measured and stored in the TRC tag in the monitor profile.

Prior to characterization, a monitor may be calibrated to a "standard" gamma. To do this, the inherent, factory response of the system is determined. Then the software asks the user

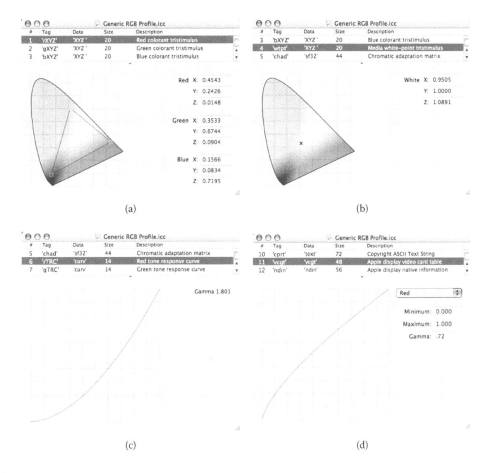

**FIGURE 1.13**
XYZ tags are used to store the monitor colorants (a), and monitor white point data (b), A tone reproduction curve tag is used to store the monitor gamma value (c), and the video card gamma correction (d).

for the required gamma. A correction is calculated and stored in a profile tag called the vcgt (video card gamma tag) (Figure 1.13d). Upon selection of a monitor profile, the data from the vcgt tag is downloaded to the video card, and the vcgt tag data in conjunction with the factory response cause the monitor to exhibit the user-requested gamma. We see that the shape of the vcgt tag data is "opposite" to the normal gamma, as it often acts to change the factory standard gamma of 3.0 to the more common gamma of 1.8 or 2.2.

### 1.5.3 Printer Characterization

The process of making a printer profile can be described in terms of calibration and characterization [17]. On inkjet printers, calibration may involve self-calibration, where the printer prints a test chart and measures it as it is being printed. Ink limiting and linearization are procedures routinely used with inkjet printers prior to characterization. Consumer desktop printers often have no explicit calibration of the printing mechanism. In this instance, calibration refers to agreeing to use particular materials, such as Epson Premium Glossy Photo paper and Epson ink. For a printing press, we may calibrate many stages of the process, such as the imagesetter, the plate exposure, dot gain characteristics, and so on. Whatever the device, calibration refers to establishing a fixed, known printing condition and some way of returning to that condition.

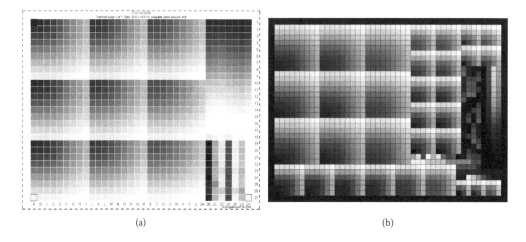

(a)　　　　　　　　　　　　　　　　(b)

**FIGURE 1.14**
A printer may be characterized with a test target such as (a) the proprietary TC9.18 GretagMacbeth RGB target or (b) the ECI 2002 CMYK Visual target.

The next step in making a printer profile is characterization. The most accurate way of studying the printer response would be to print and measure every CMYK combination. This would give us a direct CMYK–LAB transformation for every CMYK combination. However, this would run into millions of measurements and is largely impractical. Therefore, profiling vendors ask us to print and measure a target that contains a subset of CMYK combinations. A printer test chart is a digital, usually a TIFF, file containing patches of known RGB/CMYK values. The target may be standardized or a proprietary test target. Figure 1.14a shows a proprietary RGB target, and Figure 1.14b depicts the ECI 2002 CMYK test target. From the printing and measuring of this target, vendors create a model of the device behavior. The model is then used to calculate data for the lookup table that is stored in the printer profile tags. The accuracy of the characterization will depend on the sophistication of the internal model developed by each vendor and the accuracy with which they populate the lookup table.

Some vendors may use a procedure called "LAB linearization" to help increase the accuracy of the lookup table used within a profile. In printer profiling, we are trying to create a relationship between LAB and CMYK, and we would like to store this relationship in a lookup table. During printer profiling, a CMYK test chart is printed, and the LAB values of the patches are measured. Output charts tend to be designed in CMYK, and therefore, they have regular increments in CMYK, such as CMYK pixel values (10, 0, 0, 0), (20, 0, 0, 0), (30, 0, 0, 0), and so forth. When these patches are measured, they do not produce regularly spaced LAB values. The LAB values will be bunched up in some areas and spaced out in others. Although this is a truthful representation of the situation, that is, it demonstrates the response of the printer — it does not help us build accurate profiles, because it leads to inaccuracies in the LAB areas where we have scarce data. It is possible to linearize this process. A vendor may ask the user to print and measure a preprofiling chart. Based on the response of the print process, the software alters the CMYK values and calculates a new profiling test chart. In the new test chart, the CMYK values are not uniformly distributed, but their LAB measurements are. When the new profiling test chart is printed and measured, it generates LAB measurements that are more uniformly distributed, with the aim of deriving a more accurate printer profile.

### 1.5.3.1 *Printer Lookup Table*

To understand how a printer profile works, we can use a profile inspector to look inside the contents of a printer profile lookup table tag. A color management system specifies in LAB the color that is needed in part of an image. The role of the output profile is to convert this color specification into device instructions that can be sent to the printer to generate this color. A printer profile contains a LAB-to-CMYK lookup table, so that for a given LAB color, the output profile tells us what CMYK values should be sent to this particular printer to create this color.

In ColorSync Profile Inspector (Mac OS 9), it is easy to analyze the content of a lookup table. Figure 1.15a shows the lookup table for the B2A1 tag of an Epson Stylus 5000 printer profile. This table provides the LAB-to-CMYK mapping for the absolute colorimetric intent of a printer profile. It is possible to look up any LAB value using the three columns on the left in Figure 1.15a and read the corresponding CMYK (Output Values) at the right of the figure. The first column on the left in Figure 1.15a is the $L*$ value. The scale goes from 0 to 100 $L*$, and thus, this color has about 50 $L*$. The next two columns are for $a*$ and $b*$. The scale on these columns ranges from $-128$ to $+128$. The example shown has $a*$ and $b*$ values of 0, 0. The LAB for the color shown is thus 50, 0, 0, that is, a neutral mid-gray color. The corresponding CMYK values are shown as the four output values at the right of Figure 1.15a. In this case, the four channels refer to CMYK. Here, the output values are scaled from 0 to 65535. This lookup table suggests that to obtain a mid-gray color of LAB of 50, 0, 0, it is necessary to send to this Epson printer CMYK pixel values of 40, 40, 37, 0. So, to use this lookup table, any LAB value is looked up from the columns on the left, and the CMYK value necessary to create this color (on this printer) is available from the data on the right.

Now consider the corresponding profile lookup table for an HP Designjet 20ps, shown in Figure 1.15b. Let us look at the entry in this lookup table for the same LAB values considered in the previous example. To reproduce LAB of 50, 0, 0 on this printer, the lookup table suggests that the printer be sent CMYK values of 45, 48, 44, 0. The lookup table encapsulates the characteristics of each device so we see that to get the same neutral gray color

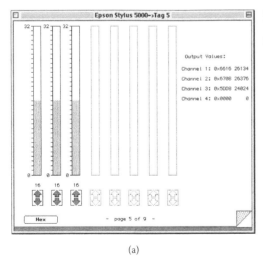
(a)

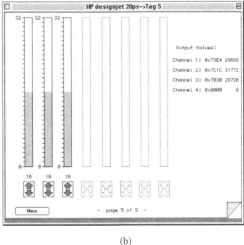
(b)

**FIGURE 1.15**
(a) The Mac OS 9 Profile Inspector allows for easy decoding of the LAB-to-CMYK lookup table of an Epson 5000 printer profile. (b) The same values in the Epson printer example are now looked up via the LAB-to-CMYK lookup table of an HP Designjet 20ps.

(LAB of 50, 0, 0), it is necessary to send CMYK values of 40, 40, 37, 0 to the Epson 5000, but CMYK values of 45, 48, 44, 0 must be sent to the HP Designjet. Based on printing and measurement of a test target, each lookup table contains instructions tailored to a specific device. This is how a color management process can reproduce the same color on different devices.

### 1.5.3.2   Color Gamut

One of the main reasons for inaccuracies produced in color imaging is gamut limitations. Because imaging devices work in totally different ways, additive or subtractive color [18], and with different colorants, they are not able to create an identical range of colors. Scanners, monitors, and printers employ different imaging technologies and, therefore, have different color capabilities. We can make a broad distinction between devices in the RGB (additive) and CMYK (subtractive) category based on the underlying technology of the devices. An accepted generalization is that RGB systems have a larger color gamut and can cope with more colors than CMYK systems (Figure 1.16). This means that sometimes you can see a color on your screen, but your CMYK printer will not be able to reproduce that color. The gamut of a device is measured during the characterization process. Measurement of the test target data in LAB directly provides information regarding the color gamut of the device. Thus, every profile contains information about the device gamut, and profile viewers can extract this information and allow comparison, for example, of a monitor and printer color gamut as shown in Figure 1.16. As images are passed into and out of the PCS, they may be sent to a device with a small color gamut. In such instances, we have to deal with colors that are out-of-gamut of the destination process. Color management provides a number of ways to deal with out-of-gamut colors.

If a color cannot be printed, the user can select from several different approaches to finding a replacement color. As described earlier, the ICC specified four standard color-replacement schemes, called rendering intents: perceptual, relative colorimetric, absolute colorimetric, and saturation.

Perceptual rendering is used to process photographic-type images. This intent processes the colors in an image so that the printed reproduction is pleasing. This process tends to alter color from the original, and therefore, there is no guarantee that the reproduction will

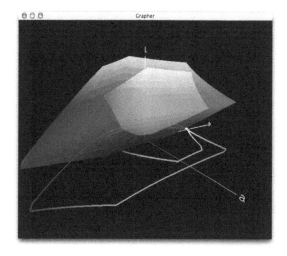

**FIGURE 1.16  (See color insert.)**
A CIE LAB gamut volume diagram showing the color gamut of a monitor (larger volume) compared to the much smaller color gamut of a printer.

be accurate when compared to the original. In fact, perceptual rendering is very likely to change the color of an image from original to reproduction. In perceptual rendering, the relationship between colors is retained, and this creates visually pleasing images. The ICC does not define the precise mechanism for perceptual mapping. Each profiling vendor is free to provide a mapping of colors that is most appropriate for their clients and the sorts of images that their clients use.

In colorimetric rendering, colors that are outside the gamut of the destination process are clipped and forced to the gamut boundary. More than one color in the original can be mapped to the same color in the reproduction. There are two versions of the colorimetric intent, relative colorimetric and absolute colorimetric. Consider an example in which the white of the paper used for the original image is slightly yellow, while the color of the paper used in the reproduction image is slightly blue.

On its own, the difference in the color of the substrate is not a problem. When we separately view each image, our eye adjusts to the paper white in each image. When we look at the original, we adjust to its yellow white point, and after a few moments this appears "white." When we view the bluish substrate, after a few moments our eye adapts, and we see the blue highlights as "white." Via chromatic adaptation, our eye will naturally adjust to the white that it finds in each image, and we will see any light point as white. Images can be reproduced on slightly different paper types, and as long as the images are viewed separately, we will not notice if the white that was in the original is different from the white in the reproduction. Relative colorimetry takes into account the white point of the destination substrate and displays or prints the image relative to the new white point. Relative colorimetric maps the white of the source to the white of the destination and adjusts other colors accordingly [19]. Thus, if there is an area of CMYK of 0, 0, 0, 0 in the original, this remains the same in the reproduction, and the image area assumes the color of the substrate.

Use of the absolute colorimetric intent in image processing does not let the white point change from source white to destination white. Absolute colorimetric intent creates exactly the colors that were in the original (where possible). Thus, if the original had a yellowish white point, the absolute colorimetric intent would ensure that the reproduction has a yellowish white point, too. The absolute colorimetric intent will create the yellow look of the original in the clear areas of the blue paper using an appropriate amount of yellow ink. Absolute colorimetry is used in proofing scenarios where we would like to simulate the output of one device on a second device and do a side-by-side comparison.

It is useful to note that if the paper color in the original matches the color of the paper used in the reproduction, then it does not matter which intent you use — relative colorimetric and absolute colorimetric give the same result. Relative and absolute colorimetry only differ when the white point in the original differs from that of the reproduction. The absolute and relative colorimetric intents are not confined to printer profiles but are used in other profile types, including monitor profiles.

## 1.6 Conclusions

A fundamental issue with color imaging is that each device has its own unique characteristics. These characteristics include device-to-device variation and gamut limitations. In order to achieve accurate color imaging, we must take into account each device's characteristics. In this chapter, we showed that the closed-loop system that existed in the past relied on a fixed workflow, and it is very difficult to extend that model to today's workflows. We described how an open-loop, ICC color management system provides a way of dealing with many different sources for images and many different destinations for printing. The principle of an ICC color managed workflow is to relate device-dependent RGB or device-dependent CMYK values to device-independent CIE LAB values. We described the PCS, which serves to provide a common link or interchange space for digital images. To process an image from RGB to CMYK, color management works by relating RGB to LAB (i.e., device-dependent to device-independent color) and then LAB to CMYK. We saw that the use of the PCS greatly reduces the number of transformations needed, while still maintaining that ability to communicate color instructions between devices.

In this chapter, we saw that color management is totally reliant on various CIE color specification systems. We saw that the CIE systems incorporate a basic calculation that takes into account the light source, the sample, and the human observer. The basic calculation produces XYZ tristimulus values for a measured color. It was shown that other CIE color spaces like Yxy and LAB are all transformations of the XYZ calculation. CIE systems meet all technical requirements of a color specification system and provide the primary framework for color management today.

We also described the ICC specification, which is responsible for much of the success of ICC color management. ICC profiles are vendor and platform independent, and the structure of a profile is strictly regulated so that a wide range of software can open a profile and interpret its contents. Via the ICC specification, the ICC provides a vital mechanism for the communication of color information today. We reviewed the current ICC specification and the tags required for scanner, monitor, and printer profiles. The two parts of an ICC profile — the header and the profile tags — were described in this chapter. We looked at the required tags for each profile class that must be present to create a valid ICC profile and saw that the tag requirements were different for scanner, monitor, and printer profiles. Also described were some of the changes that have occurred in the new Version 4 ICC profile.

It is useful in practical implementation to divide the color management process into calibration, characterization, and conversion. We saw that calibration involves establishing a fixed, repeatable condition for a device. Calibration thus involved establishing some known starting condition and some means of returning the device to that state. After a device has been calibrated, we described how the characteristic color response is studied in a process known as characterization. We saw that characterization refers to the process of making a profile and involves establishing the relationship between device values (RGB or CMYK) and device-independent values. The characterization process is equally applicable to scanner, monitor, and printer, though it is achieved in slightly different ways in each case. Via characterization, the typical behavior (gamut and characteristics) of the device are ascertained, and this information is stored in the device profile. After a device has been calibrated and characterized, the profile can be used during the scanning, printing, or display of images. The final color management process is conversion, a process in which images are converted from one color space to another using a color management module.

Toward the end of the chapter, an explanation is provided for how a lookup table works. Lookup tables are found in ICC profiles and are used to do most image conversions. Lookup tables represent a concept fundamental to many color management operations; thus, a practical example is presented to clearly demonstrate the operation of a lookup table and, thus, the primary function of an ICC profile.

For the first time, via the ICC, we have a system that is accepted and supported by the whole prepress and imaging industry. This universal color management system puts enormous power in the hands of the end user and allows functionality that was inconceivable in older ways of working. If used carefully, color management gives you a very close color match, very quickly. This saves time, money, and materials and provides an architecture that can be used in all emerging prepress and imaging technologies.

# References

[1] A. Sharma, *Understanding Color Management*, Thomson Delmar, Clifton Park, NY, 2004.

[2] B. Fraser, C. Murphy, and F. Bunting, *Real World Color Management*, 2nd Edition, Peachpit Press, Berkeley, CA, 2004.

[3] E. Giorgianni and T. Madden, *Digital Color Management*, Addison-Wesley, Reading, MA, 1998.

[4] T. Johnson, An effective colour management architecture for graphic arts, in *Proceedings of the Technical Association of the Graphic Arts*, 2000, p. 88.

[5] H. Lee, *Introduction to Color Imaging Science*, Cambridge University Press, London; New York, 2005, pp. 89–131.

[6] R. Berns, *Billmeyer and Saltzman's Principles of Color Technology*, John Wiley & Sons, New York, 2000.

[7] G. Wyszecki and W. Stiles, *Color Science: Concepts and Methods, Quantitative Data and Formulae*, Wiley-Interscience, New York, 2000.

[8] M. Fairchild, *Color Appearance Models*, 2nd Edition, Wiley-Interscience, New York, 2005.

[9] D. Walner, ch. Color management and transformation through ICC profiles, *Colour Engineering: Achieving Device Independent Colour* (edited by Phil Green and Lindsay Macdonald), John Wiley & Sons, New York, 2002, pp. 247–261.

[10] H. Kang, *Color Technology for Electronic Imaging Devices*, The International Society for Optical Engineering (SPIE), Bellingham, WA, 1997, p. 55.

[11] G. Sharma and H. Trussell, Digital color imaging, *IEEE Trans. Image Processing*, 6, 901, 1997.

[12] A. Sharma, M. Gouch, and D. Rughani, Generation of an ICC profile from a proprietary style file, *J. Imag. Sci. Tech.*, 46, 26, 2002.

[13] H. Kang, Color scanner calibration, *J. Imag. Sci. Tech.*, 36, 162, 1992.

[14] A. Sharma, Measuring the quality of ICC profiles and color management software, *Seybold Report*, 4, 10, January 2005.

[15] R. Berns, R. Motta, and M. Gorzynski, CRT colorimetry, part I: Theory and practice, *Color Res. App.*, 18, 299, 1993.

[16] R. Berns, Methods for characterizing CRT displays, *Displays*, 16, 173, 1996.

[17] R. Bala and R. Klassen, ch. Efficient color transformation implementation, *Digital Color Imaging Handbook*, G. Sharma, Ed., pp. 687–726. CRC Press, Boca Raton, FL, 2003.

[18] R. Hunt, *The Reproduction of Colour*, 6th Edition, John Wiley & Sons, New York, 2004.

[19] International Color Consortium, *Specification ICC.1:2004-10 (Profile version 4.2.0.0) Image technology colour management — Architecture, profile format, and data structure*, 2004.

# 2

## Versatile Gamut Mapping Method Based on Image-to-Device Concept

Hiroaki Kotera and Ryoichi Saito

**CONTENTS**

## 2.1 Introduction

As the year 2000 marked the 600th anniversary of Johannes Gutenberg's birth, we should reflect on the historical significance of letterpress technology and take a step forward into the new age of color imaging. In our daily lives, we encounter a variety of color images in print, television, computer displays, photographs, and movies. Now, digital imaging technology plays a leading role in visual communication, though subject to severe assessment for satisfying human vision. During the past decade, the color management system (CMS) has evolved to communicate device-independent colors across multimedia and is now introducing certain aspects of human vision for standardization. CMS for color reproduction systems has evolved as follows:

- *First generation*: colorimetric color reproduction based on device-dependent closed systems
- *Second generation*: cross-media color reproduction based on device-independent open systems
- *Third generation*: color appearance reproduction based on a human visual color appearance model (CAM)

Because each media has its own achievable color gamut, frequently some colors cannot be reproduced to precisely match the original. The gamut mapping algorithm (GMA) is one of the key technologies employed to match appearance in third-generation CMS. Various GMAs have been developed [1], [2], [3]. Most of these GMAs are designed to work on two-dimensional (2-D) lightness-chroma (LC) planes, based on the device-to-device (D-D) concept instead of the image-to-device (I-D) concept [4], [5], [6], [7], [8], [9], [10], [11], [12]. Moreover, much work has been done to describe the three-dimensional (3-D) gamut [13], [14], [15], [16], [17], [18], [19], [20], [21], [22], [23], [24], [25], [26], [27], mainly focusing on characterizing the device gamut but not the image gamut. GMA is now evolving from 2-D to 3-D [5], [9], [21], [23], [24], [28], [29], and I-D is expected to produce a better rendition than D-D.

The design concept of the 3-D I-D GMA will be introduced in this chapter using a compact gamut boundary descriptor (GBD) and its extension into a bidirectional versatile GMA with gamut compression from *wide to narrow* or gamut expansion from *narrow to wide*, depending on image color distribution. Section 2.2 describes how to extract GBD and its coding in a compact form. Section 2.3 and Section 2.4 describe gamut compression mapping for wide gamut images using GBD and gamut expansion for narrow gamut images. Finally, Section 2.5 introduces an advanced approach to a versatile GMA depending on image color distribution.

## 2.2 Gamut Boundary Descriptor

To perform the 3-D I-D GMA effectively, a simple and compact image GBD is necessary. Until now, a variety of GBDs have been presented that mainly addressed the device gamut, not the image gamut. Herzog proposed an analytical method for a compact GBD, whereby the kernel gamut of a unit cube is deformed to match the device gamut [14]. He represented the gamut surface by using the maximum chroma as a function of lightness and hue. Thus, the gamut surface for the printer is visualized as chromatic mountains over the lightness-hue plane. Braun and Fairchild also presented cathode-ray tube (CRT) device GBDs by using cylindrical CIELAB coordinates, where chroma $C_{ab}^*$ on a gamut surface is given by triangle grid points on the lightness-hue $L^* - h_{ab}$ plane and visualized as a mountain range similar to the chromatic mountains [16]. Cholewo and Love determined a printer GBD using an alpha-shape method, which generates convex hulls in 2-D triangular grids [17]. Morovic and Luo introduced the segment maxima GBD (SMGBD) that is described by a matrix containing the most extreme colors for each segment of color space, and they applied this method to practical images [25]. These methods have primarily been applied to device GBDs, such as for a printer or CRT. This section presents a new compact GBD with *r-image* attached to the original image in a very compact format. A key factor is extracting the 3-D image gamut shell from random color distributions quickly, and describing its boundary surface with a small number of data. Here, a constant division in discrete polar angle $(\theta, \varphi)$ is introduced to extract the image gamut surface. The gamut shell is described by using a set of maximum radial vectors different from the maximum chroma in chromatic mountains, and then transformed into a 2-D monochrome image, which we call *r-image* [20], [22].

The *r-image* method has the following distinct advantages over the previous work: 3-D GBD is given as a simple 2-D monochrome image, the *r-image* is suitable for data compression due to its strong spatial correlations, and 3-D I-D GMA is easily performed through direct pixel-to-pixel comparison between the *r-image* of the device and image. Though the *r-image* is compact, for a GBD of higher precision, by using smaller steps of segmentation, it can be further compressed by conventional JPEG, singular value decomposition (SVD) [20], [22], or JPEG2000 wavelet transform picture coding methods. The image gamut shell shape is quickly reconstructed from the compressed *r-image* and used for I-D mapping. Thus, flexible gamut mapping using the image GBD on the user side is our ultimate goal.

### 2.2.1 Description of Image Gamut Shell

In general, the image color center $[L_0^*, a_0^*, b_0^*]$ should be defined as the center of gravity by

$$\vec{r}_0 = [L_0^*, a_0^*, b_0^*] = \left[\frac{1}{N}\sum_{i=1}^{N}(L_i^*), \frac{1}{N}\sum_{i=1}^{N}(a_i^*), \frac{1}{N}\sum_{i=1}^{N}(b_i^*)\right] \qquad (2.1)$$

However, to perform the GMA, $\vec{r}_0$ must be placed at the same point for both the printer and images. One safe way is to set $\vec{r}_0$ at a neutral gray point $[L_0^*, a_0^*, b_0^*] = [50, 0, 0]$. If the printer and an image have different centers, then gamut mapping will lead to shifts in hue. Radial vector $\vec{r}_i$ toward arbitrary pixel $\vec{c}_i = [L_i^*, a_i^*, b_i^*]$ from image center $\vec{r}_0$ is given by

$$\vec{r}_i = \vec{c}_i - \vec{r}_0; \quad 1 \le i \le N \qquad (2.2)$$

The polar angle of each radial vector $\vec{r}_i$ is defined as follows:

$$\theta_i = \arctan\left(\frac{b_i^* - b_0^*}{a_i^* - a_0^*}\right); \quad 0 \le \theta_i \le 2\pi \qquad (2.3)$$

$$\varphi_i = \frac{\pi}{2} + \arctan\left(\frac{L_i^* - L_0^*}{[(a_i^* - a_0^*)^2 + (b_i^* - b_0^*)^2]^{\frac{1}{2}}}\right); \quad 0 \le \varphi_i \le \pi \qquad (2.4)$$

Here, we define a radial matrix *r-image* with its element given by the maximum radial vector in each polar angle segment as follows:

$$\mathbf{r}_{gamut} = [r_{jk}] = [\max\{\|\vec{r}_i\|\}]$$
$$\text{for} \quad (j-1)\Delta\theta \le \theta_i \le j\Delta\theta \quad \text{and} \quad (k-1)\Delta\varphi \le \varphi_i \le k\Delta\varphi \qquad (2.5)$$
$$\Delta\theta = {}^{2\pi}/_J; \ 1 \le j \le J \quad \text{and} \quad \Delta\varphi = {}^{\pi}/_K; \ 1 \le k \le K$$

Figure 2.1 shows the image gamut surface as described by radial matrix *r-image*.

Figure 2.2a and Figure 2.2b show a sRGB test image "wool" and its color map in CIELAB color space, respectively. Figure 2.2c and Figure 2.2d illustrate the extracted maximum

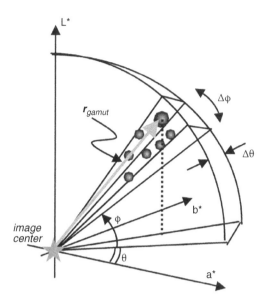

**FIGURE 2.1**
Maximum radial vectors in segmented polar angle spaces.

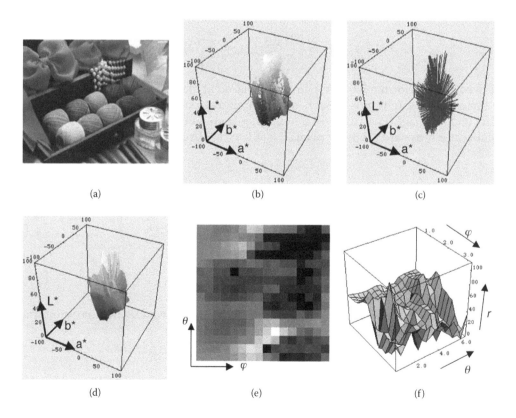

(a)            (b)            (c)

(d)            (e)            (f)

**FIGURE 2.2**
Extraction of image gamut by maximum radial vectors and *r-image*: (a) test Wool image, (b) color distribution, (c) extracted radial vectors, (d) polygon gamut shell, (e) 2-D *r-image*, and (f) 3-D view of *r-image*.

radial vectors and the polygonal gamut shell rendered by connecting these radial vectors, respectively. We proposed to replace the 3-D radial vectors with a 2-D distance array (named *r-image*) arranged at rectangular lattice points $(j, k)$. The magnitude of radial vector $\vec{r}_{jk}$ is given by the norm as follows:

$$\|\vec{r}_{jk}\| = \left[ \left( L_{jk}^* - L_0^* \right)^2 + \left( a_{jk}^* - a_0^* \right)^2 + \left( b_{jk}^* - b_0^* \right)^2 \right]^{\frac{1}{2}} \tag{2.6}$$

Here, $J \times K$ rectangular matrix $\vec{r}$ is defined as follows:

$$\vec{r} = [\|\vec{r}_{jk}\|]; \quad 1 \le j \le J, \ 1 \le k \le K \tag{2.7}$$

Matrix $\vec{r}$ (which we call *r-image*) represents a monochromatic 2-D image with pixels that denote the radial vector magnitude arranged at a discrete integer $(j, k)$ address. Although the *r-image* is a 2-D grayscale image, it reflects the 3-D gamut shell shape pointed to by the radial vectors in discrete polar angle space. Once image color distribution is converted into the *r-image*, each $[L^*, a^*, b^*]$ value on the gamut surface is approximately reconstructed from the corresponding element of matrix $\vec{r}$ for the integer values of $i$ and $j$, including quantizing errors with half of $\theta$ and $\varphi$ as follows:

$$\hat{a}_{jk}^* = \|\vec{r}_{jk}\| \cos(j - 0.5)\Delta\theta \cdot \sin(k - 0.5)\Delta\varphi + a_0^*$$

$$\hat{b}_{jk}^* = \|\vec{r}_{jk}\| \sin(j - 0.5)\Delta\theta \cdot \sin(k - 0.5)\Delta\varphi + b_0^* \tag{2.8}$$

$$\hat{L}_{jk}^* = L_0^* - \|\vec{r}_{jk}\| \cos(k - 0.5)\Delta\varphi$$

Figure 2.2e shows the *r-image* represented as a 2-D grayscale image segmented in $16 \times 16$ discrete angles. Figure 2.2f shows its 3-D representation in Cartesian coordinates. The gamut volume is intelligibly visualized in this 3-D view. This simple presentation makes it easy to compare the point-to-point gamut sizes between the image and device, and to calculate the mapping function directly.

## 2.2.2 Compact GBD by Compression of *r*-Image

The *r-image* is a grayscale image. If the gamut shell has a smooth 3-D surface, the *r-image* will have a high degree of spatial correlation. It can be compressed by applying orthogonal transform coding. To obtain a more compact GBD, the image compression technique is applied to *r-image*.

### 2.2.2.1 Compression of r-Image by DCT

A forward discrete cosine transform (DCT) is used to transform the *r-image* into spatial frequency components $\vec{R}_{DCT}$ as follows:

$$\vec{R}_{DCT} = [R_{jk}] = \vec{A}^t \vec{r} \vec{A} \tag{2.9}$$

$$\vec{A} = [a_{jk}], \ a_{jk} = \begin{cases} \dfrac{1}{\sqrt{M}}; & \text{for } k = 1 \\[2mm] \dfrac{2}{\sqrt{M}} \cos\left( \dfrac{(2j-1)(k-1)\pi}{2M} \right); & \text{for } k = 2, 3, \ldots, M, \ j = 1, 2, \ldots, M \end{cases} \tag{2.10}$$

The inverse DCT (IDCT) is given by the same formula:

$$\vec{r} = \vec{A} \vec{R}_{DCT} \vec{A}^t \tag{2.11}$$

Because the DCT power spectra are concentrated in the lower frequency components of $\vec{R}_{DCT}$, the *r-image* is approximately reconstructed from the reduced $m \times m$ matrix, for $m < M$, by cutting the higher frequency components as follows:

$$\vec{r} \cong \vec{A}\vec{R}_{DCT}^m\vec{A}^t, \ \vec{R}_{DCT}^m = \left[R_{jk}^m\right], \ R_{jk}^m = \begin{cases} R_{jk} & \text{for } j, k \leq m \\ 0 & \text{for } j, k > m \end{cases} \tag{2.12}$$

### 2.2.2.2 Compression of r-Image by SVD

DCT is easy to use, because its basis function is prefixed independent of the image. However, the image has its own shell shape, so the image-dependent basis function may be better suited for the gamut description. Here, compression by using singular value decomposition (SVD) has been tested. The *r-image* can be expressed by SVD as follows:

$$\vec{r} = [r_{jk}] = \vec{U}\vec{\Lambda}\vec{V}^t \tag{2.13}$$

where the columns of $\vec{U}$ and $\vec{V}$ are the eigenvectors of $\vec{r}\vec{r}^t$ and $\vec{r}^t\vec{r}$, and $\vec{\Lambda}$ is the diagonal matrix containing the singular values of $\vec{r}$ along its diagonal axis. Because $\vec{U}$ and $\vec{V}$ are orthogonal we obtain the following:

$$\vec{\Lambda} = \vec{U}^t\vec{r}\vec{V} = \begin{bmatrix} \lambda_1 & 0 & \cdots & \cdots & 0 \\ 0 & \lambda_2 & 0 & \cdots & 0 \\ \vdots & & \ddots & & \vdots \\ 0 & \cdots & \cdots & 0 & \lambda_M \end{bmatrix} \tag{2.14}$$

The *r-image* is approximately reconstructed from the reduced numbers of singular values and eigenvectors as

$$\vec{r} = [\hat{r}_{jk}] \cong \vec{U}_m\vec{\Lambda}_m\vec{V}_m^t \tag{2.15}$$

Thus, the $M \times M$ matrix $\vec{r}$ can be restored from $m$, $(m < M)$, singular values, and the corresponding vectors of $\vec{U}$ and $\vec{V}$ as follows:

$$\vec{\Lambda}_m = \begin{bmatrix} \lambda_1 & 0 & \cdots & \cdots & 0 \\ 0 & \lambda_2 & 0 & \cdots & 0 \\ \vdots & & \ddots & & \vdots \\ 0 & \cdots & \cdots & 0 & \lambda_m \end{bmatrix} \tag{2.16}$$

$$\vec{U}_m = \begin{bmatrix} U_{11} & U_{12} & \cdots & \cdots & U_{1m} \\ U_{21} & U_{22} & \cdots & \cdots & U_{2m} \\ \vdots & & \ddots & & \vdots \\ U_{N1} & \cdots & & \cdots & U_{Nm} \end{bmatrix}, \ \vec{V}_m = \begin{bmatrix} V_{11} & V_{12} & \cdots & \cdots & V_{1N} \\ V_{21} & V_{22} & \cdots & \cdots & V_{2N} \\ \vdots & & \ddots & & \vdots \\ V_{m1} & \cdots & & \cdots & V_{mN} \end{bmatrix} \tag{2.17}$$

### 2.2.2.3 Compression of r-Image by Wavelets

Although SVD provides a best-fit basis function dependent on a given image, the sets of eigenvectors should be transmitted together with singular values, in which case, more parameters may be needed than for fixed basis functions. Similar to Fourier series analysis (where sinusoids are chosen as the basis function), wavelet analysis is also based on the decomposition of a signal by typically (though not necessarily) using an orthogonal family of basis functions. Unlike a sinusoidal wave, a wavelet function is localized in terms of both time (or space) and frequency. Thus, sinusoids are useful in analyzing periodic and time-invariant phenomena, while wavelets are well suited for the analysis of transient, time-varying signals. Here, a forward discrete wavelet transform (DWT) is used to transform the *r-image* into spatial frequency components $\vec{R}_{DWT}$ by regarding time as space as follows:

$$\vec{R}_{DWT} = [R_{jk}] = \vec{W}^t \vec{r} \vec{W} \tag{2.18}$$

The inverse DWT (IDWT) is given by the same formula:

$$\vec{r} = \vec{W} \vec{R}_{DWT} \vec{W}^t \tag{2.19}$$

Here, we applied the well-known Daubechies filter as the discrete wavelet scaling function. Wavelet-based image compression is now a popular coding method standard-ized as JPEG2000. The *r-image* has been compressed and evaluated in accordance with JPEG2000.

### 2.2.3  Quantization Error in *r*-Image by Segmentation

Because each pixel of *r-image* carries the magnitude of the maximum radial vector in the discrete polar angle segment, it includes a quantization error in the reconstruction of color value [$L*, a*, b*$] on the gamut surface from the discrete segment as given by Equation 2.8. Thus, the GBD accuracy provided by the *r-image* method initially depends on the polar angle step ($\Delta\theta, \Delta\varphi$) in the $J \times K$ segmentations. It is estimated by the surface color reproduction error on the gamut shell and gives the necessary number ($M, N$) of segmentations for GMA design. The color difference between the maximum radial vector before and after reconstruction has been estimated for changing segmentation number $M$ when $M = N$ [30]. The error reached $\Delta E94_{SEG}(rms) = 0.98$ for "bride" and $\Delta E94_{SEG}(rms) = 1.51$ for "wool" when $J \times K = 32 \times 32$, and was reduced to $\Delta E94_{SEG}(rms) = 0.57$ for "bride" and $\Delta E94_{SEG}(rms) = 0.90$ for "wool" when $J \times K = 48 \times 48$. These errors reflect the gamut boundary accuracy in the process of reconstructing the image gamut shell shape. Because the *r-image* represents the most saturated colors located on the gamut surface, $\Delta E94_{SEG}(rms)$ should be less than gamut mapping errors when using GMA. At the very least, $J \times K = 32 \times 32$ segmentation is necessary for practical use, and $\Delta E94_{SEG}(rms) < 1.0$ when using $J \times K = 48 \times 48$ may be enough for high-precision GMA.

### 2.2.4  Image Gamut Reconstruction from Reduced DCT and SVD Parameters

The test images were converted into *r-image* and transformed to DCT and SVD coefficients. The reconstructed gamut shell shapes from the reduced coefficients were compared with the originals. Figure 2.3a shows the original sRGB test image "bride" in standard image database SHIPP, with its *r-image* segmented to $48 \times 48$ discrete polar angles in ($\theta, \varphi$), and the gamut shell shape in the wire frame. Figure 2.3b shows the reconstructed *r-image* from the DCT coefficients reduced to $J \times K = 4 \times 4, 8 \times 8$, and $16 \times 16$. Figure 2.3c shows the corresponding gamut shell shapes recovered from the reconstructed *r-image*. Figure 2.3d and Figure 2.3e show similar results of reconstruction from the reduced SVD parameters. The gamut shell shape reconstructed from reduced $4 \times 4$ or $8 \times 8$ DCT coefficients loses too much detail due to the lack of higher spatial frequency components and remains insufficient even when using $16 \times 16$ DCT. Conversely, the gamut shell shape was roughly reconstructed from $4 \times 4$ SVD and almost perfectly reconstructed from $16 \times 16$ SVD.

### 2.2.5  SVD Parameters for Reconstruction

The *r-image* is decomposed by orthogonal eigenvectors $\vec{U}$ and $\vec{V}$ through singular value $\vec{\Lambda}$. The information energy of *r-image* is known to be mainly concentrated at the lower order

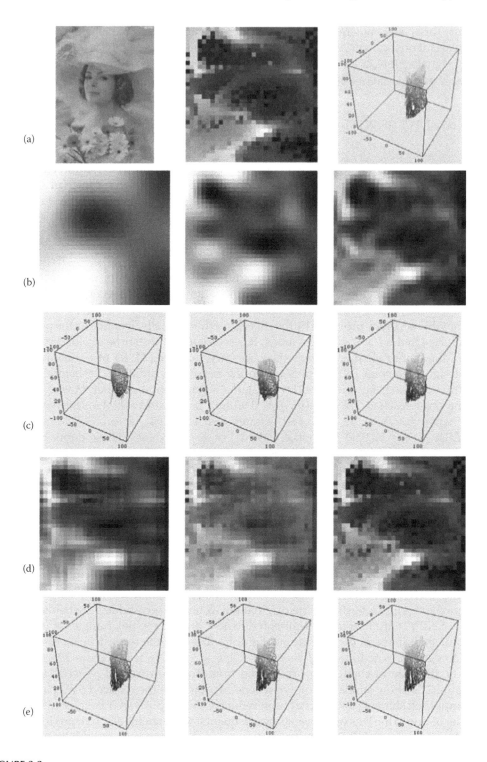

**FIGURE 2.3**
Reconstructed *r-image* and gamut shell from reduced DCT and SVD coefficients: (a) original *Bride* image (left) and the corresponding *r-image* (middle) and gamut shell (right), (b) DCT *r-image*, (c) DCT gamut shell, (d) SVD *r-image*, and (e) SVD gamut shell. Note that the results shown in parts b–e correspond to $4 \times 4$ (left), $8 \times 8$ (middle), and $16 \times 16$ (right).

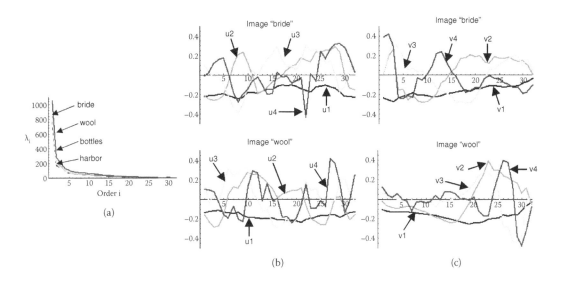

**FIGURE 2.4**
SVD parameters: (a) distribution of eigenvalues, (b) first four eigenvectors in matrix **U**, and (c) first four eigen-vectors in matrix **V**.

of eigenvectors as weighted by $\vec{\Lambda}$. Figure 2.4a shows the distribution of $\vec{\Lambda}$ for four different sRGB test images. Singular value $\vec{\Lambda} = [\lambda_i]$ drops off rapidly as order $i$ becomes larger. The singular values are mainly concentrated at lower orders less than 4 or 5. Figure 2.4b and Figure 2.4c, respectively, show the first four eigenvectors of matrix $\vec{U}$ and $\vec{V}$ for the images "bride" and "wool." These complicated shapes of the first four eigenvectors reflect that the lower order of basis functions almost carry the image-dependent gamut shell shapes. They also show that the gamut shell shape obtained by *r-image* can be roughly reconstructed from products of the first four row vectors of $\vec{U}$, four singular values of $\vec{\Lambda}$, and four column vectors of $\vec{V}$.

### 2.2.6　*r*-Image for GBD

The image gamut shell shape was simply represented by a set of radial vectors (which we call *r-image*) in the segmented polar angles. The *r-image* could be compactly approximated using a smaller number of singular values by SVD than by DCT. Thus, the larger the number of segmentations, the better the GBD accuracy, and the higher the compression rate, the more system memory required. In SVD compression using $m$ singular values for the $M \times M$ *r-image*, $M \times m$ column vectors $\vec{U}_m$, $m \times M$ row vectors $\vec{V}_m$, and $m$ singular values are needed for *GBD* in order to simply estimate compression rate $C$ as follows:

$$C = \frac{(2M+1)m}{M^2} \tag{2.20}$$

When $M \ll m$, the rate $C$ is approximately given by $C \cong 2m/M$. For example, we get $C \cong \frac{1}{4}$ in the case of ($m = 4, M = 32$), and $C \cong \frac{1}{8}$ in the case of ($m = 4, M = 64$). Of course, the larger the number $M$, the more detailed the description of gamut shell shape. In practice, the compact GBD obtained by $M \times M = 32 \times 32$ segmentations may be applied for gamut mapping to render commercial image quality (such as for color printers or copiers), and the *r-image* obtained by $M \times M = 48 \times 48$ or more segmentations is recommended for higher quality images. Because the *r-image* is a grayscale image and shows high spatial correlation, it could be efficiently compressed by applying wavelet coding (JPEG2000).

Although a set of SVD parameters (singular value $\vec{\Lambda}$, eigenvectors $\vec{U}$ and $\vec{V}$) should be computed and transmitted for every image with more bits than by DCT or wavelet coding, SVD can directly restore the *r-image* without a decoding process and reconstruct the gamut shell shape quickly, once these parameters have been received. The proposed *r-image* GBD makes it possible to easily detect the out-of-gamut segments without comparing all the pixels, instead by simply comparing the representative maximum radial vectors between the image and device. This facilitates efficient computation of the 3-D I-D GMA.

## 2.3 Compression-Based GMA

In the process of cross-media color reproduction under CMS, a key feature is the use of gamut mapping techniques to adjust color gamut differences between displays and printers. The 3-D I-D GMA is an ideal way to map a display image to within the printer gamut, while minimizing the loss in color information [12]. Conversely, the 3-D I-D GMA requires much time to calculate the intersecting points on the image and device gamut surfaces along each mapping line. Section 2.2 introduced a new simple and easy method of comparing the color gamut between the image and device, whereby the maximum radial vectors for the image and device are extracted, and then compared in each segment. The key point in the proposed GMA is using the relationship between only two vectors in each divided segment. The image quality after mapping is influenced by the focal point location and surface shape of the device gamut shell. In this section, we will first discuss the two types of focal points (single-focal and multifocal), and then the two types of gamut shell shapes formed by polygon meshes and *Overhauser spline functions*. Also described is an assessment of color appearance in psychophysical experiments involving typical combinations of these different types of focal points and shell shapes.

### 2.3.1 Focal Point

In GMA design [31], the mapping direction to a focal point is very important. A simple way is to place the focal point at the center of image color distribution. Figure 2.5a shows an

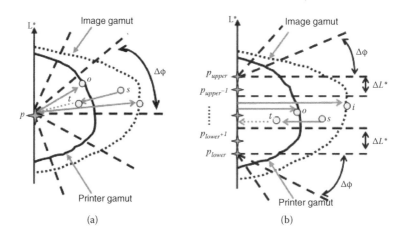

**FIGURE 2.5**
Overview of two types of focal points: (a) single-focal point, and (b) multifocal point.

overview of the single focal point method, where both hue angle $\theta$ and sector angle $\varphi$ are uniformly divided by $\Delta\theta$ and $\Delta\varphi$ toward image center $p$. Because the image center should be placed at the same location as that of the device, here the image center of a printer is decided beforehand. While mapping to a single-focal point used in the typical 2-D GMA, the change in lightness after mapping causes fatal degradation in image quality. Herzog and Buring proposed to move the focal point along the mapping line toward negative chroma by employing a relative lightness change technique [27]. Kang et al. introduced two convergent focal points determined by the lightness $L^*$ of the original medium's cusp [26]. These ideas are intended to be applied to the 2-D $L^*$–$C^*$ plane, and have reportedly shown good effects.

To maintain a natural appearance in lightness, mapping to the multifocal points is desirable. We took control parameters $p_{lower}$ and $p_{upper}$ into account when setting the multifocal points. Here, $p_{lower}$ and $p_{upper}$ are placed at the minimum and maximum $L^*$ points where the gamut boundary slope changes from high to low and low to high, respectively. Image and printer lightness are divided by polar angles under $p_{lower}$ and over $p_{upper}$, and by the parallel segments between $p_{lower}$ and $p_{upper}$. In most cases, $p_{lower}$ and $p_{upper}$ are placed at the points that divide the lightness histogram of the printer gamut equally into thirds. Figure 2.5b shows an overview of the multifocal point method with two convergent lightness points ($p_{lower}$ and $p_{upper}$) and parallel points divided by $L^*$ between them. For the ink-jet printer used in the experiment, $p_{lower}$ and $p_{upper}$ were set to $[L_0^*, a_0^*, b_0^*] = [45, 0, 0]$ and $[L_0^*, a_0^*, b_0^*] = [58, 0, 0]$, respectively.

### 2.3.2 Printer GBD

Although an accurate image GBD is obtained from a sufficient number of samples in the original color distribution, the printer GBD must be obtained from measurements of the color chips. Because the number of chips is limited in practice, the lack of color points in a segment makes the GBD inaccurate. In order to form the printer GBD by using the same radial vectors as those of the image GBD, it is necessary to first form the printer gamut shell, making it as smooth as possible, and again extract the equally divided surface points (in terms of polar angle) by calculating the intersecting points. To shape the printer gamut surface smoothly with a limited number of color samples, we developed a nonuniform segmentation method to include constant samples [7], [8], where no empty segments exist even when using a small number of color chips. In many cases, about 1000 color chips are used to characterize the printer GBD. Here, to obtain a precise printer GBD, $9261(= 21^3$; 21 gray steps for each C, M, Y ink) color chips were printed on coated paper. The approach based on Overhauser spline functions was introduced to generate a smoothed and seamless gamut shell [12], [32]. Overhauser spline surface $P(u, v)$ is calculated based on double parameters $u$ and $v$ as given by Equation 2.21 through Equation 2.23 as follows:

$$P(u, v) = \sum_{i=0}^{3} \sum_{j=0}^{3} N_i^3(u) N_j^3(v) V_{ij}, \qquad 0 \le u < 1; \quad 0 \le v < 1 \tag{2.21}$$

$$N^3(x) = [x^3 \quad x^2 \quad x \quad 1] \cdot \vec{M}_{CR}, \qquad x = u, v \tag{2.22}$$

$$\vec{M}_{CR} = \frac{1}{2} \begin{bmatrix} -1 & 3 & -3 & 1 \\ 2 & -5 & 4 & -1 \\ -1 & 0 & 1 & 0 \\ 0 & 2 & 0 & 0 \end{bmatrix} \tag{2.23}$$

where $\vec{V}_{i,j}$, for $i = 1, 2, 3, 4$ and $j = 1, 2, 3, 4$ represents the matrix element of 16 control points. The term $\vec{M}_{CR}$ is called a Catmull-Rom basic matrix that defines the edges located

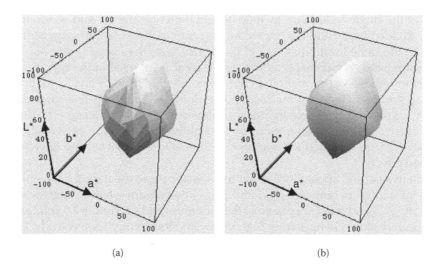

(a)          (b)

**FIGURE 2.6** (See color insert.)
Comparison of two types of printer gamut shell surfaces: (a) polygon mesh, and (b) Overhauser spline functions.

between two adjacent segmented surfaces for smooth contact. Figure 2.6b shows a gamut shell formed by the Overhauser spline functions. Its gamut surface is clearly smoother than that obtained by the polygon mesh, as shown in Figure 2.6a.

Regardless of whether the polygon mesh or Overhauser spline is selected to form the gamut surface, intersecting points must be calculated to obtain a printer GBD. The printer maximum radial vector $\vec{r}_{gamut}$ is calculated by finding the intersecting points on the surface corresponding to the same segments as those of the image in the discrete polar angle $(\theta_j, \varphi_k)$.

### 2.3.3 Application to I-D GMA

Figure 2.5 shows the basic concept of the 3-D I-D GMA using *r-image*. In the segmented CIELAB space, source color $s$ is mapped to target $t$ along the mapping line toward focal point $p$ by referencing image radial vector $\overrightarrow{pi}$ and output device radial vector $\overrightarrow{po}$. In our GMA using *r-image* GBD, all source colors included in the same segment are mapped by using the common single mapping equation computed from only two representative vectors ($\overrightarrow{pi}$ and $\overrightarrow{po}$) as follows:

$$\overrightarrow{pt} = \overrightarrow{po} \cdot \left( \frac{\overrightarrow{ps}}{\overrightarrow{pi}} \right)^{\gamma} \tag{2.24}$$

where $\gamma$ represents the $\gamma$-compression coefficient [9]. The GMA works as linear compression for $\gamma = 1$, and as nonlinear compression for $0 < \gamma < 1$.

### 2.3.4 Psychophysical Experiment

In true color hard copies, color correction is indispensable for converting RGB image data into CMY printer drive signals. In this study, a color masking technique using third-order polynomials was applied to RGB-to-CMY conversion for colorimetric color reproduction, with high-quality hard copies printed out on an ink-jet printer. A psychophysical experiment was conducted to compare matching color appearance between the original CRT image and printed image after gamut mapping. A monitor's white point was set near

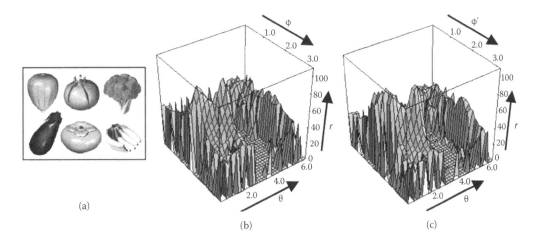

**FIGURE 2.7**
Difference in *r-image* of CG-image produced by two types of focal points: (a) CG image "fruits and vegetables," (b) *r-image* with single-focal points, and (c) *r-image* with multifocal points.

CIE illuminant D65 (with peak luminance of 80 $cd/m^2$) based on sRGB standard observation conditions. Hard copies were viewed in a light booth at the same color temperature and peak luminance as the monitor settings. A team of 21 observers employed a paired-comparison method to appraise both images in dim viewing surroundings with ambient illumination of about 64 lx. Data from the psychophysical experiment were analyzed using Thurstone's law of comparative judgment to generate interval scales (mean values of z-scores). One unit on the interval scale equals $\sqrt{2}\sigma$. Z-score values were plotted with a 95% confidence limit, that is, $\pm 1.96 \frac{\sigma}{\sqrt{N}} = \pm 1.96 \frac{1}{\sqrt{2N}} = \pm 0.302$ units [33], [34], where $N = 21$ denotes the number of observers for a sample. This means that two models are equivalent when the difference between corresponding z-score values is less than 0.302 unit.

### 2.3.5 Experimental Test for Location of Focal Point

The experiment was conducted for testing GMAs with different focal points. Figure 2.7a through Figure 2.7c show examples of *r-image* for typical test images with wide gamuts. Figure 2.7a shows the CG-image "fruits and vegetables," whereas Figure 2.7b and Figure 2.7c, respectively, show the *r-image* of the image with single-focal and multifocal points. The $32 \times 32$ segments in $(\theta_j, \varphi_k)$ at the image center $[L^*, a^*, b^* = 50, 0, 0]$ are used to construct the *r-image*. The *r-image* using multifocal points is also constructed with 32 divisions at polar hue angle $\theta$, with 10 segments over $p_{upper}$ and under $p_{lower}$, and 12 segments in the middle parallel zone. Small differences between the single-focal and multifocal models are observed in the *r-image*.

Three kinds of test images (i.e., one CG image, two sRGB images) were used for the psychophysical experiment (Figure 2.8). In our I-D GMA experiments, three different mapping conditions were set (as shown in Figure 2.8): (1) single-focal with $\gamma = 0.8$, (2) multifocal with $\gamma = 0.8$, and (3) multifocal with $\gamma = 0.5$. The proposed I-D GMA was compared with (4) the clipping GMA and (5) the D-D GMA. Because this experiment evaluates the performance of gamut compression mainly from very wide gamut images into printer images, the clipping GMA was selected for comparison because it is known to work very well for these wide gamut images. Both the D-D GMA and clipping GMA were also used under the same conditions as those of the proposed I-D GMA in 3-D CIELAB space. In the D-D GMA,

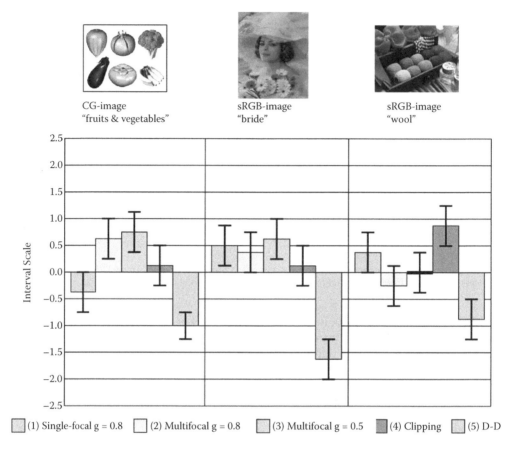

**FIGURE 2.8**
Psychophysical experimental results from the mapping method.

a set of $[L^*, a^*, b^*]$ data was generated at equal intervals [6], with the maximum radial vectors being extracted to create a CRT monitor gamut that matches the printer gamut. Both printer and monitor radial vectors were compared, and the D-D GMA was performed using single-focal points. Conversely, the clipping maps out-of-gamut colors on the printer gamut boundary surface toward $[L^*, a^*, b^*] = [50, 0, 0]$.

The evaluation results for test images are shown in Figure 2.8. For each picture, the D-D GMA obviously showed the worst result. The opinion test is summarized as follows: For the CG-image "fruits and vegetables," the single-focal I-D GMA did not work well, whereas the multifocal I-D GMA exhibited the best performance. Because the CG-image has the largest gamut and includes many out-of-gamut colors, the loss of gradation in highly saturated, continuous tone areas often causes unacceptable artifacts as seen in the clipping GMA. The proposed multifocal I-D GMA worked best for this test image. Conversely, for the sRGB image "bride," both single-focal and multifocal I-D GMAs resulted in better appearance, because the image includes small amounts of out-of-gamut colors. Thus, the single-focal I-D GMA could reproduce better gradation without artifacts as well as could the multifocal I-D GMA.

Conversely, for the image "wool," the clipping GMA showed the best performance. The clipping GMA generally meets the maximum loss in gradation for continuous color-tone objects but maintains the minimum loss in chromatic saturation or colorfulness. The reason why the clipping GMA worked best for the "wool" image can be explained as follows:

The image has uniformly spread, wide gamut color distributions, with most located just out of the printer gamut (not far from the gamut boundary), so that the clipping GMA apparently gives a better color appearance by preserving the maximum chroma in spite of a small loss in gradation.

In this chapter, a novel image-to-device 3-D GMA was proposed by introducing the quick gamut comparison method using a simple GBD called *r-image*. A complicated 3-D image gamut shell shape is simply described by using an array of maximum radial vectors rearranged along the 2-D discrete polar angle coordinates. The known device gamut shell shape is fixed before mapping and simply formed by using a polygonal surface, but it is not smooth when using insufficient sample points. The Overhauser spline function approach was introduced to shape the printer gamut shell surface more smoothly. The 3-D I-D GMA is easily executed by simply comparing the two representative radial vectors in each *r-image* of the image and device.

Figure 2.9a through Figure 2.9c compare image and printer gamuts. By overlaying the *r-image* of the test image on that of the ink-jet printer, the out-of-gamut colors are easily visualized. The gray area denotes the inside of the printer gamut. The colored bars are the image's radial vectors higher than those of the printer, thus denoting the outside of the gamut. The psychophysical experiment clearly shows that mapping to the multifocal points generally results in a better image appearance. For the image "wool," however, the clipping GMA got the better score. This image has a wider gamut throughout the entire color space than that of the printer, but the out-of-gamut colors are located just a bit outside the printer gamut, as shown in Figure 2.9c. This is why the clipping GMA worked best, because only these out-of-gamut colors are mapped on the printer gamut surface, while maximum chroma are maintained and only a little gradation is lost. The gamut of the CG-image in the red to yellow-green and blue violet zones is noticeably larger than the printer gamut (Figure 2.9a), while that of the image "bride" is a little larger in the skin color and dark hair regions (Figure 2.9b). Like the CG-image, when the source image has a large mean value and standard deviations (S.D.) for the out-of-gamut pixels, the I-D GMA will work better in avoiding noticeable false contours with gradation loss. Conversely, like the image "wool," when the mean value and S.D. are small, then the clipping GMA works better in terms of producing few false contours, without degrading gradation as much as by gamut compression. Although the sRGB-image "bride" has a high mean value, the out-of-gamut colors are mostly located at relatively inconspicuous areas of low lightness.

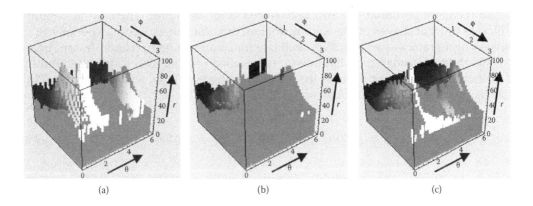

(a)   (b)   (c)

**FIGURE 2.9**
Comparison of image and printer gamuts with overlay: (a) CG image "fruits and vegetables," (b) sRGB image "bride," and (c) sRGB image "wool."

In conclusion, the multifocal I-D GMA works better when applied to wider gamut images, like CG-images or high dynamic range (HDR) outdoor images. Conversely, the clipping GMA is effective for images with color distributions located just outside the printer gamut. The Overhauser spline functions make it possible to form a smooth and seamless device gamut surface, resulting in a better rendition in terms of mapped image gradation than the polygonal GBD. However, there are high computation costs required to execute the 3-D I-D GMA by using a spline GBD. By segmenting the *r-image* with resolution higher than $32 \times 32$, the GBD obtained by this simple *r-image* method will never be inferior to the Overhauser spline GBD. Montag and Fairchild pointed out that a GMA that produces pleasing results for one image might not work well for another image [35]. The selection of GMA types with optimal mapping parameters is dependent on image content, and a fully automatic process poses a challenge to be addressed by future work.

## 2.4    Expansion-Based GMA

The current gamut mapping GMA is primarily used to compress out-of-gamut colors to within the printer gamut. Such highly saturated gamut images as CG-images on a monitor must be compressed to match appearance for printing. However, the printer gamut has recently been further expanded along with improvements made to printing media and devices. In general, source images do not always fill the entire device gamut but are distributed in the narrow color space for pictures taken under bad weather conditions, insufficient illumination, or that have faded after long preservation. Hence, the color gamut must sometimes be expanded to obtain a better color rendition [10], [11]. This section introduces an expansion-based GMA [36] applied to images with a much smaller gamut than that of devices. In the expansion GMA, the image gamut is used for specifying or stretching the histograms in terms of the lightness or chroma of the source toward the gamut boundary of target devices.

### 2.4.1    Gaussian Histogram Specification for Image

The histogram equalization (HE) method is useful for expanding the reduced dynamic ranges of monochrome images [37]. However, HE cannot be applied to tricolor images, because it causes an unnatural and unbalanced color rendition. There is no definitive solution as to what shapes of the color histogram are best suited. In our experiments, the Gaussian histogram was an effective candidate for creating a natural and pleasant image. First, an arbitrary histogram in lightness $L$ is specified for Gaussian distribution through HE as shown below. HE transforms the original lightness ($L$) to $g$ and histogram $p_1(L)$ is equalized to constant $p_c(g)$ as follows:

$$g = F(L) = \int_0^Y p_1(x)\,dx, \; p_c(g) = constant \tag{2.25}$$

where $p_1(L)$ denotes the probability density of value $L$ occurrence. Now, our target histogram $p_2(z)$ is Gaussian as follows:

$$p_2(z) = \frac{1}{\sqrt{2\pi}\,\sigma} \exp\left\{ -\frac{1}{2\sigma^2 (z - \bar{z})^2} \right\} \tag{2.26}$$

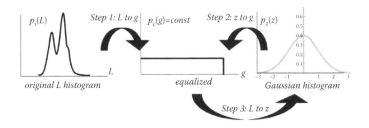

**FIGURE 2.10**
Histogram specification for Gaussian distribution.

with $z$ also being equalized to constant $p(g)$ by HE as follows:

$$g = G(z) = \int_0^z p_2(x)dx, \quad p_c(g) constant \qquad (2.27)$$

Thus, connecting the two $g$'s after HE from $L$ to $g$ and $z$ to $g$, the objective transformation from $L$ to $z$ is given by the inverse as follows:

$$Z = G^{-1}(g) = G^{-1}\{F(L)\} \qquad (2.28)$$

After the histogram specification [38] of $L$, the chrominance components are divided into $m$ segments by $\Delta H$ at hue angle $H$. Then, the Gaussian histogram specification (HS) and $L$ are used to expand the histogram of chroma $C$ in each division without changing the color hue. For example, whole pixels are totally divided into $m = 16$ segments, each of which is expanded by individual Gaussian HS. Figure 2.10 shows the Gaussian HS process for gamut expansion. Here, the histogram for lightness $L$ is specified to match a combination of Gaussian distributions with multiple peaks that are naturally stretched to cover a wide range.

In practice, the $L^*$ histogram does not always have a single peak but sometimes has multiple peaks. In such cases, the histogram may be specified for a mixed Gaussian distribution. Figure 2.11a to Figure 2.11d show an improved $L^*$ of image "stairs" by gamut expansion using Gaussian HS. In this sample, a mixed Gaussian HS (Figure 2.11d) obtains a satisfactory image with brighter color than single Gaussian (Figure 2.11b and Figure 2.11c). However, it is difficult to preserve the shape of the original histogram (Figure 2.11a) by using Gaussian HS; thus, the atmosphere of original color distribution may be lost.

### 2.4.2 Histogram Stretching for Image

Gaussian HS is an effective gamut expansion method of creating a natural and pleasant image but does not reflect the color atmosphere of original scene. To maintain the shape of the original histogram, a method based on *histogram stretching* has been successfully introduced [36]. The histogram stretching method simply stretches the original shape of color distribution through linear scaling to maintain geometrical similarity by referring the gamut boundary of the devices.

Most simply, the variable $x$ in original histogram $p_1(L)$ distributed between lowest value $a$ and highest value $b$ is stretched to the predetermined range of $[0, b_m]$ for $b_m > b$ as follows:

$$x' = b_m \left( \frac{x - a}{b - a} \right) \qquad (2.29)$$

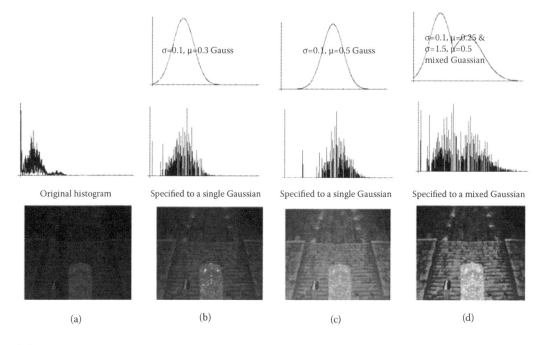

**FIGURE 2.11**
Improved $L^*$ of image "stairs" by gamut expansion using histogram specification. Images in the bottom row: (a) original image, (b) expanded by single Gaussian HS with $\sigma = 0.1$ and $\mu = 0.3$, (c) expanded by single Gaussian HS with $\sigma = 0.1$ and $\mu = 0.5$, and (d) expanded by mixed Gaussian HS.

Figure 2.12 shows that by assigning $x$ to lightness $L$, the original histogram $p_1(L)$ is expanded to $p_2(L')$. After the histogram stretching for lightness $L$, the chrominance components are segmented into $m$ divisions by $\Delta H$ at hue angle $H$. Then chroma $x = C$ of each division is expanded to $x' = C$ by histogram stretching, the same as for $L$ without changing the color hue.

Figure 2.13a through Figure 2.13c shows an improved image "room" by gamut expansion using histogram stretching. The chroma was segmented by 16 $\Delta H$ division and expanded after lightness (see Figure 2.13c). The image "room" taken in dim light was dramatically improved to achieve a satisfactory image with bright and vivid colors. Well-designed histogram stretching can automatically expand a shrunken gamut to an appropriate wider gamut, thus restoring visibility in terms of the color and tone of the degraded image.

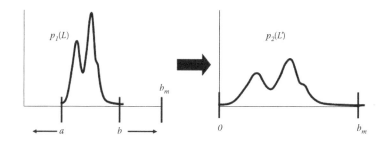

**FIGURE 2.12**
Gamut expansion by histogram stretching.

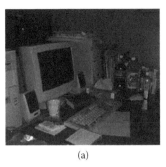
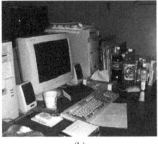
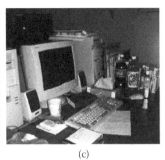

(a)           (b)           (c)

**FIGURE 2.13** (See color insert.)
Improved image "room" by gamut expansion using histogram stretching. (a) original image (b) lightness stretching image (c) lightness and chroma stretching image.

## 2.5 Versatile GMA

The latest imaging devices strive for *realistic color reproduction* with HDR and a wide color gamut, in addition to high resolution. The advent of various flat panel displays (FPDs) has raised the curtain on a new display age during which the CRT will be replaced. Because such new devices as the LCD or PDP (plasma display panel) create a different and wider color gamut from that of the CRT, the GMA again represents a key technology to make more effective and flexible use of the display gamut for advanced color imaging. Because a source image has its own color gamut, pleasant color is reproduced by applying an adaptive GMA depending on whether the image gamut is wider or narrower than that of the display. Because digital camera images of our daily lives rarely fulfill the display gamut, gamut expansion is useful in rendering more vivid colors.

Hence, a versatile GMA that maps colors bidirectionally between the narrow-to-wide and wide-to-narrow gamuts is necessary [39], [40]. The previous section presented both methods of image-dependent gamut compression using *r-image* and image-dependent gamut expansion using histogram stretching. In this chapter, a generalized histogram stretching method is introduced for a versatile GMA through automatic gamut comparison using the GBD of the image and device.

### 2.5.1 Histogram Rescaling Method

To perform natural and pleasant gamut mapping automatically, the histogram stretching method is generalized to rescale the image gamut. The *histogram rescaling* method can easily adapt an image gamut to an objective target device gamut by simply setting the lowest and highest source values corresponding to the endpoints of the destination. Figure 2.14 illustrates an explanatory model for gamut mapping based on histogram rescaling. In the original histogram, $p_1(L)$, lowest value $a$, and highest value $b$ are flexibly expanded or compressed for adaptation to the histogram of the target device gamut using Equation 2.30 as follows:

$$x' = k(x - a) + a'; \quad k = \frac{b' - a'}{b - a} \tag{2.30}$$

where $b'$ and $a'$ denote the highest and lowest endpoints to be rescaled matching the gamut boundaries of target device, and $k$ means a scaling factor working compression for $0 < k < 1$

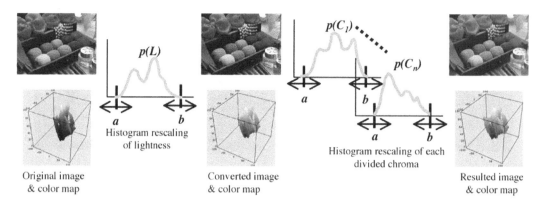

**FIGURE 2.14**
Schema of gamut mapping model based on histogram rescaling.

or expansion for $k > 1$. Under the following conditions,

$$\int_a^b p_1(x)dx = \int_{a'}^{b'} p_2(x')dx' = 1; \quad p_2(x')dx' = p_1(x)dx; \quad dx' = kdx \qquad (2.31)$$

the histogram $p_2(x')$ after rescaling is given by

$$p_2(x') = k^{-1}p_1\{k^{-1}x' + (a - k^{-1}a')\} \qquad (2.32)$$

First, the lightness rescaling is performed by assigning the variables $x'$ and $x$ to $L$ and $L'$ before and after, and next the chroma is rescaled by setting $x'$ and $x$ to $C$ and $C'$ before and after as well. After the histogram rescaling of lightness $L$, the chroma components are divided into $m$ segments by $\Delta H$ at hue angle $H$. Then, chroma $C$ of each segment is expanded or compressed by histogram rescaling as well as $L$ without changing the color hue. The hue $H$ is segmented to $m = 16$ in this experiment.

### 2.5.2 Wide Color Gamut Devices

Recently, the printer gamut has been significantly widened along with improvements made in printing media and devices. Figure 2.15a through Figure 2.15c show the measured results of various printer color gamuts in CIELAB space. There, the color gamuts for two types of ink-jet printers and a toner printer are compared with the wire frame of the sRGB color

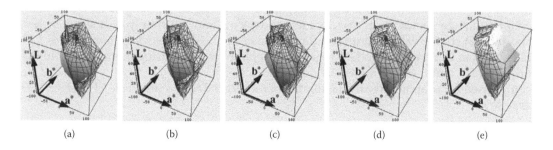

|         (a)          |         (b)          |         (c)          |         (d)          |         (e)          |

**FIGURE 2.15 (See color insert.)**
Printer and display gamuts compared with sRGB gamut (wire frame) in CIELAB space. (a) six-color dye ink-jet printer (b) four-color pigment ink-jet printer (c) four-color toner printer (d) CRT display (e) LC display.

**TABLE 2.1**

Volume of Device Color Gamut

| Device | Volume |
|---|---|
| 6-color dye ink-jet printer | 381666 |
| 4-color pigment ink-jet printer | 266361 |
| 4-color toner-based printer | 428113 |
| sRGB | 765008 |
| CRT | 563564 |
| LCD | 667682 |

gamut. The printer gamut is obtained by using a Gretag spectrophotometer to measure the XYZ tristimulus values of the printed chips on coated paper. The sRGB gamut is first generated by using a set of $a^*$, $b^*$, $L^*$ data with equal intervals of $\Delta a^* = 5$ and $\Delta b^* = 5$ in the range of $-120 < a^* < 120$, $-120 < b^* < 120$, and $0 < L^* < 100$, respectively, and then is limited to the range between 0 and 1. On the other hand, LCDs are becoming commonly used as computer color displays due to their compact size and low power consumption [41]. Here, the LCD and CRT gamuts were evaluated through an experimental study. A large number of spatially uniform color patches were displayed in the central region on screen and measured using a Specbos 1200 spectroradiometer. All measurements were made at a 0 degree viewing angle in a dark room with minimal stray light.

Figure 2.15d and Figure 2.15e show the measured results for the color gamuts of both displays in CIELAB space. Table 2.1 lists these gamut volumes in CIELAB space. The volume is calculated in the following steps [7], [8]:

1. The entire color gamut is divided by a discrete polar angle, where nonuniform steps are determined to include the constant color chips in each segmented sector.
2. The points farthest from the center are extracted.
3. The gamut surface is constructed by joining the triangles according to the ordered points, where the surfaces are deemed outward or inward.
4. The inward triangle is assigned a minus volume, and the entire color gamut is calculated by summing up the volume of each tetrahedron.

Most printer gamuts are obviously smaller than the sRGB gamut and slightly larger in part of the cyan region. The measured CRT gamut is similar to the sRGB gamut, though a little bit smaller. The LCD gamut is also a bit smaller than the sRGB gamut, but wider (especially in the red-to-orange region), and clearly wider than that of the CRT.

### 2.5.3   Gamut Rescaling to Destination Device

Figure 2.16 shows a test image "glass and lady" in JIS standard SCID-II, but with a narrow gamut in Figure 2.16a and the histogram rescaling results in Figure 2.16b to Figure 2.16f, along with the CIELAB color maps. The image was expanded to just inside each destination device gamut. The results show the extent to which the image gamut is expandable by the histogram rescaling GMA and how it changes image appearance in terms of chroma. The "red sofa and wine" of the test image displayed on the LCD is obviously more saturated than that displayed on the CRT due to color gamut differences.

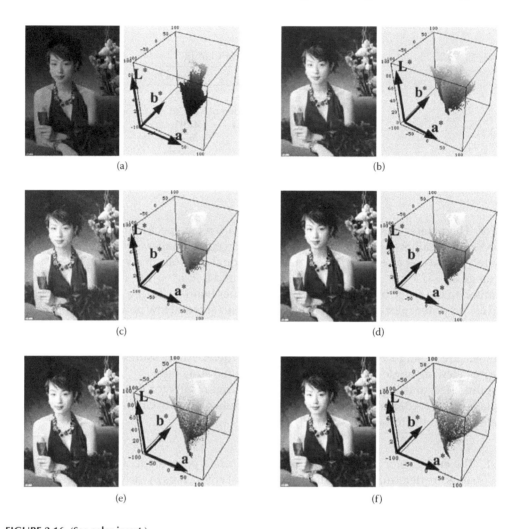

**FIGURE 2.16 (See color insert.)**

Test image "glass and lady" and GMA results with color maps: (a) original image, (b) six-color dye ink-jet printer, (c) four-color pigment ink-jet printer, (d) four-color toner-based printer, (e) CRT display, and (f) LCD display.

Figure 2.17 introduces other results by histogram rescaling GMA applied to test image "musicians" with very wide color gamut, just corresponding to the results shown in Figure 2.16a through Figure 2.16f. In this sample, the histogram rescaling algorithm works as wide-to-narrow gamut compression GMA for printers. For CRT or LCD, it partly expands narrow-to-wide in the higher lightness range but partly compresses wide-to-narrow in the lower lightness range. These two samples tell us how the histogram rescaling GMA works well automatically adapted to the gamut sizes between image and device.

In this section, we introduced an approach to a versatile GMA adapted to various devices. We proposed a histogram rescaling algorithm as a simple but practical method for gamut mapping in reference to each GBD of the image and device. This model is applied to automatic expansion for desaturated images and automatic compression for highly saturated, wide gamut images. We compared the color gamuts of certain printers and monitors with that of sRGB. The proposed GMA worked very well to reproduce a pleasant image appearance through the experiments.

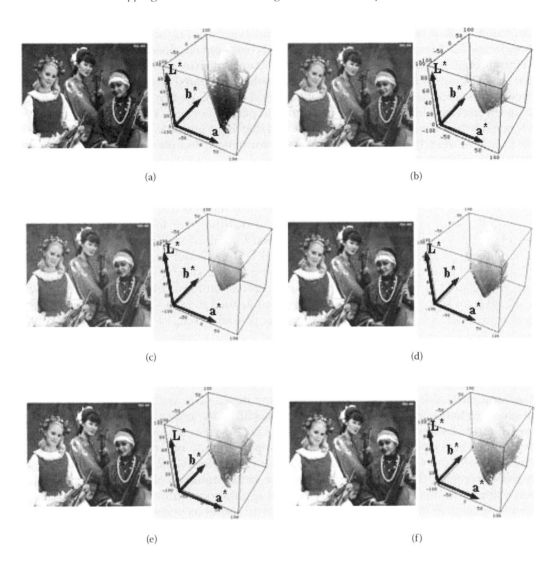

**FIGURE 2.17**

Test image "musicians" and GMA results with color maps: (a) original image, (b) six-color dye ink-jet printer, (c) four-color pigment ink-jet printer, (d) four-color toner-based printer, (e) CRT display, and (f) LCD display.

## 2.6   Conclusion

Most GMAs have been developed for 2-D L-C planes based on the D-D concept. The D-D GMA has a drawback in that some color information is lost after mapping, because the image color distributions do not always fill the entire device gamut. Conversely, because the I-D GMA can use the image gamut up to the boundary, it can minimize such color loss. The 3-D I-D GMA is an ideal way to map the display image to inside the printer gamut, while minimizing the loss of color information. To perform the 3-D I-D GMA effectively, a simple and compact GBD is necessary. A simple and compact GBD called *r-image* can be applied to any type of GMA. Multifocal I-D GMA using *r-image* worked better when applied to wider gamut images. The major objective of gamut expansion is to recover the degraded colors taken under insufficient illumination or colors faded after long preservation. It is difficult to fully restore the lost original colors, but it is possible to recover pleasant colors through gamut expansion. Sometimes, pictures taken by even the highest-grade digital camera only fill the narrow gamut ranges when compared with modern wide-gamut media, thus necessitating correction to obtain vivid colors. Gaussian histogram specification is an effective candidate for creating natural and pleasant images. However, the target histogram does not always have a single peak and may have multiple peaks. A method based on histogram stretching is simple but suitable for natural and pleasant gamut expansion, while preserving the original color atmosphere.

Until now, the GMA was mainly employed to map wide gamut images on display into the narrow printer gamut. However, with the advent of HDR cameras or wide-gamut FPD devices, a versatile GMA will be necessary for the effective and full use of the device color gamut to achieve more pleasant and realistic color imaging. We proposed a simple yet practical histogram rescaling method for gamut mapping in reference to the GBD of each image and device. The proposed GMA worked very well to reproduce a pleasant and good image appearance for most images tested. It is desirable that gamut mapping should be performed in the best perceptual, uniform color space. Although the CIELAB color space recommended by CIE was intended to map Munsell colors regularly and correct MacAdam's ellipses as uniform as possible, complete uniformity has yet to be achieved [29]. Significant shifts in perceived hue are observed depending on chroma compression and expansion. The most notable phenomenon occurs in the "blue-shift" from chromatic "blue" to chromatic "purple" when mapped along a line with a constant CIELAB metric hue angle [42]. The CIECAM97s color appearance model was proposed to extend the traditional color spaces. CIE Technical Committee 8-01 recently proposed a single set of revisions to the color appearance model. The CIECAM02 color appearance model was based on the basic structure and form of the CIECAM97s color appearance model [43]. It achieved better performance for gamut mapping than in other color spaces [44]. The color space of the CIECAM02, however, is not a complete color space, and this model is rather complex. Thus, it is necessary to use better optimal color space for the GMA according to the image content and objective of applications. Future work should focus on finding a solution to how to reproduce real-world scenes as perceived by human vision.

# References

[1] J. Morovic and M.R. Luo, Evaluating gamut mapping algorithms for universal applicability, *J. Imaging Sci. Tech.*, 45, 283–290, July 2001.

[2] J. Morovic and M.R. Luo, The fundamentals of gamut mapping: A survey, *Color Res. Appl.*, 26, 85–102, January 2001.

[3] L.W. MacDonald and M.R. Luo, *Color Imaging*, John Wiley & Sons, New York, 1999.

[4] H.S. Chen and H. Kotera, Adaptive gamut mapping method based on image-to-device, in *Proceedings of IS&T's 15th NIP*, IS&T, Springfield, VA, 1999, pp. 346–349.

[5] H.S. Chen and H. Kotera, Three-dimensional gamut mapping method based on the concept of image-dependence, in *Proceedings of IS&T's 16th NIP*, IS&T, Springfield, VA, 2000, pp. 783–786.

[6] J. Morovic and P.L. Sun, The influence of image gamut on cross media color image reproduction: A survey, in *Proceedings of the 8th IS&T/SID Color Imaging Conference*, IS&T, Springfield, VA, 2000, pp. 324–329.

[7] R. Saito and H. Kotera, Extraction of image gamut surface and calculation of its volume, in *Proceedings of IS&T's 16th NIP*, IS&T, Springfield, VA, 2000, pp. 566–569.

[8] R. Saito and H. Kotera, Extraction of image gamut surface and calculation of its volume, in *Proceedings of the 8th IS&T/SID Color Imaging Conference*, IS&T, Springfield, VA, 2000, pp. 330–333.

[9] H.S. Chen, M. Oomamiuda, and H. Kotera, Gamma-compression gamut mapping method based on the concept of image-to-device, *J. Imaging Sci. Tech.*, 45, 141–151, April 2001.

[10] H. Kotera, T. Mita, H.S. Chen, and R. Saito, Image-dependent gamut compression and extension, in *Proceedings of the PICS'01 Conference*, IS&T, Springfield, VA, 2001, pp. 288–292.

[11] H. Kotera, M. Suzuki, T. Mita, and R. Saito, Image-dependent gamut color mapping for pleasant image rendition, in *Proceedings of the AIC Color'01*, Rochester, NY, 2001, pp. 227–228.

[12] H.S. Chen and H. Kotera, Three-dimensional gamut mapping method based on the concept of image-dependence, *J. Imaging Sci. Tech.*, 46, 44–63, January 2002.

[13] G. Marcu and S. Abe, Ink jet printer gamut visualization, in *Proceedings of IS&T's 11th NIP*, IS&T, Springfield, VA, 1995, pp. 459–462.

[14] P.G. Herzog, Analytical color gamut representations, *J. Imaging Sci. Tech.*, 40, 516–521, 1996.

[15] M. Mahy, Calculation of color gamut based on the Neugebauer model, *Color Res. Appl.*, 22, 365–374, 1997.

[16] G.J. Braun and M.D. Fairchild, Techniques for gamut surface definition and visualization, in *Proceedings of the 5th IS&T/SID Color Imaging Conference*, IS&T, Springfield, VA, 1997, pp. 147–152.

[17] T.J. Cholewo and S. Love, Gamut boundary determination using alpha-shapes, in *Proceedings of the 7th IS&T/SID Color Imaging Conference*, IS&T, Springfield, VA, 1999, pp. 200–203.

[18] R.L. Reel and M. Penrod, Gamut visualization tools and metrics, in *Proceedings of the 7th IS&T/SID Color Imaging Conference*, IS&T, Springfield, VA, 1999, pp. 247–251.

[19] R. Saito and H. Kotera, Dot allocations in dither matrix with wide color gamut, *J. Imaging Sci. Tech.*, 43, 345–352, 1999.

[20] H. Kotera and R. Saito, Compact description of 3D image gamut surface by SVD, in *Proceedings of IS&T's 17th NIP*, IS&T, Springfield, VA, 2001, pp. 446–449.

[21] R. Saito and H. Kotera, 3d gamut comparison between image and device for gamut mapping, in *Proceedings of IS&T's 17th NIP*, IS&T, Springfield, VA, 2001, pp. 454–457.

[22] H. Kotera and R. Saito, Compact description of 3d image gamut by singular value decomposition, in *Proceedings of the 9th IS&T/SID Color Imaging Conference*, IS&T, Springfield, VA, 2001, pp. 56–61.

[23] R. Saito and H. Kotera, 3d image-to-device gamut mapping using gamut boundary descriptor, in *Proceedings of IS&T's 18th NIP*, IS&T, Springfield, VA, 2002, pp. 608–611.

[24] R. Saito and H. Kotera, 3d gamut mapping by comparison between image and device gamut description, in *Proceedings of ICIS'02*, Tokyo, Japan, 2002, pp. 407–408.

[25] J. Morovic and M.R. Luo, Calculating medium and image gamut boundaries for gamut mapping, *Color Res. Appl.*, 25, 394–401, 2000.

[26] B.H. Kang, M.S. Cho, J. Morovic, and M.R. Luo, Gamut compression algorithm development on the basis of observer experimental data, in *Proceedings of the 8th IS&T/SID Color Imaging Conference*, IS&T, Springfield, VA, 2000, pp. 268–272.

[27] P.G. Herzog and H. Buring, Optimizing gamut mapping: Lightness and hue adjustments, in *Proceedings of the 7th IS&T/SID Color Imaging Conference*, IS&T, Springfield, VA, 1999, pp. 160–166.

[28] K.E. Spaulding, R.N. Ellson, and J.R. Sullivan, Ultra color; a new gamut mapping strategy, in *Proceedings of SPIE*, vol. 2414, 1995, pp. 61–68.

[29] N. Katoh, M. Ito, and S. Ohno, Three-dimensional gamut mapping using various color difference formulae and color spaces, *J. Electron. Imaging*, 8, 4, 365–379, 1999.

[30] H. Kotera and R. Saito, Compact description of 3d image gamut by r-image method, *J. Electron. Imaging*, 12, 345–352, October 2003.

[31] R. Saito and H. Kotera, Image-dependent three-dimensional gamut mapping using gamut boundary descriptor, *J. Electron. Imaging*, 13, 630–638, July 2004.

[32] J.D. Foley, A. van Dam, S. Feiner, and J. Hughes, *Interactive Computer Graphics: Principles and Practice*, Addison-Wesley, Reading, MA, 1996.

[33] K.M. Braun, M.D. Fairchild, and P.J. Alessi, Viewing techniques for cross-media image comparisons, *Color Res. Appl.*, 21, 6–17, January 1996.

[34] T.C. Hseue, Y.C. Shen, P.C. Chen, W.H. Hsu, and Y.T. Liu, Cross-media performance evaluation of color models for unequal luminance levels and dim surround, *Color Res. Appl.*, 23, 169–177, 1998.

[35] E.D. Montag and M.D. Fairchild, Gamut mapping: Evaluation of chroma clipping techniques for three destination gamuts, in *Proceedings of 6th IS&T/SID Color Imaging Conference*, IS&T, Springfield, VA, 1998, pp. 57–61.

[36] R. Saito and H. Kotera, Adaptive 3d gamut mapping using based on color distribution, in *Proceedings of IS&T's 19th NIP*, IS&T, Springfield, VA, 2003, pp. 812–815.

[37] W.K. Pratt, *Digital Image Processing*, John Wiley & Sons, New York, 1978.

[38] R.C. Gonzalez and R.E. Woods, *Digital Image Processing*, Addison-Wesley, Reading, MA, 1993.

[39] R. Saito and H. Kotera, A versatile 3d gamut mapping adapted to image color distribution, in *Proceedings of the IS&T's 20th NIP*, IS&T, Springfield, VA, 2004, pp. 647–651.

[40] R. Saito and H. Kotera, A versatile gamut mapping for various devices, in *Proceedings of the IS&T's 21th NIP*, IS&T, Springfield, VA, 2005, pp. 408–411.

[41] G. Sharma, Lcds versus CRTs-color-calibration and gamut considerations, in *Proceedings of the IEEE*, 90, April 2002, pp. 605–622.

[42] G.J. Braun and M.D. Fairchild, Gamut mapping for pictorial images, in *TAGA Proceedings*, 1999, pp. 645–660.

[43] N. Moroney, M.D. Fairchild, C. Li, M.R. Luo, R.W.G. Hunt, and T. Newman, The ciecam02 color appearance model, in *Proceedings of the 10th IS&T/SID Color Imaging Conference*, IS&T, Springfield, VA, 2002, pp. 23–27.

[44] R. Saito and H. Kotera, Gamut mapping adapted to image contents, in *Proceedings of AIC Color'05*, Granada, Spain, 2005, pp. 661–664.

# 3

# Three-, Two-, One-, and Six-Dimensional Color Constancy

Graham D. Finlayson

## CONTENTS

## 3.1   Introduction

The light reaching our eye is a function of surface reflectance and illuminant color. Yet, the colors that we perceive depend mostly on surface reflectance. The dependency due to illuminant color is removed through *color constancy* computation. We have a good solution to color constancy: the white page of this book looks white whether viewed under blue sky or under a yellow artificial light. However, the processes through which color constancy is achieved are not well understood: the mechanisms of Human visual color constancy processing are not known, and most camera manufacturers do not disclose how they calculate the camera white point for a scene (essentially the same as solving for color constancy). In this chapter, we will consider in detail the computational approaches that have been developed and comment on their strengths, weaknesses, and general applicability.

Let us begin by considering the outcome of color constancy processing. The image shown in Figure 3.1a is quite yellow, and this is because this image is the raw captured image of a scene taken on a sunny day: the sun is yellowish, and this biases the color captured. Figure 3.1b shows the output of the automatic color constancy processing that is carried out in the camera. After processing, the image looks more realistic; certainly, the T-shirt, which was white, looks whiter than the original. Of course, this is not to say that from a preference point of view the right image is optimally balanced. But, rather, the colors are a truer representation of the colors of the surfaces independent of the light.

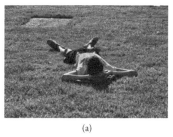 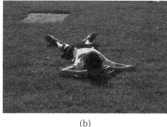 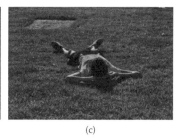

(a)                             (b)                             (c)

**FIGURE 3.1 (See color insert.)**
Unbalanced camera image (a), image after constancy processing by the camera (b), and image after gray world processing (c).

It is, of course, not known to us how the camera determines or removes the color bias due to illumination. But, a simple approach incorporated to some extent in cameras is to use the scene average as a measure of illuminant color. That is, we calculate the average in the red channel, the average in the green, and the average of the blue giving the triplet $[\mu(R), \mu(G), \mu(B)]$. This triplet is taken to be an estimate of the color of the light. In solving for color constancy, we wish to remove color bias due to illumination, so we divide by the white point estimate in order to cancel out the light color.

It has been proposed that the following

$$R \Rightarrow \frac{R}{\mu(R)}, \quad G \Rightarrow \frac{G}{\mu(G)}, \quad B \Rightarrow \frac{G}{\mu(B)} \tag{3.1}$$

should work, because the RGB (red, green, blue) of a gray surface must, by the physics of image formation, be proportional to the color of the light [1]. Assuming the scene average is an accurate estimate of illumination, then Equation 3.1 will make the RGB of a gray surface lie in the direction [1, 1, 1] (i.e., it will look gray, which is what we wish). Moreover, it is often the case that if we make achromatic colors look correct in images, then the other colors in the image are also correct (e.g., see Reference [2]). Even when Equation 3.1 does not hold, the RGBs can be transformed to a new coordinate frame where it does hold [3]. Unless otherwise stated, we will adopt the simple three-scalar adjustment as the means to remove illuminant color bias from images.

The result of gray world processing is shown in Figure 3.1c, where we see that it works poorly. Gray world fails here, because, by definition, the average scene color is mapped to gray. As there is a lot of grass in the scene, then this green will be mapped to gray. This is the wrong answer.

Interestingly, we can tell instantaneously that the gray world algorithm has failed, because we recognize the scene content. We might wonder, therefore, whether the gray world algorithm failed because it did not take account of higher-order cues. Is color constancy a high- or low-level phenomenon? In computer vision, Healey and Slater [4] assume the former and define constancy relative to the task of object recognition (a high-level task). In their algorithm, they, in the first stage, find relations between image colors that by construction are illuminant independent, and they then use these relations to recognize scene content. Assuming that objects and surfaces can be correctly identified, it is a simple matter, in a second step, to balance image colors to remove color bias due to illumination. As an example, if the white page of a book is imaged under yellow Tungsten light, then the captured image is yellowish. However, because we know that the image content should be whitish (i.e., the image contains the white page of a book), then the yellowness is easily removed from the image.

Of course, there is no guarantee that any scene we see contains a known object. So, it is interesting to consider color constancy independent of object recognition (i.e., color constancy as a low-level phenomenon). In psychophysical experiments, stimuli are designed for which there are no known object identities. The most common stimuli used are the so-called Mondrians. A Mondrian is a patchwork of variably sized and arbitrarily colored matte rectangular patches. It is well established that constancy performance for the Mondrian world is good [5]. Moreover, constancy is achieved in the blink of an eye (i.e., in a few milliseconds). Taking these results together, we might reasonably conclude that color constancy is, in the first instance, a low-level function. This is not to say that we discount the importance of higher-level processing — a wide range of experiments show that slightly improved performance can be achieved given more realistic, real-world, stimuli (e.g., scenes with objects and shapes [6]) — but that the bulk of the processing is based on low-level cues such as image color distribution. Taking this viewpoint is also pragmatic. In computer vision, we know a good deal about image color distributions but have found it difficult to say much about the range of objects or surfaces in images (the general image interpretation problem is a long way from being solved). For the rest of this chapter, we will consider the low-level, or Mondrian world, view of the constancy problem.

The gray world approach failed to solve the constancy problem, because it is based on the heuristic that the average color in every scene is gray (which is not the case). Perhaps other statistical assumptions work better? It is often assumed that the maximum R, G, and B values can be used as an estimate of the light color, and, moreover, that this estimate is generally thought to be more accurate than the gray world algorithm. Alternately, we might seek to impose harder physical constraints. Forsyth [7] observed that the bluest blue RGB cannot occur under the reddest light. That is, the range, or gamut, of colors depends on the illumination. Forsyth proposed that we can solve the Mondrian color constancy problem if camera RGBs for surfaces seen under an unknown illuminant can be mapped to corresponding RGBs under a known reference light [7]. Of course, this constraint seems reasonable, yet it is intuitively clear that there might be many ways to map a given set of image colors inside the gamut for the reference light. While Forsyth provides means for selecting among potential candidate lights, these are, like gray world, based on heuristics.

But, perhaps the three-dimensional (3-D) problem is actually too hard to solve? Maloney and Wandell argued that the 3-D problem is insoluble, as there is an intrinsic ambiguity between the brightness of an illuminant and the lightness of a surface. Thus, dark surfaces viewed under bright lights reflect the same spectral power distribution as highly reflective surfaces under dimmer light [8], [9]. This argument is taken on board in almost all modern color constancy algorithms: modern algorithms attempt only to recover reference chromaticities. Even the 3-D gamut mapping algorithm is generally used only to recover the orientation but not the magnitude of the light color.

The chromaticity constancy problem has proved to be much more tractable. Finlayson [10] made two important observations. The first was that the gamut of possible image chromaticities depends on the illuminant color (this result follows from Forsyth's work on 3-D RGB gamuts [7]). The second is that the illuminant color is limited. The chromaticities of real illuminants tend to be tightly clustered around the Planckian locus. In Finlayson's algorithm, an image chromaticity is said to be consistent with a particular light if it is within the gamut of all possible chromaticities observable under that light. Typically, a single chromaticity will be consistent with many lights; but, different chromaticities are consistent with different sets of lights. Intersecting all the illuminant sets results in an overall set of feasible illuminants: illuminants that are consistent with all image chromaticities together and at the same time. Typically, the set of feasible illuminants is small, and selecting the mean [11] or median [12] illuminant from the feasible set leads to good color constancy. Unfortunately, when color diversity is small, the feasible set can be large. In this case, it is possible that an incorrect illuminant will be selected, and when this happens, poor color constancy results. Effectively, we are back in the same position as Forsyth. We can tell which lights are plausible but not which one is present, and so heuristics are applied to determine the final illuminant estimate.

In more recent work, the ill-posed nature of the color constancy problem has been tackled using the tool of Bayesian probability theory [13], [14], [15], [16]. Given knowledge of typical scenes, it is possible to calculate the probability of observing a particular chromaticity under a particular light. This prior information can then be used to calculate the likelihood of lights given the chromaticities in an image [14]. While this approach delivers much more accurate illuminant estimates and much better color constancy, the problem of low color diversity, though certainly diminished, remains. For scenes containing small numbers of surfaces (one, two, three or four), many illuminants might be equally likely [11].

Perhaps, like the 3-D constancy problem, the two-dimensional (2-D) problem is too difficult to solve? In recent work [17], Finlayson, Hordley, and Morovic take the reductionist approach a little further. They ask if there is a single color coordinate, a function of image chromaticities, for which the color constancy problem can be solved. The idea here is that we take our RGB image, convert it in some way to a grayscale image, and then attempt to map the image gray values to those observed under reference lighting conditions. Not only does there exist a color coordinate at which color constancy computation is easy, there exists a coordinate at which no computation actually needs to be done. By construction, this invariant image factors out all dependencies due to light intensity and light color.

While this result is elegant, it probably, in truth, goes against what most people mean by color constancy. The ambiguity between light brightness and surface lightness is one thing, but we clearly cannot think of color as a one-dimensional (1-D) phenomenon. Yet, we can solve the 1-D but not the 2-D or 3-D problem. Recently, we revisited the color constancy formulation and asked if viewing the same scene twice, where the second picture is taken through a colored filter, might help. This idea is an old one, and the old reasoning goes something like this: if we have six measurements per pixel, we have twice the number of knowns to solve for the unknowns (light and surface) and so the constancy problem is easier to solve [17].

Unfortunately, this assertion is not true. By placing a filter in front of a camera, it is difficult to measure RGBs that are independent from the unfiltered counterparts. In *chromagenic* theory, this dependency is turned to our advantage, and we choose a filter so that filtered RGBs depend on unfiltered counterparts but the nature of the dependency varies with illumination. Given a set of RGBs with and without filtering, we simply check which (pre-computed) dependency exists, and this is used to determine the illuminant. This simple approach, evaluated using standard tests, is the current best algorithm. Moreover, we argue there is some plausibility of this approach in relation to human vision.

In Section 3.2, we discuss color image formation and the 3-D RGB constancy problem. The problem is seen to be difficult due to brightness/lightness indeterminacy. The 2-D chromaticity constancy problem is set forth in Section 3.3. Chromaticity constancy is possible for many scenes but remains difficult for scenes with few colors. The 2-D problem is reduced to a 1-D counterpart in Section 3.4. Here, a 1-D color coordinate is derived for which color constancy is easy to solve. By construction, the derived 1-D coordinate is independent of illumination change (no computation is necessary). As a by-product of this work, we show that it is possible to take a scene in which there are many distinct light sources present and relight the scene with one light. We must do this before we can find out the surface color at each point in a scene. Section 3.5 presents the chromagenic approach, and we see that we can solve the constancy problem more accurately if we make six measurements. In Section 3.6, we present a brief discussion of how constancy algorithms are evaluated and compared. Some conclusions are presented in Section 3.7.

## 3.2 Three-Dimensional Color Constancy

Light strikes a surface, the light is reflected, and then this reflected light enters the camera, where it is sampled by red, green, and blue sensitive receptors. This is illustrated in Figure 3.2. The function $E(\lambda)$ is a spectral power distribution. This strikes a surface that reflects a fraction $S(\lambda)$ of the incoming light. Therefore, the light entering the camera is proportional to the product $E(\lambda)S(\lambda)$. The three camera functions are functions of wavelength, and they record the sensitivity of the camera to light. Examples of light, surface, and sensor are shown in Figure 3.3.

To translate these spectral functions into the three scalar RGB values, we must integrate across the visible spectrum. In effect, the RGB is the weighted average of the light entering the camera in the red (long), green (medium), and blue (short) wave parts of the visible spectrum:

$$R = \int_{\omega} R(\lambda)E(\lambda)S(\lambda)d\lambda$$

$$G = \int_{\omega} G(\lambda)E(\lambda)S(\lambda)d\lambda \qquad (3.2)$$

$$B = \int_{\omega} B(\lambda)E(\lambda)S(\lambda)d\lambda$$

where $E(\lambda)$ is the spectral power distribution of the viewing illuminant; $S(\lambda)$ is the reflectance function of the surface; and $R(\lambda)$, $G(\lambda)$, and $B(\lambda)$ are the spectral sensitivities of the R, G, and B camera sensors. The integrals are taken over the visible spectrum $\omega$.

One of the key messages that Equation 3.2 conveys is that the responses induced in a camera depend on the spectral characteristics of the light and the surface. Color constancy algorithms attempt to remove this dependency:

$$\underline{p}_1, \underline{p}_2, \cdots, \underline{p}_k \;\rightarrow\; \boxed{\text{Color constancy}} \;\rightarrow\; \underline{d}_1, \underline{d}_2, \cdots, \underline{d}_k \qquad (3.3)$$

In the above expression, the three-vector $\underline{p}_i$ denotes the $i$th illuminant dependent R, G, and B camera response triplet that is measured in a camera image. These RGB triplets are processed by a color constancy algorithm that produces illuminant independent descriptors, $\underline{d}_i$, as output.

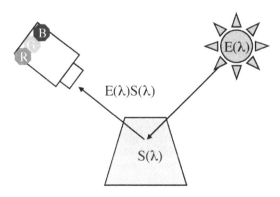

**FIGURE 3.2**
Light strikes a surface, is reflected, and the reflected light enters the camera, where it is sampled by the red, green, and blue sensors.

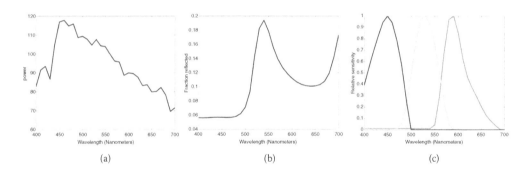

(a)                                    (b)                                    (c)

**FIGURE 3.3**
Blush light spectrum (a), dark green surface (b), and typical camera sensitivities (c).

In this chapter, we are considering constancy in the Mondrian world — a Mondrian is a random patchwork of colors (see Figure 3.4 for a Mondrian) — so there is no significance to the relationship between $\underline{p}_i$ and $\underline{p}_j$. As such, the input to color constancy processing is more properly an unordered set $\{\underline{p}_1, \underline{p}_2, \cdots, \underline{p}_k\}$ defined as follows:

$$\{\underline{p}_1, \underline{p}_2, \cdots, \underline{p}_k\} \rightarrow \boxed{\text{Color constancy}} \rightarrow \underline{d}_1, \underline{d}_2, \cdots, \underline{d}_k \qquad (3.4)$$

Intuitively, the color constancy problem expressed in this way appears to be hard. The input is an unordered set of three-vectors, and these are mapped to corresponding three-vector descriptors. However, there does not seem to be any constraint that might be used to determine the mapping. But, it is this mapping determination that is the central problem in computational color constancy research. There are two parts to the "which mapping?" question: what is the mathematical form of the mapping, and how do we estimate the parameters of the map.

Let us consider the form of the mapping. In the introduction, we considered the gray world algorithm. There we saw that the mapping that takes image colors that are biased

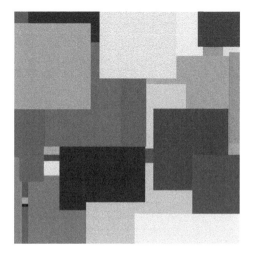

**FIGURE 3.4**
A Mondrian is a random patchwork of colors.

by the light color to those which are not is a diagonal matrix with diagonal terms equal to the reciprocal of the averages. Equation 3.1 can be rewritten as

$$
\begin{bmatrix} R \\ G \\ B \end{bmatrix} \rightarrow \begin{bmatrix} \dfrac{1}{R^e} & 0 & 0 \\ 0 & \dfrac{1}{G^e} & 0 \\ 0 & 0 & \dfrac{1}{B^e} \end{bmatrix} \begin{bmatrix} R \\ G \\ B \end{bmatrix} \tag{3.5}
$$

Note that we use the general notation $R^e$, $G^e$, and $B^e$ to denote the RGB of the light source. In the gray world algorithm, $R^e = \mu(R)$, $G^e = \mu(G)$, and $B^e = \mu(B)$. The general applicability of Equation 3.5 is discussed in detail in References [2] and [3].

Henceforth, we adopt the diagonal map shown in Equation 3.5. As such, the main problem in color constancy is estimating the illuminant color. In the literature, two approaches are followed. First, we might adopt a statistical criterion like the gray world algorithm described in the introduction. Second, we also might bring to bear additional information we have about the physics of image formation. This latter approach often includes properties such as specular highlights [18] and interreflections [19]. We will not discuss these approaches here, as we are in the Mondrian world where there are neither specular highlights nor interreflections.

The statistical approach has the advantage in that it is a simple strategy for estimating the light color, and pragmatically, it often works. The gray world algorithm gives reasonable results much of the time, especially for images in which there are no human subjects or strong memory colors. Of course, it is easy to think of images where the average is not gray (see the boy on the grass in Figure 3.1), and so it is easy to find images for which gray world processing fails.

Barnard et al. [1] wondered whether the gray world algorithm fails not because the idea is flawed but because the average in scenes is not gray but some other quantity. Because they tune the average to a given database of images, they call this approach database gray world. In database gray world, we can solve for $R^e$, $G^e$, and $B^e$ by calculating the diagonal transform, taking the average image color to the average for a white reference light. Then the reciprocal of the diagonal terms are the estimated light color. Of course, this approach may improve the gray world performance for a particular data set, but the idea that all scenes integrate to the same average color is still, in general, not true.

An alternative to the the gray world assumption is the MAX RGB algorithm. Here the illuminant color is estimated to be proportional to the maximum R, G, and B in a scene: $R^e = max(R)$, $G^e = max(G)$, and $B^e = max(B)$. This estimate has been found to be, on average, more accurate than either gray world or database gray world. Though, it is fairly easy to come across scenes for which this approach does not work (the magnitude of failure shown in Figure 3.1c is possible for the MAX RGB algorithm). Moreover, in real scenes, the scene physics often confound MAX RGB light estimation. For example, in images, specular highlights are often the brightest points, yet these highlights may have nothing to do with the color of the light: highlights for gold jewelry are typically gold, irrespective of the viewing illuminant. Estimating that the light color for a scene containing gold jewelry to be gold renders the jewelry achromatic after processing (whereas it should be gold). The MAX RGB approach also fails when images contain strong aperture colors (direct view of the light source). Even if the sky is the brightest thing in a scene, we do not wish to map blue sky to white.

Fortunately, even in the Mondrian world, we can still make an appeal to the physics of image formation in order to arrive at a more principled algorithm. Let us begin with the observation that under yellowish and bluish illuminants, camera responses are, respectively,

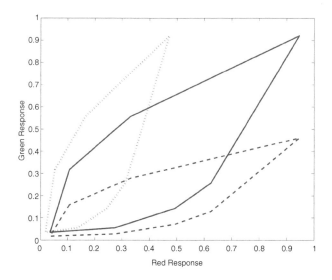

**FIGURE 3.5**
The solid line corresponds to gamut of $(R, G)$ responses under white light. The dotted line corresponds to gamut for bluish light. Dashed lines correspond to gamut for yellow light.

biased in the yellowish and bluish color directions. This idea that the gamut or range of camera measurements depends on illumination is exploited in Forsyth's gamut mapping color constancy algorithm [7]. Figure 3.5 shows the gamut — the convex hull — of the $R$ and $G$ coordinates of the camera sensitivities shown in Figure 3.3 for the 24 colors found on a Macbeth color checker[1] [20]. The solid line demarcates the responses observed under a white light. The dashed gamut shows the set of responses observable under a yellowish light, and the dotted line gamut is for blue illumination.

It is clear that the gamut of recorded colors is significantly different under different illuminations. Moreover the intersection of gamuts for illuminant pairs is small, indicating that the likelihood of observing images that are consistent with more than one light is also small. Moreover, the situation is even more favorable when viewed in three dimensions. Figure 3.5 shows a single 2-D projection (of the 3-D gamuts) that tends to overestimate the real overlap of the gamuts.

Let us now consider how Forsyth estimates the color of the light. Let $\mathcal{C}$ be the set of all RGBs that are measurable under a canonical reference light. Forsyth proved that $\mathcal{C}$ is bounded and convex. Let $\mathcal{I} = \{\underline{p}_1, \underline{p}_2, \cdots, \underline{p}_k\}$ denote the set of image colors. Now let us assume that for an illuminant $E_k(\lambda)$ there exists a mapping, $f^k()$ such that $f^k(\underline{p}_{i,k}) = \underline{d}_i$, that is $f^k()$ takes an RGB captured under $E_k(\lambda)$ onto its descriptor. Suppose now that there are $m$ illuminants, and each illuminant is characterized by its mapping function: $\mathcal{F} = \{f^1(), f^2(), \cdots, f^m()\}$. Forsyth observed that $f^k()$ is a possible solution to color constancy if and only if

$$\forall \underline{p} \in \mathcal{I} \quad f^k(\underline{p}) \in \mathcal{C} \tag{3.6}$$

Of course, many mapping functions (i.e., many lights) might satisfy this constraint. In order to choose a single overall answer to color constancy, a heuristic must be used. Forsyth chose the mapping that made the corrected image as colorful as possible (the derived descriptor gamut would be as large as possible). Here, and in Forsyth's work, the form of

---

[1] This chart, though containing few surfaces, broadly represents the important colors we see in the world and is often used as a reference chart in color science and allied disciplines.

the mapping function is chosen to be a diagonal map. Importantly, when the mapping form is diagonal, Forsyth showed that it is possible to calculate the set of all diagonal maps (a continuous bounded set).

To be consistent with the MAX RGB and gray world algorithms, we might wonder how Forsyth's notion of diagonal map relates to the estimate of $R^e$, $G^e$, and $B^e$. It is straightforward to show that, assuming that the canonical light is white ($R = G = B$), the diagonal terms of the inverse of the diagonal map comprise the RGB of the light color.

Forsyth's algorithm, though quite ingenious, suffers from two problems. First, the algorithm is not easy to implement: $C$ and $I$ are 3-D convex sets, and the mapping functions $f(\cdot)$ are also parameterized by three numbers. In the 3-D case, the set of maps taking an image gamut to reference lighting conditions is also a 3-D convex set. Computing the continuous map set is a fairly laborious task and involves intersecting many convex sets. The second, and more serious, problem is that it is not obvious that the 3-D problem can be solved. It is clear that

$$R = \int_\omega R(\lambda)E(\lambda)S(\lambda)d\lambda = \int_\omega R(\lambda)\alpha E(\lambda)\frac{S(\lambda)}{\alpha}d\lambda$$

$$G = \int_\omega G(\lambda)E(\lambda)S(\lambda)d\lambda = \int_\omega G(\lambda)\alpha E(\lambda)\frac{S(\lambda)}{\alpha}d\lambda \quad (3.7)$$

$$B = \int_\omega B(\lambda)E(\lambda)S(\lambda)d\lambda = \int_\omega B(\lambda)\alpha E(\lambda)\frac{S(\lambda)}{\alpha}d\lambda$$

That is, there is an indeterminacy between the power of the incident illumination and the reflectivity, or lightness, of a surface [8]. Finlayson and Hordley [11] proved that in the face of brightness indeterminacy, the 3-D computation was equivalent to a 2-D computation.

## 3.3 Two-Dimensional Chromaticity Constancy

To reduce the 3-D color constancy problem to two dimensions, RGBs are mapped to chromaticities. For the purposes of this chapter, we define a chromaticity to be any 2-D function of a 3-D RGB such that it is possible to reconstruct the original RGB up to an unknown scalar. The most common form of chromaticity, the *rg* chromaticity space, is defined as $(\frac{R}{R+G+B}, \frac{G}{R+G+B})$. Note that $b = \frac{B}{R+G+B}$ so $b = 1 - r - g$; that is, $r$ and $g$ uniquely parameterize the magnitude normalized vector $[rgb]$.

Denoting an *rg* chromaticity as a two-vector $\underline{q}$, the chromaticity constancy problem becomes

$$\{\underline{q}_1, \underline{q}_2, \cdots, \underline{q}_k\} \rightarrow \boxed{\text{2-D-constancy}} \rightarrow \underline{c}_1, \underline{c}_2, \cdots, \underline{c}_k \quad (3.8)$$

where the outputs of constancy processing are now the 2-D chromaticity descriptors $\underline{c}_i$.

The "color in perspective" chromaticity constancy algorithm of Finlayson works in analogous manner to Forsyth's 3-D solution. Given reference and image chromaticity gamuts $C^c$ and $I^c$, the aim is to find the set of mapping functions taking all the 2-D points $I^c$ into $C^c$ (where the superscript $c$ denotes 2-D chromaticity):

$$\forall \underline{q} \in I^c \quad f^k(\underline{q}) \in C^c \quad (3.9)$$

As before, many mapping functions (i.e., many lights) might be possible. In order to choose a single overall answer to color constancy, a heuristic is used. Mean and median mapping

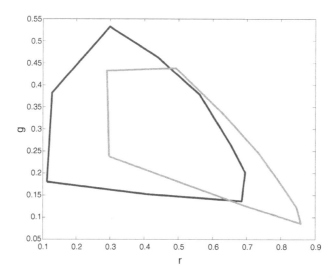

**FIGURE 3.6**
How an RGB is mapped to its RG chromaticity coordinate: see text for detailed description.

functions were found to deliver reasonable color constancy performance [11]. If the chromaticity transform maps RGB to [R/G and G/B], then $f^k$ is a 2-D diagonal map, and as before, a continuous mapping set can be estimated.

However, chromaticity constancy was found to be not so accurate when the number of maps satisfying Equation 3.9 was large (and this was sometimes true even for images with a fairly large number of colors). Moreover, in chromaticity space, the overlap between gamuts is exaggerated. Figure 3.6 shows the *rg* gamut for the Macbeth color checker viewed under whitish light and delimited by a solid blue line. The gamut under a more yellowish light is shown in red (these are for the same lights as used in Figure 3.5). Notice that now, in chromaticity space, the size of the intersection is proportionally much bigger. The intuition for what is happening here can be explained by appealing to our own vision. The mapping that takes a 3-D world and projects to a 2-D image is a perspective mapping and is the same mathematically as a chromaticity transform. Suppose we take a picture of a person standing in front of an arch (say L'Arc de Triumphe). Then the person is inside the arch in the photo. A person in front of the arch does not intersect the arch in 3-D but is inside the arch in the photo (viewed in 2-D). Similarly, the two 3-D convex bodies may not overlap greatly, yet viewed in perspective, in chromaticity space, the overlap is exaggerated.

In order to tease the gamuts apart (and in so doing make the gamut idea more powerful), various authors [13], [14], [16] have proposed looking not at the gamuts under different lights but at the chromaticity probability distributions. These are easy to compute. Images are taken of a representative set of reflectances, and the RGBs in these images are converted to chromaticities. Figure 3.7 shows the probability distributions for the whitish and yellowish lights (assuming a normal distribution). Note that bright areas indicate higher probability. Because colors occur with different probabilities, the distributions shown in Figure 3.7 look more separate than the gamuts shown in Figure 3.6.

Probability distributions calculated in this way are then used as priors in constancy computation. Under assumptions of surface reflectance independence (true for the Mondrian world),

$$Pr(E(\lambda)|\underline{q}_1, \underline{q}_2, \cdots, \underline{q}_k) \propto \sum_{i=1}^{n} log(Pr(q_i|E(\lambda))) \tag{3.10}$$

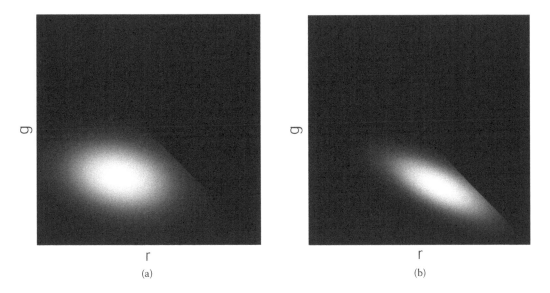

**FIGURE 3.7**
Probability distribution of *rg* chromaticities for (a) whitish light (brighter means more probable) and (b) yellowish light.

The probability that the light was $E(\lambda)$ given a set of image chromaticities is proportional to the sum of the log of the probabilities that given chromaticities $q_i$ appear under $E(\lambda)$. Under the assumptions that each surface reflectance is independent (true for the Mondrian world), choosing the maximally probable illuminant is the Bayes optimal estimate of illumination. Given an accurate estimate, it is then a simple matter to map chromaticities to the reference illuminant, thereby solving the chromaticity constancy problem.

As evident from Figure 3.7, the probability distributions for chromaticities are fairly smooth. So while different illuminants have different probability distributions, it is not hard to envisage scenes that might make a pair of illuminants equally probable. This is even more likely when the presence of image noise is taken into account, because noise can strongly perturb the true position of chromaticities calculated in dark image regions. For scenes with small numbers of distinct surfaces, even the Bayes optimal chromaticity constancy is sometimes far from the correct answer.

## 3.4 One-Dimensional Scalar Constancy

If it is not possible to reliably estimate the illuminant, and so recover chromaticities, then perhaps a 1-D analogue of the color constancy problem might still be soluble? To reduce the 2-D chromaticity constancy problem to one dimension, chromaticities are mapped to scalars: $\alpha_i = h(\underline{q}_i)$ according to the function $h(\cdot)$.

The 1-D scalar constancy problem (sometimes called color invariance) is defined as

$$\{\alpha_1, \alpha_2, \cdots, \alpha_k\} \rightarrow \boxed{\text{Scalar constancy}} \rightarrow s_1, s_2, \cdots, s_k \qquad (3.11)$$

Let us suppose that $[a\ b]$ is a chromaticity for a reflectance $S(\lambda)$ viewed under the reference illuminant $E(\lambda)$. Now, suppose that the same surface is viewed under $E'(\lambda)$ giving a second chromaticity $[a + \Delta\ b]$. Clearly, in this case, the function $h([x\ y]) = y$ would solve the

1-D scalar constancy problem ($h([a \quad b]) = b$ and $h([a + \Delta \quad b]) = b$. Rather remarkably, Finlayson and Hordley [21] showed that for most typical illuminants and for most typical cameras, there exists a chromaticity space where a change in illumination color affects only one of the two coordinates. The coordinate that is invariant to illumination color change has the following form:

$$\alpha(\ln R - \ln G) + \beta(\ln R + \ln G - 2 \ln B) \tag{3.12}$$

The second coordinate is in the direction orthogonal to the first:

$$\alpha(\ln R - \ln G) - \beta(\ln R + \ln G - 2 \ln B) \tag{3.13}$$

with $\ln R - \ln G = \ln \frac{R}{G}$.

The scalars $\alpha$ and $\beta$ depend on the spectral characteristics of the camera. To give some intuition of why Equation 3.12 and Equation 3.13 work, we begin by considering the definition of typical illuminants. Photographers know that the color temperature of an illuminant gives a good characterization of its color. A temperature of 2900 K is a very yellowish illuminant, 5500 K is white, and 10,000 K is blue. These temperatures are not arbitrary but rather relate to the physics of black-body radiation. If a black-body radiator is heated to 2900 K, 5500 K, and 10,000 K temperatures, then yellowish, whitish, and bluish spectra result. The importance of all of this is that illumination might be approximately characterized by two numbers: its color temperature and its average power.

If we look at the $rg$ chromaticity coordinates of illuminants across a temperature range, we end up with a crescent locus. A surface seen with respect to this range of illuminants also induces a crescent, and different surfaces induce different crescents with many different sizes and orientations. Opponent type color differences in log chromaticity space straighten out these lines. Figure 3.8a shows the $rg$ chromaticites for nine surfaces viewed under a set of Planckian lights (varying from 3000 K to 10,000 K; each line represents a single surface). In Figure 3.8b, we show a log chromaticity plot (note the opponent type axes), and we see that these crescents are substantially straightened. The red line shows an axes approximately perpendicular to the direction of light variation ($\alpha \approx \frac{1}{\sqrt{6}}$ and $\beta \approx \frac{-2}{\sqrt{6}}$) (projecting to this line is the definition of $h(\cdot)$). Notice that the lines are not completely straight and parallel. For this to occur, the sensors in the camera would need to be sensitive only to a single wavelength of light [21] which is not the case here. The log chromaticity plot for a camera with sensitivity only at 450, 540, and 610 nm is shown in Figure 3.8.

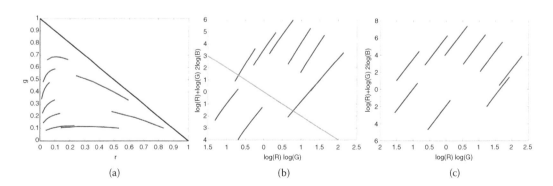

(a)　　　　　　　　　　(b)　　　　　　　　　　(c)

**FIGURE 3.8**

(a) RG chromaticities for nine checker colors under a variety of Planckian lights. (Each line denotes the color of a single light as a function of light color.) (b) In log chromaticity space, these lines become approximately straight and parallel. The red line is orthogonal to the direction of light variation. (c) Perfectly straight lines result if a camera with narrow band sensitivities is used.

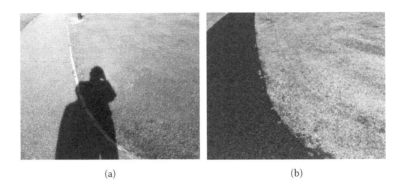

(a)                            (b)

**FIGURE 3.9 (See color insert.)**
(a) Input color image. (b) 1-D coordinate transform coded as a grayscale; notice how the shadow disappears.

What are the implications of this 1-D constancy in practical applications? Generally, when we talk about color constancy, we assume that input RGBs are mapped to output RGBs; that is, we look at an output image. Here, by definition, the output images must be grayscale, because the color constant coordinate is a single number. To illustrate these ideas further, consider the picture of an outdoor scene shown in Figure 3.9a. We see that there is a pronounced shadow area. The light striking the shadow is bluish (from a blue sky), and the light striking the nonshadow area is less blue, as there is a direct contribution from the sun. If, as we claim, 1-D color constancy works at a pixel, then coding the 1-D coordinate as a grayscale should result in an image in which the shadow magically disappears. This is the case, as can be seen in Figure 3.9b.

It is a simple matter to code this invariant 1-D coordinate as a grayscale. It follows then that in an image where there are two distinctly colored lights — for example, sun and shadow — the corresponding grayscale image will be shadow free. We show an input image that has a shadow (Figure 3.9a) and the corresponding shadow-free counterpart (Figure 3.9b). Moreover, we have shown two important further results. First, we can use the shadow-free grayscale image to remove shadows in full color images [22]. Second, we can find the invariant coordinate using only the image statistics [23].

We acknowledge that the application of this 1-D invariant does not really solve the color constancy problem as it is generally defined. Even when we remove the shadow (even in a color image), we still do not know the overall white point. Yet, discovering the illumination field is a prerequisite for solving the color constancy problem for multiple lights. That is, that we can find a 1-D coordinate independent of light color might in due course make it possible to recover the full color of surfaces across an image.

## 3.5 Six-Dimensional Constancy

Rather than reduce the dimensionality of the color constancy problem, maybe one can solve for color constancy if more measurements are available, not fewer. This is the starting point for the chromagenic theory of color constancy [17]. A chromagenic camera captures two images of every scene. The first is taken using a conventional camera. The second is captured using the same camera, but a specially chosen chromagenic filter is placed in front of the camera. The filter is chosen so that the relationship between filtered and unfiltered RGBs depends on the illumination. In short, by assessing how RGBs are related to filtered counterparts, we can recover the light color. One embodiment of a chromagenic camera is shown in Figure 3.10.[2]

Abstractly, this six-dimensional (6-D) chromagenic constancy can be written as

$$\{\underline{p}_1, \underline{p}_2, \cdots, \underline{p}_k, \underline{p}_1^F, \underline{p}_2^F, \cdots, \underline{p}_k^F\} \rightarrow \boxed{\text{Color constancy}} \rightarrow \underline{d}_1, \underline{d}_2, \cdots, \underline{d}_k \qquad (3.14)$$

where the superscript $F$ denotes dependence on the chromagenic filter.

To understand the chromagenic approach to illuminant estimation, let us consider again Equation (3.2) governing the formation of unfiltered and filtered sensor responses. We can write the RGBs captured through a chromagenic filter $F(\lambda)$ as

$$\underline{p}^F = R = \int_\omega R(\lambda)E(\lambda)F(\lambda)S(\lambda)d\lambda$$

$$G = \int_\omega G(\lambda)E(\lambda)F(\lambda)S(\lambda)d\lambda \qquad (3.15)$$

$$B = \int_\omega B(\lambda)E(\lambda)F(\lambda)S(\lambda)d\lambda$$

We can think of $\underline{p}$ and $\underline{p}^F$ as the sensor responses to a single surface under two different lights (because the filter effectively introduces a change of lighting). Now, suppose that we model a change of illumination by a linear transform. This implies that the two pairs of chromagenic camera responses are related:

$$\underline{\rho}^F = T_E^F \underline{\rho} \qquad (3.16)$$

Here, $T_E^F$ is a $3 \times 3$ linear transform that depends on the chromagenic filter $F(\lambda)$ and the scene illuminant $E(\lambda)$. Equation 3.16 implies that for a known chromagenic filter, and given sensor responses under a known illuminant, we can predict the corresponding filtered sensor responses. In the context of illumination estimation, we are given both the filtered and unfiltered sensor responses, and our task is to determine the illuminant or, equivalently, its corresponding transform $T_E^F$. The chromagenic algorithm [17] determines the appropriate transform in a two-step algorithm: a preprocessing step, applied once for a given chromagenic camera, and a second operation, applied to a given pair of images for which we wish to estimate the scene illuminant.

### 3.5.1 Preprocessing

We choose *a priori* a set of $m$ plausible scene illuminants with SPDs (spectral power distribution) $E_i(\lambda)$, $i = 1, \ldots, m$. In addition, we select a set of $n$ surface reflectances $S_j(\lambda)$ representative of the surfaces that occur in the world. Now, for the $i$th illuminant, we define a $3 \times n$ matrix $Q_i$ with a $j$th column that contains $(R_{ij}, G_{ij}, B_{ij})$: the sensor response to the $j$th surface imaged under the $i$th illuminant. Similarly, we define $Q_i^F$, also a $3 \times n$ matrix with a $j$ column that contains $(R_{ij}^F, G_{ij}^F, B_{ij}^F)$, the sensor response to the $j$th surface imaged under the $i$th illuminant and filtered by a chromagenic filter $F(\lambda)$. Then, for each plausible illuminant, we define a $3 \times 3$ transform matrix:

$$T_i = Q_i^F Q_i^+ \qquad (3.17)$$

where $+$ denotes the pseudo-inverse operator. That is, $T_i$ is the $3 \times 3$ transform that best maps unfiltered sensor responses, imaged under illuminant $i$ to the corresponding filtered sensor responses, in a least-squares sense.

---

[2] The object is taken from Powerpoint clip art.

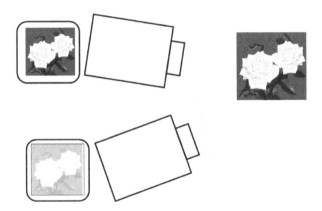

**FIGURE 3.10**
A chromagenic camera takes two pictures of a scene, with and without a colored filter.

### 3.5.2 Operation

Now, suppose we are given a pair of chromagenic images captured under an unknown scene illuminant. Let us suppose that each image of the pair consists of $p$ pixels, and let $\mathcal{Q}$ and $\mathcal{Q}^F$ denote the $3 \times p$ matrices of unfiltered and filtered sensor responses, respectively. For each plausible scene illuminant, we can calculate a fitting error:

$$e_i = \|\mathcal{T}_i \mathcal{Q} - \mathcal{Q}^F\| \tag{3.18}$$

under the assumption that $E_i(\lambda)$ is the scene illuminant. We then hypothesize that the scene illuminant is the illuminant corresponding to the transform $\mathcal{T}_i$ that best describes the relationship between filtered and unfiltered RGBs. That is, we choose the illuminant with minimum fitting error so that our estimate of the scene illuminant is $E_{est}(\lambda)$, where

$$est = \min_i(e_i) \quad (i = 1, 2, \cdots, m) \tag{3.19}$$

As we will see in the next section, the chromagenic algorithm delivers very good constancy performance. While this is good news for computer vision, it does not, at first glance, seem to shed light on human visual processing. However, in Reference [24], it is argued that the chromagenic approach may be relevant. It is well known that in front of the central part of the retina (but not elsewhere), there is yellow macular pigment. Prefiltered light striking our central vision appears yellow. Moreover, in seeing the world, we make many rapid fixation points (three to four per second), and so it is plausible that the visual system has access to both normal cone responses and those that were prefiltered by the yellow macular pigment.

In the context of color science, this idea seems even more plausible. For small color targets, the CIE (Committee Internationale d'Eclairage) suggests using the XYZ 2 degree observer [25][3] (2 degrees of visual angle). For large samples, the 10-degree observer [25] should be used. These sets of observer curves are significantly different in shape from one another, and this difference might be explained by the presence of the macular pigment. Experiments were carried out where the 2- and 10-degree observer curves were used to generate the six

---

[3] Observer curves are linear combinations of cone responses.

RGBs used in the chromagenic algorithm. Excellent color constancy was delivered by this color science chromagenic algorithm [17], [26].

---

## 3.6 Evaluation

Most color constancy algorithms work by estimating the color of the light defined in the RGB space — $R^e$, $G^e$, and $B^e$ — and then using this estimate to remove the color bias due to illumination. It is generally assumed that the correct estimate is the measured RGB of a white reflectance under a given light source. Let us denote the estimated RGB as $\underline{P}$ and the measured RGB of the actual light as $\underline{Q}$. Then the angle between these vectors is often used to measure the error in the estimate:

$$angle(\underline{P}, \underline{Q}) = cos^{-1} \left( \frac{\underline{P} \cdot \underline{Q}}{|\underline{P}||\underline{Q}|} \right) \tag{3.20}$$

Thus, we might say that for a given camera and a given set of test images, the average recovery error for an algorithm is 10 degrees.

To evaluate color constancy performance, we use the Simon Fraser [1] set of 321 images (of 31 scenes under up to 11 different lights). This set is particularly useful as, along with each image, there is a measurement of the RGB from a white patch (a measurement of the color of the light), which makes the process of calculating the angular error straightforward. We ran five of the algorithms discussed in this chapter, and the results are summarize in Table 3.1.

If we look at the mean statistics, it looks as though gamut mapping works better than anything else. However, in Reference [27], the error distribution for the different algorithms was found to be highly skewed, and, as such, it was argued that the median statistic is a better summary statistic for algorithm performance. Here, we see that the probabilistic and gamut mapping approaches appear to work equally well, and even the venerable MAX RGB looks competitive.

To more formally decide whether one algorithm delivers better constancy than another, we can use the tools of significance testing. Given a median statistic, we should use the Wilcoxon rank sum test to determine whether one algorithm is significantly better than another [27]. Accordingly, gamut mapping and the probabilistic approach are found to work better than the Max RGB and gray world (either one), and, in turn, Max RGB was found to deliver better results than gray world. But, it was not found that gamut mapping delivered significantly better performance than the probabilistic approach.

**TABLE 3.1**

Mean and Median Angular Recovery Error for Five Color Constancy Algorithms

| Color Constancy Algorithm | Mean Angular Error | Median Angular Error |
|---|---|---|
| Gray world | 14.32 | 8.85 |
| Database gray world | 12.25 | 6.58 |
| Max RGB | 8.77 | 4.02 |
| Gamut mapping | 5.46 | 2.92 |
| Probabilistic (color by correlation) | 9.93 | 2.93 |

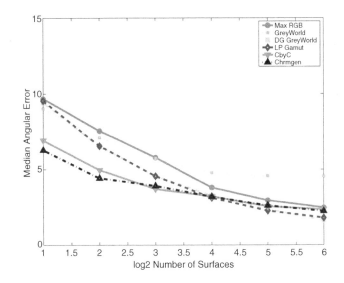

**FIGURE 3.11**
Median angular error for six algorithms as a function of the number of surfaces in a scene.

Unfortunately, the Simon Fraser set of real images did not allow us to test the chromagenic algorithm (because it comprises only RGB images and does not have filtered counterparts). However, given measured lights, surfaces, and camera sensitivities, it is possible to generate synthetic images. With respect to these, we can test how well the chromagenic approach works. In Reference [1], a methodology is proposed for generating synthetic images containing 2, 4, 8, 16, 32, and 64 surfaces, where the surfaces are illuminated with one of a large number of measured lights. Importantly, algorithms such as chromagenic and the probabilistic set are not trained on the set of all test lights but on a smaller subset, and so these algorithms must estimate the RGB of the light source for lights that are not part of the training set. An advantage of the synthetic approach is that we can generate many thousands of images and arrive at stable statistical measures of algorithm performance.

Figure 3.11 shows the median angular error recorded for all the algorithms discussed in this chapter for the Simon Fraser synthetic image protocol. It is clear that all algorithms improve as the number of surfaces increase. Notice also that the chromagenic algorithm delivers the best performance for small surface numbers. In terms of statistical significance, the chromagenic approach was found to perform the same as the probabilistic method.

We believe that the chromagenic algorithm performance is impressive, especially because the only information that is exploited is the relationship between RGBs and filtered counterparts. Of course, one might argue that we might expect this performance increment, because we now have additional information not available in conventional constancy processing. However, there have been many previous attempts to solve for constancy with greater than three measurements (see [17] for a discussion) that have not delivered the performance increment shown here. In Reference [17], a hybrid gamut mapping plus chromagenic approach was proposed. Here, we exploit the gamut constraint to rule out implausible lights and then choose among those that are plausible using the chromagenic algorithm. In Figure 3.12, we compare the performance of chromagenic and chromagenic plus gamut mapping algorithms. We see that applying a gamut constraint improves performance. Moreover, this hybrid algorithm was also found to deliver results that were

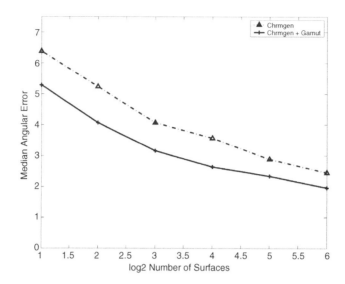

**FIGURE 3.12**
Median angular error for the chromagenic algorithm compared with chromagenic plus gamut mapping.

significantly better than all other algorithms tested. The hybrid chromagenic algorithm is, to our knowledge, the current leading algorithm evaluated using the synthetic image testing protocol.

## 3.7   Conclusion

The hard part of color constancy computation is estimating the light color. Simple statistical strategies often deliver reasonably accurate estimates: the simple mean RGB or Max RGB in an image are often the same color as the prevailing light. But, these simple methods can also fail catastrophically. To try and ameliorate the failures, additional constraints can be brought to bear. In gamut mapping, we exploit the constraint that the set of colors we measure shifts with illumination, and so we can easily tell which lights were not present. Similarly, in the probabilistic approach, we can calculate the likelihood of observing particular colors under given lights. Then, given image RGBs, we can use Bayes rule to infer the most likely light.

However, it would be fair to say that all of these approaches leave the constancy problem open: even gamut mapping and the probabilistic approach can fail. However, we showed that it is possible to solve an easier yet related subconstancy problem. For typical viewing conditions, there exists a single color coordinate that can be computed that depends only on reflectance. This is a remarkable result, as the presence of different lights disappears in the single-coordinate reflectance-only image: images with shadows can be rendered shadow free.

We also presented the chromagenic approach to color constancy. Here, two images are taken of every scene. The first is a normal image. The second is a normal image taken with a specially chosen colored filter placed in front of the camera. The chromagenic algorithm, though very simple in its operation, delivers constancy that is comparable to advanced probabilistic or gamut mapping approaches. Combining chromagenic theory with gamut mapping currently gives the best performance when evaluated on an established testing procedure. We also presented some speculative preliminary evidence that chromagenic theory might be relevant to our own visual processing.

## Acknowledgments

My own work on color constancy has been developed with several coauthors over the years, and I acknowledge their contributions. Special thanks to Dr. Steven Hordley who has been my main research collaborator in this area. I am grateful to Hewlett Packard for grant support between 1996 to 2002. The chromagenic color constancy research was funded by the U.K. government: EPSRC grant GR/R65978.

## References

[1] K. Barnard, V. Cardei, and B. Funt, A comparison of computational color constancy algorithms — part i: Methodology and experiments with synthesized data, *IEEE Transactions on Image Processing*, 11, 972–984, September 2002.

[2] J. Worthey and M. Brill, Heuristic analysis of von Kries color constancy, *J. Opt. Soc. Am. A*, 3, 10, 1708–1712, 1986.

[3] G. Finlayson, M. Drew, and B. Funt, Spectral sharpening: Sensor transformations for improved color constancy, *J. Opt. Soc. Am. A*, 11, 1553–1563, May 1994.

[4] G. Healey and D. Slater, Global color constancy: Recognition of objects by use of illumination invariant properties of color distributions, *J. Opt. Soc. Am. A*, 11, 3003–3010, November 1994.

[5] E. Land, The retinex theory of color vision, *Sci. Am.*, 237, 6, 108–129, 1977.

[6] D. Brainard, W. Brunt, and J. Speigle, Color constancy in the nearly natural image. 1. Asymmetric matches, *J. Opt. Soc. Am. A*, 14, 2091–2110, 1997.

[7] D. Forsyth, A novel algorithm for color constancy, *Int. J. Comput. Vis.*, 5, 5–36, 1990.

[8] L. Maloney and B. Wandell, Color constancy: A method for recovering surface spectral reflectance, *J. Opt. Soc. Am. A*, 3, 29–33, 1986.

[9] B. Wandell, The synthesis and analysis of color images, *IEEE Trans. Patt. Anal. and Mach. Intell.*, PAMI-9, 18, 2–13, 1987.

[10] G. Finlayson, Color in perspective, *IEEE Trans. Patt. Anal. and Mach. Intell.*, 18, 1034–1038, October 1996.

[11] G. Finlayson and S. Hordley, A theory of selection for gamut mapping colour constancy, *Im. and Vis. Comput.*, 17, 597–604, June 1999.

[12] G. Finlayson and S. Hordley, A theory of selection for gamut mapping color constancy, in *IEEE Conference on Computer Vision and Pattern Recognition*, 60–65, June 1998.

[13] G. Sapiro, Bilinear voting, in *IEEE International Conference on Computer Vision*, 1998, pp. 178–183.

[14] M. D'Zmura and G. Iverson, Probabalistic color constancy, in *Geometric Representations of Perceptual Phenomena: Papers in Honor of Tarow Indow's 70th Birthday*, R. Luce, M.M. D'Zmura, D. Hoffman, G. Iverson, and K. Romney, Eds., Laurence Erlbaum Associates, Mahweh, NJ, 1994, pp. 187–202.

[15] D.H. Brainard and W.T. Freeman, Bayesian color constancy, *J. Opt. Soc. Am.*, 14, 7, 1393–1411, 1997.

[16] G. Finlayson, S. Hordley, and P. Hubel, Colour by correlation: A simple unifying theory of colour constancy, in *IEEE International Conference on Computer Vision*, 1999, pp. 835–842.

[17] G. Finlayson, S. Hordley, and P. Morovic, Colour constancy using the chromagenic constraint, in *IEEE Conference on Computer Vision and Pattern Recognition*, 2005, pp. I, 1079–1086.

[18] S. Shafer, Using color to separate reflection components, *Color Res. Appl.*, 10, 210–218, 1985.

[19] B. Funt, M. Drew, and J. Ho, Color constancy from mutual reflection, *Int. J. Comp. Vis.*, 6, pp. 5–24, 1991.

[20] C. McCamy, H. Marcus, and J. Davidson, A color-rendition chart, *J. App. Photog. Eng.*, 95–99, 1976.

[21] G. Finlayson and S. Hordley, Color constancy at a pixel, *JOSA-A*, 18, 253–264, February 2001.

[22] G.D. Finlayson, S.D. Hordley, C. Lu, and M.S. Drew, On the removal of shadows from images, *IEE Transactions on Pattern Analysis and Machine Intelligence*, 28, 1, 59-68, 2006.

[23] G. Finlayson, M. Drew, and C. Lu, Intrinsic images by entropy minimization, in *European Conference on Computer Vision*, Vol III, 2004, pp. 582–595.

[24] G. Finlayson and P. Morovic, Human visual processing: Beyond 3 sensors, in *IEE International Conference on Visual Information Engineering*, 2005, pp. 1–7.

[25] G. Wyszecki and W.S. Stiles, *Color Science, Concepts and Methods, Quantitative Data and Formulas*, 2nd Edition, John Wiley, N.Y., 1982.

[26] G. Finlayson, P. Morovic, and S. Hordley, Chromagenic colour constancy, in *10th Congress of the International Colour Association AIC Colour'05*, 2005, pp. 547–551.

[27] S. Hordley and G. Finlayson, Re-evaluating colour constancy algorithms, in *17th International Conference on Pattern Recognition*, 2004, pp. I: 76–79.

# 4

# *Noise Reduction and Edge Detection in Color Images*

Bogdan Smolka and Anastasios N. Venetsanopoulos

## CONTENTS

## 4.1 Introduction

In this chapter, the emphasis is placed on vectorial noise reduction and edge detection methods, which play a crucial role in many tasks of computer vision, as the efficient noise suppression and reliable edge detection enable the success of the subsequent color image analysis and its understanding [1], [2], [3].

The earliest, component-wise methods, based on the transformations commonly applied in grayscale imaging, process each channel of the color image independently. By neglecting the correlation that exists between the color channels of a natural image, component-wise noise suppression and edge detection solutions produce an image that contains color shifts and other serious artifacts.

To address this problem, recent color image processing solutions utilize the spectral interrelation of the neighboring color samples in an attempt to eliminate color artifacts and to increase the accuracy of the edge detection process. Because a natural red-green-blue (RGB) image exhibits strong spectral correlation among its color planes, vectorial processing of color images is beneficial in most applications [2].

The topics covered in this chapter are organized as follows. Section 4.2 begins with the presentation of noise sources that degrade the quality of color images and presents the basic concepts used for the restoration of color images. Then the family of vector median-based filters, fuzzy, and switching filters are discussed. Also, in this section, the application of anisotropic diffusion to color image denoising is considered.

Section 4.3 focuses on the problem of edge detection in color images. In the first part, a class of edge detection operators based on various definitions of the image gradient is presented. Section 4.3.2 describes a more advanced approach, in which the color image is treated as a vector field. Then the powerful class of operators based on the vector order statistics, described in Section 4.2, is reviewed, and Section 4.3.4 outlines an interesting approach based on hypercomplex convolution. Finally, we compare the presented edge detectors and give some concluding remarks.

## 4.2 Noise Reduction in Color Images

Noise, arising from a variety of sources, is inherent to all electronic image sensors. There are many types of noise sources that decrease the quality of color images, including the following

- *Cross color noise* that is caused by the mixing of the signals of adjacent color image samples
- *False color noise* that is an inherent weakness of single-plate sensor cameras and produces colors not actually present in the image scene
- *Color phase noise* that produces color blotches in dark gray areas or generates color shifts
- *Quantization noise* that is inherent in the amplitude quantization process and occurs in the analog-to-digital converter
- *Banding noise* that is introduced by the camera, when it reads data from the digital sensor
- *Fixed pattern noise* that includes the so-called "hot" and "dead" pixels
- *Random noise*, like *photon noise*, *dark current noise*, and *read out noise*, among many others

Additionally, transmission errors, periodic or random motion of the camera system during exposure, electronic instability of the image signal, electromagnetic interferences, sensor malfunctions, optic imperfections, or aging of the storage material all degrade the image quality [4]. Therefore, the noisy signal has to be processed by a filtering algorithm that removes the noise component but retains the original image features.

In this chapter, the color image is treated as a mapping $\mathbb{Z}^2 \to \mathbb{Z}^3$ that assigns to a point $\chi = (\chi_1, \chi_2)$ on the image plane a three-dimensional vector $x_\chi = (x_\chi^1, x_\chi^2, x_\chi^3)$, where the superscripts correspond to the red, green, and blue color image channel. In this way, a color image will be considered as a two-dimensional vector field of dimension, equal to the number of color channels (see Figure 4.1).

Color images are nonstationary; therefore, the filtering operators work on the assumption that the local image features can be extracted from a small image region called a *sliding filtering window*. The size and shape of the window influence the properties and efficiency of the image processing operations and are therefore application dependent. Mostly, a $3 \times 3$ window, as depicted in Figure 4.2, is used to process the central pixel surrounded by its neighbors. The *filter window* denoted as $W$ of length $n$ is a set of vectors $\{x_1, x_2, \ldots, x_n\}$, and the sample $x_1$ determines its position on the image domain.

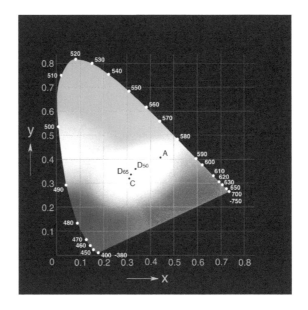

**COLOR FIGURE 1.5**
On the 1931 CIE *x, y* chromaticity diagram, the locus is labeled with the wavelength of the dominant hue. (Courtesy of X-Rite Incorporated.)

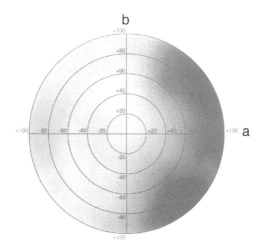

**COLOR FIGURE 1.6**
A slice through the CIE 1976 CIE L*a*b* diagram shows colors arranged on a red/green ($a^*$) and yellow/blue ($b^*$) axis.

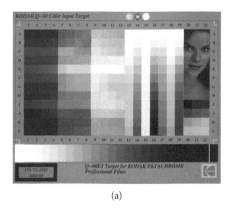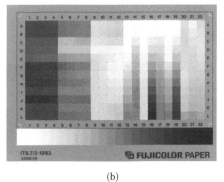

(a)                                             (b)

**COLOR FIGURE 1.11**
(a) The IT8.7/1 is a transparency scanner target, and (b) the IT8.7/2 is for reflection prints.

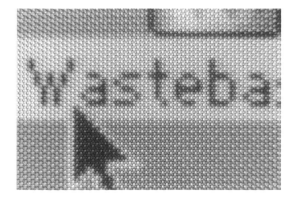

**COLOR FIGURE 1.12**
CRT displays create color using red, green, and blue phosphor dots. The "color" of the monitor phosphors is measured in terms of XYZ. The phosphor dot pitch is 0.2 mm.

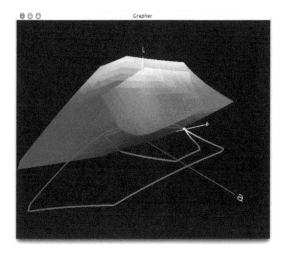

**COLOR FIGURE 1.16**
A CIE LAB gamut volume diagram showing the color gamut of a monitor (larger volume) compared to the much smaller color gamut of a printer.

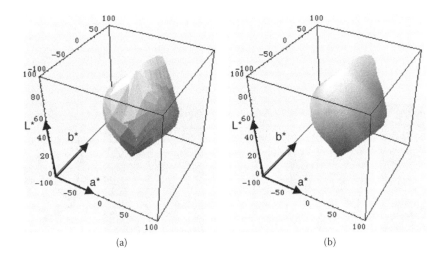

(a)

(b)

**COLOR FIGURE 2.6**
Comparison of two types of printer gamut shell surfaces: (a) polygon mesh, and (b) Overhauser spline functions.

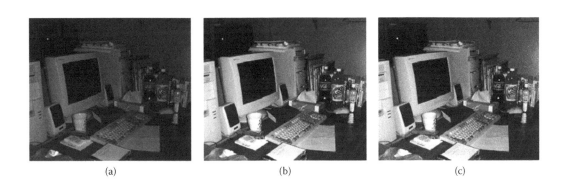

(a)

(b)

(c)

**COLOR FIGURE 2.13**
Improved image "room" by gamut expansion using histogram stretching: (a) original image (b) lightness stretching image (c) lightness and chroma stretching image.

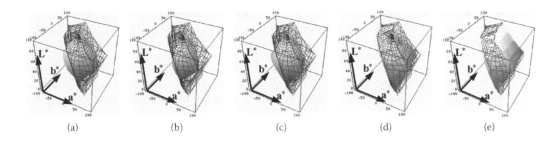

(a)

(b)

(c)

(d)

(e)

**COLOR FIGURE 2.15**
Printer and display gamuts compared with sRGB gamut (wire frame) in CIELAB space. (a) six-color dye ink-jet printer (b) four-color pigment ink-jet printer (c) four-color toner printer (d) CRT display (e) LC display.

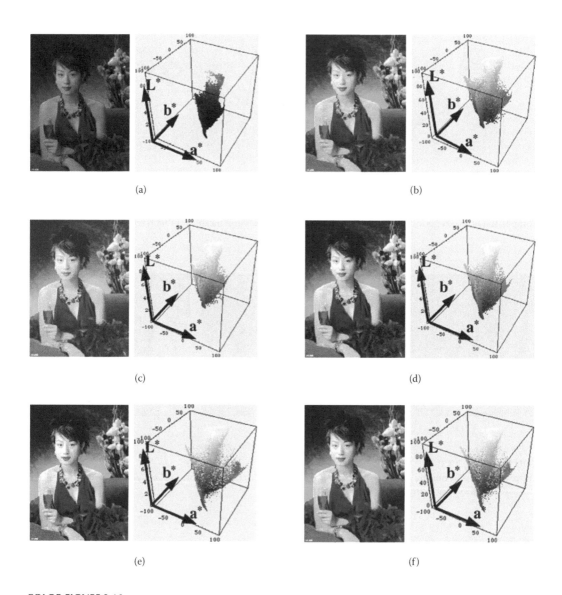

**COLOR FIGURE 2.16**
Test image "glass and lady" and GMA results with color maps: (a) original image, (b) six-color dye ink-jet printer, (c) four-color pigment ink-jet printer, (d) four-color toner-based printer, (e) CRT display, and (f) LCD display.

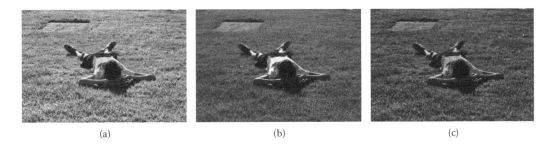

(a)            (b)            (c)

**COLOR FIGURE 3.1**
Unbalanced camera image (a), image after constancy processing by the camera (b), and image after gray world processing (c).

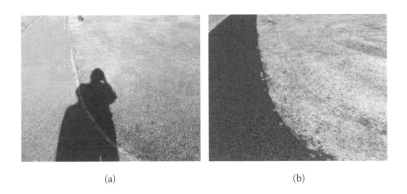

(a)            (b)

**COLOR FIGURE 3.9**
(a) Input color image. (b) 1-D coordinate transform coded as a grayscale; notice how the shadow disappears.

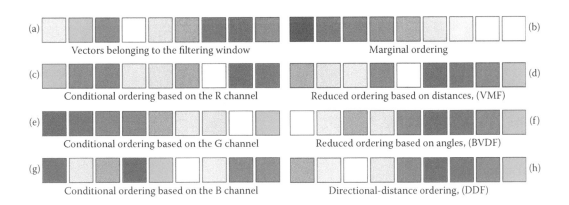

(a)   Vectors belonging to the filtering window     Marginal ordering   (b)

(c)   Conditional ordering based on the R channel     Reduced ordering based on distances, (VMF)   (d)

(e)   Conditional ordering based on the G channel     Reduced ordering based on angles, (BVDF)   (f)

(g)   Conditional ordering based on the B channel     Directional-distance ordering, (DDF)   (h)

**COLOR FIGURE 4.5**
Ordering of color samples according to various criteria.

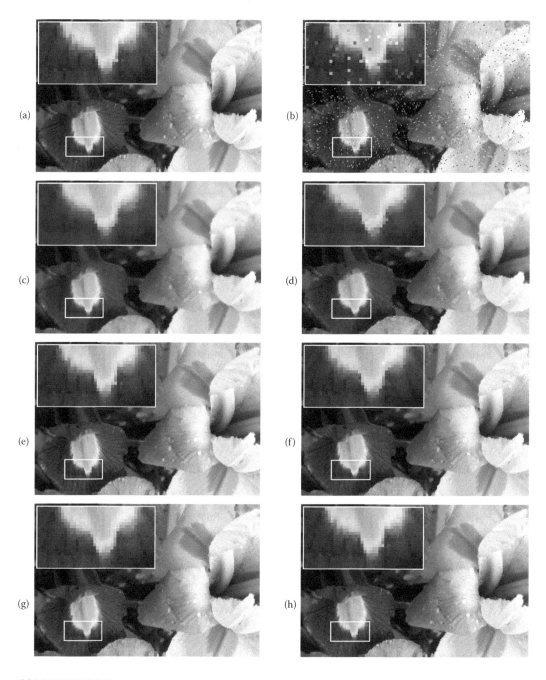

**COLOR FIGURE 4.10**
The effectiveness of the described switching filters: (a) color test image, (b) image distorted by 10% impulsive noise, (c) output of the VMF, (d) BDF, (e) SVMF (see Lukac, R. et al., *J. Intell. and Robotic Syst.*, 42, 361, 2005), (f) AVMF (see Lukac, R., *Pattern Recognition Lett.*, 24, 1889, 2003), (g) FPGF (see Smolka, B., and Chydzinski, A., *Real-Time Imaging*, 11, 389, 2005), and (h) SF (see Smolka, B., et al., *Pattern Recognition*, 35, 1771, 2002).

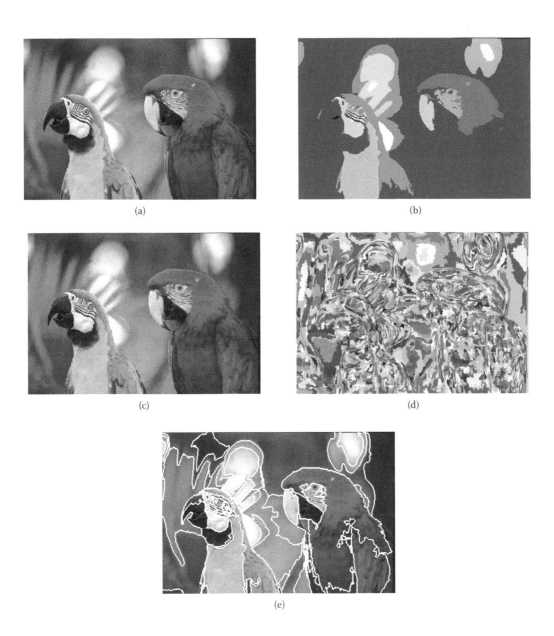

**COLOR FIGURE 5.2**

*Parrots* image and segmentation results: (a) original image, (b) segmentation into 48 regions (undersegmentation), (c) segmentation into 3000 regions (oversegmentation), (d) segmentation into 3000 regions presented in pseudo-colors, and (e) segmentation into 62 white-bordered regions.

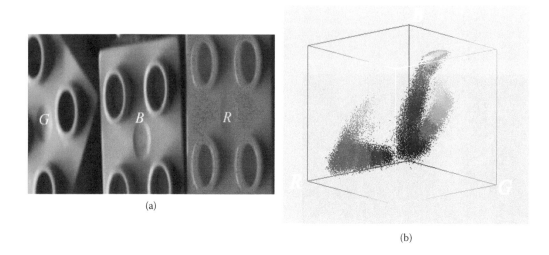

**COLOR FIGURE 5.3**

(a) Color image *Blocks1*, and (b) its clusters formed in RGB color space.

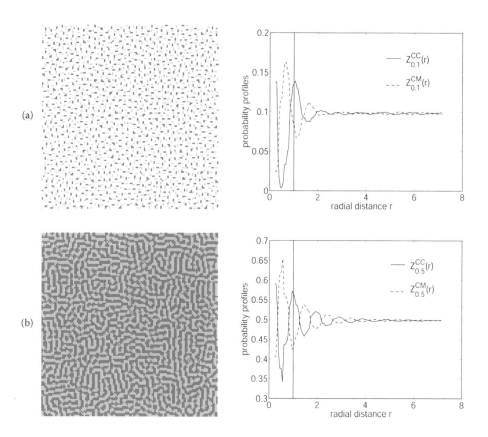

**COLOR FIGURE 7.5**

Performance of optimum color donut multifilters for (a) $g = 10\%$ and (b) $g = 50\%$; (left) cyan-magenta halftones, and (right) computed spatial probability profiles for the cyan color plane. The vertical line indicates the location of $\lambda_g$.

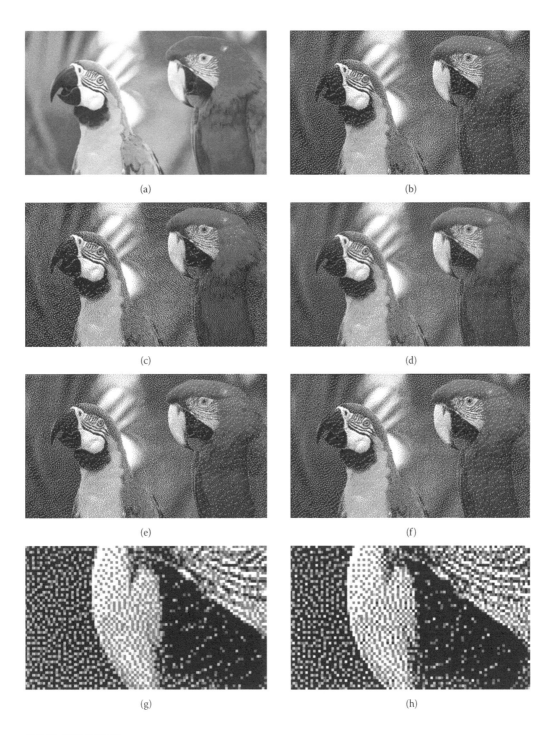

(a)

(b)

(c)

(d)

(e)

(f)

(g)

(h)

**COLOR FIGURE 7.10**

Comparison of various color error diffusion algorithms: (a) continuous tone *toucan* color image, (b) separable Floyd–Steinberg error diffusion, (c) optimum matrix-valued error filter, (d) vector error diffusion in XYZ space, (e) boundary artifact reduction of (d), (f) MBVC error diffusion, (g) detail of MBVC halftone, and (h) detail of Floyd–Steinberg error diffusion. Note the significant reduction in color halftone noise in parts (c) through (f) over separable FS error diffusion in part (b).

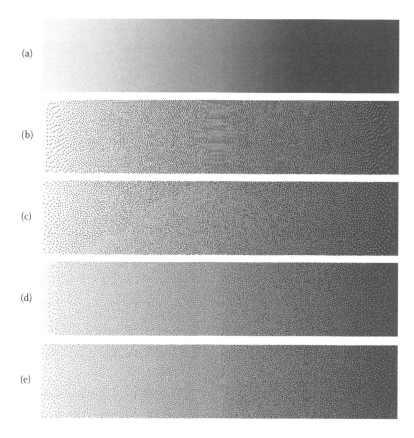

**COLOR FIGURE 7.13**

A color ramp and its halftone images: (a) original color ramp image, (b) Floyd–Steinberg error diffusion, (c) separable application of grayscale TDED, (d) color TDED, and (e) colorant-based direct binary search. The halftone in part (c) is courtesy of Prof. Jan P. Allebach and Mr. Ti-Chiun Chang at Purdue University. The halftone in part (e) is courtesy of Dr. Je-Ho Lee at Hewlett-Packard and Prof. Jan P. Allebach at Purdue University.

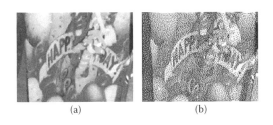

(a)    (b)

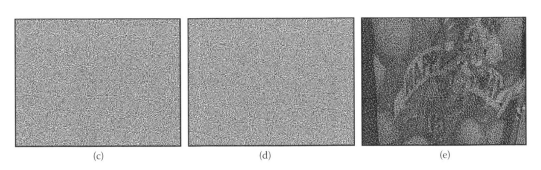

(c)    (d)    (e)

**COLOR FIGURE 8.4**
Secure color imaging using {2, 2}-VSS scheme: (a) 120 × 160 color secret image, (b) 120 × 160 halftone image produced using Floyd–Steinberg filter, (c, d) 240 × 320 binarized color shares, and (e) 240 × 320 decrypted color image.

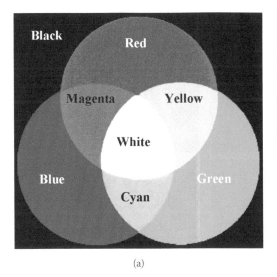

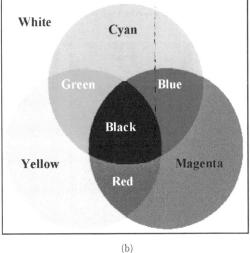

(a)    (b)

**COLOR FIGURE 8.5**
Two of the most common color models: (a) additive model and (b) subtractive model.

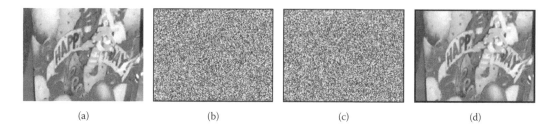

(a)  (b)  (c)  (d)

**COLOR FIGURE 8.10**

Secure color imaging using {2, 2}-ISS scheme: (a) 120 × 160 color secret image, (b,c) 120 × 160 full-color shares, and (d) 120 × 160 decrypted color image.

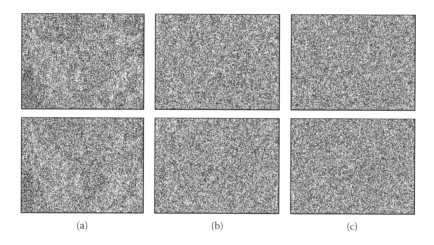

(a)  (b)  (c)

**COLOR FIGURE 8.11**

Color shares obtained using the nonexpansive ISS solution when cryptographic processing is performed for a reduced set of binary levels: (a) $b = 1$, (b) $b = 1, 2$, and (c) $b = 1, 2, 3$.

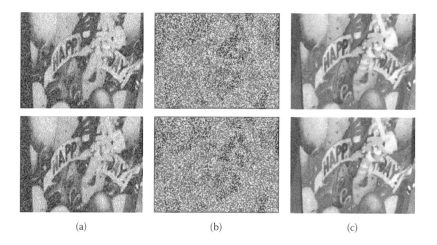

(a)  (b)  (c)

**COLOR FIGURE 8.12**

Color shares obtained using the nonexpansive ISS solution when cryptographic processing is performed for a single color channel: (a) R channel with $c = 1$, (b) G channel with $c = 2$, and (c) B channel with $c = 3$.

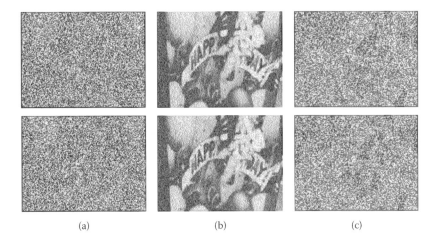

(a)          (b)          (c)

**COLOR FIGURE 8.13**
Color shares obtained using the nonexpansive ISS solution when cryptographic processing is performed for two color channels: (a) RG channels with $c = 1$ and $c = 2$, (b) RB channels with $c = 1$ and $c = 3$, and (c) GB channels with $c = 2$ and $c = 3$.

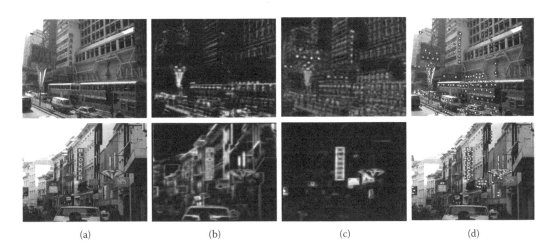

(a)        (b)        (c)        (d)

**COLOR FIGURE 9.8**
In columns, respectively, (a) input image, (b) RGB-gradient-based saliency map, (c) color-boosted saliency map, and (d) the results with red dots (lines) for gradient-based method and yellow dots (lines) for salient points after color saliency boosting.

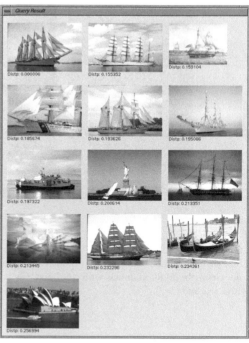

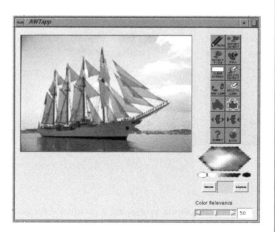

**COLOR FIGURE 10.14**
A query by image example (left), and the corresponding retrieval set (right).

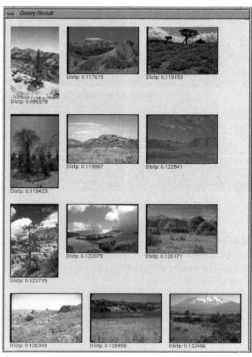

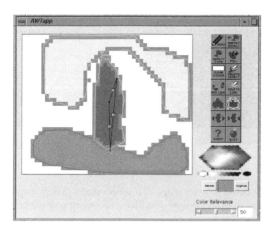

**COLOR FIGURE 10.15**
A query by sketch (left), and the corresponding retrieval set (right).

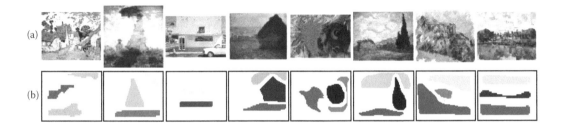

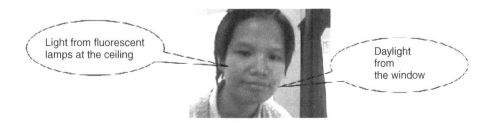

**COLOR FIGURE 10.19**
(a) The target images used in the test; and (b) a user's query sketches for the eight images.

Light from fluorescent
lamps at the ceiling

Daylight
from
the window

**COLOR FIGURE 12.4**
The face is illuminated by the nonuniform illumination field, and the white balancing partially fails. The color appearance of the face varies at different parts of the light field.

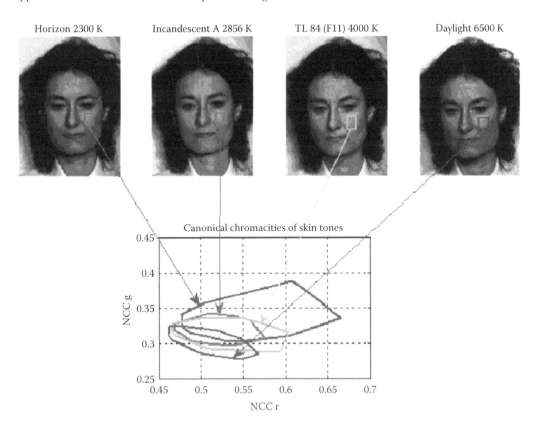

**COLOR FIGURE 12.7**
The skin tone appearance difference can be clearly observed in the four images taken with the Sony camera (see Figure 12.2). From the selected area marked with a box, the RGB values were taken and converted to NCC color space. As shown in the graph below the images, the areas of canonical chromaticities more or less overlap.

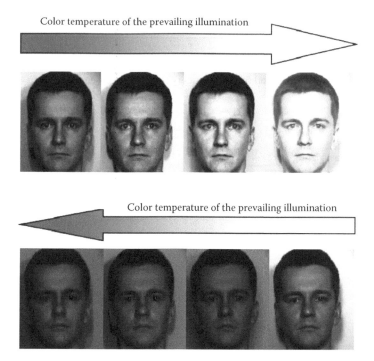

**COLOR FIGURE 12.8**
The color appearance shift. The color temperature of the light sources increases from left to right. The arrow indicates the change in the color of the light. The limited dynamic response range causes distortion in color: pixels can saturate to a maximum value (the rightmost image at the upper row) or be underexposed to zero (the leftmost image at the lower row).

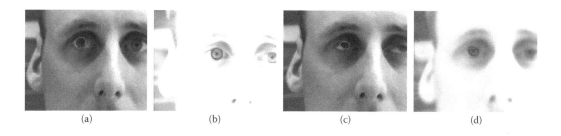

(a)  (b)  (c)  (d)

**COLOR FIGURE 13.8**
Tracking the iris while staying outdoors and additionally changing the illumination conditions by altering between IR to non-IR lighting. Notice how light conditions change when switching between IR and non-IR light emission (greenish looking images are IR "night vision").

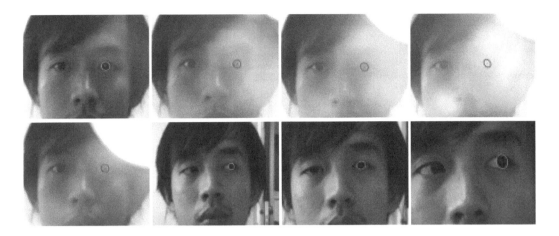

**COLOR FIGURE 13.9**
Tracking the iris of Asians under scale changes and heavy light disturbances.

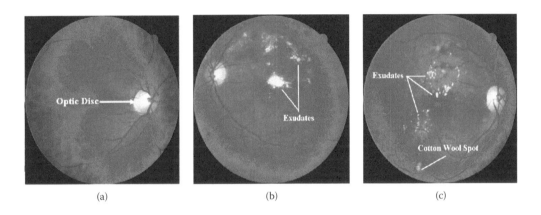

(a)                    (b)                    (c)

**COLOR FIGURE 14.1**
Normal and abnormal images: (a) a typical normal image with optic disc region, (b) severe retinopathy, with large plaques of exudates, and (c) diabetic retinopathy including retinal exudates and a cotton wool spot.

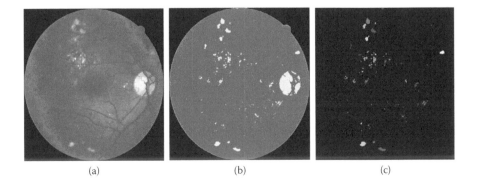

(a)                    (b)                    (c)

**COLOR FIGURE 14.7**
Connected component labeling and boundary tracing algorithms results: (a) a typical retinal image, (b) FCM segmented image, and (c) labeled regions using connected component approach.

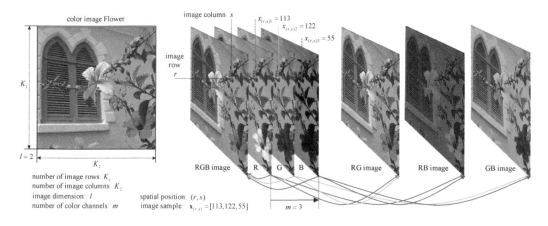

**COLOR FIGURE 16.1**
Color image representation in the RGB color domain.

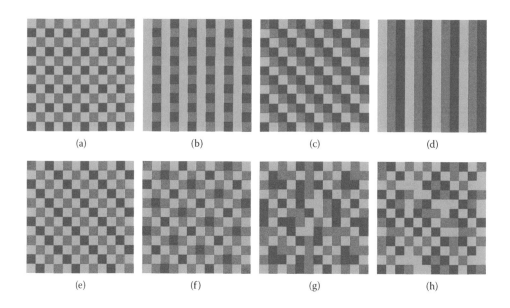

**COLOR FIGURE 16.6**
Examples of RGB CFAs: (a) Bayer pattern, (b) Yamanaka pattern, (c) diagonal stripe pattern, (d) vertical stripe pattern, (e) diagonal Bayer pattern, (f,g) pseudo-random patterns, and (h) HVS-based pattern.

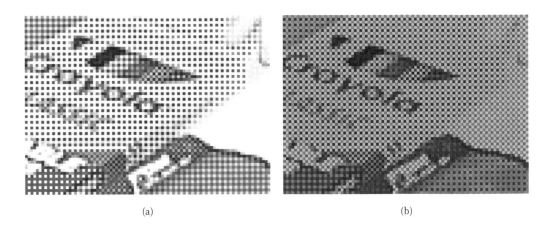

(a)                                                         (b)

**COLOR FIGURE 16.9**

CFA image obtained using a well-known Bayer CFA with the GRGR phase in the first row: (a) acquired grayscale CFA image and (b) CFA image rearranged as a color image.

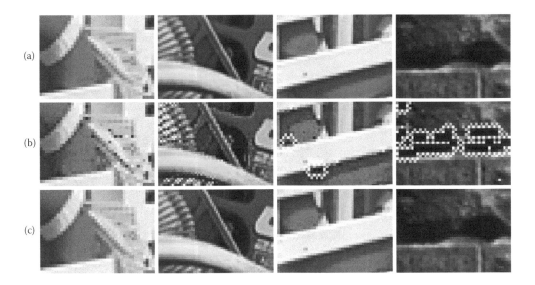

**COLOR FIGURE 16.16**

Performance improvements obtained by changing the SM: (a) original image, (b) Kimmel algorithm based on the color-ratio model (Kimmel, R., *IEEE Trans. on Image Process.*, 8, 1221, 1999), and (c) Kimmel algorithm based on the normalized color-ratio model (Lukac, R., and Plataniotis, K.N., *IEEE Trans. on Consumer Electron.*, 50, 737, 2004).

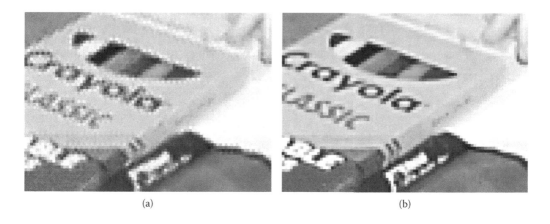

(a)                                         (b)

**COLOR FIGURE 16.17**
Demosaicking process: (a) restoration of the image shown in Figure 16.9a using the demosaicking solution and
(b) image shown in Figure 16.17a enhanced using the demosaicked image postprocessor.

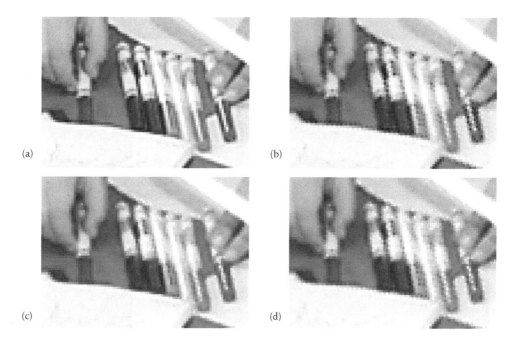

(a)                                         (b)

(c)                                         (d)

**COLOR FIGURE 16.18**
Influence of the ESM and SM on the quality of the demosaicked image: (a) used both ESM and SM, (b) omitted
ESM, (c) omitted SM, and (d) omitted both ESM and SM.

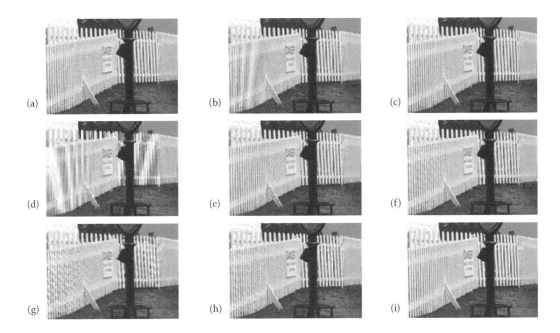

**COLOR FIGURE 16.19**
Influence of the CFA on the quality of the demosaicked image demonstrated using the same processing solution: (a–h) demosaicked image respectively corresponding to the RGB CFAs shown in Figure 16.6a to Figure 16.6h and (i) original image.

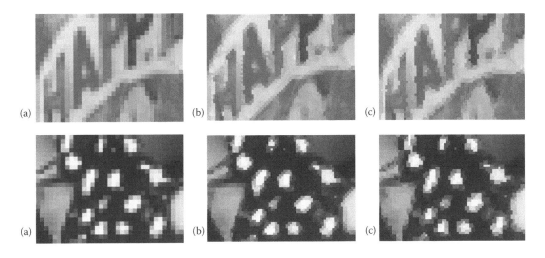

**COLOR FIGURE 16.24**
Median filtering based spatial interpolation (R. Lukac, K.N. Plataniotis, B. Smolka, and A.N. Venetsanopulos, in *Proceedings of the I.E.E.E. International Symposium on Industrial Electronics*, III, 1273, 2005). The cropped patterns correspond to: (a) original (small) images, and (b, c) upsampled images obtained using (b) component-wise processing and (c) vector processing.

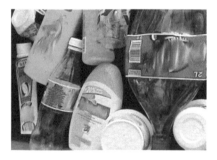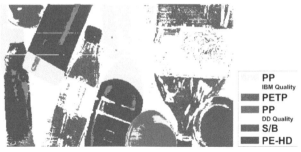

**COLOR FIGURE 17.12**

Classification of polymer waste: (left) input image and (right) after classification. The classification image shows the assignment of each pixel to the material PP (injection blow molding [IBM] quality), PETP, PP (deep drawing [DD] quality), S/B (styrenebutadiene copolymer), and PE-HD.

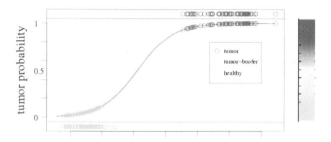

**COLOR FIGURE 17.15**

Binomial prediction of tumor probability in a one-dimensional subspace resulting from a dimension reduction step (compare densities of Figure 17.14). The predicted tumor probabilities can be mapped out using the color bar shown on the right, see Figure 17.16.

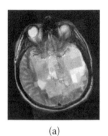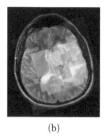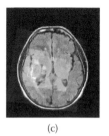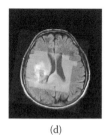

| (a) | (b) | (c) | (d) |

**COLOR FIGURE 17.16**

Color maps indicating the tumor probability computed automatically from MR spectral images (a, c), superimposed onto morphologic MR images (b, d). The color mapping used is defined on the right-hand side of Figure 17.15.

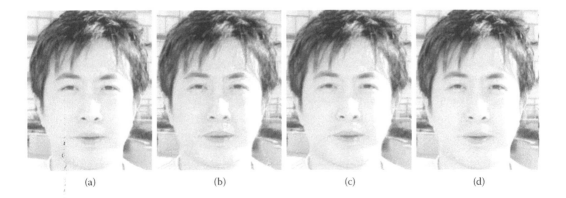

(a)            (b)           (c)           (d)

**COLOR FIGURE 18.5**
Simulation of dynamic false contours: (a) original image, (b) simulation with [1 2 4 8 16 32 48 48 48 48], (c) simulation with [1 2 4 8 16 32 42 44 52 54], and (d) simulation with error diffusion.

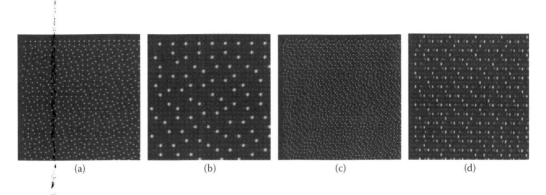

(a)            (b)           (c)           (d)

**COLOR FIGURE 18.13**
Constant image with 8-bit coded fraction = 32 by error diffusion-based technique: (a, b) result of conventional error diffusion and its enlarged version, and (c, d) result of described technique and its enlarged version.

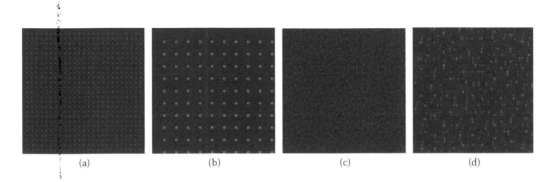

(a)            (b)           (c)           (d)

**COLOR FIGURE 18.18**
Constant image with 4-bit coded fraction = 1 by dithering-based technique: (a, b) result of conventional error diffusion and its enlarged version, and (c, d) result of described technique and its enlarged version.

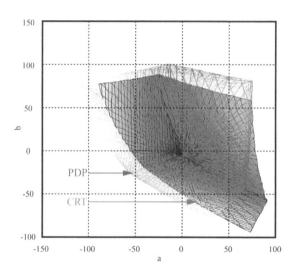

**COLOR FIGURE 18.20**
Gamut difference between PDP and CRT.

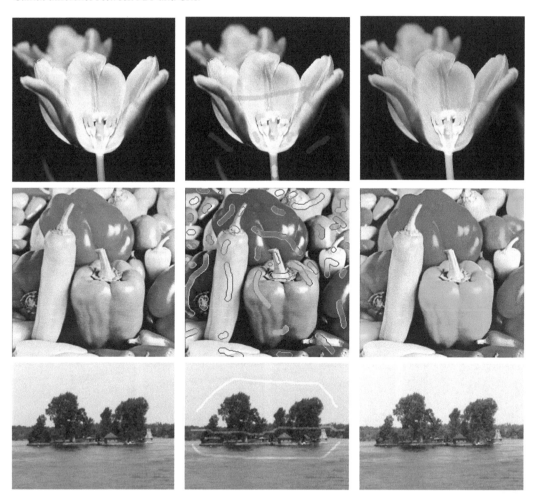

**COLOR FIGURE 20.1**
Still image colorization examples. Given a grayscale image (left), the user marks chrominance scribbles (center), and our algorithm provides a colorized image (right). The image size/run-times top to bottom are $270 \times 359$/less than 0.83 seconds, $256 \times 256$/less than 0.36 seconds, and $400 \times 300$/less than 0.77 seconds.

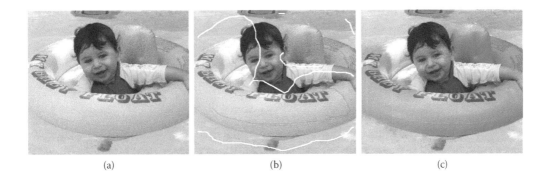

(a)         (b)         (c)

**COLOR FIGURE 20.6**

Recolorization example. (a) Original color image, (b) shows the scribbles placed by the user, where white is a special scribble used in recolorization that preserves the original colors of the image in selected regions of the image, and (c) is the recolored image. Note that only a few scribbles were used. Applying more scribbles would increase the quality of the result image.

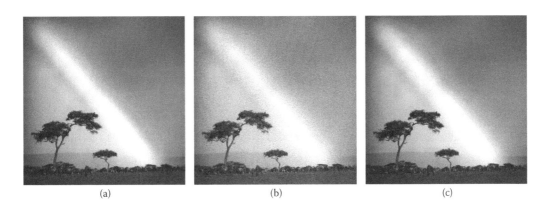

(a)         (b)         (c)

**COLOR FIGURE 20.7**

Recolorization example using the $Cr$ channel for measurement ($M$) rather than the intensity channel. (a) is the original color image, and (b) is the intensity channel of the image. It can be clearly seen that the intensity image does not contain significant structural information on the red rainbow strip (this is a unique example of this effect). On the other hand, both the $Cb$ and $Cr$ change significantly between the stripes and therefore can be used for recolorization. (c) Recolored image in which the red stripe of the rainbow was replaced by a purple one.

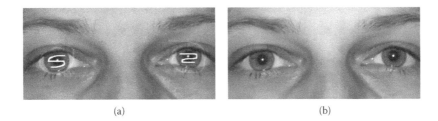

(a)         (b)

**COLOR FIGURE 20.9**

Using the described technique to remove color from certain image regions: (a) original image, and (b) only the eyes from the original image are preserved.

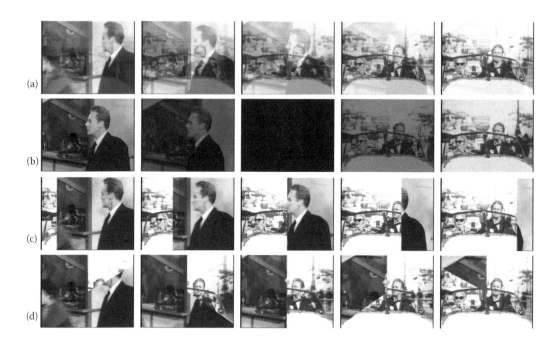

**COLOR FIGURE 23.2**
Examples of gradual transitions: (a) dissolve, (b) fade, (c) a classical wipe, and (d) a wipe of the "curtain" variety.

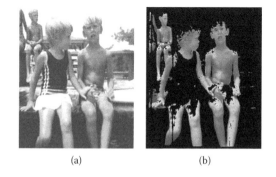

(a)             (b)

**COLOR FIGURE 24.7**
Example of color-based skin detection/segmentation: (a) original image, and (b) image after skin detection.

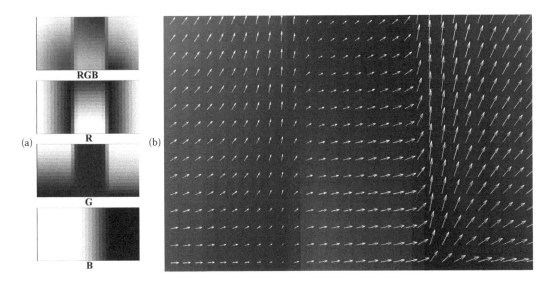

**FIGURE 4.1**
A color image is treated as a vector field: (a) the test image and its three RGB components and (b) the test image intensity and the directions of vectors in the normalized *rg* color space.

It is clear that there are some significant aspects that influence the design and selection of an appropriate filtering technique. An efficient filter suitable for the processing of color images should be designed mainly with respect to its *trichromatic nature*, its *nonlinear characteristics*, and the *statistics of noise corruption*.

The color image processing techniques are commonly divided into two main classes:

- *Marginal (component-wise) methods* that operate on each color channel separately (Figure 4.3). Because the independent processing ignores the correlation that exists between the color channels, the projection of the separate outputs into the color image usually results in perceivable color artifacts.

- *Vector methods* that process the input samples as a set of vectors. Because no new colors are introduced into the image, this kind of filtering is much more effective and is adequate in color image processing applications.

An example of a distortion caused by component-wise processing is shown in Figure 4.4, where impulsive noise has been added to a signal component, and then the channels were separately processed by a median filter of length five [5]. The filtering removes the impulses

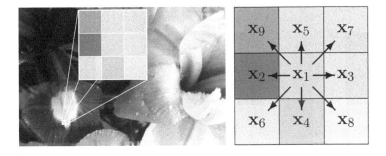

**FIGURE 4.2**
Sliding filtering window.

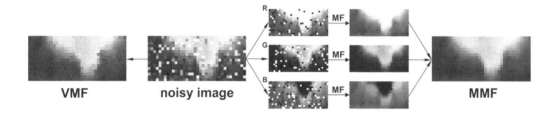

**FIGURE 4.3**
The marginal median filtering (MMF) with the median filter (MF) and the vector filtering using the vector median filter (VMF).

in flat signal areas but causes the edge shift to the left, if there is an impulse in front of it. As a result of the edge shift, the output color sample will not be one of the inputs, and color shifts like those visible in Figure 4.3 for marginal median filtering (MMF) are generated.

If the noise corrupting the image is of impulsive nature, filtering approaches based on the order statistics theory are often employed. The most popular color filtering class operating on a window, sliding over the image domain, is based on sample ordering. When performing the scalar ordering operation on a grayscale image, the atypical image samples are moved to the borders of the ordered set. Thus, the center of the ordered sequence known as a median represents the sample, which has the largest probability to be noise free. The direct application of the median filter to the RGB color channels — known as *marginal median filtering* — leads, however, to visible color artifacts (Figure 4.3 and Figure 4.4).

In the vectorial case, outliers are associated with the extremes of the aggregated distances to other input samples in the sliding window. For this reason, the output of the vector filters based on ranking is defined according to a specific ordering scheme as the lowest-ranked vector in the sliding window. Because the lowest-ranked vector is the sample of the input set, vector filters do not generate new color samples (color artifacts), and such behavior is beneficial due to the inherent correlation that exists between the RGB channels of natural images.

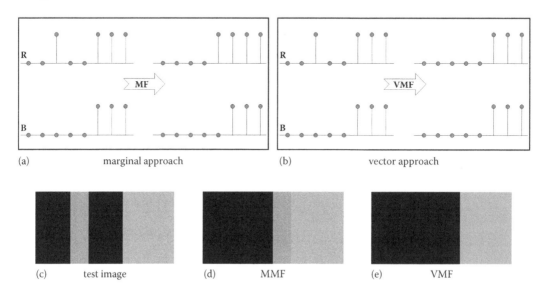

**FIGURE 4.4**
The difference between the marginal median filtering and vector median filtering in the one-dimensional case (window length 5) and below the corresponding difference between the MMF and VMF using a window of size $5 \times 5$.

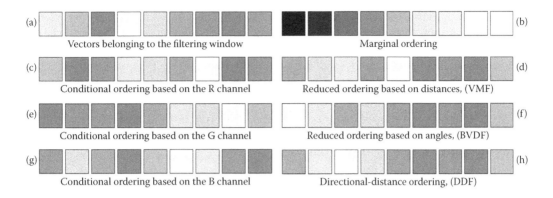

(a) Vectors belonging to the filtering window

(b) Marginal ordering

(c) Conditional ordering based on the R channel

(d) Reduced ordering based on distances, (VMF)

(e) Conditional ordering based on the G channel

(f) Reduced ordering based on angles, (BVDF)

(g) Conditional ordering based on the B channel

(h) Directional-distance ordering, (DDF)

**FIGURE 4.5 (See color insert.)**
Ordering of color samples according to various criteria.

The ordering of scalar data, such as samples of grayscale images, is naturally defined, and it was extensively studied [6], [7]. However, it cannot be extended in a straightforward way to multidimensional data, as there is no unambiguous, universal way of multivariate data ordering. Nevertheless, a number of multivariate subordering schemes are often applied in the processing of color images. Their aim is to detect the outliers, as the samples that occupy the highest ranks in the ordered set.

The ordering schemes can be divided into the following four main types:

- *Marginal ordering*, where the color samples are ordered along each channel independently. If the ordered set of the scalar data $\{x_1, x_2, \ldots, x_n\}$ is denoted as $\{x_{(1)}, x_{(2)}, \ldots, x_{(n)}\}$, where $x_{(1)}$ and $x_{(n)}$ signify the lowest- and highest-ranked sample, then the marginal ordering applied independently to each color channel of the samples $\{x_1, x_2, \ldots, x_n\}$ belonging to $W$ yields the ordered set of the channel components: $\{x_{(1)}^k, x_{(2)}^k, \ldots, x_{(n)}^k\}$, where $k$ denotes the color image channel. In this way, the lowest-ranked vector is $[x_{(1)}^1, x_{(1)}^2, x_{(1)}^3]$, and the highest rank is occupied by $[x_{(n)}^1, x_{(n)}^2, x_{(n)}^3]$. Because of the independent ordering performed separately in each channel, the vectors $[x_{(j)}^1, x_{(j)}^2, x_{(j)}^3]$, $j = 1, 2, \ldots, n$ are generally different from the original vectors contained in $W$, because new color values are generated, (Figure 4.5).

- *Conditional ordering*, where the samples are ordered conditional on one of its marginal sets of observations. In this kind of ranking, vectors are ordered according to the ranked values of one of the color image components. In this way, three main schemes of conditional ordering based on the R, G, and B channel can be constructed. This ordering scheme privileges one channel, which leads to a loss of information contained in other channels, when performing the ranking of vectors.

- *Partial ordering*, where the input data are partitioned into smaller groups using the concept of a convex hull. The samples are then ranked according to the so-called *peeling* principle [6].

- *Reduced* or *aggregated ordering*, where each vector sample is associated with a scalar value that serves as the ordering criterion. According to the kind of relationship between the sample vectors, we can differentiate techniques operating on the *vector distance domain* [5], [8], *angular domain* [9], [10], or their combinations [1], [11], [12], (Figure 4.5).

The most popular filtering approaches are based on the *reduced vector ordering* scheme defined through the sorting of *aggregated distance functions* or *dissimilarity measures* [1], [13]. The aggregated distance measure assigned to the sample $x_k$ is defined as

$$R_k = \sum_{j=1}^{n} \rho(x_k, x_j) \tag{4.1}$$

where $\rho(\cdot)$ denotes the chosen distance or dissimilarity function [2]. The scalar quantities $R_1, R_2, \ldots, R_n$ are then sorted in the order of their value, and the associated vectors are correspondingly ordered as follows (Figure 4.5):

$$R_{(1)} \leq R_{(2)} \leq \ldots \leq R_{(n)} \;\Rightarrow\; x_{(1)} \prec x_{(2)} \prec \ldots \prec x_{(n)} \tag{4.2}$$

This ordering scheme focuses on the relationships between the color samples, because it determines dissimilarity between all pairs of the samples belonging to $W$. The output of the ranking procedure depends on the type of data used for the determination of the aggregated distance $R$ in Equation 4.1 and on the function $\rho$ selected to evaluate the dissimilarity (distance) between the vectors.

### 4.2.1  Vector Median-Based Filters

In Reference [5], a powerful family of nonlinear filters for noise removal based on the reduced ordering principle, utilizing the distance between the vectors in the filtering window was proposed [1], [6], [14], [15]. Assuming that each input color sample $x_k$ is associated with an aggregated distance

$$R_k = \sum_{j=1}^{n} \|x_k - x_j\|_\gamma, \quad k = 1, 2, \ldots, n \tag{4.3}$$

where $\|x_k - x_j\|_\gamma$ quantifies the distance among two color vectors $x_k$ and $x_j$ using the Minkowski metric, with $\gamma$ characterizing the used norm.

The sample $x_{(1)} \in W$ associated with the minimal aggregated distance $R_{(1)}$ constitutes the output of the *vector median filter* (VMF), which minimizes the distance to other samples inside the sliding filtering window $W$ [5]. Thus, the output of the VMF is the pixel $x_{(1)} \in W$, for which the following condition is satisfied:

$$\sum_{j=1}^{n} \|x_{(1)} - x_j\|_\gamma \leq \sum_{j=1}^{n} \|x_k - x_j\|_\gamma, \quad k = 1, 2, \ldots, n \tag{4.4}$$

In this way, the construction of VMF consists of comparing the values of $R_k$, and the output is the vector $x_{(1)}$, which minimizes $R$ in Equation 4.3. The construction of the VMF is illustrated in Figure 4.6, where the Euclidean distance is used.

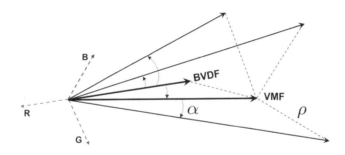

**FIGURE 4.6**
The VMF filter minimizes the sum of aggregated distances and BVDF the sum of angles.

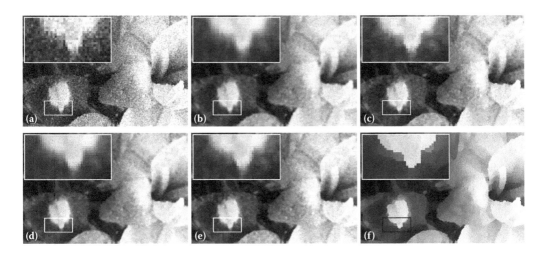

**FIGURE 4.7**
Filtering results obtained using a test image distorted by a strong Gaussian noise: (a) color test image distorted by Gaussian noise of $\sigma = 30$; (b) output of AMF; (c) $\alpha$VMF for $\alpha = 6$; (d) result of a fuzzy weighted filter (FWAF) with the weighting function $\psi_k = \exp\{-R_k^c/\beta\}$, with $c = 0.15$ and $\beta = 1.2$; (see Plataniotis, K.N. Androutsos, D., and Venetsanopoulos, A.N., *Signal Process. J.*, 55, 93, 1996); (e) output of ANNF; (f) result of the generalized anisotropic diffusion (GAD) (see Smolka, B., *Comput. and Graphics*, 27, 503, 2003).

It has been observed that the VMF discards impulses and preserves, to some extent, image edges. However, its performance in the suppression of additive Gaussian noise, which is frequently encountered in color images, is significantly inferior to the linear *arithmetic mean filter* (AMF). If a color image is corrupted by both additive Gaussian and impulsive noise, an effective filtering scheme should make an appropriate compromise between the AMF and VMF (see Figure 4.7).

The so-called $\alpha$-*trimmed vector median filter* ($\alpha$VMF) exemplifies this trade-off [8]. In this filtering design, the $\alpha$ samples closest to the vector median output are selected as inputs to an averaging filter. The output of the $\alpha$VMF is defined as $\hat{x}_\alpha = (\sum_{k=1}^{\alpha} x_{(k)})/\alpha$. The trimming operation guarantees good performance in the presence of impulsive noise, whereas the averaging operation causes the filter to perform well in the presence of short-tailed noise. The drawback of this filter is that it generates new colors that were not present in the noisy image.

Another technique that is a compromise between the output of the AMF ($\hat{x}$) and VMF ($x_{(1)}$) and that is capable of reducing both the impulsive and short-tailed noise was proposed in the literature [5]. The rule for choosing the estimate of the central pixel in $W$ is

$$y = \begin{cases} \hat{x}, & \text{if } \sum_{j=1}^{n} \|\hat{x} - x_j\| \leq \sum_{j=1}^{n} \|x_{(1)} - x_j\|, \\ x_{(1)}, & \text{otherwise} \end{cases} \tag{4.5}$$

In Reference [8], the VMF concept was generalized, and the so-called *weighted vector median filter* (WVMF) was proposed. Using the WVMF approach, the filter output is the vector $x_{(1)}$ in $W$, for which the following condition holds:

$$\sum_{j=1}^{n} \psi_j \|x_{(1)} - x_j\|_\gamma < \sum_{j=1}^{n} \psi_j \|x_k - x_j\|_\gamma, \quad k = 1, \ldots, n \tag{4.6}$$

The WVMF output is a function of the weight vector $\psi = \{\psi_1, \psi_2, \ldots, \psi_n\}$, and it can be expressed as the sample from $W$ minimizing the aggregated weighted distances. Each setting of the weight coefficients represents a unique filter that can be used for specific purposes. Using an optimization scheme and incorporating the directional information, the weight coefficients can follow the noise statistics and structural context of the original signal [12], [16].

If $\psi_1 > 1$ and $\psi_k = 1$ for $k = 2, \ldots, n$, $(\psi = \{\psi_1, 1, 1 \ldots, 1\})$, then the simplified *central weighted VMF* (CWVMF) is obtained. The difference between the VMF and CWVMF is that the distance between the central pixel $x_1$ and its neighbors is multiplied by the weighting coefficient $\psi_1$, which privileges the central pixel $x_1$.

Within the framework of the ranked-type nonlinear filters, the orientation difference between vectors can also be used to remove samples with atypical directions. The *basic vector directional filter* (BVDF) is a ranked-order filter that employs the angle between two vectors as the distance measure. In the directional processing of color images [9], [10], [16], [17], each input vector $x_k$ is associated with the aggregated angles

$$A_k = \sum_{j=1}^{n} a(x_k, x_j), \quad k = 1, 2, \ldots, n, \quad a(x_k, x_j) = \arccos\left(\frac{x_k \cdot x_j}{\|x_k\| \|x_j\|}\right) \quad (4.7)$$

where $a(x_k, x_j)$ denotes the angle between vectors $x_k$ and $x_j$ (see Figure 4.6).

The sample $x_{(1)}$ associated with the minimal angular distance $A_{(1)}$ (i.e., the sample minimizing the sum of angles with other vectors) represents the output of the BVDF [9]. A drawback of the BVDF is that because it uses only information about vector directions (chromaticity information), it cannot remove achromatic noisy pixels.

To improve the efficiency of the directional filters, another method called *directional-distance filter* (DDF) was proposed [11]. The DDF is a combination of VMF and BVDF and is derived by simultaneous minimization of their aggregated distances:

$$D_k = R_k^{1-\kappa} \cdot A_k^{\kappa} = \left(\sum_{j=1}^{n} \|x_k - x_j\|_\gamma\right)^{1-\kappa} \cdot \left(\sum_{j=1}^{n} a(x_k, x_j)\right)^{\kappa}, \quad k = 1, 2, \ldots, n \quad (4.8)$$

where the first term is defined by Equation 4.1 and the second by Equation 4.7. The parameter $\kappa$ regulates the influence of the distance and angular components. For $\kappa = 0$, we obtain the VMF, and for $\kappa = 1$, the BVDF. The DDF is defined for $\kappa = 0.5$, and its usefulness stems from the fact that it combines the criteria used in both VMF and BVDF [10], [12], [16].

### 4.2.2 Fuzzy Adaptive Filters

The performance of various nonlinear filters based on order statistics depends heavily on the type of noise contaminating the color image. To overcome difficulties caused by the uncertainty associated with the image data, adaptive designs based on local features were introduced [18], [19]. Such filters utilize fuzzy transformations based on the samples from the filtering window. The general form of the fuzzy adaptive filters is given as a nonlinear transformation of a weighted average of the input vectors inside the processing window:

$$y = f\left(\sum_{k=1}^{n} \psi_k^* x_k\right) = f\left(\sum_{k=1}^{n} \psi_k x_k \bigg/ \sum_{k=1}^{n} \psi_k\right) \quad (4.9)$$

where $f(\cdot)$ is a nonlinear function that operates on the weighted average of the input set. The weighting coefficients are transformations of the distance between the central vector and its neighbors inside $W$ and can be considered as membership functions.

Within the general fuzzy adaptive filtering framework, numerous designs may be constructed by changing the form of the nonlinear function $f(\cdot)$, as well as the way the fuzzy weights are determined [20], [21]. The *fuzzy weighted average filter* (FWAF) is an example of a scheme derived from the general nonlinear fuzzy framework. The output of this filter is a fuzzy weighted average of the ordered input set:

$$y = \sum_{k=1}^{n} \psi_k^* x_{(k)}, \quad \text{with} \quad \sum_{k=1}^{n} \psi_k^* = 1 \tag{4.10}$$

where the weighting coefficients are decreasing functions of the aggregated distances assigned to the samples of $W$ (Figure 4.7d).

Another possible choice of the nonlinear function $f(\cdot)$ is the maximum selector. In this case, the output of the nonlinear function is the input vector that corresponds to the maximum fuzzy weight. Using the maximum selector concept, the output of the filter is a part of the original input set. If the vector angle criterion is used to calculate distances, the fuzzy filter delivers the same output as the BVDF [1], [19], whereas the Minkowski distance provides the output of the VMF. In this way, utilizing an appropriate distance function, diverse filters can be obtained, and filters such as VMF or BVDF can be seen as special cases of this specific class of fuzzy filters.

The *adaptive nearest neighbor filter* (ANNF) [1] employs a scheme in which the value of the weight $\psi_k$ in Equation 4.9 is determined according to the rule $\psi_k = R_{(n)} - R_{(k)}$, where $R_{(n)}$ is the maximal accumulated distance in the filtering window. The highest value of $\psi_k$ is assigned to the output of the VMF, and the smallest is assigned to the vector sample with the highest rank, so that when the coefficients $\psi_k$ are normalized, the corresponding weights are 1 and 0, respectively (Figure 4.7d).

A filtering scheme similar to the fuzzy weighted average described in Equation 4.10 can be obtained utilizing the nonparametric approach. Based on the samples from $W$, an adaptive multivariate kernel density estimator can be employed to approximate the sample's probability density function $\Psi(x)$:

$$\Psi(x) = \frac{1}{n} \sum_{k=1}^{n} \frac{1}{h_k^m} \mathcal{K} \left\{ \frac{\|x - x_k\|}{h_k} \right\} \tag{4.11}$$

where $m$ denotes the dimensionality of the measurement space, and $h_k$ is the data-dependent smoothing parameter that regulates the shape of the kernel function $\mathcal{K}$.

The adaptive nonparametric filter based on the available noisy samples is defined as

$$y = \sum_{k=1}^{n} \frac{h_k^{-3} \mathcal{K} \left\{ \frac{\|x_1 - x_k\|}{h_k} \right\}}{\sum_{j=1}^{n} h_j^{-3} \mathcal{K} \left\{ \frac{\|x_1 - x_j\|}{h_j} \right\}} x_k = \sum_{k=1}^{n} \psi_k^* x_k \tag{4.12}$$

where $\psi_k$ are the weighting coefficients. Usually, instead of the noisy sample, the VMF output $\tilde{x}$ is chosen, and the resulting design has the following form:

$$y = \sum_{k=1}^{n} \frac{h_k^{-3} \mathcal{K} \left\{ \|\tilde{x}_1 - x_k\| / h_k \right\}}{\sum_{j=1}^{n} h_j^{-3} \mathcal{K} \left\{ \|\tilde{x}_1 - x_j\| / h_j \right\}} \tilde{x}_k = \sum_{k=1}^{n} \psi_k^* \tilde{x}_k \tag{4.13}$$

This filter can be viewed as a double-window, two-stage estimator. First, the original image is denoised by the VMF in order to reject possible outliers, and then an adaptive nonlinear filter with data-dependent coefficients is utilized to provide the final output.

### 4.2.3 Switching Filters

The main drawback of the widespread vector filters, such as the VMF, BVDF, and DDF, lies in introducing too much smoothing, which results in an extensive blurring of the output

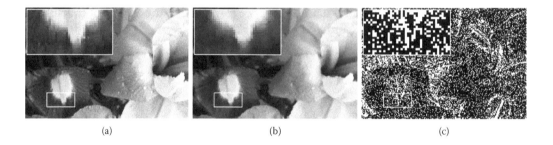

(a)                                   (b)                                   (c)

**FIGURE 4.8**
Excessive smoothing of the VMF: (a) color test image, (b) output of the VMF, and (c) changes introduced by the VMF to the original image (black pixels denote samples that were treated as noise and were replaced by one of its neighbors).

image (Figure 4.8). This undesired property is caused by the unnecessary filtering of the noise-free samples that should be passed to a filter output without any change.

To alleviate the problem of oversmoothing, several switching mechanisms were proposed in the literature to improve the efficiency of the standard smoothing filters. Such switching filters detect if the central pixel in $W$ is affected by the noise process, and if it is found to be noisy, then it is replaced by the output of some robust filter, otherwise, it is left unchanged (Figure 4.9).

In References [22] and [23], an efficient switching scheme called the *sigma vector median filter* (SVMF) changes between the nonlinear mode, which smooths out noisy samples, and the identity operation, which leaves the uncorrupted samples unchanged, was presented. The SVMF is based on the robust order statistics theory and on the approximation of the local multivariate dispersion, determined using the input color samples contained in $W$. In this scheme, the input central sample is considered to be noisy if it lies outside the range $r$, formed by the approximated multivariate dispersion of the input multichannel samples, expressed as $r = R_{(1)}/(n-1)$, where $R_{(1)}$ is the minimal accumulated sum of distances: $R_{(1)} = \sum_{j=1}^{n} \left\| x_{(1)} - x_j \right\|_\gamma$. The local variance approximation $r$ represents the mean distance between the vector median $x_{(1)}$ and all other samples contained in $W$. The output $y$ of the SVMF is defined as

$$y = \begin{cases} x_{(1)}, & \text{for } R_1 \geq \lambda, \\ x_1, & \text{otherwise} \end{cases} \tag{4.14}$$

where $R_1$ is the cumulated distance from the central pixel $x_1$ to all other pixels contained in $W$, and $\lambda$ is a threshold value given by $\lambda = R_{(1)} + \varrho r$, where $\varrho$ is a tuning parameter used to adjust the smoothing properties of the SVMF (Figure 4.10e).

Another efficient scheme that aims to preserve the desired image features, while suppressing the impulsive noise, was proposed in Reference [24]. The decision rule is expressed

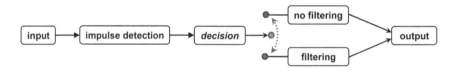

**FIGURE 4.9**
Switching filtering scheme.

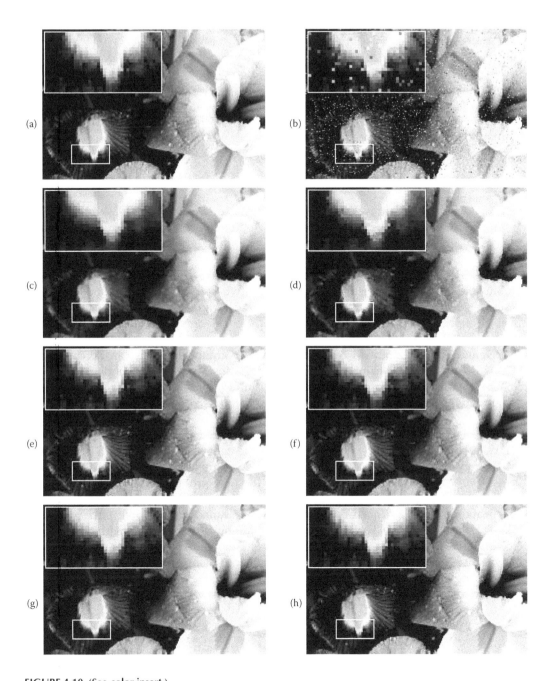

**FIGURE 4.10 (See color insert.)**

The effectiveness of the described switching filters: (a) color test image, (b) image distorted by 10% impulsive noise, (c) output of the VMF, (d) BDF, (e) SVMF (see, Lukac, R. et al., *J. Intell. and Robotic Syst.*, 42, 361, 2005), (f) AVMF (see Lukac, R., *Pattern Recognition Lett.*, 24, 1889, 2003), (g) FPGF (see Smolka, B., and Chydzinski, A., *Real-Time Imaging*, 11, 389, 2005), and (h) SF (see Smolka, B., et al., *Pattern Recognition*, 35, 1771, 2002).

as follows:

$$y = \begin{cases} x_{(1)}, & \text{for } \Omega \geq \lambda, \\ x_1, & \text{otherwise,} \end{cases} \qquad (4.15)$$

where $\Omega$ is the output of a noise detection operation utilizing the samples in the filtering window, and $\lambda$ is a local or global threshold value. If the central pixel $x_1$ is detected as being corrupted by noise, then it is replaced by the output of the VMF, otherwise, it is left unchanged. In Reference [24], the *adaptive VMF* (AVMF) utilizes the following rule for obtaining the $\Omega$ value in Equation 4.15:

$$\Omega = \|x_1 - \hat{x}_{(\alpha)}\|_\gamma, \quad \hat{x}_{(\alpha)} = \left( \sum_{k=1}^{\alpha} x_{(k)} \right) \Big/ \alpha \qquad (4.16)$$

where $\hat{x}_{(\alpha)}$ denotes the arithmetic mean of the first $\alpha$ ordered vectors ($\alpha$VMF). For moderate impulsive noise intensity $\alpha = 5$ and $\lambda = 60$ guarantees good performance of the proposed noise cancellation scheme (Figure 4.10f). In Reference [25], a generalized rule for determining the value of $\Omega$ was introduced: $\Omega = \sum_{k=u}^{u+\tau} \|x_1 - y_k\|_\gamma$, where $y_k$ is the output of the CWVMF with a weight assigned to the central pixel equal to $n - 2k + 2$. The $\tau$ and $u$ parameters gave optimal results when equal to two with a threshold value $\lambda = 80$. In Reference [26] instead of the Euclidean distance, the angular distance between the central pixel and the outputs of the *central weighted vector directional filter* (CWVDF) were utilized.

In Reference [27], a modified concept of the peer group introduced in Reference [28] and extensively used in various filtering designs, mostly under the name of extended spatial neighborhood, was proposed. The peer group $\mathcal{P}(x_i, m, r)$, denotes the set of $m$ pixels belonging to the filtering window $W$ centered at the pixel $x_i$, which satisfy the condition: $\|x_i - x_j\| \leq r$, $x_j \in W$. In other words, the peer group $\mathcal{P}$ associated with the central pixel of $W$ is a set of pixels, with distance to the central pixel that does not exceed $r$. If we calculate the distances $\rho(x_i, x_j)$ between the central pixel $x_i$ and all other pixels from $W$, then when the distances are ordered, a corresponding set of ordered vectors is obtained: $x_i = x_{(1)}, x_{(2)}, \ldots, x_{(m)}, \ldots, x_{(n)}$. Then the peer group is a set of $m$ first vectors: $\{x_{(1)}, x_{(2)}, \ldots, x_{(m)}\}$, with $\rho(x_{(1)}, x_{(m)}) \leq r$.

The proposed impulsive noise detection algorithm, called *fast peer group filtering* (FPGF), works as follows: if there exists a peer group containing at least $k$ pixels with a distance to the central pixel that is less than $r$, then the pixel $x_i$ is treated as not corrupted by noise, otherwise, it is declared to be noisy and has to replaced by an appropriate filter.

If $y_i$ denotes the output of the filtering operation, then the following filtering algorithm is constructed:

$$y_i = \begin{cases} x_i & \text{if} \quad m \geq k, \\ \hat{x} & \text{if} \quad m < k \quad \text{and} \quad \tau \geq 1, \\ x_{(1)} & \text{if} \quad m < k \quad \text{and} \quad \tau = 0 \end{cases} \qquad (4.17)$$

where $k$ is a parameter that determines the minimal size of the peer group, $\tau$ is the number of undisturbed pixels in $W$, and $\hat{x}$ is the average of the pixels in $W$ that were found to be not corrupted by the noise process. If the pixel is found to be noisy ($m < k$), then it is replaced by the mean of its neighbors that are not disturbed by noise. When the image is noisy there may be no undisturbed pixels in $W$, and then the central pixel is replaced by the vector median of the samples in $W$.

It is easy to observe that the proposed algorithm is extremely fast. The low computational complexity stems from the fact that when the peer group parameter $k$ is low, for example, $k = 4$, then if the algorithm finds three pixels that are close enough to the central pixel $x_i$, it is declared to be noise free, and the sliding window moves to the adjacent pixel. Often, only a few calculations of distances are needed to classify a pixel as being undisturbed by noise. In Reference [27], the following parameter settings gave satisfying results: $k = 3$ or 4, $r = 50$ (see Figure 4.10g).

Instead of the distance function $\rho(x_j, x_k)$, various measures that quantify the similarity or closeness of the vectors can be designed to obtain filters with desired properties. A similarity function $\psi : [0, \infty) \to \mathbb{R}$, like in the fuzzy techniques, should satisfy $\psi(0) = 1$, $\psi(\infty) = 0$. Applying the similarity concept, we can build the following cumulated similarities:

$$\Psi(x_1) = \sum_{j=2}^{n} \psi(\rho\{x_1, x_j\}), \quad \Psi(x_k) = \sum_{j=2, j \neq k}^{n} \psi(\rho\{x_k, x_j\}) \tag{4.18}$$

The omission of the similarity value $\psi(x_k, x_1)$ when calculating $\Psi(x_k)$, privileges the central pixel $x_1$, as $\Psi(x_1)$ contains $(n-1)$ similarities $\psi(x_1, x_k)$ and $\Psi(x_k)$, for $k > 1$ has only $(n-2)$ similarity values, as the central pixel $x_1$ is excluded from the calculation of the sum $\Psi(x_k)$ in Equation 4.18 [29], [30], [31].

In the construction of the *similarity filter* (SF), the reference pixel $x_1$ in $W$ is replaced by one of its neighbors if $\Psi(x_1) < \Psi(x_k)$, $k > 1$. If this is the case, then $x_1$ is substituted by that $x_j$ for which $j = \arg \max \Psi$. Applying the linear similarity function, $\psi(x_j, x_k) = 1 - \rho(x_j, x_k)/h$ for $\rho(x_j, x_k) < h$ and $\psi(x_j, x_k) = 0$ otherwise, we obtain the following expression [32]:

$$\Psi(x_1) - \Psi(x_k) \geq 0 \quad \text{if} \quad h \geq \sum_{j=2}^{n} [\rho(x_1, x_j) - \rho(x_k, x_j)], \quad k = 2, \ldots, n \tag{4.19}$$

If this condition is satisfied, then the central pixel $x_1$ is considered as not being disturbed by the noise process, otherwise, the pixel $x_k$ for which the cumulative similarity value $\Psi$ attains maximum replaces the central noisy pixel (Figure 4.10h).

It is easy to observe that the construction of this switching filter, when applying the linear kernel function, is similar to the standard VMF [32]. To achieve the rule in Equation 4.19, instead of the function $R_k$ in Equation 4.1, a modified cumulative distance function has to be used: $R_1' = -h + \sum_{j=2}^{n} \rho(x_1, x_j)$, $R_k' = \sum_{j=2}^{n} \rho(x_k, x_j)$ for $k > 1$, and in the same way as in the VMF, the central vector $x_1$ in $W$ is being replaced by $x_j$ such that $j = \arg \min R'$. Now, instead of maximizing the cumulative similarity $\Psi$, the modified cumulative distance $R'$ is minimized. In this way, the condition for retaining the original image pixel is $R_1' \leq R_k'$, $k > 1$, which leads to the rule of retaining $x_1$:

$$R_1' \leq R_k' \quad \text{if} \quad h \geq \sum_{j=2}^{n} [\rho(x_1, x_j) - \rho(x_k, x_j)], \quad k = 2, \ldots, n \tag{4.20}$$

The illustration of the efficiency of the switching filters as compared with the standard VMF and BDF is shown in Figure 4.10a through Figure 4.10h. As can be easily noticed, the switching scheme enables efficient impulsive noise cancellation with the preservation of image details and edges.

### 4.2.4 Application of Anisotropic Diffusion to Color Images

Recently, growing attention has been given to the nonlinear processing of vector-valued noisy image signals through the *anisotropic diffusion* (AD) technique. This filtering method was introduced in Reference [33] in order to selectively enhance image contrast and reduce noise, using a modified diffusion concept [34]. The main idea of AD is based on the modification of the isotropic diffusion, so that smoothing across image edges can be inhibited. This modification is done by introducing a conductivity function that encourages intraregion over interregion smoothing.

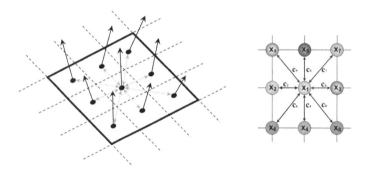

**FIGURE 4.11**
Anisotropic diffusion scheme on the vector field.

If $x(\chi_1, \chi_2) = [x^1(\chi_1, \chi_2), x^2(\chi_1, \chi_2), x^3(\chi_1, \chi_2)]$ denotes a color image pixel at a position $(\chi_1, \chi_2)$, the partial derivative equation of vector-valued anisotropic diffusion [33], [34] is

$$\frac{\partial x(\chi_1, \chi_2, t)}{\partial t} = \nabla \left[ c(\chi_1, \chi_2, t) \nabla x(\chi_1, \chi_2, t) \right] \qquad (4.21)$$

where $t$ denotes time, $c(\chi_1, \chi_2, t) = f(\|\nabla x\|)$ is the conductivity function, the same for each image channel, which couples the color image planes [35], [36].

The conductivity function $c$ is a space-varying, monotonically decreasing function of the image gradient magnitude and usually contains a free parameter $\beta$, which determines the amount of smoothing introduced by the nonlinear diffusion process. This function is chosen to be large in relatively homogeneous regions to encourage smoothing, and small in regions with high gradients to preserve image edges.

Various conductivity functions were suggested in the literature [34], however, the most popular are those introduced in Reference [33]:

$$c_1(\chi_1, \chi_2) = \exp \left( -\frac{\|\nabla x(\chi_1, \chi_2)\|^2}{2\beta^2} \right), \quad c_2(\chi_1, \chi_2) = \left( 1 + \frac{\|\nabla x(\chi_1, \chi_2)\|^2}{\beta^2} \right)^{-1} \qquad (4.22)$$

The discrete, iterative version of Equation 4.21 can be written as

$$x_1(t+1) = x_1(t) + \lambda \sum_{k=2}^{n} c_k(t) \left[ x_k(t) - x_1(t) \right], \quad \text{for stability} \quad \lambda \le 1/(n-1) \qquad (4.23)$$

where $t$ denotes discrete time, (iteration number), $c_k(t)$, $k = 2, \ldots, n$ are the diffusion coefficients in the $n-1$ directions (Figure 4.11), $x_1(t)$ denotes the central pixel of the filtering window and $x_k(t)$ are its neighbors. The equation of anisotropic diffusion (Equation 4.23) can be rewritten as follows:

$$x_1(t+1) = x_1(t) \left[ 1 - \lambda \sum_{k=2}^{n} c_k(t) \right] + \lambda \sum_{k=2}^{n} c_k(t) x_k(t), \quad \lambda \le 1/(n-1). \qquad (4.24)$$

If we set $[1 - \lambda \sum_{k=2}^{n} c_k(t)] = 0$, then we can switch off to some extent the influence of the central pixel $x_1(t)$ in the iteration process. In this way, the central pixel is not taken into the weighted average, and the anisotropic smoothing scheme reduces to a weighted average of the neighbors of the central pixel $x_1$: $x_1(t+1) = \sum_{k=2}^{n} c_k(t) x_k(t)$. Such a design is efficient, especially in the case of images distorted by impulsive or Gaussian noise of high $\sigma$, as it diminishes the influence of the central pixel $x_1$, which ensures the suppression of the outliers injected by the noise process. This effect can be observed when evaluating

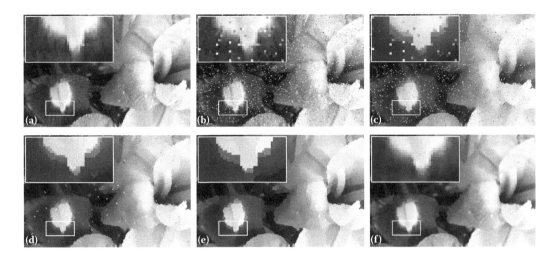

**FIGURE 4.12**
Efficiency of the AD diffusion schemes: (a) color test image, (b) noisy image distorted by 10% impulsive noise, (c) AD, ($c_1$, $\lambda = 0.1$), (d) AD with rejected central pixel, (e) GAD (see Smolka, B., Plataniotis, K.N., and Venetsanopoulos, A., *Nonlinear Signal and Image Processing: Theory, Methods, and Applications*, CRC Press, Boca Raton, FL, 2004; Smolka, B., *Comput. and Graphics*, 27, 503, 2003), and (f) VMF.

the smoothing achieved using the conventional AD scheme, shown in Figure 4.12, with the smoothing result obtained when rejecting the central pixel from the weighted average ($\lambda \sum_{k=2}^{n} c_k(t) = 1$). As can be seen in Figure 4.12c, the impulsive noise is preserved by the anisotropic diffusion, as it is treated as an edge. The filtering efficiency is improved in Figure 4.12d, however, clusters of impulses are preserved. This effect can be alleviated by applying the *generalized anisotropic diffusion* (GAD) scheme, which is based on the digital paths and fuzzy adaptive filtering [3], [37]. Instead of using a fixed window, this method exploits the similarity of pixels and the concept of fuzzy connectedness. According to the proposed methodology, image pixels are grouped together, forming paths that reveal the underlying structural dynamics of the color image. In this way, small clusters of impulsive noise are discarded, and image edges are preserved and even enhanced (Figure 4.12e). These properties can be used for efficient edge detection in images contaminated by impulsive noise and, as will be shown in Figure 4.20, also by the Gaussian noise contaminating the color image.

## 4.3 Edge Detection in Color Images

Color is a key feature describing the contents within an image scene, and it is found to be a highly reliable attribute that should be employed in the edge detection. The primary assumption used in color edge detection is that there is a change in chromaticity or intensity of pixels at the boundaries of objects. Hence, boundary detection can be accomplished by searching for abrupt discontinuities of the color features.

The major performance issues concerning edge detectors are their ability to precisely extract edges, their robustness to noise, and their computational complexity. An optimal edge detector should address the following issues [38]:

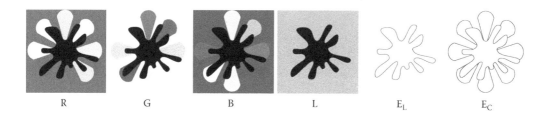

**FIGURE 4.13**

Test image with its $R, G, B$ channels and the luminance $L$. $E_L$ depicts the edges found utilizing only the luminance, and $E_C$ shows the detected edges when the color information is also considered.

- *Detection* — none of the image edges should be missed, and nonexisting edges should not be detected
- *Localization* — the edges should be well localized, which means that the distance between real and detected edges should be minimized
- *Response* — an optimal edge detector should have only one response to a single edge

In many cases, edge detection based only on the intensity of the image may not be sufficient, because no edges will be detected when neighboring objects have different chromaticity but the same luminance (see Figure 4.13). Because the capability of distinguishing between different objects is crucial for applications such as object recognition and image segmentation, the additional boundary information provided by color is of great importance. Therefore, there is a strong motivation to develop efficient color edge detectors that provide high-quality edge maps.

In monochrome grayscale imaging, edges are commonly defined as sharp intensity discontinuities, as physical edges often coincide with places of strong illumination and reflection changes. The definition of an edge in color imagery is much more challenging. In the case of color images, represented in the three-dimensional (3-D) color space, edges may be defined as discontinuities in the vector field representing the color image (Figure 4.1). In this way, edges split image regions of different color, and the variation in color has to be taken into account, as shown in an exaggerated form in Figure 4.13.

In the low-level processing of grayscale images, edge detection methods are mostly based upon differential operators. Unfortunately, the extension of the grayscale techniques into color imaging is not a trivial task, and the effectiveness of an edge detector depends on how the gradients obtained from the separate channels are fused to obtain a map of the edge strength.

According to the definition of an edge as an abrupt change of the intensity in a grayscale image, the first derivative operation is often used for the detection of intensity discontinuities. The first derivative informs about the rate of the changes of a function and allows points to be localized where large changes of the intensity function are present. Extending this concept to the two-dimensional (2-D) case enables the rate of image intensity changes to be traced, which leads to the creation of the edge strength map.

The straightforward approaches to color edge detection are based on the extensions of monochrome operators. These techniques are applied to the three color channels independently, performing the grayscale edge detection on each color channel. The results are then combined to provide a single edge map (Figure 4.14) [39]. In general, to achieve color edge detection, the intensity-based techniques are extended by taking the maximum of the gradient magnitudes, their weighted sum, the root mean square of the sum of squared

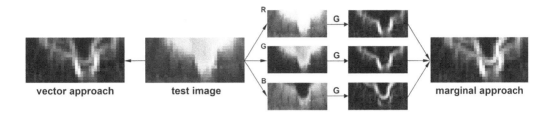

**FIGURE 4.14**
The marginal and vector approach to edge detection.

intensities of the edge maps, or by performing other transformations of the individual outputs.

Another group of gradient-based edge operators locates an edge by finding the zero crossing of the second derivative of the image intensity function. The zero crossing carries the information about the local extremum of the first derivative and indicates a point of rapid change of the intensity function. By detecting zero crossings, edges of one pixel thickness can be obtained, which is hardly possible for the first derivative-based methods. The most commonly used operator based on the second partial derivatives is the Laplacian, which coupled with the Gaussian is used in the so-called LoG or Marr-Hildreth operator.

The extension of the Laplacian of Gaussian method to the color case is complex. In Reference [40], a technique based on the detection of the zero crossing of the sum of the Laplacians determined separately in each image channel was described. However, such an extension generates spurious edges and is sensitive to noise. Mathematically rigorous discussion of the problem of finding zero crossings in color images is provided in Reference [41].

### 4.3.1 Vector Gradient Operators

There are many ways of implementing the vector-gradient-based edge detectors that utilize color information contained in the samples belonging to the local window $W$ (Figure 4.14). One of the simplest approaches is to employ a $3 \times 3$ window centered at each pixel and then to obtain eight gradient magnitudes by computing the Euclidean distance between the center sample and its eight neighbors (Figure 4.15). The magnitude of the *vector gradient* $\Gamma$, denoted as VG, is then defined as $\Gamma = \max \Gamma_k, k = 2, \ldots, 9$, where $\Gamma_k = \rho(x_1, x_k)$, according to the notation used in Figure 4.2. A similar scheme was used in the pioneering work [42] on color edge detection, in which 24 directional derivatives (8 neighbors, 3 channels) were calculated, and the one with the largest magnitude was chosen as the gradient.

The operators based on the first derivative, commonly applied in the grayscale imaging, can be generalized into the multidimensional case. For example, the Prewitt ($c = 1$) or Sobel

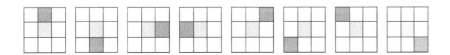

**FIGURE 4.15**
The structuring masks used for the construction of the vector gradient (VG).

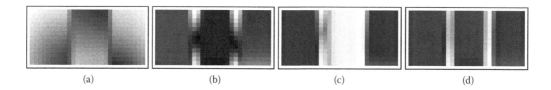

(a)       (b)       (c)       (d)

**FIGURE 4.16**
Edge detection using the artificial image shown in Figure 4.1: (a) test color image, (b) edge map obtained using the Sobel operator applied to the image luminance, (c) result of the independent edge detection on separate channels, and (d) VDG output.

($c = 2$) operator, with the following horizontal and vertical masks,

$$X_1 = \begin{bmatrix} -1 & 0 & 1 \\ -c & 0 & c \\ -1 & 0 & 1 \end{bmatrix}, \qquad X_2 = \begin{bmatrix} -1 & -c & -1 \\ 0 & 0 & 0 \\ 1 & c & 1 \end{bmatrix} \qquad (4.25)$$

can be extended by constructing the vectors: $\Gamma_1^+ = x_7 + c\,x_3 + x_8$, $\Gamma_1^- = x_9 + c\,x_2 + x_6$, $\Gamma_2^+ = x_6 + c\,x_4 + x_8$, $\Gamma_2^- = x_9 + c\,x_5 + x_7$ (Figure 4.2). The magnitude of the *vector directional gradient* (VDG) can be calculated from $\|\Gamma_1^+ - \Gamma_1^-\|$, $\|\Gamma_2^+ - \Gamma_2^-\|$ using an appropriate metric (Figures 4.20b and 4.21c). Figures 4.14 and 4.16a through Figure 4.16d show the difference between the marginal and vector approach using the gradient defined by the Sobel mask. The superiority of the vectorial approach over the marginal one is evident.

If larger convolution masks are employed, we obtain the following structures: $X_1 = [X_1^+ \ 0 \ X_1^-]$, $X_2 = [X_2^- \ 0 \ X_2^+]^T$. The components are convolution kernels with outputs that are vectors corresponding to the local, weighted average. In order to estimate the gradient at the image sample, the outputs of the following operators are calculated [43]:

$$\Gamma_1^+ = \sum_{u,v \in X_1^+} c_{u,v}\, x_{u,v}, \quad \Gamma_1^- = \sum_{u,v \in X_1^-} c_{u,v}\, x_{u,v}, \quad \Gamma_2^+ = \sum_{u,v \in X_2^+} c_{u,v}\, x_{u,v}, \quad \Gamma_2^- = \sum_{u,v \in X_2^-} c_{u,v}\, x_{u,v}, \qquad (4.26)$$

where $c_{u,v}$ are the weighting coefficients like in Equation 4.25. In order to estimate the local variation in the vertical and horizontal directions, the following vector differences are determined: $\Delta\Gamma_1 = \Gamma_1^+ - \Gamma_1^-$, $\Delta\Gamma_2 = \Gamma_2^+ - \Gamma_2^-$. The output of the *generalized vector directional gradient* (GVDG) can be determined by fusing the two gradients using a chosen vector metric.

This approach was extended in Reference [44], where it was assumed that edges occur when there are local statistical differences in the distribution of color image samples. To locate edges, a circular operation mask, called a compass, which measures the difference between the distribution of the pixels between two halves of a circular window,

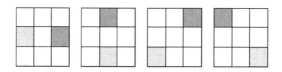

**FIGURE 4.17**
The structuring masks used for the definition of the difference vector (DV) operator.

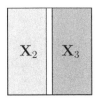 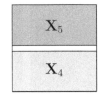 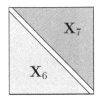 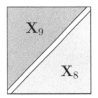

**FIGURE 4.18**
Subwindows corresponding to the DV operator.

is utilized. The orientation producing the maximum difference is the direction of the edge, and the difference between the distributions yields a measure of the edge strength (Figure 4.21d).

The class of difference vector (DV) operators frequently used for edge detection in color images is based on the first derivatives working on vectorial inputs. Using this approach, each pixel represents a vector in the color space and a gradient is obtained in each of the four directions by applying appropriate convolution masks (Figure 4.17). Then, a thresholding technique is applied to the edge map constructed from the maximal gradients to locate edges. The gradient values are defined as $\Gamma_k = \rho(x_{2k+1}, x_{2k})$, and the DV operator chooses the gradient of maximal magnitude, $DV = \max \Gamma_k$, $k = 1, \ldots, 4$ (Figure 4.20c and Figure 4.21e).

The DV operator is very fast; however, it is sensitive to impulsive and Gaussian noise [1]. The sensitivity to noise can be decreased be applying convolution masks of larger size and then dividing the masks into a set of subwindows $X_k$, $X_{k+1}$, $k = 2, \ldots, 8$, as depicted in Figure 4.18.

Depending on the type of noise one wishes to attenuate, different filters can be applied to the pixels belonging to the subwindows, to obtain the outputs that can then be used by the DV operator. In case of impulsive noise affecting the image, the application of the vector median filter to the set of pixels belonging to each of the subwindows yields satisfactory results (Figure 4.19b).

If we denote by $\tilde{x}_k$ the VMF output of the samples belonging to the subwindow $X_k$ from Figure 4.18, we obtain a set of gradients $\Gamma_{k+1,k} = \tilde{x}_{k+1} - \tilde{x}_k$, $k = 2, \ldots, 8$, and the DV operator chooses as output the gradient with the highest magnitude (Figure 4.19 and Figure 4.20).

In case of the Gaussian noise, the application of the *arithmetic mean filter* (AMF) is advantageous. In this way, the output of the DV operator in a specific direction is a distance between the means of the vector samples from the respective subwindows. As the $\alpha$-trimmed VMF is a compromise between the VMF and AMF, this filter can improve the detector performance in the presence of both Gaussian and impulsive noise (Figure 4.21g).

The drawback of the technique based on the subwindows is the high computational load. To alleviate this problem, image prefiltering can be applied, and the DV operator working in a $3 \times 3$ window can be employed (Figure 4.19c and Figure 4.20d through Figure 4.20f).

This approach yields good results, as the edge detection is performed on an image with significantly decreased noise intensity. However, care must be taken when applying a specific filtering design, as the choice of the filter can significantly influence the accuracy of the edge detection step.

### 4.3.2 Vector Field Approach

The difference between two color samples at positions $\chi_1$ and $\chi_2$ of a vector field, called a local contrast, is given by $\Delta x = x_{\chi_1} - x_{\chi_2}$. When the distance between the two vectors tends

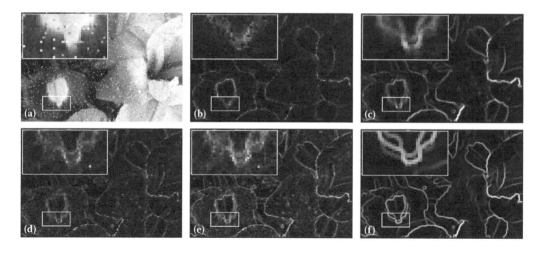

**FIGURE 4.19**
Edge detection results for an image distorted by impulsive noise: (a) test color image contaminated by 10% impulsive noise, (b) edge map obtained using the DV operator with the VMF subfilters in a 7 × 7 window, (c) result of DV using prefiltering with the VMF, (d) output of the MVDD with $\alpha$ and $k$ equal to 6, (e) edge map of the NNMVD for $k = 6$, and (f) output of the VDG applied on the image filtered with the generalized anisotropic diffusion (GAD).

to zero, the difference becomes $dx = \sum_{j=1}^{2} \frac{\partial x}{\partial \chi_j} d\chi_j$, with its squared norm given by [45]

$$dx^2 = \sum_{k=1}^{2} \sum_{l=1}^{2} \frac{\partial x}{\partial \chi_k} \cdot \frac{\partial x}{\partial \chi_l} d\chi_k d\chi_l = \sum_{k=1}^{2} \sum_{l=1}^{2} g_{kl} d\chi_k d\chi_l = \begin{bmatrix} d\chi_1 \\ d\chi_2 \end{bmatrix}^T \begin{bmatrix} g_{11} & g_{12} \\ g_{21} & g_{22} \end{bmatrix} \begin{bmatrix} d\chi_1 \\ d\chi_2 \end{bmatrix} \quad (4.27)$$

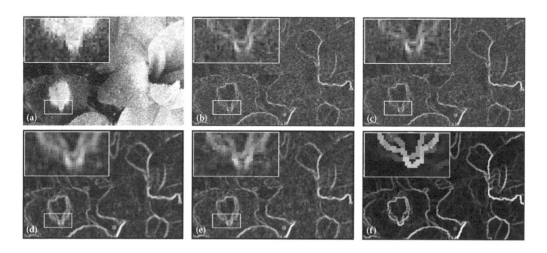

**FIGURE 4.20**
Edge detection results for an image distorted by strong Gaussian noise: (a) color test image contaminated by noise of $\sigma = 30$, (b) output of the vectorial Sobel operator, (c) difference vector (DV) operator output, (d) DV after the AMF prefiltering, (e) DV after $\alpha$ VMF prefiltering ($\alpha = 6$), and (f) DV after GAD (Smolka, B., Platoniotis, K.N., and Venetsanopoulos, A., *Nonlinear Signal and Image Processing: Theory, Methods, and Applications*, CRC Press, Boca Raton, FL, 2004; Smolka, B., *Comput. and Graphics*, 27, 503, 2003.)

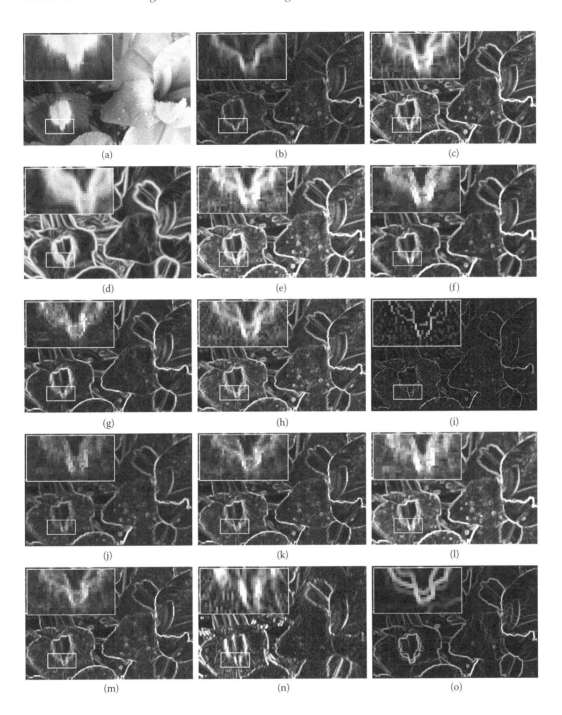

**FIGURE 4.21**

Comparison of various color edge detection methods: (a) color test image; (b) output of the Sobel edge detector working on the image intensity; (c) VDG output using Sobel operator; (d) method of Ruzon (Ruzon, M.A., and Tomasi, C., *IEEE Trans. on PAMI*, 23, 1281, 2001); (e) DV; (f) VG after filtering with VMF; (g) DV ($5 \times 5$) with $\alpha$-trimmed mean subfilter; (h) method of di Zenzo (Zenzo, S.D., *Comput. Vision, Graphics and Image Process.*, 33, 116, 1986); (i) $\lambda^+$ (Zenzo, S.D., *Comput. Vision, Graphics and Image Process.*, 33, 116, 1986); (j) VRD; (k) MVDD, $\alpha = 6$, $k = 3$, (l) NNVRD; (m) NNMVD, $k = 3$; (n) method of Sangwine (Sangwine, S.J., *Electron. Lett.*, 34, 969, 1998; Sangwine, S.J., and Ell, T.A., *IEE Proc. — Vision, Image and Signal Process.*, 147, 89, 2000); and (o) VDG applied after anisotropic diffusion.

where

$$g_{kl} = \frac{\partial \mathbf{x}}{\partial \chi_k} \cdot \frac{\partial \mathbf{x}}{\partial \chi_l} = \sum_{j=1}^{3} \frac{\partial x^j}{\partial \chi_k} \frac{\partial x^j}{\partial \chi_l} \tag{4.28}$$

For a unit vector $\mathbf{n} = (\cos\theta, \sin\theta)$, $d\mathbf{x}^2(\mathbf{n})$ indicates the rate of change of the image in the direction of $\mathbf{n}$:

$$d\mathbf{x}^2 = \mathcal{E} \cos^2\theta + 2\mathcal{F} \cos\theta \sin\theta + \mathcal{G} \sin^2\theta = \{\mathcal{E} + \mathcal{G} + \mathcal{H} \cos 2\theta + 2\mathcal{F} \sin 2\theta\}/2 \tag{4.29}$$

with $\mathcal{E} = g_{11}$, $\mathcal{F} = g_{12} = g_{21}$, $\mathcal{G} = g_{22}$, $\mathcal{H} = g_{11} - g_{22}$. The corresponding eigenvalues and eigenvectors are

$$\lambda_{\pm} = \frac{1}{2}\left(\mathcal{E} + \mathcal{G} \pm \sqrt{\mathcal{H}^2 + 4\mathcal{F}^2}\right), \quad \mathbf{n}_{\pm} = (\cos\theta_{\pm}, \sin\theta_{\pm}), \quad \theta_{+} = \frac{1}{2}\arctan\left\{\frac{2\mathcal{F}}{\mathcal{H}}\right\} \tag{4.30}$$

with $\theta_{-} = \theta_{+} \pm \pi/2$. These two solutions correspond to the maximum and minimum of $d\mathbf{x}^2$, and $\theta_{+}, \theta_{-}$ define two directions: along one of them $\mathbf{x}$ attains its maximal rate of change, along the other one it reaches its minimum.

Instead of using trigonometric functions, the eigenvector $\mathbf{n} = [n^1, n^2]$ can be computed using the vector $v = [\mathcal{H}, 2\mathcal{F}]$, with the nice property $\|v\| = \lambda_{+} - \lambda_{-}$ [41], [46]. Then,

$$\mathbf{n} = \left[\sqrt{(1+b)/2}, \; \text{sign}\{\mathcal{F}\}\sqrt{(1-b)/2}\right], \quad \text{with} \quad b = \mathcal{H}/\|v\| \tag{4.31}$$

The strength of an edge in a vector valued case can be described by $\lambda^+$ (see Figure 4.21i) by the difference between the extrema: $\lambda^+ - \lambda^- = (\mathcal{E} + \mathcal{G})/2$, and also by its sum: $\lambda^+ + \lambda^- = \sqrt{\mathcal{H}^2 + 4\mathcal{F}^2}$ [35], [47], [48].

### 4.3.3    Vector Order-Statistics Edge Operators

Order-statistics-based operators play an important role in image processing and have been used extensively in monochrome and color image processing. The class of color edge detectors based on order statistics is constructed as a linear combination of the ordered vector samples belonging to the processing window. Different sets of coefficients of the linear combination generate edge detectors that vary in performance and efficiency.

The simplest edge detection operator based on order statistics is the *vector range detector* (VRD). This operator determines the deviation between the vector median $x_{(1)}$ and the vector with the highest rank $x_{(n)}$: VRD $= \rho(x_{(n)}, x_{(1)})$. Its computational speed and performance are satisfactory in the case of images that are not affected by noise (Figure 4.21j). In the noisy environments, however, the impulses present in the image are falsely detected as edges. To alleviate this drawback, dispersion measures known as robust estimates in the presence of noise can be applied.

The *vector dispersion detector* (VDD) is defined as VDD $= \|\sum_{j=1}^{n} \psi_j x_{(j)}\|$, where $\psi_j$, $j = 1, \ldots, n$ are the weighting coefficients. It is worth noticing that VRD is a special case of VDD with $\psi_1 = -1$, $\psi_n = 1$, and $\psi_j = 0$ for $j = 2, \ldots, n - 1$. This definition can be generalized by employing a set of $k$ coefficients and combining the resulting vector magnitudes in a desired way. For example, the *generalized vector dispersion detector* (GVDD) employs a minimum operator that attenuates the effect of impulsive noise and is defined as [1]

$$\text{GVDD} = \min_{j} \left\|\sum_{l=1}^{n} \psi_{jl} x_{(l)}\right\|, \quad j = 1, 2, \ldots, k \tag{4.32}$$

where $k$ is the parameter of the detector.

Specific color edge detectors can be obtained from GVDD by selecting the set of coefficients $\psi_{jl}$. A special member of the GVDD family is the *minimum vector dispersion detector* (MVDD), defined as

$$\text{MVDD} = \min_j \rho(x_{(n-j+1)}, \hat{x}_{(\alpha)}), \quad j = 1, 2, \ldots, k, \quad \alpha < n \tag{4.33}$$

where $\hat{x}_{(\alpha)}$ is the arithmetic mean of the first $\alpha$ ordered vectors ($\alpha$VMF), and the parameters $k$ and $\alpha$ control the trade-off between the computational complexity and noise suppression efficiency (Figure 4.19d and Figure 4.21k).

As the high-ranked vectors are likely to represent pixels disturbed by noise, fixing the parameter $j$ leads to an edge detector robust to impulsive noise: $\text{MVDD}^* = \rho(x_{(n-k+1)}, \hat{x}_{(\alpha)})$, $k < n$, which is also immune to the influence of the Gaussian noise, due to the averaging operation performed in $\hat{x}_{(\alpha)}$.

An alternative design of the GVDD operator utilizes the adaptive nearest-neighbor filtering concept. The *nearest-neighbor vector range detector* (NNVRD) is defined as

$$\text{NNVRD} = \rho\left(x_{(n)}, \sum_{j=1}^{n} \psi_j x_{(j)}\right), \quad \psi_j = \frac{1}{n}\frac{R_{(n)} - R_{(j)}}{R_{(n)} - \hat{R}_{(n)}} \tag{4.34}$$

where the weighting coefficients $\psi_j$ are determined adaptively, and $\hat{R}_{(n)}$ denotes the arithmetic mean value of the aggregated distances $R_j$, $j = 1, \ldots, n$ (see Figure 4.21l).

The MVDD operator can also be combined with the NNVRD operator to improve its performance in the presence of impulse noise. The *nearest-neighbor minimum vector dispersion detector* (NNMVDD) is defined as

$$\text{NNMVD} = \min_j \rho\left(x_{(n-j+1)}, \sum_{l=1}^{n} \psi_l x_{(l)}\right), \quad \text{for} \quad j = 1, \ldots, k, \quad k < n \tag{4.35}$$

where the weights $\psi_l$ are given by Equation 4.34 (see Figure 4.19e and Figure 4.21m).

### 4.3.4 Edge Detection Based on Hypercomplex Convolution

There is a growing interest in the applications of *quaternions* to color image processing tasks. Quaternions can be thought of as an extension of the complex numbers and are usually written as $Q = q_0 + q_1 i + q_2 j + q_3 k$, where $q_l$, $l = 0, \ldots, 3$ are real numbers, and i, j, and k are symbolic elements with the properties that $i^2 = j^2 = k^2 = -1$, and $ij = k, ji = -k, jk = i, kj = -i, ki = j$, and $ik = -j$.

The quaternion $Q = q_0 + q_1 i + q_2 j + q_3 k$ can be interpreted as having a real part $q_0$ and a vector part $(q_1 i + q_2 j + q_3 k)$. The subspace $Q_v = (0 + i q_1 + j q_2 + k q_3)$ may be regarded as being equivalent to the ordinary vectors, $Q_v = v = (i q_1 + j q_2 + k q_3)$.

The conjugate of a quaternion is defined as $\bar{Q} = q_0 - q_1 i - q_2 j - q_3 k$, the norm as $|Q| = \sqrt{\sum_{l=0}^{3} q_l^2}$, $(\bar{Q}Q = Q\bar{Q} = |Q|^2)$ and the inverse $Q^{-1}$ is $\bar{Q}/|Q^2|$. The subspace $Q_u$ of a unit quaternion that satisfies the condition $|Q_u| = 1$ has a useful property: $Q_u = \cos\phi + \mu\sin\phi$, where $\mu$ is a vector unit quaternion parallel to the vector part of $Q_u$, and $\phi$ is a real number.

The operator $Q_u v \bar{Q}_u$ performs a rotation of $v$ by an angle $2\phi$ about an axis parallel to $Q_u$, ($\bar{Q}_u v Q_u$ reverses the rotation). This operation has been employed in the construction of filters working on color images, as the color image $x$ can be treated as a system of vector quaternions: $x(\chi_1, \chi_2) = [x^1(\chi_1, \chi_2)i + x^2(\chi_1, \chi_2)j + x^3(\chi_1, \chi_2)k]$, where $x^l$, $l = 1, 2, 3$ are the RGB channels of a pixel at position $(\chi_1, \chi_2)$. If $\mu = (iR, jG, kB)/\sqrt{3}$ is the gray line axis of the RGB color space, then $Q_u x_i \bar{Q}_u$ rotates the pixel $x_i$ of a color image in a plane normal to this axis [49], [50]. The convolution of the image $x$ with a quaternion $Q$ is given as $x * Q = x^1 * Q \cdot i + x^2 * Q \cdot j + x^3 * Q \cdot k$, where $x^l$ denotes the color image channel.

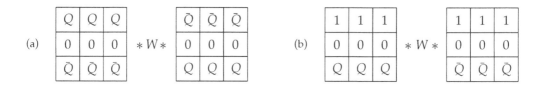

**FIGURE 4.22**
Convolution masks used in: (a) Sangwine, S.J., *Electron. Lett.*, 34, 969, 1998 and (b) Sangwine, S.J., and Ell, T.A., *IEE Proc. — Vision, Image and Signal Process*, 147, 89, 2000.

In Reference [51], an edge detector based on the rotation about the gray axis was proposed. The first convolution, as depicted in Figure 4.22a, operates in the vertical direction using the unit operator $Q = S\exp\{\mu\pi/4\} = S\{\cos(\pi/4) + \mu\sin(\pi/4)\}$. The $QW\bar{Q}$ and $\bar{Q}WQ$ perform the rotation about the gray line axis to $\pi/2$ and $-\pi/2$, respectively. Thus, if the filtering window contains pixels of similar color, the rotations in opposite directions will cause the cancellation of the chromaticity because of the vector addition incorporated in the convolution. If, however, the rows of the filtering window contain pixels of different colors, which signifies the existence of an edge, then the canceling effect does not occur, and the convolution operation detects an edge. This kind of edge detector is working on the chromaticity components and is insensitive to the intensity of the pixels, as the pixels are rotated in the RGB cube, and their magnitude is preserved.

In Reference [49], the operator presented in Figure 4.22b has been used, and the quaternion operator performed the rotations through $\pi$ radians. In this paper, the edge detector has also been extended using the Sobel and Kirsch masks. The resulting edge map depends to some extent on the kind of chromatic thresholding. Following the discussion in Reference [49], the edge map shown in Figure 4.21n was obtained performing the operation $E = (R + G + B)/3 - \min(R, G, B)$.

In Reference [52], a similar edge detection technique was formulated. The proposed edge detector is based on the difference of two operators $QW\bar{Q}$ and $\bar{Q}WQ$, which rotate the pixels of $W$ in opposite directions through the angle of $\pi/2$. In this work, the following conversion of the RGB space was applied: $r = (B - G)/I'$, $g = (R - B)/I'$, $b = (G - R)/I'$, where $I' = (R + G + B)/\sqrt{3}$. It interesting to notice that such a conversion was found to be very favorable for color edge detection in Reference [53].

### 4.3.5  Evaluation of the Edge Detection Efficiency

The major performance issues concerning edge detectors are their ability to precisely extract edges, robustness to noise, and computational complexity. In order to objectively evaluate the performance of the edge detectors for color images, quantitative and qualitative measures are used.

The quantitative performance measures can be grouped into two types: *statistical measures* based on the statistics of correctly and falsely detected edges and *distance measures* based on the deviation of the detected edges from the true edges. The first type of quality measure can be adopted to evaluate the accuracy of edge detection by measuring the percentage of correctly and falsely detected edges. Because a predefined edge map (ground truth) is needed, synthetic images are used for this evaluation. The second type of measure can be adopted to evaluate the performance of edge detectors by measuring the spatial deviation from true edges caused by the noise process [1], [54].

Because numerical measures do not correlate well with the perception of the human visual system, qualitative subjective tests are necessary in many image processing applications.

Edge operators can be rated in terms of several criteria, such as the precision of edge detection, continuity of edge-map lines, thinness of edges, performance in a noisy environment, and in terms of overall visual appeal.

The objective and subjective tests show that the performance of the Sobel, VR, and DV operators are similar in that they all produce good edge maps for images not affected by noise. The MVD and NNMVD operators are more robust to noise and are less sensitive to texture variations because of the averaging operation that smooths out small color variations.

The family of difference vector operators with subfiltering and prefiltering demonstrate good performance for noise-corrupted images (Figure 4.19). The operator utilizing the AMF performs best when detecting edges in images contaminated by Gaussian noise, the VMF yields good results in the case of impulsive noise degrading the color image, and operators based on $\alpha$-trimmed filters perform well on images disturbed by mixed noise. Very good results are also obtained by first performing the generalized anisotropic diffusion (GAD) [37] and then using any of the fast methods of vector gradient estimation (Figure 4.19f and Figure 4.20f).

## 4.4  Concluding Remarks

Vector image processing methods continue to grow in popularity, and the advances in computing performance have accelerated the process of moving from theoretical explorations to practical implementations. As a result, many effective methods of color noise suppression and edge detection have been proposed. Their aim is to efficiently remove various kinds of noise contaminating the color image, while preserving original image features. As edge information is very important for human perception, its preservation and possibly enhancement is a very important aspect of the performance of color image noise reduction filters.

In case of the impulsive noise, the switching filters, presented in Section 4.2.3, are a good choice. For the suppression of Gaussian noise, the fuzzy filters described in Section 4.2.2 and filters utilizing the anisotropic diffusion scheme (Section 4.2.4) yield good results. The attenuation of mixed (Gaussian and impulsive) noise is the most difficult task. For its removal, filters based on modifications of the anisotropic diffusion technique have been very effective.

The choice of an edge detector for a specific task is also image and noise dependent. Images containing textured regions or contaminated by Gaussian noise, should be processed utilizing a fuzzy averaging concept or order-statistics-based detectors with incorporated smoothing mechanisms. Another possibility is to employ, before the edge detection step, a suitable noise reduction technique. Performing an appropriate noise suppression prior to the actual edge detection generally gives good results and can be preferred in many edge detection tasks.

The results of the objective and subjective evaluations of the effectiveness of the edge detection algorithms lead to the conclusion that there is no universal method for edge detection [1], [54]. Figure 4.21 shows examples of the edge strength maps achieved using various edge detection techniques. As can be observed, the evaluation of the results is difficult, and the type of detector should be chosen according to the requirements posed by a particular image processing task. It is worth noticing that the quality of the edge detection will be significantly increased when performing the nonmaxima suppression on the edge strength maps and afterwards a binarization utilizing the thresholding with hysteresis.

The authors hope that the brief overview of the state-of-the-art of the challenging field of low-level color image processing methods will be useful for practitioners working on various applications in which noise removal and edge detection are of vital importance. For a deeper investigation of the presented methods, a representative bibliography was prepared.

## Acknowledgment

The contribution of M.A. Ruzon who evaluated the approach presented in Reference [44] on the test color image used in this chapter is gratefully acknowledged (Figure 4.21d). The authors are also grateful to S.J. Sangwine for the comments on the application of hypercomplex convolutions for edge detection and for the image presented in Figure 4.21n that was obtained using the algorithm presented in Reference [49].

B. Smolka has been supported by grant 3T11C 016 29 from the Polish Ministry of Science and Information Society Technologies.

## References

[1] K.N. Plataniotis and A.N. Venetsanopoulos, *Color Image Processing and Applications*, Springer–Verlag, Heidelberg, 2000.

[2] R. Lukac, B. Smolka, K. Martin, K.N. Plataniotis, and A.N. Venetsanopoulos, Vector filtering for color imaging, *IEEE Signal Process. Mag. Spec. Issue on Color Image Process.*, 22, 74–86, 2005.

[3] B. Smolka, K.N. Plataniotis, and A.N. Venetsanopoulos, *Nonlinear Signal and Image Processing: Theory, Methods, and Applications*, ch. Nonlinear techniques for color image processing, K.E. Barner and G.R. Arce, Eds., CRC Press, Boca Raton, FL, 2004, pp. 445–505.

[4] J. Zheng, K.P. Valavanis, and J.M. Gauch, Noise removal from color images, *J. Intelligent and Robotic Syst.*, 7, 257–285, 1993.

[5] J. Astola, P. Haavisto, and Y. Neuvo, Vector median filters, *Proceedings of the IEEE*, 78, 678–689, 1990.

[6] I. Pitas and A.N. Venetsanopoulos, *Nonlinear Digital Filters, Principles and Applications*, Kluwer, Boston, MA, 1990.

[7] J. Astola and P. Kuosmanen, *Fundamentals of Nonlinear Digital Filtering*, CRC Press, Boca Raton, FL, 1997.

[8] T. Viero, K. Oistamo, and Y. Neuvo, Three-dimensional median-related filters for color image sequence filtering, *IEEE Trans. on Circuits and Syst. for Video Technol.*, 4, 129–142, 1994.

[9] P.E. Trahanias and A.N. Venetsanopoulos, Vector directional filters: A new class of multichannel image processing filters, *IEEE Trans. on Image Process.*, 2, 528–534, 1993.

[10] P.E. Trahanias, D.G. Karakos, and A.N. Venetsanopoulos, Directional processing of color images: Theory and experimental results, *IEEE Trans. on Image Process.*, 5, 868–881, 1996.

[11] D. Karakos and P.E. Trahanias, Generalized multichannel image filtering structures, *IEEE Trans. on Image Process.* 6, 1038–1045, 1997.

[12] R. Lukac, B. Smolka, K.N. Plataniotis, and A.N. Venetsanopulos, Selection weighted vector directional filters, *Comput. Vision and Image Understanding, Spec. Issue on Colour for Image Indexing and Retrieval*, 94, 140–167, 2004.

[13] K. Tang, J. Astola, and Y. Neuvo, Nonlinear multivariate image filtering techniques, *IEEE Trans. on Image Process.*, 4, 788–798, 1995.

[14] I. Pitas and P. Tsakalides, Multivariate ordering in color image processing, *IEEE Trans. on Circuits and Syst. for Video Technol.*, 1, 247–256, 1991.

[15] I. Pitas and A.N. Venetsanopoulos, Order statistics in digital image processing, *Proceedings of the IEEE*, 80, 1893-1921, 1992.

[16] R. Lukac, K.N. Plataniotis, B. Smolka, and A.N. Venetsanopoulos, Generalized selection weighted vector filters, *EURASIP J. on Appl. Signal Process., Spec. Issue on Nonlinear Signal and Image Process.*, 12, 1870–1885, 2004.

[17] N. Nikolaidis and I. Pitas, Multivariate ordering in color image processing, *Signal Process.*, 38, 299–316, 1994.

[18] K.N. Plataniotis, D. Androutsos, S. Vinayagamoorthy, and A.N. Venetsanopoulos, Color image processing using adaptive multichannel filters, *IEEE Trans. on Image Process.*, 6, 933–949, 1997.

[19] K.N. Plataniotis, D. Androutsos, and A.N. Venetsanopoulos, Fuzzy adaptive filters for multi-channel image processing, *Signal Process. J.*, 55, 93–106, 1996.

[20] R. Lukac, K.N. Plataniotis, B. Smolka, and A.N. Venetsanopoulos, cDNA microarray image processing using fuzzy vector filtering framework, *J. Fuzzy Sets and Syst. Spec. Issue on Fuzzy Sets and Syst. in Bioinformatics*, 152, 17–35, 2005.

[21] R. Lukac, K.N. Plataniotis, B. Smolka, and A.N. Venetsanopoulos, A multichannel order-statistic technique for cDNA microarray image processing, *IEEE Trans. on Nanobioscience*, 3, 272–285, 2004.

[22] R. Lukac, K.N. Plataniotis, A.N. Venetsanopoulos, and B. Smolka, A statistically-switched adaptive vector median filter, *J. Intell. and Robotic Syst.*, 42, 361–391, 2005.

[23] R. Lukac, B. Smolka, K. Plataniotis, and A.N. Venetsanopoulos, Vector sigma filters for noise detection and removal in color images, *J. Visual Commun. and Image Representation*, 17, 1–26, 2006.

[24] R. Lukac, Adaptive vector median filtering, *Patt. Recognition Lett.*, 24, 1889–1899, 2003.

[25] R. Lukac, V. Fischer, G. Motyl, and M. Drutarovsky, Adaptive video filtering framework, *Int. J. Imaging Syst. and Technol.*, 14, 223–237, 2004.

[26] R. Lukac, Adaptive color image filtering based on center-weighted vector directional filters, *Multidimensional Syst. and Signal Process.*, 15, 2, 169–196, 2004.

[27] B. Smolka and A. Chydzinski, Fast detection and impulsive noise removal in color images, *Real-Time Imaging*, 11, 389–402, 2005.

[28] C. Kenney, Y. Deng, B.S. Manjunath, and G. Hewer, Peer group image enhancement, *IEEE Trans. on Image Process.*, 10, 326–334, 2001.

[29] B. Smolka, A. Chydzinski, K. Wojciechowski, K.N. Plataniotis, and A.N. Venetsanopoulos, On the reduction of impulsive noise in multichannel image processing, *Optical Eng.*, 40, 902–908, 2001.

[30] B. Smolka, K.N. Plataniotis, A. Chydzinski, and M. Szczepanski, Self-adaptive algorithm of impulsive noise reduction in color images, *Patt. Recognition*, 35, 1771–1784, 2002.

[31] S. Morillas, V. Gregori, G. Peris-Fejarnés, and P. Latorre, A fast impulsive noise color image filter using fuzzy metrics, *Real-Time Imaging*, 11, 417–428, 2005.

[32] B. Smolka, R. Lukac, A. Chydzinski, K.N. Plataniotis, and K. Wojciechowski, Fast adaptive similarity based impulsive noise reduction filter, *Real-Time Imaging, Spec. Issue on Spectral Imaging*, 9, 261–276, 2003.

[33] P. Perona and J. Malik, Scale space and edge detection using anisotropic diffusion, *IEEE Trans. on PAMI*, 12, 629–639, 1990.

[34] B. R. ter Haar, *Geometry-Driven Diffusion in Computer Vision*, Kluwer, Boston, MA, 1994.

[35] G. Sapiro and D.L. Ringach, Anisotropic diffusion of multivalued images with applications to color filtering, *IEEE Trans. on Image Process.*, 5, 1582–1586, 1996.

[36] G. Gerig, R. Kikinis, O. Kuebler, and F. Jolesz, Nonlinear anisotropic filtering of mri data, *IEEE Trans. on Medical Imaging*, 11, 221–232, 1992.

[37] B. Smolka, On the new robust algorithm of noise reduction in color images, *Comput. and Graphics*, 27, 503–513, 2003.

[38] J.F. Canny, A computational approach to edge detection, *IEEE Trans. on PAMI*, 8, 679–698, 1986.

[39] A. Koschan, A comparative study on color edge detection, in *Proceedings of the Second Asian Conference on Computer Vision (ACCV'95)*, Singapore, Vol. III, December 1995, pp. 574–578.

[40] S.J. Sangwine and R.E.N. Horne, (eds), *The Colour Image Processing Handbook*, Chapman & Hall, London; New York, 1998.

[41] A. Cumani, Edge detection in multispectral images, *Comp. Vision Graphics and Image Process.: Graphical Models and Image Process.*, 53, 40–51, 1991.

[42]  G.S. Robinson, Color edge detection, *Optical Eng.*, 16, 479–484, 1977.

[43]  J. Scharcanski and A.N. Venetsanopoulos, Edge detection of color images using directional operators, *IEEE Trans. Circuits and Syst. for Video Technol.*, 7, 397–401, 1997.

[44]  M.A. Ruzon and C. Tomasi, Edge, junction, and corner detection using color distributions, *IEEE Trans. on PAMI*, 23, 1281–1295, 2001.

[45]  S.D. Zenzo, A note on the gradient of a multi-image, *Comput. Vision, Graphics and Image Process.*, 33, 116–125, 1986.

[46]  A. Cumani, Efficient contour extraction in color images, in *Proceedings of the Third Asian Conference on Computer Vision (ACCV'98)*, Hong Kong, Vol. 1351, January 1998, pp. 582–589.

[47]  D. Tschumperle and R. Deriche, Diffusion pde's on vector-valued images: Local approach and geometric viewpoint, *IEEE Signal Process. Mag.*, 5, 15–25, 2002.

[48]  P. Blomgren and T.F. Chan, Color tv: Total variation methods for restoration of vector-valued images, *IEEE Trans. on Image Process.*, 7, 304–309, 1998.

[49]  S.J. Sangwine and T.A. Ell, Colour image filters based on hypercomplex convolution, *IEE Proceedings — Vision, Image and Signal Processing*, 147, 89–93, April 2000.

[50]  S. Pei and C. Cheng, Color image processing by using binary quaternion-moment-preserving thresholding technique, in *IEEE Trans. Image Process.*, 8, 614–628, September 1999.

[51]  S.J. Sangwine, Colour image edge detector based on quaternion convolution, *Electron. Lett.*, 34, 969–971, 1998.

[52]  C. Cai and S.K. Mitra, A normalized color difference edge detector based on quaternion representation, in *Proceedings of International Conference on Image Processing*, Vancouver, Canada, Vol. II, September 2000, pp. 816–819.

[53]  S. Wesolkowski, M.E. Jernigan, and R.D. Dony, Comparison of color image edge detectors in multiple color spaces, in *Proceedings of International Conference on Image Processing*, Vancouver, Canada, Vol. II, September 2000, pp. 796–799.

[54]  P. Androutsos, D. Androutsos, K.N. Plataniotis, and A.N. Venetsanopoulos, Color edge detectors: A subjective analysis, in *Proceedings of IS&T/SPIE Conference on Nonlinear Image Processing IX*, San Jose, CA, Vol. 3304, January 1998, pp. 260–267.

# 5

# Color Image Segmentation: Selected Techniques

Henryk Palus

## CONTENTS

## 5.1 Introduction

In different applications of color image processing, great importance is attached to the techniques used for image segmentation. The results of the further steps of image processing depend on the segmentation quality (e.g., the object recognition and tracking, the retrieval in image databases, etc.). The goal of image segmentation is partitioning of the image into homogeneous and connected regions without using additional knowledge on objects in the image. Homogeneity of regions in color image segmentation involves colors and sometimes also color textures [1]. In the segmented image, the regions have, in contrast to single pixels, many interesting features, like shape, texture, and so forth. A human being recognizes objects in the environment using the visual system and segmenting color images.

The first state-of-the-art papers in the field of color image segmentation date back to the 1990s [2], [3], [4], [5]. In the first color image processing handbooks, we can find separate chapters devoted to color image segmentation [6], [7]. Almost all the image segmentation techniques, for grayscale images developed earlier [8], have also been applied to the segmentation of color images. Each such expansion into color images is connected with a choice of some color space. The segmentation techniques use very different mathematical tools, but no method that is effective for each color image has been developed so far.

Segmentation of some objects from the background often requires processing of their color images. An example of such a situation is presented in Figure 5.1a through Figure 5.1f, showing color and grayscale versions of the image *Flowers1*. Both versions of the image have been segmented by the technique of seeded region growing, described in Section 5.3. The goal of the example segmentation task is to segment out blue petals of flower placed

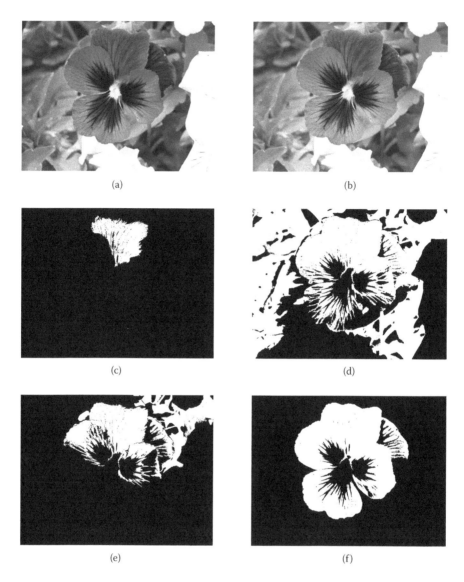

**FIGURE 5.1**

Example segmentation results: (a) color image *Flowers1*, (b) grayscale image *Flowers1*, (c) segmented grayscale image (parameter $d = 30$), (d) segmented grayscale image (parameter $d = 50$), (e) segmented grayscale image (parameter $d = 70$), and (f) segmented color image (parameter $d = 100$).

in the center of the image. The segmentation for both image versions (Figure 5.1a and Figure 5.1b) starts from a seed located in the same point on the upper petal of the flower. All attempts to segment out the blue petals from the grayscale image, consisting in changing a parameter $d$ (Figure 5.1c through Figure 5.1e), have failed. In contrast to grayscale image, the segmentation of a color image with the same technique gives a good result (Figure 5.1f) and shows the potential of color image processing.

If an image after segmentation contains many small regions corresponding to the homogeneous objects in the original image, we can use a new term: *oversegmentation*. On the other hand, if an image after segmentation contains few large regions, and each region corresponds to several objects in the original image, the case can be named *undersegmentation*.

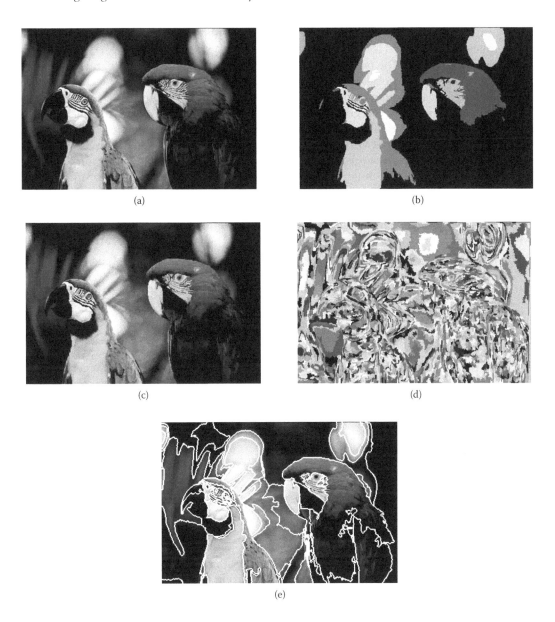

**FIGURE 5.2 (See color insert.)**

*Parrots* image and segmentation results: (a) original image, (b) segmentation into 48 regions (undersegmentation), (c) segmentation into 3000 regions (oversegmentation), (d) segmentation into 3000 regions presented in pseudocolors, and (e) segmentation into 62 white-bordered regions.

Figure 5.2a through Figure 5.2e show the color image *Parrots* and examples of oversegmented and undersegmented images. Pseudocolors have been used for better visualization of the oversegmentation effect (Figure 5.2d). Erroneous image segmentation (e.g., oversegmentation, undersegmentation) is a source of error in further image analysis and recognition. However, oversegmentation is more convenient in further processing, as by using suitable postprocessing techniques, we can decrease the number of regions in the image. Figure 5.2e shows a relatively good segmentation result (62 regions) for the color image *Parrots*. The white contours have been superimposed on the original image to distinguish the segmentation results.

Among many existing methods of color image segmentation, four main categories can be distinguished: pixel-based techniques, region-based techniques, contour-based techniques, and hybrid techniques. The last category is comprised of methods that integrate two techniques from former categories, for example, pixel-based and region-based techniques [9], as well as methods simultaneously using both regions and contours [10]. Sometimes in such taxonomies, separate categories for the techniques that use special mathematical tools (e.g., graph techniques, mathematical morphology, fuzzy techniques [5], [8], or techniques based on artificial neural networks [3], [5]) are created.

Because the color image acquisition devices are sources of noise, it is important to apply different noise reduction techniques as preprocessing algorithms before color image segmentation. The general task of preprocessing is to suppress noise and preserve edges at the same time. Unfortunately, most commonly used linear smoothing filters smooth images but blur the edges as well. Therefore, the best performance of preprocessing is obtained with nonlinear filters that work in the spatial domain. They preserve edges and details and remove Gaussian and impulsive noise. Good examples of such filters are the symmetric nearest neighbor filter described in Reference [11], the Kuwahara-Nagao filter proposed in the 1970s [12], [13], or the peer group filter presented in Reference [14]. The application of such filters may significantly improve segmentation results. Comparing such filters is most often based on visual evaluation or calculation of different quality factors. The other possibility is to evaluate filters according to the segmented images. Palus [15] suggests an evaluation function, resulting from research work on image segmentation. The performance of preprocessing depends on the method of color image segmentation; generally, it is more effective for simpler pixel-based segmentation than for region-based segmentation.

In this chapter, two classical image segmentation techniques are presented: the $k$-means clustering technique and the region growing technique in application to the color images.

## 5.2   Clustering in the Color Space

Clustering is the process of partitioning a set of objects (pattern vectors) into subsets of similar objects called clusters. Pixel clustering in three-dimensional color space on the basis of color similarity is one of the popular approaches in the field of color image segmentation. Clustering is often seen as an unsupervised classification of pixels. Generally, *a priori* knowledge of the image is not used during the clustering process. Colors, dominated in the image, create dense clusters in the color space in a natural way. Figure 5.3a and Figure 5.3b show three "pixel clouds" representing clusters in the RGB (red, green, blue) color space. Many different clustering techniques, proposed in the pattern recognition literature [16], can be applied to color image segmentation. One of the most popular and fastest clustering techniques is the $k$-means technique.

The $k$-means technique was proposed in the 1960s [17] and was described in many pattern recognition handbooks (e.g., Reference [18]). The first step of this technique requires determining a number of clusters $k$ and choosing initial cluster centers $C_i$:

$$C_1, C_2, \ldots, C_k \quad \text{where} \quad C_i = [R_i, G_i, B_i], \; i = 1, 2, \ldots, k \tag{5.1}$$

The necessity of determining input data is the drawback of the $k$-means technique. During the clustering process, each pixel $x$ is allocated to cluster $K_j$ with the closest cluster center using a predefined metric (e.g., the Euclidean metric, the city-block metric, the Mahalanobis metric, etc.). For pixel $x$, the condition of membership to the cluster $K_j$ during the $n$th

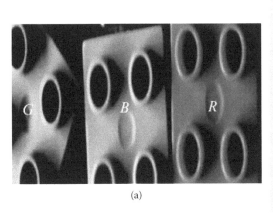

(a)

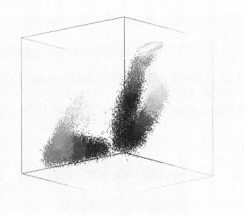

(b)

**FIGURE 5.3 (See color insert.)**
(a) Color image *Blocks1*, and (b) its clusters formed in RGB color space.

iteration can be formulated as follows:

$$x \in K_j(n) \iff \forall i = 1, 2, \ldots, j-1, j+1, \ldots, k \quad \|x - C_j(n)\| < \|x - C_i(n)\| \quad (5.2)$$

where $C_j$ is the center of the cluster $K_j$.

The main idea of $k$-means is to change the positions of cluster centers as long as the sum of distances between all the points of clusters and their centers will be minimal. For cluster $K_j$, the minimization index $J$ can be defined as follows:

$$J_j = \sum_{x \in K_j(n)} \|x - C_j(n+1)\|^2 \quad (5.3)$$

After each allocation of the pixels, new positions of cluster centers are computed as arithmetical means. Starting from Equation 5.3, we can calculate color components of the center of the cluster $K_j$ formed after $n+1$ iterations as arithmetical means of color components of the pixels belonging to the cluster:

$$C_{jR}(n+1) = \frac{1}{N_j(n)} \sum_{x \in K_j(n)} x_R \quad (5.4)$$

$$C_{jG}(n+1) = \frac{1}{N_j(n)} \sum_{x \in K_j(n)} x_G \quad (5.5)$$

$$C_{jB}(n+1) = \frac{1}{N_j(n)} \sum_{x \in K_j(n)} x_B \quad (5.6)$$

where $N_j(n)$ is the number of pixels in cluster $K_j$ after $n$ iterations. Because this kind of averaging based on Equation 5.4 to Equation 5.6 is repeated for all $k$ clusters, the clustering procedure can be named the $k$-means technique.

In the next step, a difference between new and old positions of the centers is checked. If the difference is larger than some threshold $\delta$, then the next iteration is starting, and the distances from the pixels to the new centers, pixels membership, and so forth, are calculated.

If the difference is smaller than $\delta$, then the clustering process is stopped. The smaller the value of $\delta$, the larger is the number of iterations. This stop criterion can be calculated as follows:

$$\forall i = 1, 2, \ldots, k \quad \|C_i(n+1) - C_i(n)\| < \delta \tag{5.7}$$

It can also be realized by limiting the number of iterations. During the last step of the $k$-means technique, the color of each pixel is turned to the color of its cluster center. The number of colors in the segmented image is reduced to $k$ colors. The $k$-means algorithm is converged, but it finds a local minimum only [19].

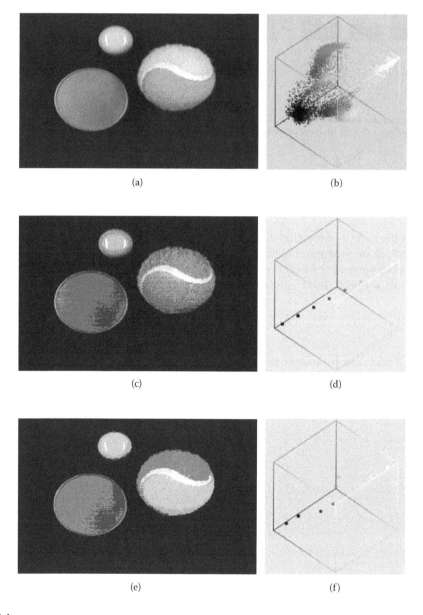

**FIGURE 5.4**
Development of the iterative clustering process: (a) color image *Objects*, (b) distribution of the pixels, (c) segmented image after the first iteration, (d) distribution of the cluster centers after the first iteration, (e) segmented image after the second iteration, and (f) distribution of the cluster centers after the second iteration.

The results of segmentation by $k$-means depend on the position of the initial cluster centers. In the case of a semiautomated version of $k$-means, the input data can be defined by the human operator. In the case of the automated version of $k$-means, the initial centers can be chosen randomly from all the colors of the image. There are also other possibilities for the choice of centers, including $k$ colors from the first pixels in the image and $k$ gray levels from the gray line uniformly partitioned into $k$ segments. Figure 5.4a through Figure 5.4e and Figure 5.5a through Figure 5.5f depict the results obtained for the color image *Objects* in individual iterations in the image domain as well as in RGB color space. This image was

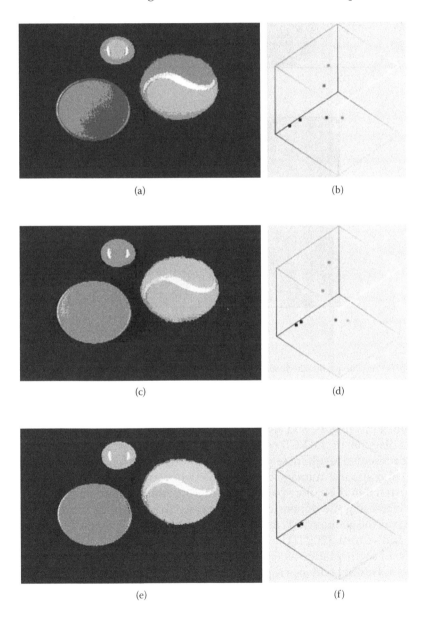

(a)                                             (b)

(c)                                             (d)

(e)                                             (f)

**FIGURE 5.5**
Continuation of Figure 5.4: (a) segmented image after the third iteration, (b) distribution of the cluster centers after the third iteration, (c) segmented image after the fifth iteration, (d) distribution of the cluster centers after the fifth iteration, (e) segmented image after the seventh iteration, and (f) distribution of the cluster centers after the seventh iteration.

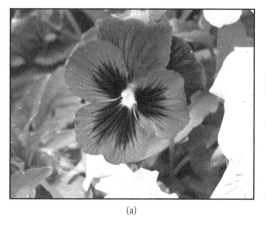
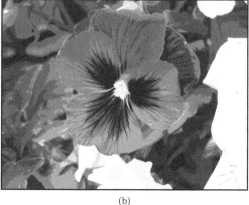

(a)                                                            (b)

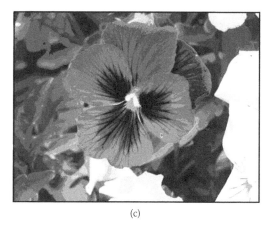

(c)

**FIGURE 5.6**

Segmentation of *Flowers1* image into 20 clusters: (a) original *Flowers1* image, (b) example segmented image (R component, 26 iterations), and (c) example segmented image (R component, 18 iterations).

clustered into eight clusters, and eight initial cluster centers were located on the gray-level axis (i.e., the diagonal of the RGB cube).

The above presented results of segmentation were obtained by $k$-means technique applied in the RGB color space. An image can be converted from RGB space to a new color space and then clustered in this color space. Other modifications of this clustering technique are realized by increasing the dimension of the feature space through introducing additional features, such as the geometrical coordinates of the pixel in the image, the gradient of color, the texture, and so forth [20], [21].

The results of segmentation as well as the number of iterations are dependent on initial cluster centers. This dependence is presented in Figure 5.6a through Figure 5.6c. Images in Figure 5.6b and Figure 5.6c were obtained when randomly choosing 20 initial centers. The program has stopped, dependent on initial centers, after 26 iterations (Figure 5.6b) and 18 iterations (Figure 5.6c). The difference between both segmented images is observable in the color segmented images: in the first segmented image, there are two yellow regions that do not exist in the second segmented image.

In the segmented image, the pixels that belong to one cluster can belong to many different regions. The larger the number of clusters $k$, the more regions are obtained after image segmentation. The processing of pixels without taking into consideration their neighborhoods is inherent to the nature of clustering techniques. It often results in sensitivity to noise and, therefore, needs to be postprocessed (Section 5.4) to eliminate oversegmentation.

## 5.3  Region Growing for Color Images

Region-based techniques group pixels into homogeneous regions. In this family of techniques, we can find the following: region growing, region splitting, region merging, and others. The region growing technique, proposed for grayscale images so long ago [22], is constantly popular in color image processing. In this section, we will examine the region growing technique.

The region growing technique is a typical bottom-up technique. Neighboring pixels are merged into regions, if their attributes, for example, colors, are sufficiently similar. This similarity is often represented by a homogeneity criterion. If a pixel satisfies the homogeneity criterion, then the pixel can be included in the region, and the region attributes (a mean color, an area of region, etc.) are updated. The region growing process, in its classical version, starts from chosen pixels called *seeds* and is continued as long as all the pixels are assigned to the regions. Each of these techniques varies in homogeneity criteria and methods of seed location. The advantages of region growing techniques result from taking into consideration two important elements: color similarity and pixel proximity in the image.

If the color in the image is described by RGB components, then the homogeneity criterion based on the Euclidean metric has the following form:

$$\sqrt{(R - \overline{R})^2 + (G - \overline{G})^2 + (B - \overline{B})^2} \leq d \qquad (5.8)$$

where $R, G, B$ are color components of the tested pixel; $\overline{R}, \overline{G}, \overline{B}$ are color components of the mean color of the creating region; and $d$ is the parameter that is very important for segmentation results. The homogeneity criterion in RGB space can be formulated as a conjunction of a few inequalities:

$$\overline{R} - T_1^R \leq R \leq \overline{R} - T_2^R \quad \wedge \quad \overline{G} - T_1^G \leq G \leq \overline{G} - T_2^G \quad \wedge \quad \overline{B} - T_1^B \leq B \leq \overline{B} - T_2^B \quad (5.9)$$

where $T_1^R, \ldots, T_2^B$ denote thresholds.

A similar growing process is sometimes realized in other color spaces, for example, in the HSI (Hue, Saturation, Intensity) cylindrical color space [23]. This space better represents the human perception of colors than does the RGB color space. In this case, Equation 5.8 must be modified to

$$\sqrt{(I - \overline{I})^2 + S^2 + \overline{S}^2 - 2S\overline{S}\cos(H - \overline{H})} \leq d \qquad (5.10)$$

where $H, S, I$ denote, respectively, hue, saturation, and intensity of the tested pixel, whereas $\overline{H}, \overline{S}, \overline{I}$ denote color components of the mean color of the creating region. The homogeneity criterion can also be based on variances of the color components of the creating region. This approach was applied to the HSV (Hue, Saturation, Value) space in the literature [24]:

$$\gamma = \frac{A_1}{\sigma_H^2} + \frac{A_2}{\sigma_S^2} + \frac{A_3}{\sigma_V^2} \qquad (5.11)$$

where $A_1, A_2, A_3$ represent constants; and $\sigma_H^2, \sigma_S^2, \sigma_V^2$ denote, respectively, the variances of hue, saturation, and value in the region after pixel-candidate inclusion. In this case, a pixel may be included in the region when the criterion's value $\gamma$ increases after this operation.

Sometimes in the literature (see, for example, Reference [25]), a need for a real color difference between the pixel candidate and the mean color of the creating region is stressed. This means that it is necessary to use a perceptually uniform color space [23], for example, CIE $L^*a^*b^*$ space. In this case, the homogeneity criterion has the following form:

$$\sqrt{(L^* - \overline{L}^*)^2 + (a^* - \overline{a}^*)^2 + (b^* - \overline{b}^*)^2} \leq d \qquad (5.12)$$

where $L^*, a^*, b^*$ are color components of the tested pixel; and $\overline{L}^*, \overline{a}^*, \overline{b}^*$ are color components of the mean color of the creating region.

If a tested pixel fulfills the homogeneity criterion, the following recurrent formula can be used to update the mean color of the region. Here is the example version for intensity $I$ only:

$$\overline{I}_n = \frac{(n-1)\overline{I}_{n-1} + I_{ij}}{n} \qquad (5.13)$$

where $I_{ij}$ is the intensity of the pixel with coordinates $ij$, the term $\overline{I}_{n-1}$ is the intensity of the region with $(n-1)$ pixels, and $\overline{I}_n$ denotes the intensity of the region with $n$ pixels, after the merging of the tested pixel. Similar recurrent formulas can be derived for other region descriptors (e.g., variance):

$$\sigma_n^2 = \frac{(n-1)(\sigma_{n-1}^2 + \overline{I}_{n-1}^2) + I_{ij}^2}{n} - \overline{I}_n^2 \qquad (5.14)$$

where $\sigma_{n-1}^2$ is the variance of intensity in the region with $n-1$ pixels, and $\sigma_n^2$ is the variance of intensity in the region with $n$ pixels, after pixel-candidate merging. It is necessary to know that during the segmentation process, the values of the above-described statistics of the region are only approximately known, because not all the pixels (members of region) are known.

In the region growing process, we can use a four-connectivity or an eight-connectivity concept [20]. A pixel that satisfies the requirements of four-connectivity or eight-connectivity is merged into the creating region, if its color fulfills the homogeneity criterion.

### 5.3.1 Seeded Region Growing

In the 1990s, two versions of the seeded region growing (SRG) algorithm for grayscale images were proposed [26], [27]. The seeds in this technique are often chosen in the regions of interest (ROI). One good example is an image *Sign* shown in Figure 5.7a to Figure 5.7d that contains six characters but, simultaneously, eight separate regions. For complete segmentation of the image *Sign* into $N$ regions, one seed in each potential region should be chosen, and a proper value of parameter $d$ should be selected.

The distribution of seeds is presented in Figure 5.7a, and the result of segmentation by the SRG technique in the RGB color space with color component values from the range [0, 255] and the value of the parameter $d = 50$ is shown in Figure 5.7b. It should be pointed out that for each image, there is a range of values of the parameter $d$, which is necessary for good segmentation. The use of out-of-range values of the parameter $d$ results in incomplete segmentation (Figure 5.7c) or in character deformation (Figure 5.7d). The background of the segmented image was removed for simplification purposes. The regions that grow around the seeds can be parallel segmented from the rest of the image. The SRG technique with application of a manual location of seeds works properly if the image contains a limited number of objects [28].

However, the SRG technique results depend on the positions of seeds. Figure 5.8a to Figure 5.8e present images segmented by using seeds placed in two different places.

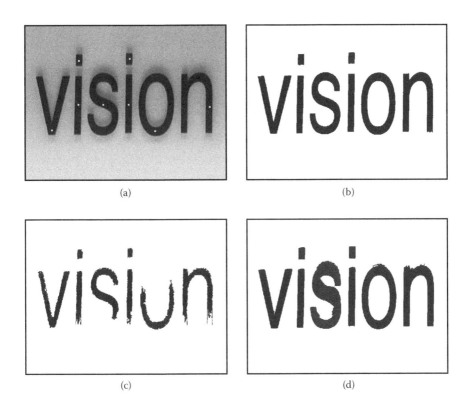

**FIGURE 5.7**
Seeded region growing for color image *Sign*: (a) original *Sign* image with the seeds, (b) segmented image using $d = 50$, (c) segmented image using $d = 10$, and (d) segmented image using $d = 90$.

Figure 5.8d proves that the position of seed is essential to the segmentation results. Using two seeds placed on one object (i.e., a blue flower), results in two regions instead of one (Figure 5.8e). In the postprocessing step, both regions can be merged into one. The influence of seed size, from 1 pixel to $20 \times 20$ pixels, on the results of the segmentation was tested. It is definitely smaller than the influence of seed position in the image. The difference image between the segmented images that were segmented based on both the small and large seeds, contains a few dozens of single pixels by the image resolution $640 \times 480$ pixels.

The seeds can be located in the image manually, randomly, or automatically. An operator uses his or her knowledge of the image for seed location. The random choosing of seeds is particularly risky in the case of a noisy image, because a seed can also be located on a noisy pixel. The seeds can be also found using the color histogram peaks. Additional edge information is sometimes also applied to the location of seeds inside closed contours. Sinclair [29] proposed a position of seeds on the peaks in the Voronoi image. His method, first of all, requires that the edges in the original image be found. A binarized edge image is a base for generating the Voronoi image. The gray level in the Voronoi image is the function of distance from the pixel to the closest edge. The larger this distance, the brighter is the pixel in the Voronoi image. Therefore, the seeds are located in the brightest pixels of a Voronoi image (Figure 5.9a and Figure 5.9b).

Ouerhani et al. [30] applied the so-called attention points coming from a visual attention model as natural candidates to fulfill the role of seeds. Ikonomakis et al. [31] determined the seeds for chromatic regions by checking the variance of hue in the symmetrical masks.

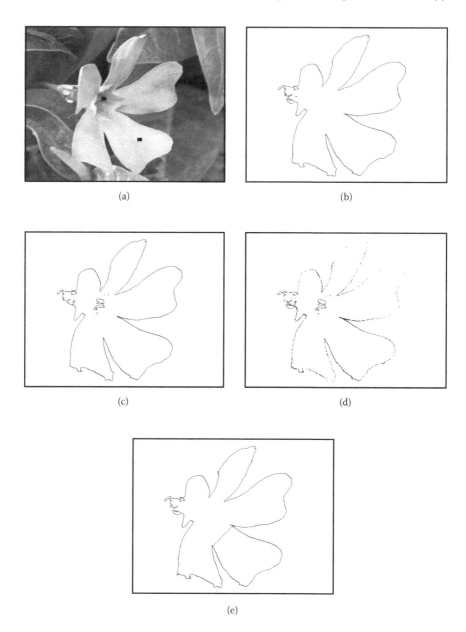

**FIGURE 5.8**
Seeded region growing for color image *Flowers2*, parameter $d = 150$: (a) original *Flowers2* image with two marked locations for one seed, (b) result of segmentation using seed in the middle of the flower, (c) results of segmentation using the seed on the petal of the flower, (d) difference of images (b) and (c), and (e) result of segmentation using two seeds located as in image (a).

If this variance is smaller than some threshold, a seed in the mask is located. In practical applications, knowledge about processed images is used for seed location. For example, a mobile robot equipped with a vision system should find all doors in the interior rooms. In images from the robot's camera, the seeds are automatically placed at some distance from the corners of doors that have been found with the help of the Harris method [32].

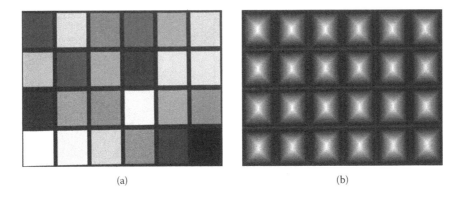

**FIGURE 5.9**
(a) Color image *Chart* and (b) Voronoi image obtained from image (a).

## 5.3.2 Unseeded Region Growing

This technique can also be named as a region growing technique by the pixel aggregation. It is based on the concept of region growing without needing the seeds to start the segmentation process. At the beginning of the algorithm, each pixel has its own label (one-pixel regions). A pixel is included in a region if it is four-connected or eight-connected to this region and has a color value in the specified range from the mean color of an already constructed region. After each inclusion of the pixel in the region, the region's mean color is updated. For this updating, recurrent formulas are used. One or two simple raster scans of the color image are applied: One pass from the left to the right and from the top to the bottom can be followed by an additional reverse pass over the image [33]. In the case of four-connectivity, four neighbors of the tested pixel are checked during both scans. In the case of eight-connectivity, two pixels are checked additionally during each scan (Figure 5.10a and Figure 5.10b). The pixel aggregation process results in a set of regions characterized by their mean colors, their sizes, and lists of pixels that belong to proper regions. The regions in this process are generated sequentially. The basic version of the algorithm works in the RGB color space.

During the tests, it was observed that if the value of the parameter $d$ increased, the number of regions $R$ in the segmented image simultaneously decreased. The results for color image *Flowers2* are shown in Figure 5.11a to Figure 5.11d. Too low a value of the parameter $d$ leads to oversegmentation, and too high a value causes undersegmentation.

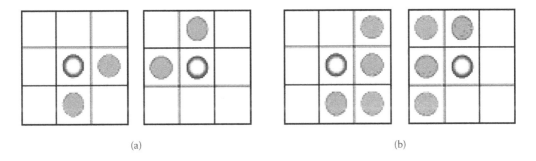

(a)                    (b)

**FIGURE 5.10**
Masks used in the segmentation process: (a) mask for four-connectivity and (b) mask for eight-connectivity.

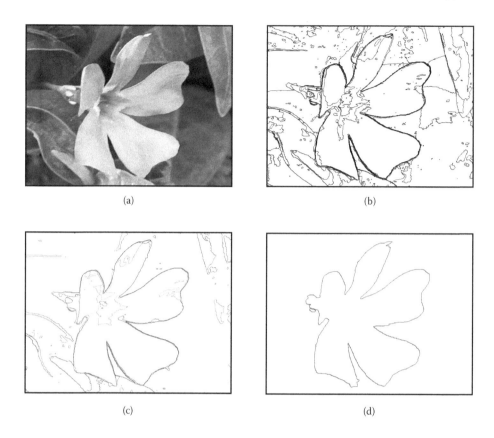

**FIGURE 5.11**
Edge representation of segmentation results of the color image *Flowers2* — different values of the parameter $d$:
(a) original *Flowers2* image; (b) segmented image, $d = 40$ (2194 regions); (c) segmented image, $d = 70$ (413 regions);
and (d) segmented image, $d = 180$ (3 regions).

The described technique demonstrates a sensitivity to the direction of the scanning process. Several images were also segmented using a reverse direction (i.e., from the bottom right pixel to the top left pixel). The numbers of regions obtained for images scanned in both direct and reverse directions differ slightly. For each pair of images segmented in this way, a difference image can be generated. Figure 5.12a to Figure 5.12c show the results of such an experiment for the image *Flowers2*. The negative of the difference image (Figure 5.12c) is not a white image, which means that the result of the proposed segmentation technique is dependent on the order of merging pixels into the regions. The independence of segmentation results from the order of merging pixels requires that the growing algorithm be explicated. The idea of such an approach used for grayscale images is described as the ISRG algorithm in the literature [27].

Region techniques are inherently sequential and, hence, the significance of the used order of the pixel and region processing. We can easily notice that the SRG technique is very useful for cases where an image should be segmented to a small number of regions. On the other hand, unseeded region growing is suitable for application in the complete image segmentation. Information on edges obtained with the use of the gradient can help control the region growing process. Such an approach was proposed for grayscale images in the work [34]. Many hybrid techniques, where region and edge information complement each other in the image segmentation process have been developed [35]. The idea of region growing was also applied in watershed segmentation and was used for the color images for

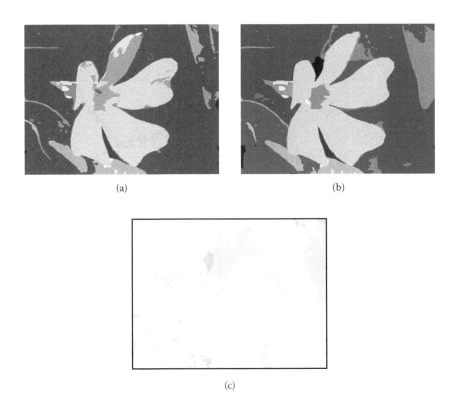

(a)                                                    (b)

(c)

**FIGURE 5.12**
Segmentation results of the color image *Flowers2* — different scanning directions, parameter $d = 70$: (a) segmentation based on the direct scanning direction (413 regions), (b) segmentation based on the inverse scanning direction (411 regions), and (c) negative image of difference image between images (a) and (b).

the first time by Meyer [36]. Sometimes the region growing technique is used as an initial segmentation before the main segmentation process [37].

## 5.4   Postprocessing

One of the reasons for oversegmentation can be the presence of noise contained in the image before the segmentation. The segmentation of good-quality images also results in a large number of small regions on the edges of the objects. It is possible to remove these regions from the segmented image by postprocessing. Application of postprocessing to the region growing based on the pixel aggregation is shown below.

One of the most effective methods of postprocessing is to remove the small regions from the image and to merge them into the neighboring regions with the most similar color. It is not a difficult task, because after the region-based segmentation, we have at our disposal a list of regions that can be sorted according to their areas. A threshold value of the area of the small region $A$ depends on the image. In one image, the same threshold $A$ allows unnecessary artifacts (e.g., highlights or noises) to be removed, while in the other, it removes necessary details. After the merging of the pixels, the mean color of the new region is computed, and the label of the pixel, which shows that it lies in the defined region, is changed. Due to such postprocessing, the number of regions in the segmented image significantly decreases.

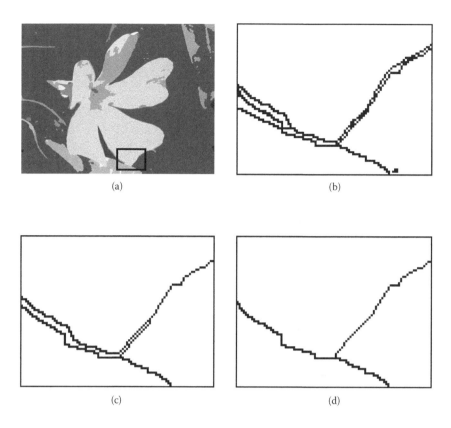

**FIGURE 5.13**
Results of postprocessing step on the segmented image *Flowers2* (parameter $d = 70$): (a) segmented image with marked window, (b) enlarged edge representation of the window (26 regions), (c) result of postprocessing — parameter $A = 100$, and (d) result of postprocessing — parameter $A = 1000$.

In Figure 5.13b an enlarged part of the segmented image (Figure 5.13a) is presented; we can see the small regions on the edges of objects. In our case, there are regions on the edge of the flower petal. In Figure 5.13b, we can see that the image contains 26 small regions. After the application of postprocessing, which is based on removing the regions of the area smaller than 100 pixels, the number of regions in this part of the image has been decreased to four. Among them is one small region located along the edges (Figure 5.13c). The expansion of the definition of a small region to the maximal value $A = 1000$ pixels causes the removal of all the small regions, leaving one region of petal and two regions of leaves (Figure 5.13d).

The results of postprocessing obtained for the whole tested image *Flowers2* (Figure 5.14a to Figure 5.14d) are presented below. We can observe that the postprocessing procedure can be used not only for the removal of small regions, but also for the merging of adjacent regions, after introducing a large value of the parameter $A$. In Figure 5.14d we can see an effect of the merging of regions into one homogeneous region of the background for the value of parameter $A = 10,000$.

The merging of small regions into large ones with similar color does not have to be based on defining the threshold value for the area of the small region. Sometimes it is assumed that, for example, 90% of all the pixels in the image belong to the essential regions. Next, all regions are sorted according to size, the large regions containing 90% pixels

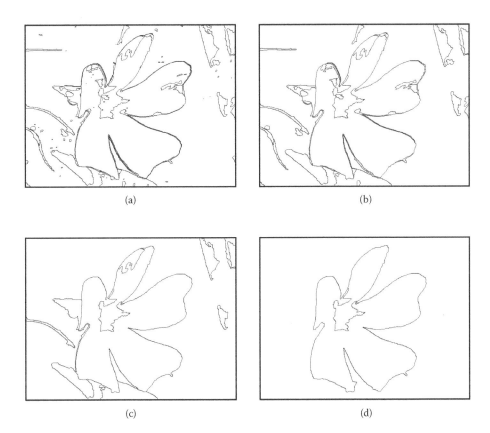

**FIGURE 5.14**

Results of the postprocessing step on the segmented image *Flowers2* (parameter $d = 70$): (a) segmented image (413 regions), (b) result of postprocessing — parameter $A = 100$ (47 regions), (c) result of postprocessing — parameter $A = 1000$ (12 regions), and (d) result of postprocessing — parameter $A = 10,000$ (3 regions).

are chosen, and the remaining regions are treated as small regions [38]. Yagi et al. [39] proposed that the merging of the colors of regions by means of the distance in the HSV color space and a variable value of threshold depending inversely proportionally on the area of the region be analyzed. Along with a small area of the region, additional indicators for the region merging can be proposed (e.g., a low value of color variance of the region, expressed by the trace of covariance matrix or the location of the region near the image border).

The color similarity of neighboring regions can be evaluated independently by area. Region similarity can be measured by means of the difference between mean colors determined using Equation 5.8 to Equation 5.12 or by more computationally complicated features:

- Color histograms of the regions [40] with color similarity being evaluated through the histogram intersection technique [41]

- Formula dependent on mean color gradient calculated for the pixels included in these regions [42]

- Fisher distance between adjacent regions for one color component [43], [44]:

$$F D_{12} = \frac{\sqrt{(n_1 + n_2)}|\hat{\mu}_1 - \hat{\mu}_2|}{\sqrt{n_1\hat{\sigma}_1^2 + n_2\hat{\sigma}_2^2}} \qquad (5.15)$$

where $n_1, n_2, \hat{\mu}_1, \hat{\mu}_2, \hat{\sigma}_1{}^2, \hat{\sigma}_2{}^2$ denote the number of pixels, a sample mean, and sample variance of color of the first and the second regions. A maximal value of Fisher distance chosen among the distances calculated for all three color components can be used as a final measure of color similarity between regions.

Since the first publications on the region growing technique [22], attention was called to the length of the common part of contours of the neighboring regions. An additional condition for the merging of neighboring regions is often formulated: some minimal value of length of a common part of their contours should be exceeded [45]:

$$\frac{B_{ij}}{B_i + B_j} > T \tag{5.16}$$

where $B_i$, $B_j$ denote the lengths of the contours of regions $R_i$, $R_j$; the term $B_{ij}$ represents the length of the common parts of contours $R_i$, $R_j$; and $T$ is the threshold (e.g., 0.05).

The graph methods [46], [47] headed by a region adjacency graph (RAG) [48] and defined in many handbooks [49] are applied for determining the relations between regions and for fixing the order of regions in the merging process. The nodes of the RAG represent regions. An arc in the graph links two nodes that represent two adjacent regions. For each arc, a cost of region merging can be calculated. The main idea of RAG-based region merging is to remove arcs with the lowest cost and to connect the corresponding nodes.

The order of region merging has an influence on the final result of segmentation [50]. A methodical approach to operating on the list of regions by means of a metric from Equation 5.12 as the color difference between the regions was described in the literature [51]. The final goal of region merging is to garner a segmented image that contains the most possible homogeneous regions.

## 5.5    Shadows and Highlights in the Image Segmentation Process

In practical applications of color image processing, it is often important to have a segmentation technique that is robust to shadows and highlights in the image. This problem is presented below for the case of the region growing by pixel aggregation. The shadows in the image can be so large that during the postprocessing it is not possible to remove them without simultaneously removing some other essential regions. We can see such a situation in the color image *Blocks2* (Figure 5.15a). The application of the Euclidean metric, defined in the RGB space, results in the segmented image with the large regions of shadow (Figure 5.15b). The selection of a suitable color space and metric to be used in the homogeneity criterion together with suitable parameter values $(d, A)$ enables the removal of the shadow regions from the segmented image. Required for such an operation is an early nonlinear transformation from the RGB color space to the HSI or the CIE $L^*a^*b^*$ color spaces. After omitting the luminance component in Equation 5.10 and Equation 5.12, the technique can segment objects from their images (Figure 5.15c and Figure 5.15d). We can avoid time-consuming color space transformations by using an angle between the color vectors in the RGB space instead of the Euclidean metric [52].

Let us assume that a mean color of the creating region and the color of the tested pixel are represented by the following vectors:

$$c_1 = [R_1, G_1, B_1], \qquad c_2 = [R_2, G_2, B_2] \tag{5.17}$$

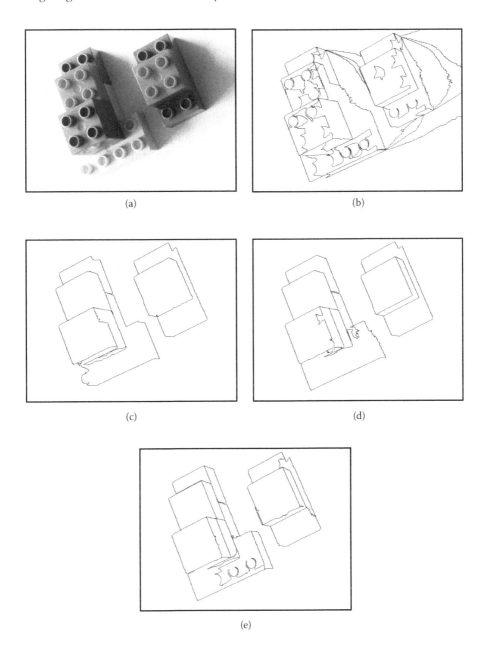

**FIGURE 5.15**
Segmentation results for the color image *Blocks2*: (a) original *Blocks2* image, (b) result for Euclidean metric in the RGB space and parameters $d = 45$ and $A = 710$, (c) result for Euclidean metric on the HS plane and parameters $d = 50$ and $A = 1000$, (d) result for Euclidean metric on the $a^*b^*$ plane and parameters $d = 12$ and $A = 1800$, and (e) result for "angle between vectors" metric in the RGB space and parameters $d = 21$ and $A = 2000$.

An angle between the color vectors $c_1$ and $c_2$, denoted by $\theta$, based on the definition of the scalar product of vectors, can be written as follows:

$$\cos \theta = \frac{c_1^T \circ c_2}{\|c_1\| \|c_2\|} \tag{5.18}$$

The smaller the angle $\theta$, the closer the pixel color is to the mean color of the region. Hence, the sine function can be used as a measure of color similarity, and on its base, we can formulate the following homogeneity criterion:

$$255 \cdot \sqrt{1 - \left( \frac{c_1^T \circ c_2}{\|c_1\| \|c_2\|} \right)^2} \leq d \qquad (5.19)$$

The application of Equation 5.19 in the region growing process results in a robust image segmentation, which is shown in Figure 5.15e. The angular data, like an angle between the color vectors $\theta$ and a hue $H$, need, due to the periodicity, special methods of statistical analysis (e.g., directional statistics) [53]. The integration of the shadows into the image background results in a growth of a bluish color in the background (Figure 5.15c to Figure 5.15e).

Highlights, produced by smooth surfaces of the objects in the scene and specular reflections, may also impede the image segmentation process (Figure 5.16a). In general, the highlights occur in the image as the separate regions, with the colors similar to the color of the light source (e.g., white color) (Figure 5.16b). The highlight regions can be removed by the postprocessing (Figure 5.16c). It is possible, because the size of the highlight is definitely smaller than the size of the object.

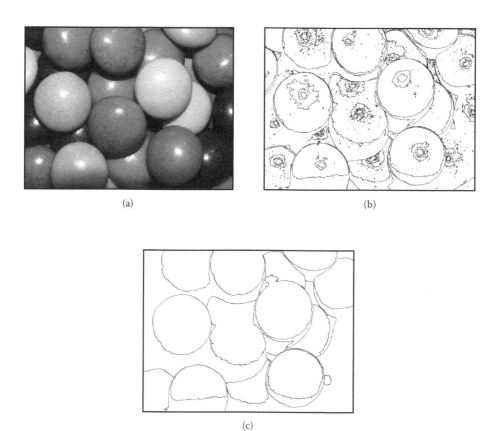

(a)      (b)

(c)

**FIGURE 5.16**

Segmentation results for the color image *Candies*: (a) original *Candies* image, (b) result for Euclidean metric in the RGB space and parameter $d = 60$, and (c) result for Euclidean metric in the RGB space and parameters $d = 60$ and $A = 5000$.

## 5.6 Quantitative Evaluation of the Segmentation Results

Nowadays there are many color image segmentation techniques, but there are few results in the field of evaluation of the segmented images. The reason is a lack of generally accepted criteria and a deficiency of the uniform procedures for the evaluation of the segmentation results. In the literature, there are many algorithms of segmentation presented that are tested on the small number of images.

The simplest way to evaluate a segmented image is for a human expert or experts to conduct a subjective evaluation. According to some researchers, a human is the best judge in this evaluation process [8]. In some applications of the image segmentation (e.g., in an object recognition), a recognition rate can serve as an indirect assessment of a segmentation algorithm independently of expert opinions on the segmented image. In the classical Zhang paper [54], the quantitative methods of evaluation of the segmentation results were grouped into two categories: analytical and experimental methods. The analytical methods are weakly developed, because there is no general image segmentation theory.

Among the experimental methods, two approaches predominate: the empirical goodness approach and the empirical discrepancy approach. The first does not need a reference image, and the evaluation of a segmented image is based on the original image. An example of a goodness measure can be shown in the case of region-based segmentation homogeneity of a region or a contrast between regions. In the second approach, a discrepancy measure, expressed as a difference between segmented and reference images, is computed. The reference image (also called ground truth) is an image that has been manually segmented by an expert. Generation of the reference image sometimes constitutes a difficult problem, because different people create different segmentations for the same image. The discrepancy measure is often based on a number of missegmented pixels, a position of missegmented pixels, and so forth.

In the field of data clustering, different measures for the evaluation of results have been developed. A simple measure is an intracluster distance that can be computed as a sum of the distances between the cluster points and the cluster center. This measure evaluates a compactness of clusters. A complementary measure to the intracluster distance is an intercluster distance that can be computed as a sum of distances among the centers of clusters. The value of intercluster distance estimates a separation of the clusters.

Turi and Ray [55] proposed a validity measure VM, defined for the clustering technique as a proportion of two measures described above, that characterizes the clusters:

$$VM = y(k)\frac{intra}{inter} \qquad (5.20)$$

where *intra* is a measure of cluster compactness, *inter* is a measure of distance between the clusters, and $y(k)$ is a continuous function based on the Gauss function of number of clusters $k$ with the mean value equal to two and standard deviation equal to one. If the number of clusters is larger than four, then the $y(k)$ function is one and does not influence the VM measure.

The main goal of the segmentation by clustering is the minimization of the VM measure. It means that we should minimize the distances between the elements of clusters and their centers to create compact clusters. At the same time, we should maximize the distances between the clusters for a good separation of the clusters. We can calculate the value of *intra*, used in the VM expression (Equation 5.20), with the help of the following equation:

$$intra = \frac{1}{MN} \sum_{i=1}^{k} \sum_{x \in K_i} \|x - C_i\|^2 \qquad (5.21)$$

where $M \times N$ is the number of pixels in the image, $k$ is the number of clusters , $x$ is a pixel from the cluster $K_i$, $C_i$ is the color of the cluster center $K_i$.

The distance between the centers of clusters is defined as follows:

$$\forall i = 1, 2, \ldots, k-1, \quad \forall j = i+1, \ldots, k, \quad inter = \min(\|C_i - C_j\|^2) \qquad (5.22)$$

The VM minimization can be used for the determination of the optimal value of the number of clusters $k$.

Borsotti et al. [56] proposed an empirical function $Q(I)$ designed for the evaluation of the segmentation results and checked for different clustering techniques:

$$Q(I) = \frac{\sqrt{R}}{10000(N \times M)} \cdot \sum_{i=1}^{R} \left[ \frac{e_i^2}{1 + \log A_i} + \left( \frac{R(A_i)}{A_i} \right)^2 \right] \qquad (5.23)$$

where $I$ is the segmented image, $M \times N$ is the size of the image, $R$ is the number of regions in the segmented image, $A_i$ is the area of pixels of the $i$th region, $e_i$ is the color error of the region $i$, and $R(A_i)$ is the number of regions with the area equal to $A_i$. The color error in the RGB space is calculated as a sum of the Euclidean distances between the color components of the pixels of the region and components of an average color that is an attribute of this region in the segmented image. The color errors calculated in different color spaces are not comparable; hence, their values are transformed back to the original RGB space. The formula (Equation 5.23) is a result of generalization and improvement of previous simpler formulas as described in Reference [57].

The first term of Equation 5.23 is a normalization factor; the second term penalizes results with too many regions (oversegmentation); and the third term penalizes the results with nonhomogeneous regions. The last term is scaled by the area factor, because the color error is higher for large regions. The main idea of using the $Q(I)$ function can be formulated as follows: the lower the value of $Q(I)$, the better the segmentation result. Usefulness of the $Q(I)$ function for the evaluation of unseeded region growing was presented in Reference [58].

Both VM and $Q(I)$ quality indexes aid in the determination of values of parameters that enable avoidance of oversegmentation as well as undersegmentation for some classes of images. We used the $Q(I)$ function for comparison of the segmentation results from the clustering method ($k$-means) and from the region-based method (unseeded region growing). During the comparison, all images presented in this chapter were used except two images with shadows (*Sign*, *Blocks2*) that demanded the use of another metric. For each tested image, the values of segmentation parameters $k$ and $d$ that minimize the function $Q(I)$ were found. Contained in Table 5.1 are values of the segmentation parameters and quality indexes $Q(I)$. We can see that for each image, the region-based technique gives a smaller value of $Q(I)$ (i.e., we have better segmentation results than those obtained with use of the $k$-means method).

**TABLE 5.1**

Values of Parameters and Quality Indexes

| Name | $k$ | $Q_{min}$ | $d$ | $Q_{min}$ |
|------|-----|-----------|-----|-----------|
| *Flowers1* | 24 | 3,953 | 34 | 3,675 |
| *Parrots* | 19 | 2,420 | 29 | 1,019 |
| *Blocks1* | 24 | 188 | 25 | 144 |
| *Objects* | 8 | 456 | 81 | 266 |
| *Flowers2* | 17 | 3,023 | 26 | 2,747 |
| *Chart* | 25 | 4,191 | 7 | 94 |
| *Candies* | 15 | 12,740 | 40 | 3,799 |

## 5.7 Summary

The focus of this chapter was on relatively simple image segmentation techniques ($k$-means clustering technique, region growing technique) that are easily incorporated into applications. The influences of location of initial cluster centers and number of iterations on the segmentation results obtained from the $k$-means technique were investigated experimentally. Two versions of the region growing technique — semiautomated seeded version and automated unseeded version — were described in detail. It can be concluded that there are many possibilities of reasonable choice of seeds for the seeded version. The directions used in the pixel aggregation process and an accepted concept of connectivity are important in the case of unseeded region growing. It was shown that the segmentation algorithm can be robust to shadows in the image when a special angular metric is applied. The postprocessing step eliminates the oversegmentation caused by each of the two segmentation techniques, removes the highlights, and merges regions with similar colors. The segmentation results obtained using the two techniques mentioned above were compared on the basis of the values of the quantitative quality index $Q(I)$. This comparison has unambiguously pointed to the region-based technique as being better.

The problem of impact of chosen color space on the segmentation results has not been solved. During the color image segmentation, such a color space should be chosen that gives the best results for solving task or images class, because there is no single ideal color space. In this chapter, we presented only the most popular spaces. Sometimes a color space is developed specifically for image processing tasks. For example, Ohta et al. proposed a color space intended for image segmentation and experimentally checked it during the thresholding of color images [59].

All images presented in this chapter were good-quality images. If the level of noise (impulsive noise, Gaussian, etc.) in the image is high, than the image needs to be filtered before being segmented into the regions. An appropriate filter should smooth the image and, at the same time, preserve its edges. If a noisy unfiltered image is segmented, then the number of regions in the segmented image is significantly increasing, the mean color error is increasing, and simultaneously, the value of the quality function $Q(I)$ is significantly increasing.

Finally, it should be noted that the universal technique for color image segmentation probably does not exist. The main goals of segmentation clearly depend on the art of solving the problem, for which this segmentation process is only one step. The growing computational possibilities allow for the development of more complicated segmentation techniques than the techniques presented in this chapter. It especially applies to the hybrid methods, with the use of color texture and other methods, which are important for the future development of color image processing.

## References

[1] Y.N. Deng and B.S. Manjunath, Unsupervised segmentation of color–texture regions in images and video, *IEEE Trans. on Patt. Anal. and Machine Intelligence*, 23, 800–810, August 2001.

[2] W. Skarbek and A. Koschan, Colour Image Segmentation — A Survey, Technical Report 94–32, Technical University of Berlin, Berlin, Germany, October 1994.

[3] L. Lucchese and S.K. Mitra, Advances in color image segmentation, in *Proc. IEEE Globecom'99*, Rio de Janeiro, Brazil, Vol. IV, 1999, pp. 2038–2044.

[4]   N. Ikonomakis, K.N. Plataniotis, and A.N. Venetsanopoulos, Color image segmentation for multimedia applications, *J. Intelligent and Robotic Syst.*, 28, 5–20, June 2000.

[5]   H.D. Cheng, X.H. Jiang, Y. Sun, and J. Wang, Color image segmentation: Advances and prospects, *Patt. Recognition*, 34, 2259–2281, December 2001.

[6]   S.J. Sangwine and R.E.N. Horne, *The Colour Image Processing Handbook*, Chapman and Hall, London, 1998.

[7]   K.N. Plataniotis and A.N. Venetsanopoulos, *Color Image Processing and Applications*, Springer-Verlag, Berlin, 2000.

[8]   N.R. Pal and S.P. Pal, A review on image segmentation techniques, *Patt. Recognition*, 26, 1277–1293, September 1993.

[9]   T.Q. Chen and Y. Lu, Color image segmentation — an innovative approach, *Patt. Recognition*, 35, 395–405, February 2002.

[10]  J. Freixenet, X. Munot, D. Raba, J. Marti, and X. Cuti, *ECCV 2002*, ch. Yet another survey on image segmentation: Region and boundary information integration, A. Heyden, G. Sparr, M. Nielsen, P. Johanssen, Eds., pp. 408–422. Springer-Verlag, Heidelberg, 2002.

[11]  M. Pietikainen and D. Harwood, *Advances in Image Processing and Pattern Recognition*, ch. Segmentation of color images using edge-preserving filters, V. Cappellini, R. Marconi, Eds., pp. 94–99. Elsevier, Amsterdam; New York, 1986.

[12]  M. Nagao and T. Matsuyama, Edge preserving smoothing, *Comput. Graphics and Image Process.*, 9, 374–407, 1979.

[13]  M. Kuwahara, K. Hachimura, S. Eiho, and M. Kinoshita, *Digital Processing of Biomedical Images*, ch. Processing of ri-angiocardiographic images, K. Preston, Jr., M. Onoe, Eds., pp. 187–202. Plenum Press, New York, 1976.

[14]  Y. Deng, C. Kenney, M.S. Moore, and B.S. Manjunath, Peer group filtering and perceptual color image quantization, in *Proceedings of IEEE International Symposium on Circuits and Systems (ISCAS)*, Orlando, FL, Vol. IV, 1999, IEEE, New York, pp. 21–24.

[15]  H. Palus, Estimating the usefulness of preprocessing in colour image segmentation, in *Proceedings of Second European Conference on Colour in Graphics, Imaging, and Vision (CGIV2004)*, Aachen, Germany, 2004, IS&T, Springfield, VA, USA, pp. 197–200.

[16]  A.K. Jain and R.C. Dubes, *Algorithms for Clustering Data*, Prentice Hall, Englewood Cliffs, NJ, 1988.

[17]  J. Mac Queen, Some methods for classification and analysis of multivariate observations, in *Proceedings of the Fifth Berkeley Symposium on Mathematics, Statistics, and Probabilities*, Berkeley and Los Angeles, CA, Vol. I, University of California, Berkeley, CA, USA, 1967, pp. 281–297.

[18]  M. Anderberg, *Cluster Analysis for Applications*, Academic Press, New York, 1973.

[19]  S.Z. Selim and M.A. Ismail, K-means-type algorithms, *IEEE Trans. on Patt. Anal. and Machine Intelligence*, 6, 81–87, January 1984.

[20]  L.G. Shapiro and G.C. Stockman, *Computer Vision*, Prentice Hall, Upper Saddle River, NJ, 2003.

[21]  D.A. Forsyth and J. Ponce, *Computer Vision*, Prentice Hall, Upper Saddle River, NJ, 2003.

[22]  C.R. Brice and C.L. Fennema, Scene analysis using regions, *Artif. Intelligence*, 1, 205–226, Fall 1970.

[23]  H. Palus, *The Colour Image Processing Handbook*, ch. Representations of colour images in different colour spaces, S.J. Sangwine, R.E.N. Horne, Eds., Chapman & Hall, London; New York, 1998, pp. 67–90.

[24]  A. De Rosa, A.M. Bonacchi, V. Cappellini, and M. Barni, Image segmentation and region filling for virtual restoration of art-works, in *Proceedings of IEEE International Conference on Image Processing (ICIP01)*, Thessaloniki, Greece, IEEE, New York, 2001, pp. 562–565.

[25]  H. Gao, W.C. Siu, and C.H. Hou, Improved techniques for automatic image segmentation, *IEEE Trans. on Circuits and Systems for Video Technol.*, 11, 1273–1280, December 2001.

[26]  R. Adams and L. Bischof, Seeded region growing, *IEEE Trans. on Patt. Anal. and Machine Intelligence*, 16, 641–647, June 1994.

[27]  A. Mehnert and P. Jackway, An improved seeded region growing algorithm, *Patt. Recognition Lett.*, 18, 1065–1071, October 1997.

[28]  S.W. Zucker, Region growing: Childhood and adolescence, *Comput. Graphics and Image Process.*, 5, 382–399, September 1976.

[29] D. Sinclair, Voronoi Seeded Colour Image Segmentation, Technical Report TR99–4, AT&T Laboratories, Cambridge, United Kingdom, 1999.

[30] N. Ouerhani, N. Archip, H. Huegli, and P.J. Erard, Visual attention guided seed selection for color image segmentation, in *Proceedings of the Ninth International Conference on Computer Analysis of Images and Patterns (CAIP01)*, Warsaw, Poland, W. Skarbek, Ed., Springer, Berlin, 2001, pp. 630–637.

[31] N. Ikonomakis, K.N. Plataniotis, and A.N. Venetsanopoulos, Unsupervised seed determination for a region-based color image segmentation scheme, in *Proceedings of IEEE International Conference on Image Processing (ICIP00)*, Vancouver, Canada, Vol. I, IEEE, New York, 2000, pp. 537–540.

[32] J. Chamorro-Martinez, D. Sanchez, and B. Prados-Suarez, *Advances in Soft Computing, Engineering, Design and Manufacturing*, ch. A fuzzy color image segmentation applied to robot vision, J.M. Benitez, O. Cordon, F. Hoffman, R. Roy., Eds., Springer-Verlag, Heidelberg, 2003, pp. 129–138.

[33] H. Palus and D. Bereska, Region-based colour image segmentation, in *Proceedings of the Fifth Workshop Farbbildverarbeitung*, Ilmenau, Germany, ZBS e.V., Ilmenau, Germany, 1999, pp. 67–74.

[34] S.A. Hojjatoleslami and J. Kittler, Region growing: A new approach, *IEEE Trans. on Image Process.*, 7, 1079–1084, July 1998.

[35] J. Fan, D. Yau, A. Elmagarmid, and W. Aref, Automatic image segmentation by integrating color-edge extraction and seeded region growing, *IEEE Trans. on Image Process.*, 10, 1454–1466, October 2001.

[36] F. Meyer, Color image segmentation, in *Proceedings of the IEE International Conference on Image Processing and Its Applications*, Maastricht, the Netherlands, IEE, London, UK, 1992, pp. 303–306.

[37] J. Mukherjee, MRF clustering for segmentation of color images, *Patt. Recognition Lett.*, 23, 917–929, August 2002.

[38] M. Li, I.K. Sethi, D. Li, and N. Dimitrova, Region growing using online learning, in *Proceedings of the International Conference on Imaging Science, Systems, and Technology (CISST03)*, Las Vegas, Nevada, vol. I, H.R. Arabnia, Youngsong Mun, Eds., CSREA Press, 2003, pp. 73–76.

[39] D. Yagi, K. Abe, and H. Nakatani, Segmentation of color aerial photographs using HSV color models, in *Proceedings of the IAPR Workshop on Machine Vision Applications (MVA92)*, M. Takagi, Ed., Tokyo, Japan, 1992, IEEE, New York, pp. 367–370.

[40] M.J. Swain and D.H. Ballard, Color indexing, *Int. J. Comput. Vision*, 7, 11–32, 1991.

[41] X. Jie and S. Peng-Fei, Natural color image segmentation, in *Proceedings of the IEEE International Conference on Image Processing (ICIP03)*, Barcelona, Spain, vol. I, IEEE, New York, 2003, pp. 973–976.

[42] E. Navon, O. Miller, and A. Averbuch, Color image segmentation based on adaptive local thresholds, *Image and Vision Comput.*, 23, 69–85, January 2005.

[43] R. Schettini, A segmentation algorithm for color images, *Patt. Recognition Lett.*, 14, 499–506, June 1993.

[44] S.C. Zhu and A. Yuille, Region competition: Unifying snakes, region growing and Bayes/MDL for multiband image segmentation, *IEEE Trans. on Patt. Anal. and Machine Intelligence*, 18, 884–900, September 1996.

[45] I. Grinias, Y. Mavrikakis, and G. Tziritas, Region growing colour image segmentation applied to face detection, in *Proceedings of the International Workshop on Very Low Bitrate Video Coding*, Athens, Greece, 2001.

[46] C. Garcia and G. Tziritas, Face detection using quantized skin color regions merging and wavelet packet analysis, *IEEE Trans. on Multimedia*, 1, 264–277, September 1999.

[47] S. Makrogiannis, G. Economou, and S. Fotopoulos, A graph theory approach for automatic segmentation of color images, in *Proceedings of the International Workshop on Very Low Bitrate Video Coding*, Athens, Greece, 2001, pp. 162–166.

[48] A. Trémeau and P. Colantoni, Region adjacency graph applied to color image segmentation, *IEEE Trans. on Image Process.*, 9, 735–744, September 2000.

[49] T. Pavlidis, *Structural Pattern Recognition*, Springer, New York, 1977.

[50] H.S. Park and J.B. Ra, Homogeneous region merging approach for image segmentation preserving semantic object contours, in *Proceedings of the International Workshop on Very Low Bitrate Video Coding*, Chicago, IL, 1998, pp. 149–152.

[51]  H.D. Cheng, A hierarchical approach to color image segmentation using homogeneity, *IEEE Trans. on Image Process.*, 9, 2071–2082, September 2000.

[52]  R.D. Dony and S. Wesolkowski, Edge detection on color images using RGB vector angle, in *Proceedings of the IEEE Canadian Conference on Electrical and Computer Engineering (CCECE)*, Edmonton, Canada, 1999, pp. 687–692.

[53]  K.V. Mardia and P.E. Jupp, *Directional Statistics*, John Wiley & Sons, New York, 2000.

[54]  Y.J. Zhang, A survey on evaluation methods for image segmentation, *Patt. Recognition*, 29, 1335–1346, August 1996.

[55]  R.H. Turi and S. Ray, An application of clustering in colour image segmentation, in *Proceedings of the Sixth International Conference on Control, Automation, Robotics and Vision (ICARCV00)*, IEEE, Singapore Section, Nanyang Technological University, Singapore, CD-ROM, Proceedings, Singapore, 2000.

[56]  M. Borsotti, P. Campadelli, and R. Schettini, Quantitative evaluation of color image segmentation results, *Patt. Recognition Lett.*, 19, 741–747, June 1998.

[57]  J. Liu and Y.H. Yang, Multiresolution color image segmentation, *IEEE Trans. on Patt. Anal. and Machine Intelligence*, 16, 689–700, July 1994.

[58]  H. Palus, Region-based colour image segmentation: Control parameters and evaluation functions, in *Proceedings of the First European Conference on Color in Graphics, Imaging and Vision (CGIV02)*, Poitiers, France, 2002, IS&T, Springfield, VA, USA, pp. 259–262.

[59]  Y.I. Ohta, T. Kanade, and T. Sakai, Color information for region segmentation, *Comput. Graphics and Image Process.*, 13, 222–241, July 1980.

# 6

# *Resizing Color Images in the Compressed Domain*

Jayanta Mukherjee and Sanjit K. Mitra

## CONTENTS

## 6.1 Introduction

Resizing images is the process by which an image of size $M_1 \times N_1$ is converted into an image of size $M_2 \times N_2$. A typical example of an image resizing operation is image halving when $M_2$ and $N_2$ are halves of $M_1$ and $N_1$, respectively. Likewise, for image doubling, $M_2 = 2M_1$ and $N_2 = 2N_1$. The image resizing operation is required for various purposes such as display, storage, and transmission of images. While displaying an image, the resolution of the display devices imposes constraint on the maximum size of the display screen. Sometimes, the display interface provides for the scrolling of images in the display window. However, in many cases, it is preferred to get the image displayed as a whole. The resizing of images is essential in such cases. Similarly, insufficient bandwidth of a communication channel may demand smaller sizes of images for faster transmission of data. Image resizing operations may also be required during surfing through the Internet. For the browsing and downloading of images, it may require transmission of the same image at varying resolutions for different specifications of the display and communication network at the client ends. Another important application of the image resizing operation is in the transcoding of images and videos from one data format to the other (e.g., high-definition television [HDTV] to National Television Standard Committee [NTSC]).

Usually, the resizing operation is performed in the spatial domain. However, as most images are stored in the compressed format, it is more attractive to perform the resizing operation directly in the compressed domain. This reduces the computational overhead associated with decompression and compression operations with the compressed stream. In this regard, one has the advantage of performing these operations with the images compressed by the JPEG2000 [1] scheme. In JPEG2000, multiresolutional image representation is carried out through subband decomposition, and as a result, images with different spatial resolutions can easily be obtained using a combination of different subbands. Further, interpolations and decimations of the subband components could also be performed in the same way as they are done in the spatial domain. However, this is not true for the cases of JPEG compressed images. In the usual JPEG standard, the discrete cosine transform (DCT) is used for representing images. Hence, it is necessary to exploit different properties of DCTs for performing resizing operations directly in this domain.

In this chapter, we consider image resizing in the DCT domain. To start with, we review several approaches for resizing gray-level images in the DCT domain. DCT is a linear unitary transform [2]. The transform operation also satisfies the distributive property. There are a number of image resizing approaches that have used this property by manipulating the matrix multiplications directly in the DCT domain [3], [4], [5], [6], [7], [8]. There are also resizing algorithms [9], [10], [11] that exploit the convolution–multiplication properties of trigonometric transforms [12]. The spatial relationship of the block DCTs [13] has also been used in developing image resizing algorithms [14], [15], [16], [17], [18]. In all such approaches, relationships among lower-order DCT to higher-order DCT (referred to as subband DCT computation [19]) have been exploited for the purpose of image decimation or interpolation. As color images consist of three components, all these techniques for gray-level images may be applied to each component separately. However, according to the JPEG standard, these components (namely, $Y$, $U$, and $V$) may not be the same size. Hence, one has to take care of this factor to maintain the same ratios in the resized compressed stream. In the next section, we discuss different approaches for image resizing operations for gray-level images followed by a discussion of color image resizing. We also summarize definitions and properties of DCTs in the Appendix.

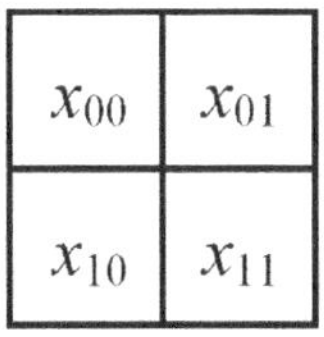

|         |          |
|---------|----------|
| $x_{00}$ | $x_{01}$ |
| $x_{10}$ | $x_{11}$ |

**FIGURE 6.1**
Four adjacent spatial domain blocks.

## 6.2 Image Resizing Techniques

A variety of resizing algorithms [3], [4], [5], [8] have been developed during the last 10 years that make use of the linear, distributive, and unitary (for Type-II DCT) properties.[1] In many such algorithms [8], [11], [14], [18], relationships among the subband DCT coefficients are implicitly assumed (by truncating higher coefficients during decimation or by padding with zero coefficients during upsampling). In some work [10], [12], the convolution–multiplication properties are used for performing the filtering operations directly in the transform domain. The resizing algorithms also address the issue of efficient computation requiring a lower number of multiplications and additions for resizing operations.

### 6.2.1 Using Linear, Distributive, and Unitary Transform Properties

As the Type-II DCT is a linear, distributive unitary transform, the following relationship holds in the transform domain:

*LEMMA 6.2.1*
*If $y = Ax + b$, $DCT(y) = DCT(A) \cdot DCT(x) + DCT(b)$.*

The above property has been used in a number of algorithms for performing the resizing operation in the transform domain. Chang et al. [4] considered the spatial domain relationship of adjacent four $8 \times 8$ blocks with the downsampled block in the following form.

Let $x_{ij}$, $0 \leq i, j \leq 1$, denote the adjacent four blocks as shown in Figure 6.1. A spatial domain downsampled block $x_d$ can be generated from these blocks according to

$$x_d = \sum_{j=0}^{1} \sum_{i=0}^{1} p_i x_{ij} p_j^T \tag{6.1}$$

where

$$p_i = \begin{bmatrix} D_{4 \times 8} \\ Z_{4 \times 8} \end{bmatrix},$$

$$p_j = \begin{bmatrix} Z_{4 \times 8} \\ D_{4 \times 8} \end{bmatrix} \tag{6.2}$$

---

[1] A summary of definitions of different types of DCTs and their properties is provided in the Appendix (Section 6.6). In our subsequent discussion, we will refer to them when necessary.

In the above equations, $Z_{4\times8}$ is a $4 \times 8$ null matrix, and $D_{4\times8}$ is defined as

$$D_{4\times8} = \begin{bmatrix} 0.5 & 0.5 & 0 & 0 & 0 & 0 & 0 & 0 \\ 0 & 0 & 0.5 & 0.5 & 0 & 0 & 0 & 0 \\ 0 & 0 & 0 & 0 & 0.5 & 0.5 & 0 & 0 \\ 0 & 0 & 0 & 0 & 0 & 0 & 0.5 & 0.5 \end{bmatrix} \tag{6.3}$$

In the transform domain, Equation 6.1 is given by

$$DCT(x_d) = \sum_{j=0}^{1}\sum_{i=0}^{1} DCT(p_i)DCT(x_{ij})DCT\left(p_j^T\right) \tag{6.4}$$

Equation 6.4 provides the computational framework for directly performing downsampling operations in the transform domain. Even though the $p_i$ matrices are sparse in the spatial domain, their DCTs are not at all sparse. Hence, there is little incentive in performing these tasks in the compressed domain, considering the fact that fast DCT (and inverse DCT [IDCT]) algorithms [20] are employed in spatial domain approaches. However, as many of the DCT coefficients turn out to be nearly zero in practice, there is some improvement in computations in the compressed domain.

### 6.2.2 Using Convolution–Multiplication Properties

In this approach, low-pass filtering is applied directly in the compressed domain, exploiting the convolution–multiplication properties of DCTs — see Equation 6.52 and Equation 6.53. In References [9] and [10], during the downsampling operations, low-pass filtering is applied using Equation 6.53, and the result is obtained in the Type-I DCT domain. Next, the Type-II DCT coefficients of the decimated sequence are obtained following Lemma 2 in the Appendix. Similarly, one may obtain the upsampled DCT coefficients following Lemma 3 in the Appendix, and these coefficients are filtered by a low-pass filter using Equation 6.53 directly in the Type-II DCT domain. It may be noted that impulse responses of these low-pass filters should be symmetric, and only the half responses (along positive axes in all the dimensions) are made use of during computation. For details, one may refer to the discussion in Reference [12]. Martucci [9] discussed only the downsampling and upsampling operations of the DCT coefficients. In Reference [10], the concept is further elaborated in the block DCT domain by considering the spatial relationship of adjacent blocks.

Interestingly in Reference [11], the convolution–multiplication properties of DCTs are used from the reverse perspective. In this case, downsampling and upsampling operations are shown as the sum of multiplication operations of the sample values with given windows in the spatial domain. The multiplication operations are efficiently computed in the transform domain using symmetric convolution in the DCT domain. Though convolution is apparently a costlier operation, in this case, several redundancies in the computations are identified to improve the computational efficiency.

### 6.2.3 Using Subband DCT Approximation

In several other resizing methods, the subband relationships are exploited for directly obtaining the downsampled and upsampled DCT coefficients from the input DCT blocks. It should be noted that the subband DCT approximation is equivalent to the low-pass filtering operation in the transform domain, as in this case, higher-order DCT coefficients are ignored — see Equation 6.42 and Equation 6.43. It is also observed [14], [16] that the performance of such approximations is better than the conventional low-pass filtering operations. Once these DCT coefficients are obtained, DCT blocks of desired sizes ($8 \times 8$ for JPEG-compressed images) are recomputed. There are various intuitive approaches [14], [16] for performing these computations directly in the compressed domain efficiently. One such image-doubling algorithm is presented below as a case study.

### 6.2.3.1 Image Doubling: A Case Study

For image-doubling operation, we first compute the upsampled $16 \times 16$ DCT coefficients from an $8 \times 8$ block using Equation 6.42 or Equation 6.43 and then apply the $16 \times 16$ IDCT to get the pixels in the spatial domain. Finally, these are converted to four $8 \times 8$ DCT blocks using the forward transforms. However, equivalent computations of the IDCT and the DCTs could be efficiently performed as follows.

Let $B$ be a block of DCT coefficients in the original image. Let $\tilde{B}$ be the approximated $16 \times 16$ DCT coefficients obtained from $B$ as

$$\tilde{B} = \begin{bmatrix} \hat{B} & Z_{8 \times 8} \\ Z_{8 \times 8} & Z_{8 \times 8} \end{bmatrix} \tag{6.5}$$

In Equation 6.5, $\hat{B}$ is obtained from $B$ according to Equation 6.42 or Equation 6.43, and $Z_{8 \times 8}$ is an $8 \times 8$ null matrix.

Let $C_{(16 \times 16)}$ and $C_{(8 \times 8)}$ be the DCT matrices for the 16-point and 8-point DCTs, respectively. Let us also represent the $C_{(16 \times 16)}$ matrix by its four $8 \times 8$ submatrices as follows:

$$C_{(16 \times 16)} = \begin{bmatrix} T_{16LL} & T_{16LH} \\ T_{16HL} & T_{16HH} \end{bmatrix} \tag{6.6}$$

Let $b$ be a $16 \times 16$ block of pixels in the spatial domain obtained from $\tilde{B}$. One may express its different subblocks by the transform domain operations as given below:

$$\begin{aligned}
b &= \begin{bmatrix} b_{11} & b_{12} \\ b_{21} & b_{22} \end{bmatrix} \\
&= IDCT(\tilde{B}) \\
&= C_{(16 \times 16)}^{T} \tilde{B} C_{(16 \times 16)} \\
&= \begin{bmatrix} T_{16LL}^{T} & T_{16LH}^{T} \\ T_{16HL}^{T} & T_{16HH}^{T} \end{bmatrix} \begin{bmatrix} \hat{B} & 0 \\ 0 & 0 \end{bmatrix} \begin{bmatrix} T_{16LL} & T_{16LH} \\ T_{16HL} & T_{16HH} \end{bmatrix} \\
&= \begin{bmatrix} T_{16LL}^{T} \hat{B} T_{16LL} & T_{16LL}^{T} \hat{B} T_{16LH} \\ T_{16HL}^{T} \hat{B} T_{16LL} & T_{16HL}^{T} \hat{B} T_{16LH} \end{bmatrix}
\end{aligned} \tag{6.7}$$

Hence, the four $8 \times 8$ DCT blocks could be computed by the following set of equations:

$$\begin{aligned}
B_{11} &= DCT(b_{11}) = \left( T_{16LL} C_{(8 \times 8)}^{T} \right)^{T} \hat{B} \left( T_{16LL} C_{(8 \times 8)}^{T} \right), \\
B_{12} &= DCT(b_{12}) = \left( T_{16LL} C_{(8 \times 8)}^{T} \right)^{T} \hat{B} \left( T_{16LH} C_{(8 \times 8)}^{T} \right), \\
B_{21} &= DCT(b_{21}) = \left( T_{16HL} C_{(8 \times 8)}^{T} \right)^{T} \hat{B} \left( T_{16LL} C_{(8 \times 8)}^{T} \right), \\
B_{22} &= DCT(b_{22}) = \left( T_{16HL} C_{(8 \times 8)}^{T} \right)^{T} \hat{B} \left( T_{16LH} C_{(8 \times 8)}^{T} \right)
\end{aligned} \tag{6.8}$$

The computations could be further improved by exploiting the redundancies in the inherent structure of conversion matrices as described below. Let us denote the matrices $(T_{16LL}T_8^t)$, $(T_{16LH}T_8^t)$ and $(T_{16HL}T_8^t)$ as $P$, $Q$, and $R$. They are all $8 \times 8$ matrices. It can be seen that about 50% of the terms of those matrices are either zero or an integer power of 2. One may further simplify the computation by considering $P = E + F$ and $Q = E - F$. Typically, the matrices $E$ and $F$ are as follows [15][2]:

$$
E = \begin{bmatrix}
32 & 0 & 0 & 0 & 0 & 0 & 0 & 0 \\
0 & 6.76 & 0 & 0.55 & 0 & 0.16 & 0 & 0.04 \\
0 & 0 & 0 & 0 & 0 & 0 & 0 & 0 \\
0 & 12.32 & 0 & -2.15 & 0 & -0.53 & 0 & -0.13 \\
0 & 0 & 16 & 0 & 0 & 0 & 0 & 0 \\
0 & -5.02 & 0 & 9.07 & 0 & 1.12 & 0 & 0.25 \\
0 & 0 & 0 & 0 & 0 & 0 & 0 & 0 \\
0 & 3.42 & 0 & 11.25 & 0 & -2.44 & 0 & -0.44
\end{bmatrix}
\tag{6.9}
$$

$$
F = \begin{bmatrix}
0 & 0 & 0 & 0 & 0 & 0 & 0 & 0 \\
20.40 & 0 & -1.32 & 0 & -0.28 & 0 & -0.09 & 0 \\
0 & 16 & 0 & 0 & 0 & 0 & 0 & 0 \\
-6.89 & 0 & 8.63 & 0 & 0.99 & 0 & 0.29 & 0 \\
0 & 0 & 0 & 0 & 0 & 0 & 0 & 0 \\
4.24 & 0 & 11.50 & 0 & -2.40 & 0 & -0.57 & 0 \\
0 & 0 & 0 & 16 & 0 & 0 & 0 & 0 \\
-3.15 & 0 & -4.58 & 0 & 9.20 & 0 & 1.07 & 0
\end{bmatrix}
\tag{6.10}
$$

One can see that these matrices are significantly sparse. In Table 6.1, different steps of computations (along with their computational costs) are summarized. In this table, computational costs associated with $a$ multiplications and $b$ additions are represented by $aM + bA$. One may observe that the image-doubling algorithm under present consideration requires four multiplications and 3.375 additions per pixel of the upsampled image.

It should be noted that the above approach has been adapted from the resizing algorithms proposed by Dugad and Ahuja [14]. In their approach, during downsampling, first, a four-point IDCT is applied to the $4 \times 4$ lower-frequency-terms of an $8 \times 8$ DCT block. Next, the adjacent four $4 \times 4$ blocks are transformed to $8 \times 8$ DCT blocks. On the other hand, during upsampling, an $8 \times 8$ DCT block is first inverse transformed in the spatial domain. For each of its $4 \times 4$ subblocks, $4 \times 4$ DCT coefficients are computed, which are converted to an $8 \times 8$ DCT block by zeropadding. In all these techniques, instead of computing the IDCT and forward DCT directly, equivalent computations are performed through composite matrix operations (following an approach similar to that shown in Table 6.1). Interestingly, in Dugad and Ahuja's [14] image-doubling method, most of the high-order DCT coefficients in the upsampled blocks assume zero values, while the image-doubling algorithm presented in the case study produces upsampled blocks with nonzero high-frequency DCT coefficients. This

---

[2] The elements of $E$ and $F$ are required to be scaled by a constant factor with the present definition of DCT.

**TABLE 6.1**

Computational Complexity Measures for Image Doubling

| | |
|---|---:|
| $P^t \hat{B}$ | $8(32M + 14A)$ |
| $R^t \hat{B}$ | $8(32M + 14A)$ |
| $(P^t \hat{B})E$ | $8(16M + 12A)$ |
| $(P^t \hat{B})F$ | $8(16M + 12A)$ |
| $(R^t \hat{B})E$ | $8(16M + 12A)$ |
| $(R^t \hat{B})F$ | $8(16M + 12A)$ |
| $B_{11} = P^t \hat{B} P = ((P^t \hat{B})E) + ((P^t \hat{B})F)$ | $64A$ |
| $B_{12} = P^t \hat{B} Q = ((P^t \hat{B})E) - ((P^t \hat{B})F)$ | $64A$ |
| $B_{21} = R^t \hat{B} P = ((R^t \hat{B})E) + ((R^t \hat{B})F)$ | $64A$ |
| $B_{22} = R^t \hat{B} Q = ((R^t \hat{B})E) - ((R^t \hat{B})F)$ | $64A$ |
| Subtotal | $1024M + 864A$ |
| Per pixel | $4M + 3.375A$ |

*Source*: Reproduced with permission from "Image resizing in the compressed domain using subband DCT," J. Mukherjee and S.K. Mitra, *IEEE Trans. on Circuits and Systems for Video Technol.*, 12, 7, 620–627, July 2002 © 2002 IEEE.

improves the quality of the resized images, as shown in Table 6.2. Table 6.2 presents the peak signal to noise ratio (PSNR) values obtained after halving and doubling, respectively, a gray-level image. In the table, the subband approximations are denoted by SB for Equation 6.42 and TR for Equation 6.43. The technique proposed by Dugad and Ahuja is denoted by DA. The set of images was obtained from http://vision.ai.uiuc.edu/~dugad/draft/dct.html. It may be noted, however, that though subband approximation (SB) does not show any improvement over the truncated approximation (TR) cases, the relevance of the subband theory in approximating the DCT coefficients during image resizing is of interest. It helps in understanding how these approximations work — refer to Equation 6.42 and Equation 6.43 — during image-halving and image-doubling operations.

Though all these techniques have provided elegant algorithms for performing image resizing operations, they are presented in a very special context, where resizing algorithms for arbitrary factors in the compressed domain are difficult to conceive. Hence, it is of interest to look for a more general computational framework for performing these tasks. This will also provide a better understanding for developing image resizing algorithms for arbitrary factors. In the next section, we revisit these algorithms with this general perspective.

**TABLE 6.2**

PSNR Values After Halving and Doubling a
Gray-Level Image

| Images | PSNR (dB) | | |
|---|---|---|---|
| | **DA** | **SB** | **TR** |
| Lena | 34.64 | 34.83 | 34.95 |
| Watch | 29.26 | 29.57 | 29.72 |
| Cap | 34.33 | 34.33 | 34.37 |
| F-16 | 32.43 | 32.70 | 32.82 |

*Source*: Reproduced with permission from "Image resizing in the compressed domain using subband DCT," J. Mukherjee and S.K. Mitra, *IEEE Trans. on Circuits and Systems for Video Technol.*, 12, 7, 620–627, July 2002 © 2002 IEEE.

## 6.3 Image-Halving and Image-Doubling Algorithms Revisited

In this section, we review the above image-halving and image-doubling problems in the context of more generalized approaches. Subsequently, resizing algorithms with arbitrary factors are discussed.

### 6.3.1 Image Halving

Let $b$ be an $8 \times 8$ block of an image in the spatial domain, with DCT coefficients that are encoded as an $8 \times 8$ block $B$ in the compressed domain. For performing an image-halving operation directly in the $8 \times 8$ block DCT space (adhering to JPEG standard), one needs to convert *four* adjacent DCT blocks to a *single* $8 \times 8$ DCT block. This could be done in two different ways. In the first approach, each of the $4 \times 4$ adjacent blocks are derived from the corresponding $8 \times 8$ blocks in the input image using the subband approximation of the DCT coefficients. Then they are recomposed to an $8 \times 8$ block. Consider four adjacent $8 \times 8$ blocks, $B_{00}$, $B_{01}$, $B_{10}$, and $B_{11}$ of an input image. One may compute the corresponding four-point DCT blocks $\{\hat{B}_{ij}^{(4 \times 4)}\}$, $i = 0, 1$, and $j = 0, 1$, using Equation 6.42 or Equation 6.43. Subsequently, these four $4 \times 4$ DCT blocks are combined to form an $8 \times 8$ DCT block $B_d$ as follows:

$$B_d = A_{(2,4)} \begin{bmatrix} \hat{B}_{00}^{(4 \times 4)} & \hat{B}_{01}^{(4 \times 4)} \\ \hat{B}_{10}^{(4 \times 4)} & \hat{B}_{11}^{(4 \times 4)} \end{bmatrix} A_{(2,4)}^T \qquad (6.11)$$

In the second approach, first, a *single* $16 \times 16$ DCT block is recomposed from *four* adjacent DCT blocks using

$$B^{(16 \times 16)} = A_{(2,8)} \begin{bmatrix} B_{00} & B_{01} \\ B_{10} & B_{11} \end{bmatrix} A_{(2,8)}^T \qquad (6.12)$$

and then the $8 \times 8$ block in the resulting image is derived from the composed block using subband approximations — refer to Equation 6.42 or Equation 6.43.

In the first approach (called here the *image-halving–approx-comp* [IHAC] *algorithm*), the subband approximation is followed by the composition of DCT blocks, while in the second one (called here the *image-halving-comp-approx* [IHCA] *algorithm*), composition is followed by approximation. It may be noted that the IHAC algorithm follows the same principle proposed by Dugad and Ahuja [14] or the modified version of Mukherjee and Mitra [15]. The IHCA algorithm distinctly differs from the techniques reported in References [14] and [15]. In Figure 6.2a to Figure 6.2e, we present typical examples of image-halving operations by different algorithms.

In Table 6.3, the PSNR values for an image-halving operation (computed with respect to a spatially downsampled image) are shown. From the table, it can be observed that the IHAC algorithm with TR is equivalent to the algorithm proposed by Dugad and Ahuja [14]. Similarly, MM with SB [15] is equivalent to the IHCA algorithm with SB. It may also be noted that MM with TR is the same as DA. Hence, PSNR values against it are not shown in the table. Interestingly, the IHCA algorithm with TR (as well as DA) performs better than other algorithms.

### 6.3.2 Image Doubling

For doubling an image, one may use the DCT block decomposition. In this case, there are also two approaches, namely, decomposition followed by subband approximation (called

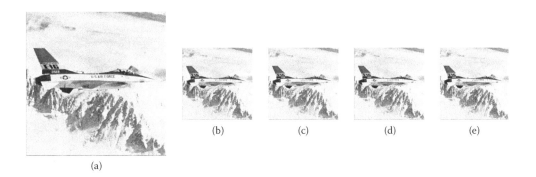

(a)  (b)  (c)  (d)  (e)

**FIGURE 6.2**
Image halving: (a) original, (b) spatially downsampled, (c) IHCA (TR), (d) IHAC (TR), and (e) DA.

*image-doubling-decomp-approx* [IDDA] *algorithm*) and subband approximation followed by decomposition (called *image-doubling-approx-decomp* [IDAD] *algorithm*). In the IDDA method, an $8 \times 8$ DCT block is decomposed to four $4 \times 4$ DCT blocks using the following expression:

$$\begin{bmatrix} B_{00}^{(4\times4)} & B_{01}^{(4\times4)} \\ B_{10}^{(4\times4)} & B_{11}^{(4\times4)} \end{bmatrix} = A_{(2,4)}^{-1} B A_{(2,4)}^{-1^T} \tag{6.13}$$

The generated $4 \times 4$ blocks are subsequently transformed into an $8 \times 8$ DCT block by using the subband approximation and zero padding.

In the IDAD algorithm, an $8 \times 8$ DCT block $B$ is transformed into a $16 \times 16$ DCT block $\hat{B}$ using the subband approximation and zero padding. Subsequently, the transformed block is decomposed into four $8 \times 8$ DCT blocks as follows:

$$\begin{bmatrix} B_{00}^{(8\times8)} & B_{01}^{(8\times8)} \\ B_{10}^{(8\times8)} & B_{11}^{(8\times8)} \end{bmatrix} = A_{(2,8)}^{-1} \hat{B}^{(16\times16)} A_{(2,8)}^{-1^T} \tag{6.14}$$

The IDDA algorithm follows the same principle of the image-doubling algorithm proposed by Dugad and Ahuja [14]. The IDAD method is similar to the algorithm proposed in Reference [15].

**TABLE 6.3**

PSNR Values of Image Halving

| | PSNR (dB) | | | | | |
| | IHCA | | IHAC | | MM | |
| Images | SB | TR | SB | TR | SB | DA |
|---|---|---|---|---|---|---|
| Lena | 37.43 | 41.72 | 38.64 | 43.01 | 38.64 | 43.01 |
| Watch | 31.52 | 35.97 | 32.93 | 37.39 | 32.93 | 37.39 |
| Cap | 38.22 | 41.44 | 40.14 | 43.33 | 40.14 | 43.33 |
| F-16 | 34.34 | 37.98 | 35.71 | 39.48 | 35.71 | 39.48 |

*Source*: Reproduced with permission from "Arbitrary resizing of images in the DCT space," J. Mukherjee and S.K. Mitra, *IEE Proc. Vision, Image & Signal Process.*, vol. 152, no.2, pp. 155–164, 2005 © IEE 2005.

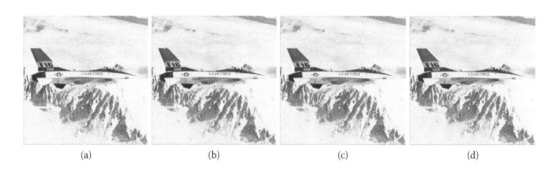

| (a) | (b) | (c) | (d) |

**FIGURE 6.3**
Image doubling with respect to Figure 6.2b: (a) IDDA (TR), (b) IDAD (TR), (c) DA, and (d) MM (TR).

For evaluating performances of the image-doubling algorithms, spatially downsampled images are taken as inputs to the algorithms, and the PSNR values are computed between the upsampled images and $I_{orig}$. Examples of image-doubling operations on spatially downsampled images (see Figure 6.2b) are shown in Figure 6.3a to Figure 6.3d.

Table 6.4 presents the PSNR values for the image-doubling operation. One can observe that in this case, DA is equivalent to IDDA with TR. On the other hand, MM and IDAD are equivalent. The later cases provide better-quality upsampled images. These are also compared with the results obtained from a spatial interpolation technique. In this case, bicubic interpolation has been employed. The PSNR values obtained by this technique are significantly lower than those obtained by compressed domain techniques.

By exploiting the sparseness and repetitions of elements in conversion matrices, these computations could be performed efficiently. For a detailed discussion, we refer to the work reported in Reference [17]. Summarized in Table 6.5 are the computational costs for different algorithms. In this table, an element $(\alpha, \beta)$ denotes $\alpha$ numbers of multiplications and $\beta$ numbers of additions. The downsampling and upsampling algorithms of DA are referred to as DS and US, respectively. Similarly, for MM, US denotes the upsampling operation.

It may be noted that in Reference [11], image halving is carried out with 3.375 multiplications and 3.75 additions per pixel of the original image, while image doubling is carried out with 3.375 multiplications and 3 additions per pixel of the upsampled image.

**TABLE 6.4**

PSNR Values of Image Doubling

| | PSNR (dB) | | | | | | | |
|---|---|---|---|---|---|---|---|---|
| | IDDA | | IDAD | | MM | | | |
| Images | SB | TR | SB | TR | SB | TR | DA | cubic |
| Lena | 34.29 | 34.85 | 34.54 | 35.19 | 34.54 | 35.19 | 34.85 | 27.21 |
| Watch | 28.10 | 28.60 | 28.43 | 29.07 | 28.43 | 29.07 | 28.60 | 24.90 |
| Cap | 33.68 | 33.88 | 33.69 | 33.91 | 33.69 | 33.91 | 33.88 | 29.68 |
| F-16 | 31.21 | 31.69 | 31.42 | 31.97 | 31.42 | 31.97 | 31.69 | 25.53 |

*Source*: Reproduced with permission from "Arbitrary resizing of images in the DCT space," J. Mukherjee and S.K. Mitra, *IEE Proc. Vision, Image & Signal Processing*, vol. 152, no. 2, pp. 155–164, 2005 © IEE 2005.

**TABLE 6.5**

Computation Costs of Different Algorithms

| IHCA (TR) | IHAC (TR) | IDDA (TR) | IDAD (TR) | MM (TR) US | DA DS | US |
|---|---|---|---|---|---|---|
| (6, 5.75) | (1, 2) | (1, 2) | (6.75, 5) | (4, 3.375) | (1.25, 1.25) | (1.25, 1.25) |

*Source*: Reproduced with permission from "Arbitrary resizing of images in the DCT space," J. Mukherjee and S.K. Mitra, *IEE Proc. Vision, Image & Signal Process.*, vol. 152, no. 2, pp. 155–164, 2005 © IEE 2005.

## 6.4 Resizing with Arbitrary Factors

Even though the IHCA and the IDAD algorithms are found to be computationally more expensive than their counterparts (i.e., the IHAC and the IDDA algorithms), they are easily adaptable for arbitrary image resizing operations. In this section, we present their extensions to more general cases.

### 6.4.1 Resizing with Integral Factors

While downsampling an image by a factor of $L \times M$ (where $L$ and $M$ are two positive integers), one may consider $L \times M$ number of $N \times N$ DCT blocks and convert them into a block of $LN \times MN$-DCT. Then, one may obtain the $N \times N$ DCT coefficients of the downsampled block from the subband relationship. In this case, we used the following subband approximation that is extended from Equation 6.43. Using the DCT coefficients $X_{LL}(k, l), 0 \leq k \leq N - 1, 0 \leq l \leq N - 1$ of a $N \times N$ block of the downsampled image, the DCT coefficients of a $LN \times MN$ block are approximated as follows:

$$X(k, l) = \begin{cases} \sqrt{LM} X_{LL}(k, l), & k, l = 0, 1, \ldots, N - 1, \\ 0, & \text{otherwise} \end{cases} \tag{6.15}$$

This method for downsampling images by $L \times M$ is referred to here as the *LM_Downsampling* (LMDS) *algorithm*.

Equation 6.15 may also be used for converting a $N \times N$ DCT block $B$ of an image to a $LN \times MN$ DCT block $\hat{B}$ of the upsampled image as follows:

$$\hat{B} = \begin{bmatrix} \sqrt{LM}B & Z_{(N,(M-1)N)} \\ Z_{((L-1)N,N)} & Z_{((L-1)N,(M-1)N)} \end{bmatrix} \tag{6.16}$$

where $Z_{(a,b)}$ is a null matrix of size $a \times b$. After conversion, one may use the DCT-block decomposition to obtain $L \times M$ numbers of $N \times N$-DCT blocks in the upsampled image using Equation 6.49. This method is referred to here as the *LM-UpSampling* (LMUS) *algorithm*. Typical examples of image resizing operations with a factor of $2 \times 3$ are shown in Figure 6.4a and Figure 6.4b.

The performances of these algorithms are observed with respect to spatially downsampled images in Table 6.6. In this case, the PSNR values between the downsampled image ($I_d^c$) from the original image ($I_{orig}$) using the LMDS and the downsampled image ($I_d^s$) obtained by bilinear operations in the spatial domain are shown. We refer to this PSNR as downsampled PSNR or DS-PSNR. Similarly, taking $I_d^s$ as input to our upsampling algorithms,

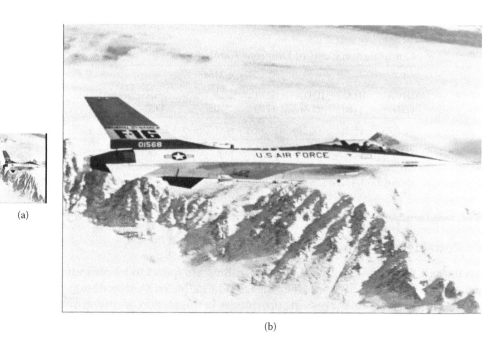

(a)

(b)

**FIGURE 6.4**
Image resizing by a factor of $2 \times 3$: (a) downsampled image and (b) upsampled image.

**TABLE 6.6**

PSNR Values for Resizing Operations

| Images | L | M | DS-PSNR (dB) (LMDS) | US-PSNR (dB) (LMUS) | DS-US-PSNR (dB) (LMDS/LUDS) | DS-US-PSNR (dB) (bilinear/bilinear) |
|---|---|---|---|---|---|---|
| Lena | 1 | 2 | 42.70 | 35.58 | 36.53 | 31.97 |
| | 2 | 2 | 41.69 | 34.41 | 35.33 | 30.29 |
| | 2 | 3 | 39.32 | 31.47 | 32.21 | 27.54 |
| | 3 | 3 | 38.69 | 30.83 | 31.54 | 26.73 |
| | 3 | 4 | 37.71 | 29.19 | 29.83 | 25.34 |
| Watch | 1 | 2 | 39.70 | 32.51 | 33.46 | 28.66 |
| | 2 | 2 | 36.03 | 28.94 | 29.92 | 25.25 |
| | 2 | 3 | 34.66 | 26.84 | 27.64 | 23.47 |
| | 3 | 3 | 33.30 | 24.92 | 25.61 | 21.85 |
| | 3 | 4 | 32.54 | 23.91 | 24.57 | 21.01 |
| Cap | 1 | 2 | 46.16 | 39.15 | 40.10 | 35.40 |
| | 2 | 2 | 41.61 | 34.00 | 34.83 | 32.19 |
| | 2 | 3 | 40.94 | 32.74 | 33.44 | 30.67 |
| | 3 | 3 | 40.45 | 31.33 | 31.86 | 29.61 |
| | 3 | 4 | 40.30 | 30.74 | 31.23 | 28.87 |
| F-16 | 1 | 2 | 41.29 | 34.99 | 36.17 | 31.48 |
| | 2 | 2 | 38.07 | 32.74 | 33.88 | 28.92 |
| | 2 | 3 | 36.54 | 30.12 | 30.98 | 26.58 |
| | 3 | 3 | 35.98 | 28.75 | 29.56 | 25.18 |
| | 3 | 4 | 35.61 | 27.47 | 28.17 | 24.12 |

*Source*:   Adapted with permission from "Arbitrary resizing of images in the DCT space," J. Mukherjee and S.K. Mitra, *IEE Proc. Vision, Image & Signal Process.*, vol. 152, no. 2, pp. 155–164, 2005 © IEE 2005.

we computed the upsampled image ($I_u^c$) using the LMUS and computed the PSNR between this image with the original ($I_{orig}$). This PSNR is referred to here as US-PSNR. In the third approach, the resulting image by downsampling followed by an upsampling operation is obtained. This computed image is again compared with the original image ($I_{orig}$). This PSNR is referred to here as DS-US-PSNR. Also, DS-US-PSNR values obtained from the spatial domain bilinear downsampling and upsampling operations are noted. Interestingly, resizing methods in the compressed domain provide greater PSNR values in all the cases. It may also be noted here that resizing operations with $8 \times 8$ block operations may result in additional zero-padded rows and columns at the right and bottom margins of the output images. That is why PSNR values in Table 6.6 are computed by ignoring those boundary blocks.

### 6.4.2 Computational Cost

For computational efficiency, we have to exploit the following properties of the conversion matrices for block composition and decomposition operations:

1. The matrices are sparse with a significant number of zeros or nearly zero elements.

2. In every row, there are repeated occurrences of elements having the same magnitudes.

Let such a sparse matrix $A$ of size $L \times N$ be multiplied with another arbitrary matrix $B$ of size $N \times M$. Let $z_i$ be the number of zero elements and $d_i$ be the number of distinct elements (of distinct magnitudes only) in the $i$th row of $A$. Hence, the total number of multiplications ($n_m(\cdot)$) and the total number of additions ($n_a(\cdot)$) are given by the following equations:

$$n_m(A; L, N, M) = M \sum_{i=1}^{L} d_i, \tag{6.17}$$

$$n_a(A; L, N, M) = M \sum_{i=1}^{L} (N - z_i - 1) \tag{6.18}$$

These computational models are used for computing the computational cost for resizing operations. Table 6.7 shows computational costs per pixel of the original image (for the LMDS) and per pixel of the upsampled image (for the LMUS). For a detailed discussion, we refer to the material presented in Reference [17].

**TABLE 6.7**

Computational Costs of LMDS and LMUS Algorithms

| L | M | LMDS (a, b) | LMUS (a, b) | L | M | LMDS (a, b) | LMUS (a, b) |
|---|---|---|---|---|---|---|---|
| 1 | 2 | (5.5, 4.5) | (5.5, 3.5) | 2 | 2 | (7, 6) | (7, 5.25) |
| 1 | 3 | (5.08, 4.54) | (5.20, 3.54) | 3 | 3 | (6, 5.5) | (6.16, 4.72) |
| 2 | 3 | (6.08, 5.54) | (6.21, 4.71) | 4 | 4 | (5.22, 7.38) | (7.88, 6.56) |
| 2 | 5 | (5.3, 6.25) | (6.65, 5.35) | 5 | 5 | (5.2, 6.42) | (6.82, 5.58) |
| 2 | 7 | (4.57, 6.25) | (6.5, 5.32) | 6 | 6 | (3.82, 6.60) | (6.93, 5.74) |
| 3 | 4 | (5.31, 6.97) | (7.47, 6.14) | 7 | 7 | (4.43, 6.39) | (6.63, 5.51) |
| 3 | 5 | (5.25, 6.23) | (6.63, 5.36) | 8 | 8 | (3.95, 7.78) | (7.93, 6.89) |

*Source*: Adapted with permission from "Arbitrary resizing of images in the DCT space," J. Mukherjee and S.K. Mitra, *IEE Proc. Vision, Image & Signal Processing*, vol. 152, no. 2, pp. 155–164, 2005 © IEE 2005.

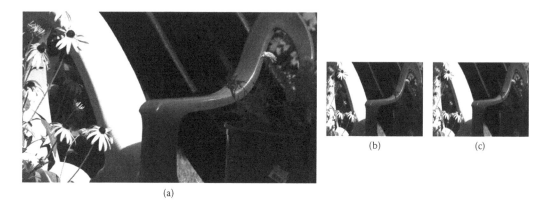

**FIGURE 6.5**
Conversion of an HDTV frame (1080 × 1920) to a NTSC frame (480 × 640): (a) HDTV, (b) NTSC (up-sampling followed by downsampling), and (c) NTSC (downsampling followed by upsampling). Reproduced with permission from "Arbitrary resizing of images in the DCT space," J. Mukherjee and S.K. Mitra, *IEE Proc. Vision, Image & Signal Process.*, vol. 152, no. 2, pp. 155–164, 2005 © IEEE 2005.

### 6.4.3    Resizing with Rational Factors

The LMDS and LMUS algorithms in tandem could be used for resizing with a factor of rational numbers. Let an image be resized by a factor of $\frac{P}{Q} \times \frac{R}{S}$, where $P$, $Q$, $R$, and $S$ are positive integers. This could be carried out by upsampling an image with the integral factor of $P \times R$, followed by a downsampling operation with the factor of $Q \times S$. One may also carry out the downsampling operation (by a factor of $Q \times S$) before the upsampling one (with $P \times R$ factor). This will speed up the computation. Figure 6.5a to Figure 6.5c present a typical example of conversion of a $1020 \times 1920$ HDTV frame[3] to a $480 \times 640$ NTSC image. We used both approaches, namely, upsampling followed by downsampling and its reverse. Though the first is computationally expensive, it usually provides a visually better-quality image than the latter. In this case ($P = 8$, $R = 1$, $Q = 17$, and $S = 3$), downsampling followed by upsampling takes $6.88M + 0.96A$ operations per pixel (of the original image), whereas upsampling followed by downsampling takes $351M + 49A$ operations per pixel (of the original image).

## 6.5    Color Image Resizing

In the DCT-based JPEG standard, color images are represented in the $YUV$ color space, where $Y$ represents the luminance part, and $U$ and $V$ represent the chrominance components, respectively. Moreover, the $U$ and $V$ components are subsampled, so that corresponding to four luminance values, there is only one pair of $UV$ values. Hence, the color images are transformed to $YUV$ space and encoded in a 4:1:1 ratio. Image resizing algorithms could be easily extended for color images by applying them independently on individual components. We present here a typical example by extending image-halving and image-doubling algorithms (DA, SB, TR). The PSNR values obtained after halving and doubling of color

---

[3] Obtained from www.siliconimaging.com/hdtv-images.htm.

**TABLE 6.8**

PSNR Values after Halving and Doubling
a Color Image

| Images | PSNR (dB) | | |
|--------|-----------|------|------|
|        | **DA**    | **SB** | **TR** |
| Lena   | 33.82     | 34.00 | 34.09 |
| Pepper | 26.39     | 26.54 | 26.59 |
| Baboon | 22.90     | 22.87 | 22.88 |

*Source*: Reproduced with permission from "Image
resizing in the compressed domain using subband
DCT," *IEEE Trans. on Circuits and systems for Video
Technology,* vol. 12, No. 7, pp. 620–627, July 2002 ©
2002 IEEE.

images are indicated in Table 6.8.[4] For color images, it has also been observed that the SB and TR algorithms perform better than the DA algorithm in most cases. Again, out of the last two, TR has the best performance. However, for the image *Baboon*, the DA algorithm has slightly higher PSNR than the other two.

The performances of the three algorithms for images compressed at different levels are also of interest. One should consider here the effect of quantizations on the approximated coefficients during image halving or image doubling. The PSNR values for different compression levels for the color image *Peppers* are plotted in Figure 6.6 for all three techniques. It can be observed that with the subband and low-pass truncated approximations, resizing algorithms exhibit improved performances over the DA algorithm. In fact, at low compression ratio, low-pass truncated approximation performs best in most of the cases. For some images, we found the DA algorithm to give the best result at low compression (e.g., *Baboon* in Table 6.8). Typical reconstructed images of *Peppers* at 0.57 bpp are shown for all three methods in Figure 6.7a to Figure 6.7c. We also demonstrated here a part of those reconstructed images zoomed for the purpose of comparison at the same compression level (Figure 6.8a to Figure 6.8c). There is hardly any noticeable difference among them at this level of compression. However, at lower compression, the differences are noticeable. One may observe an improvement in the reconstruction of the green texture of the pepper formed at 1.2 bpp by the SB and the TR compared to the method DA (Figure 6.9a to Figure 6.9c).

Similarly, the LMDS and LMUS algorithms have been extended to color images. Unfortunately, the downsampling algorithm (LMDS) suffers from dimensional mismatch problems among the downsampled components of color images. The height and width of an image may not be integral multiples of $8L$ and $8M$, respectively. As $L \times M$ blocks produce a single block in the downsampled image, boundary blocks are zero-padded during downsampling. The desired height and width information for the downsampled image is kept as a header, which is used during decompression. This works fine with gray-level images. However, usually in a JPEG-compressed color image, there are different dimensions for subsampled chromatic components (for $U$ and $V$) and luminance component ($Y$). Hence, the downsampled color image may not be able to maintain the 4:1:1 ratio in the number of blocks for $Y$, $U$, and $V$, respectively. In such situations, minimum height and minimum width among all the components determine the size of the color images. Hence, for downsampled images,

---

[4] The PSNR values are computed by converting the reconstructed images from the YUV color space to the RGB (red, green, blue) color space.

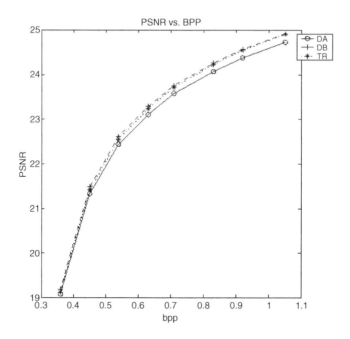

**FIGURE 6.6**

PSNR plots for different techniques at varying compression ratios for color image *Peppers*. Reproduced with permission from "Image resizing in the compressed domain using subband DCT," J. Mukherjee and S.K. Mitra, *IEEE Trans. on Circuits and Systems for Video Technol.*, vol. 12, no. 7, pp. 620–627, July 2002 © 2002 IEEE.

reconstruction quality at right and bottom boundaries is poorer. However, for the upsampling algorithm, this problem does not arise as in such a case number of output blocks is always $LM$ times of the number of input blocks. In Figure 6.10a and Figure 6.10b, typical examples of downsampled and upsampled images (by $2 \times 3$) are presented. It can be seen that the upsampled image has no problem with the reconstruction of the boundary blocks, whereas the downsampled image has colored artifacts at boundaries.

We carried out further experimentations on the reconstruction quality of the downsampled image (using LMDS), upsampled image (using LMUS), down- and upsampled image

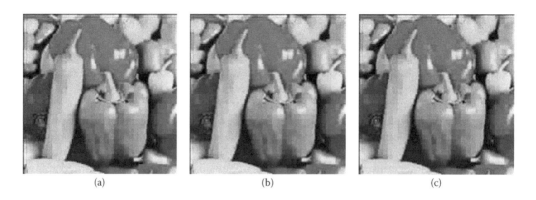

(a)                              (b)                              (c)

**FIGURE 6.7**

Reconstructed images at 0.57 bpp by (a) DA, (b) SB, and (c) TR.

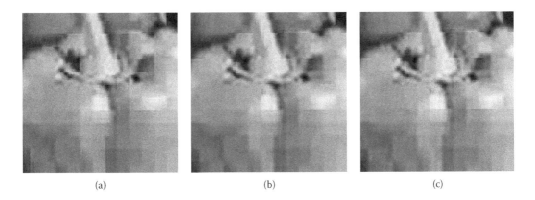

(a)            (b)            (c)

**FIGURE 6.8**
A part of reconstructed images (at 0.57 bpp) by (a) DA, (b) SB, and (c) TR.

(using LMDS followed by LMUS), and down- and upsampled images using a bilinear interpolation technique in the spatial domain. The PSNRs are computed following the same principles described in Section 6.4, and they are denoted as DS-PSNR, US-PSNR, DS-US-PSNR (for LMDS-LMUS), and DS-US-PSNR (with bilinear interpolation), respectively, and they are shown in Table 6.9. It can be seen from this table that the compressed domain techniques perform better than the spatial domain techniques in terms of PSNR measures.

During resizing color images with rational factors, the dimension-mismatch problem of the different components of downsampled images places constraints on the sequence of downsampling and upsampling operations. In this case, it is suggested that the upsampling operations be implemented before the downsampling operations to restrict the propagation of block round-off errors. Typical examples of resizing with rational factors ($\frac{2}{3} \times \frac{3}{4}$) are presented in Figure 6.11a and Figure 6.11b. The quality of reconstruction for the resizing algorithm where upsampling operations are followed by downsampling operations, is visibly much better than that obtained by employing downsampling followed by upsampling algorithm. One could clearly observe the improvement in the reconstruction for the latter approach (upsampling followed by downsampling) in Figure 6.12a and Figure 6.12b, where portions of the corresponding images in Figure 6.11a and Figure 6.11b are shown with magnification.

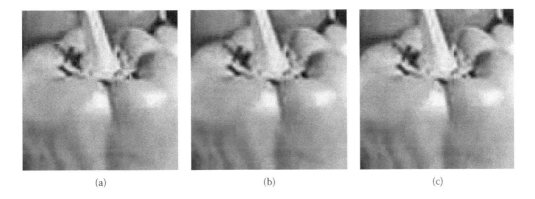

(a)            (b)            (c)

**FIGURE 6.9**
A part of reconstructed images (at 1.2 bpp) by (a) DA, (b) SB, and (c) TR.

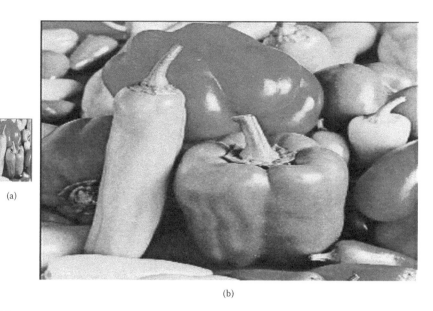

(a)

(b)

**FIGURE 6.10**
Image resizing of a color image by a factor of $2 \times 3$: (a) downsampled image and (b) upsampled image.

**TABLE 6.9**

PSNR Values for Color Image Resizing Operations

| Images | L | M | DS-PSNR (dB) (LMDS) | US-PSNR (dB) (LMUS) | DS-US-PSNR (dB) (LMDS/LUDS) | DS-US-PSNR (dB) (bilinear/bilinear) |
|---|---|---|---|---|---|---|
| Lena | 1 | 2 | 37.10 | 34.71 | 35.49 | 29.88 |
| | 2 | 2 | 35.84 | 33.61 | 34.30 | 27.75 |
| | 2 | 3 | 29.37 | 26.50 | 30.40 | 26.19 |
| | 3 | 3 | 27.00 | 24.25 | 29.04 | 25.60 |
| | 3 | 4 | 29.07 | 25.83 | 28.86 | 24.84 |
| Peppers | 1 | 2 | 30.28 | 27.92 | 28.39 | 24.84 |
| | 2 | 2 | 29.25 | 26.08 | 26.70 | 22.22 |
| | 2 | 3 | 26.01 | 22.61 | 24.15 | 21.67 |
| | 3 | 3 | 24.35 | 20.82 | 22.75 | 21.20 |
| | 3 | 4 | 25.47 | 21.60 | 22.87 | 20.35 |
| Baboon | 1 | 2 | 28.93 | 25.32 | 25.78 | 24.70 |
| | 2 | 2 | 28.40 | 22.52 | 23.07 | 21.75 |
| | 2 | 3 | 26.69 | 21.25 | 22.15 | 20.84 |
| | 3 | 3 | 25.87 | 20.10 | 22.19 | 20.05 |
| | 3 | 4 | 27.00 | 20.19 | 20.91 | 19.71 |

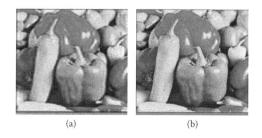

(a)      (b)

**FIGURE 6.11**
Rational resizing of a color image by $\frac{2}{3} \times \frac{3}{4}$: (a) downsampling followed by upsampling and (b) upsampling followed by downsampling.

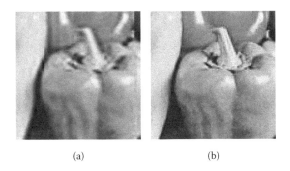

(a)                              (b)

**FIGURE 6.12**
Parts of resized images of Figure 6.11a and Figure 6.11b: (a) downsampling followed by upsampling, and (b) upsampling followed by downsampling.

## 6.6 Concluding Remarks

In this chapter, we discussed the resizing of images in the compressed domain. Different approaches for image resizing algorithms were discussed. Also presented was a discussion of a general computation framework using the spatial relationship of the block DCT coefficients and subband approximations. Extensions of these techniques are shown for color images. In particular, while downsampling color images, it is observed that the same ratio of the numbers of blocks among their color components may not be maintained. This causes mismatch among the components after decompression. It is proposed here that the minimum height and width of the components be used for reconstructing the color image. However, this problem does not arise during the upsampling of color images. Hence, during arbitrary resizing with rational factors, it is recommended that upsampling be carried out before the downsampling operation to obtain better-quality resized color images.

## Acknowledgments

This work was supported in part by a University of California MICRO grant with matching support from the Intel Corporation, National Instruments, and the NEC Corporation.

## Appendix: Mathematical Preliminaries

In this section, we briefly review some commonly used discrete cosine transforms and their properties in the context of the image resizing problem. For convenience, we first consider the one-dimensional (1-D) case. As DCTs are separable transforms, the observations made in the 1-D case are easily extended to the two-dimensional (2-D) case.

### 6.6.1 DCT: Definitions and Notations

There are different types of DCTs. The commonly used DCTs are referred to as Type-I, Type-II, Type-III, and Type-IV DCTs, as defined below. Further details about the general class of trigonometric transforms can be found in Reference [12].

Let $x(n)$, $n = 0, 1, 2 \ldots$, be a sequence of input data. Then the above four types of $N$-point DCTs are defined as follows:

$$X_I^{(N)}(k) = \sqrt{\frac{2}{N}}\alpha(k) \sum_{n=0}^{N} x(n) \cos\left(\frac{n\pi k}{N}\right), \quad 0 \leq k \leq N \tag{6.19}$$

$$X_{II}^{(N)}(k) = \sqrt{\frac{2}{N}}\alpha(k) \sum_{n=0}^{N-1} x(n) \cos\left(\frac{(2n+1)\pi k}{2N}\right), \quad 0 \leq k \leq N-1 \tag{6.20}$$

$$X_{III}^{(N)}(k) = \sqrt{\frac{2}{N}}\alpha(k) \sum_{n=0}^{N-1} x(n) \cos\left(\frac{n\pi(2k+1)}{2N}\right), \quad 0 \leq k \leq N-1 \tag{6.21}$$

$$X_{IV}^{(N)}(k) = \sqrt{\frac{2}{N}}\alpha(k) \sum_{n=0}^{N-1} x(n) \cos\left(\frac{(2n+1)\pi(2k+1)}{4N}\right), \quad 0 \leq k \leq N-1 \tag{6.22}$$

In the above equations, $\alpha(p)$ is given by

$$\alpha(p) = \begin{cases} \sqrt{\frac{1}{2}}, & \text{for } p = 0, \\ 1, & \text{otherwise} \end{cases} \tag{6.23}$$

We denote the Type-I through Type-IV DCTs of a sequence $x(n)$ by $C_{1e}\{x(n)\}$, $C_{2e}\{x(n)\}$, $C_{3e}\{x(n)\}$, and $C_{4e}\{x(n)\}$, respectively. All these transforms are linear and distributive, and invertible; that is,

$$\begin{aligned} x(n) &= C_{1e}\{C_{1e}\{x(n)\}\}, \\ x(n) &= C_{3e}\{C_{2e}\{x(n)\}\}, \\ x(n) &= C_{2e}\{C_{3e}\{x(n)\}\}, \\ x(n) &= C_{4e}\{C_{4e}\{x(n)\}\} \end{aligned} \tag{6.24}$$

It should be noted that the Type-I $N$-point DCT is defined over $N+1$ samples, whereas, the Type-II to Type-IV DCTs are defined with a length of $N$ data points. They could be shown as special cases of the generalized discrete Fourier transforms (GDFTs) of symmetrically extended sequences [12]. By symmetric extensions, the resulting periods in the above four cases become $2N$. For the Type-I DCT, the symmetric extension of $N+1$ samples takes place in the following manner:

$$\hat{x}(n) = \begin{cases} x(n), & n = 0, 1, 2, \ldots, N, \\ x(2N - n), & n = N+1, \ldots, 2N-1 \end{cases} \tag{6.25}$$

For the Type-II DCT, the symmetric extension of the input sequence is carried out as follows (before the application of the GDFT):

$$\hat{x}(n) = \begin{cases} x(n), & n = 0, 1, 2, \ldots, N-1, \\ x(2N-1-n) & n = N, N+1, \ldots, 2N-1 \end{cases} \tag{6.26}$$

We refer to the above symmetric extensions in this text as the Type-I and Type-II symmetric extensions, respectively. Subsequently, we restrict our discussions to the Type-I and Type-II DCTs only.

### 6.6.1.1 2-D DCT

The above definitions are easily extended to the 2-D case. The Type-I and Type-II 2-D DCTs of an input sequence $x(m, n)$, $m = 0, 1, 2, \ldots, n = 0, 1, 2, \ldots$, are defined as follows:

$$X_I(k, l) = \frac{2}{N}.\alpha(k).\alpha(l). \sum_{m=0}^{N}\sum_{n=0}^{N} \left( x(m, n) \cos\left(\frac{m\pi k}{N}\right) \cos\left(\frac{n\pi l}{N}\right) \right), \quad 0 \leq k, l \leq N \quad (6.27)$$

$$X_{II}(k, l) = \frac{2}{N}.\alpha(k).\alpha(l). \sum_{m=0}^{N-1}\sum_{n=0}^{N-1} \left( x(m, n) \cos\left(\frac{(2m+1)\pi k}{2N}\right) \cos\left(\frac{(2n+1)\pi l}{2N}\right) \right),$$
$$0 \leq k, l \leq N-1 \quad (6.28)$$

It should be noted that the Type-I 2-D DCT is defined over $(N+1) \times (N+1)$ samples, whereas, the Type-II 2-D DCT is defined over $N \times N$ samples. These can also be derived from the 2-D GDFT of symmetrically extended sequences, as in the 1-D case. We denote the Type-I and the Type-II 2-D DCTs of $x(m, n)$ by $C_{1e}\{x(m, n)\}$ and $C_{2e}\{x(m, n)\}$, respectively.

### 6.6.1.2 Matrix Representation

As the DCTs are linear operations, they can be conveniently represented by matrix operations. Let $C_{(N \times N)}$ denote the $N \times N$ Type-II DCT matrix, whose $(i, j)$th element (for $0 \leq i \leq N$ and $0 \leq j \leq N$) is given by $\sqrt{\frac{2}{N}}.\alpha(i) \cos(\frac{(2j+1)\pi i}{2N})$. Let us also represent the sequence $\{x(n), n = 0, 1, \ldots N-1\}$ by the $N$-dimensional column-vector $\mathbf{x}$. Then the Type-II DCT of $\mathbf{x}$ is given as follows:

$$X = C_{(N \times N)}.\mathbf{x} \quad (6.29)$$

A 2-D input sequence $\{x(m, n), 0 \leq m \leq M, 0 \leq n \leq N\}$ is represented by $M \times N$ matrix $\mathbf{x}$. Its DCT can be expressed in the following form:

$$X = DCT(x) = C_{(M \times M)}.\mathbf{x}.C_{(N \times N)}^T \quad (6.30)$$

Here we have represented the transpose of a matrix $A$ as $A^T$. As Type-II DCT is an orthonormal transform, the following relationship holds with its inverse:

$$C_{(N \times N)}^{-1} = C_{(N \times N)}^T \quad (6.31)$$

### 6.6.2 Downsampling and Upsampling Properties of the DCTs

The downsampling and upsampling properties of DCTs are useful in the context of image resizing. These properties are stated below [9]:

*LEMMA 6.6.2*
*If $X_I(k) = C_{1e}(x(n))$, $k, n = 0, 1, 2, \ldots, N$, then $x_d(n) = x(2n+1) = C_{2e}^{-1}\{\frac{X_I(k)-X_I(N-k)}{\sqrt{2}}\}$ for $k, n = 0, 1, 2, \ldots, \frac{N}{2} - 1$.*

LEMMA 6.6.3

If $X_{II}(k) = C_{2e}(x(n))$, $k, n = 0, 1, 2, \ldots, \frac{N}{2}$ then $x_u(n) = C_{1e}^{-1}\{\frac{X_{II}(k) - X_{II}(N-k)}{\sqrt{2}}\}$ for $k, n = 0, 1, 2, \ldots, N$, where

$$x_u(n) = \begin{cases} 0, & n \text{ even}, \\ x\left(\dfrac{n-1}{2}\right), & n \text{ odd} \end{cases} \tag{6.32}$$

Lemma 2 is useful for decimating signals directly in the compressed domain, while Lemma 3 is used in interpolation.

## 6.6.3 Subband Relationship of the Type-II DCT

We briefly review here the representation of the Type-II DCT of a signal in terms of its subbands [19]. In this chapter, the usual DCT operations are assumed to be for the Type-II DCT, unless otherwise mentioned. Let $x(n)$, $n = 0, 1, \ldots, N - 1$, be an $N$-point data sequence with $N$ even. Let the sequence $x(n)$ be decomposed into two subsequences $x_L(n)$ and $x_H(n)$ of length $\frac{N}{2}$ each, as follows:

$$\begin{aligned} x_L(n) &= \frac{1}{2}\{x(2n) + x(2n+1)\}, \\ x_H(n) &= \frac{1}{2}\{x(2n) - x(2n+1)\}, \quad n = 0, 1, \ldots \frac{N}{2} - 1 \end{aligned} \tag{6.33}$$

The subband computation of the DCT of $x(n)$ can be performed using the DCT and the discrete sine transform (DST) of $x_L(n)$ and $x_H(n)$, respectively. The DCT of $x(n)$ given by Equation 6.20 is rewritten as

$$X(k) = \sqrt{\frac{2}{N}}\alpha(k)\sum_{n=0}^{N-1} x(n)\cos\left(\frac{(2n+1)\pi k}{2N}\right), \quad 0 \le k \le N - 1 \tag{6.34}$$

Similarly, the DST of $x(n)$ is defined as

$$S(k) = \sqrt{\frac{2}{N}}\sum_{n=0}^{N-1} x(n)\sin\left(\frac{(2n+1)\pi k}{2N}\right), \quad 0 \le k \le N - 1 \tag{6.35}$$

Let $X_L(k)$ be the $\frac{N}{2}$-point DCT of $x_L(n)$, and $S_H(k)$ be the $\frac{N}{2}$-point DST of $x_H(n)$. Then the computation of DCT of $x(n)$ from $X_L(k)$'s and $S_H(k)$'s can be carried out as follows [19]:

$$X(k) = \sqrt{2}\cos\left(\frac{\pi k}{2N}\right)\overline{X_L}(k) + \sqrt{2}\sin\left(\frac{\pi k}{2N}\right)\overline{S_H}(k), \quad 0 \le k \le N - 1 \tag{6.36}$$

where

$$\overline{X_L}(k) = \begin{cases} X_L(k), & 0 \le k \le \dfrac{N}{2} - 1, \\ 0, & k = \dfrac{N}{2}, \\ -X_L(N-k), & \dfrac{N}{2} + 1 \le k \le N - 1 \end{cases} \tag{6.37}$$

and

$$\overline{S_H}(k) = \begin{cases} S_H(k), & 0 \leq k \leq \dfrac{N}{2} - 1, \\ \sqrt{2} \displaystyle\sum_{n=0}^{\frac{N}{2}-1} (-1)^n x_H(n), & k = \dfrac{N}{2}, \\ S_H(N-k), & \dfrac{N}{2} + 1 \leq k \leq N - 1 \end{cases} \tag{6.38}$$

### 6.6.3.1 Approximate DCT Computation

In practice, most of the energy of a signal is in the lower frequency range. Hence, Equation 6.36 can be approximated as

$$X(k) = \begin{cases} \sqrt{2} \cos\left(\dfrac{\pi k}{2N}\right) \overline{X_L}(k), & k \in \left\{0, 1, \ldots, \dfrac{N}{2} - 1\right\}, \\ 0, & \text{otherwise} \end{cases} \tag{6.39}$$

We refer to this approximation as the subband approximation of DCT. The approximation could be further simplified by removing the cosine factors as follows:

$$X(k) = \begin{cases} \sqrt{2} \cdot \overline{X_L}(k), & k \in \left\{0, 1, \ldots, \dfrac{N}{2} - 1\right\}, \\ 0, & \text{otherwise} \end{cases} \tag{6.40}$$

We refer to this approximation as the low-pass truncated approximation of DCT.

### 6.6.3.2 Approximate DCT in 2-D

The approximate DCT computation scheme can also be directly extended to the 2-D case. The low-low subband $x_{LL}(m, n)$ of the image $x(m, n)$ is obtained as

$$x_{LL}(m, n) = \frac{1}{4}\{x(2m, 2n) + x(2m+1, 2n) + x(2m, 2n+1) + x(2m+1, 2n+1)\},$$
$$0 \leq m, n \leq \frac{N}{2} - 1 \tag{6.41}$$

Let $\overline{X_{LL}}(k, l), 0 \leq k, l \leq \frac{N}{2} - 1$ be the 2-D DCT of $x_{LL}(m, n)$. Then the subband approximation of DCT of $x(m, n)$ is given by

$$X(k, l) = \begin{cases} 2\cos\left(\dfrac{\pi k}{2N}\right)\cos\left(\dfrac{\pi l}{2N}\right)\overline{X_{LL}}(k, l), & k, l = 0, 1, \ldots, \dfrac{N}{2} - 1, \\ 0, & \text{otherwise} \end{cases} \tag{6.42}$$

Similarly, the low-pass truncated approximation of the DCT is given by

$$X(k, l) = \begin{cases} 2\overline{X_{LL}}(k, l), & k, l = 0, 1, \ldots, \dfrac{N}{2} - 1, \\ 0, & \text{otherwise} \end{cases} \tag{6.43}$$

### 6.6.4 Recomposition and Decomposition of the DCT Blocks

In this section, we briefly describe the technique for the recomposition and decomposition of the DCT blocks [13]. For convenience, we first discuss the spatial relationships of the

DCT blocks in the 1-D case. Let $\{x(n)\}$, $n = 0, 1, \ldots, MN - 1$, be a sequence of length $MN$. The sequence can be partitioned into $M$ blocks (or subsequences), each containing $N$ data points. In the block DCT space, an $N$-point DCT is applied to each block of $N$ data points. Hence, the $N$-point DCT of the $p$th block can be expressed as follows:

$$X_p(k) = \sqrt{\frac{2}{N}}\alpha(k) \sum_{n=0}^{N-1} x(pN + n) \cos\left(\frac{(2n+1)\pi k}{2N}\right),$$

$$0 \le p \le M - 1, \quad 0 \le k \le N - 1$$

(6.44)

On the other hand, the $MN$-point DCT of $x(n)$ is given by

$$X(k) = \sqrt{\frac{2}{M \times N}}\alpha(k) \sum_{n=0}^{M \times N - 1} x(n) \cos\left(\frac{(2n+1)\pi k}{2 \times M \times N}\right),$$

$$0 \le k \le M \times N - 1$$

(6.45)

In both of the above two equations, $\alpha(k)$ is given by Equation 6.23.

Jiang and Feng [13] showed that a block DCT transformation as expressed by Equation 6.44 is nothing but orthonormal expansion of the sequence $\{x(n)\}$ with a set of $MN$ basis vectors, each of which is derived from the basis vectors of the $N$-point DCT. Hence, there exists an invertible linear transformation from $M$ blocks of the $N$-point DCT transform to the usual $MN$-point DCT transform. In other words, for a sequence of $N$-point DCT blocks $\{X_i^{(N)}\}$, $i = 0, 1, \ldots, M - 1$, there exists a matrix $A_{(M,N)}$ of size $MN \times MN$ such that the corresponding composite DCT $X^{(MN)}$ ($MN$-point DCT) can be generated using the relation

$$X^{(MN)} = A_{(M,N)} \left[X_0^{(N)} X_1^{(N)} \ldots X_{M-1}^{(N)}\right]^T$$

(6.46)

The matrix $A_{(M,N)}$ can be easily computed and is given by

$$A_{(M,N)} = C_{(MN \times MN)} \begin{bmatrix} C_{(N \times N)}^{-1} & Z_{(N \times N)} & Z_{(N \times N)} & \cdots & Z_{(N \times N)} & Z_{(N \times N)} \\ Z_{(N \times N)} & C_{(N \times N)}^{-1} & Z_{(N \times N)} & \cdots & Z_{(N \times N)} & Z_{(N \times N)} \\ \vdots & \vdots & \vdots & \ddots & \vdots & \vdots \\ Z_{(N \times N)} & Z_{(N \times N)} & Z_{(N \times N)} & \cdots & C_{(N \times N)}^{-1} & Z_{(N \times N)} \\ Z_{(N \times N)} & Z_{(N \times N)} & Z_{(N \times N)} & \cdots & Z_{(N \times N)} & C_{(N \times N)}^{-1} \end{bmatrix}$$

(6.47)

where $Z_{(N \times N)}$ represents the $N \times N$ null matrix.

The analysis in the 1-D case can be easily extended to the 2-D case. Here, for $L \times M$ adjacent DCT blocks, a composite DCT block can be formed as

$$X^{(LN \times MN)} = A_{(L,N)} \begin{bmatrix} X_{0,0}^{(N \times N)} & X_{0,1}^{(N \times N)} & \cdots & X_{0,M-1}^{(N \times N)} \\ X_{1,0}^{(N \times N)} & X_{1,1}^{(N \times N)} & \cdots & X_{1,M-1}^{(N \times N)} \\ \vdots & \vdots & \ddots & \vdots \\ X_{L-1,0}^{(N \times N)} & X_{L-1,1}^{(N \times N)} & \cdots & X_{L-1,M-1}^{(N \times N)} \end{bmatrix} A_{(M,N)}^T$$

(6.48)

Similarly, for decomposing a DCT block $X^{(LN \times MN)}$ to $L \times M$ DCT blocks of size $N \times N$ each, the following expression is used:

$$\begin{bmatrix} X_{0,0}^{(N \times N)} & X_{0,1}^{(N \times N)} & \cdots & X_{0,M-1}^{(N \times N)} \\ X_{1,0}^{(N \times N)} & X_{1,1}^{(N \times N)} & \cdots & X_{1,M-1}^{(N \times N)} \\ \vdots & \vdots & \ddots & \vdots \\ X_{L-1,0}^{(N \times N)} & X_{L-1,1}^{(N \times N)} & \cdots & X_{L-1,M-1}^{(N \times N)} \end{bmatrix} = A_{(L,N)}^{-1} X^{(LN \times MN)} A_{(M,N)}^{-1^T} \tag{6.49}$$

A typical example of a conversion matrix is given below:

$$A_{(2,4)} = C_{(8 \times 8)} \cdot \begin{bmatrix} C_{(4 \times 4)}^{-1} & Z_{(4 \times 4)} \\ Z_{(4 \times 4)} & C_{(4 \times 4)}^{-1} \end{bmatrix}$$

$$= \begin{bmatrix} 0.7071 & 0 & 0 & 0 & 0.7071 & 0 & 0 & 0 \\ 0.6407 & 0.294 & -0.0528 & 0.0162 & -0.6407 & 0.294 & 0.0528 & 0.0162 \\ 0 & 0.7071 & 0 & 0 & 0 & 0.7071 & 0 & 0 \\ -0.225 & 0.5594 & 0.3629 & -0.0690 & 0.225 & 0.5594 & -0.3629 & -0.069 \\ 0 & 0 & 0.7071 & 0 & 0 & 0 & 0.7071 & 0 \\ 0.1503 & -0.2492 & 0.5432 & 0.3468 & -0.1503 & -0.2492 & -0.5432 & 0.3468 \\ 0 & 0 & 0 & 0.7071 & 0 & 0 & 0 & -0.7071 \\ -0.1274 & 0.1964 & -0.2654 & 0.6122 & 0.1274 & 0.1964 & 0.2654 & 0.6122 \end{bmatrix}$$
$$\tag{6.50}$$

It may be noted that the conversion matrices and their inverses are sparse. Hence, fewer numbers of multiplications and additions of two numbers are needed than those required in the usual matrix multiplications.

### 6.6.5 Symmetric Convolution and Convolution–Multiplication Properties in DCT Domain

In this section, we briefly introduce the concept of symmetric convolution and its equivalent operation in the DCT domain. For the sake of brevity, we restrict our discussions to the operations relevant to conventional block DCT (Type-II DCT). For other cases, we refer to Martucci [12].

Symmetric convolution of two sequences of appropriate lengths is nothing but the periodic convolution of their symmetrically extended sequences (having the same periods). The resulting output of this operation is observed for a defined interval. An example relevant to our discussion is described below.

Let $x(n)$, $n = 0, 1, 2, \ldots, N - 1$, and $h(n)$, $n = 0, 1, 2, \ldots, N$, be two sequences. Let the Type-II symmetric extension of $x(n)$ be denoted as $\hat{x}(n)$, (see Equation 6.26), and the Type-I symmetric extension of $h(n)$ be denoted as $\hat{h}(n)$, (see Equation 6.25). Symmetric convolution of $x(n)$ and $h(n)$ is then defined as follows:

$$
\begin{aligned}
y(n) &= x(n)\,Sh(n) \\
&= \hat{x}(n) * \hat{h}(n) \\
&= \sum_{k=0}^{n} \hat{x}(k)\hat{h}(n-k) + \sum_{k=n+1}^{2N-1} \hat{x}(k)\hat{h}(n-k+2N), \\
&\qquad\qquad n = 0, 1, 2, \ldots, N-1
\end{aligned}
\tag{6.51}
$$

Martucci [12], discussed how convolution–multiplication properties hold for the trigonometric transforms with symmetric convolution. In particular, with respect to Equation 6.51, this property is stated as follows:

$$
C_{2e}\{x(n)\,Sh(n)\} = C_{2e}\{x(n)\}C_{1e}\{h(n)\}
\tag{6.52}
$$

One may note here that the $N$th coefficient of the Type-II DCT of $x(n)$ (denoted by $X_{II}^{(N)}(N)$) is zero, only $N$ multiplications are involved in Equation 6.52.

It should be observed that when both $x(n)$ and $h(n)$ are extended with the Type-II symmetry, the symmetric convolution operation has the following relationship in the transform domain:

$$
C_{1e}\{x(n)\,Sh(n)\} = C_{2e}\{x(n)\}C_{2e}\{h(n)\}
\tag{6.53}
$$

#### 6.6.5.1  *Extension to 2-D*

Similar convolution multiplication properties hold in the 2-D case, and, in particular, Equation 6.52 and Equation 6.53 are trivially extended in 2-D as follows:

$$
C_{2e}\{x(m, n)\,Sh(m, n)\} = C_{2e}\{x(m, n)\}C_{1e}\{h(m, n)\}
\tag{6.54}
$$

$$
C_{1e}\{x(m, n)\,Sh(m, n)\} = C_{2e}\{x(m, n)\}C_{2e}\{h(m, n)\}
\tag{6.55}
$$

The above equations involve $N \times N$ multiplications for performing the convolution operation in the transform domain.

## References

[1]  D.S. Taubman and M. Marcelin, JPEG2000: Standard for interactive imaging, *Proceedings of the IEEE*, 90, 8, 1336–1357, August 2002.

[2]  A.K. Jain, *Fundamentals of Digital Image Processing*, Prentice-Hall of India Private Limited, New Delhi, 1995.

[3]  N. Merhav and V. Bhaskaran, Fast algorithms for DCT-domain image down-sampling and for inverse motion compensation, *IEEE Trans. on Circuits and Syst. for Video Technol.*, 7, 468–476, 1997.

[4]  S.-F. Chang and D.G. Messerschmitt, Manipulation and composition of MC-DCT compressed video, *IEEE J. Selected Areas Commun.*, 13, 1–11, 1995.

[5]  B. Smith and L. Rowe, Algorithms for manipulating compressed images, *IEEE Comput. Graph. Applicat. Mag.*, 13, 34–42, September 1993.

[6]  Q. Hu and S. Panchanathan, Image/video spatial scalability in compressed domain, *IEEE Trans. on Ind. Electron.*, 45, 23–31, February 1998.

[7]  A. Neri, G. Russo, and P. Talone, Inter-block filtering and downsampling in DCT domain, *Signal Process.: Image Commun.*, 6, 303–317, August 1994.

[8] H. Shu and L. Chau, An efficient arbitrary downsizing algorithm for video transcoding, *IEEE Trans. on Circuits and Syst. for Video Technol.*, 14, 887–891, June 2004.

[9] S. Martucci, Image resizing in the discrete cosine transform domain, in *Proceedings of International Conference on Image Processing (ICIP)*, Washington, D.C., USA, 1995, pp. 244–247.

[10] G. Shin and M. Kang, Transformed domain enhanced resizing for a discrete-cosine-transform-based code, *Opt. Eng.*, 42, 11, 3204–3214, November 2003.

[11] H. Park, Y. Park, and S. Oh, L/M-image folding in block DCT domain using symmetric convolution, *IEEE Trans. on Image Process.*, 12, 1016–1034, September 2003.

[12] S. Martucci, Symmetric convolution and the discrete sine and cosine transforms, *IEEE Trans. on Signal Process.*, 42, 1038–1051, May 1994.

[13] J. Jiang and G. Feng, The spatial relationships of DCT coefficients between a block and its sub-blocks, *IEEE Trans. on Signal Process.*, 50, 1160–1169, May 2002.

[14] R. Dugad and N. Ahuja, A fast scheme for image size change in the compressed domain, *IEEE Trans. on Circuits and Syst. for Video Technol.*, 11, 461–474, 2001.

[15] J. Mukherjee and S. Mitra, Image resizing in the compressed domain using subband DCT, *IEEE Trans. on Circuits and Syst. for Video Technol.*, 12, 620–627, July 2002.

[16] J. Mukherjee and S. Mitra, Resizing of images in the DCT space by arbitrary factors, in *Proceedings of International Conference on Image Processing (ICIP)*, Singapore, October 2004, pp. 2801–2804.

[17] J. Mukherjee and S. Mitra, Arbitrary resizing of images the DCT space, *IEE Proceedings — Visual Image Signal Processing*, 152, 2, 155–164, April 2005.

[18] C. Salazar and T. Tran, On resizing images in the DCT domain, in *Proceedings of IEEE International Conference on Image Processing (ICIP)*, Singapore, October 2004, pp. 2799–2800.

[19] S.-H. Jung, S. Mitra, and D. Mukherjee, Subband DCT: Definition, analysis and applications, *IEEE Trans. on Circuits and Syst. for Video Technol.*, 6, 273–286, June 1996.

[20] C. Loeffer, A. Ligtenberg, and G. Moschytz, Practical fast 1-D DCT algorithms with 11 multiplications, in *Proceedings of IEEE International Conference on Accoustics, Speech and Signal Processing*, Glasgow, Scotland, May 1989, pp. 988–991.

# 7

# Color Image Halftoning

Vishal Monga, Niranjan Damera-Venkata, and Brian L. Evans

## CONTENTS

## 7.1 Introduction

Digital halftoning is the process of representing continuous-tone (aka, grayscale and color) images with a finite number of levels for the purpose of display on devices with finite reproduction palettes. Examples include conversion of a 24-bit color image to a 3-bit color image and conversion of an 8-bit grayscale image to a binary image. The resulting images are called halftones. Until the late 1990s, printing presses, ink-jet printers, and laser printers were only able to apply or not apply ink to paper at a given spatial location. For grayscale printing, the ink dots were black. For color printing, a cyan, magenta, and yellow ink dot is possible at each spatial location. Most color printing devices today can also produce a black ink dot. In these cases, the printer is a binary device capable of reproducing only two levels, where the presence of a dot on the paper may be indicated by level 1, and the absence of a dot may be indicated by level 0. In other applications, such as display on monochrome or color monitors, the levels available are usually more than two, but finite. In all cases, the goal of digital halftoning is to produce, via an ingenious distribution of dots, the illusion of continuous tone.

Halftoning is more complicated than simply truncating each multi-bit intensity to the lower resolution. Simple truncation would give poor image quality, because the quantization error would be spread equally over all spatial frequencies. In particular, one of the important goals of color halftoning is to shape the quantization noise because of the bit-depth reduction to frequencies and colors of least visual sensitivity. Halftoning methods in current use may be categorized as classical screening, dithering with blue noise, error diffusion, and iterative or search-based methods.

Classical screening, which is the oldest halftoning method in printing, applies a periodic array of thresholds to each color of the multi-bit image. Pixels can be converted to 0 (paper white) if they are below the threshold or 1 (black) otherwise. With the continuous-tone images taking pixel values from 0 to 1 inclusive, a mask of $M$ uniform thresholds would be a permutation of the set $\{0, \dots, \frac{M-3}{M+1}, \frac{M-1}{M+1}\}$ for $M$ odd, or the set $\{0, \dots, \frac{M-3}{M}, \frac{M-1}{M}\}$ for $M$ even. A mask of $M$ thresholds would support $M+1$ intensity levels. When applying a mask with uniform thresholds to a constant mid-gray image, half of the halftone pixels within the extent of the mask would be turned on, and half would be turned off. The ordering of the thresholds in the mask has a significant effect on the visual quality of the halftone. A clustered dot screen would cluster dots in a connected way, which helps mitigate ink spread when printed. A dispersed dot screen would spread out the dots, which is well suited for low-cost displays. Both classical clustered dot and dispersed dot screens suffer from periodic artifacts due to quantization by a periodic threshold array.

To a very rough approximation as a linear spatially invariant system, the human visual system (HVS) is low-pass to the luminance component of a color image or to a monochrome image with respect to spatial frequency. The HVS is generally less sensitive to uncorrelated high-frequency noise than uncorrelated low-frequency noise. Dithering with blue noise (i.e., high-frequency noise) [1] attempts to place the quantization noise from the halftoning process into the higher frequencies. Noise shaping is a characteristic of error diffusion as described below, but large periodic masks of thresholds (e.g., $128 \times 128$ pixels) can be designed to produce halftones with blue noise [2], [3].

Error diffusion produces halftones of much higher quality than classical screening, with the trade-off of requiring more computation and memory [4]. Screening amounts to pixel-parallel thresholding, whereas error diffusion requires a neighborhood operation and thresholding. The neighborhood operation distributes the quantization error due to thresholding to the unhalftoned neighbors of the current pixel. The term "error diffusion" refers to the process of diffusing the quantization error along the path of the image scan. In the case of a raster scan, the quantization error diffuses across and down the image. "Qualitatively speaking, error diffusion accurately reproduces the gray-level in a local region by driving the average error to zero through the use of feedback" (see page 25 in Reference [5]).

Iterative or search-based methods [6], [7], [8] produce blue-noise halftones by iteratively searching for the best binary pattern to match a given grayscale or color image by minimizing a distortion criterion. The distortion criterion typically incorporates a linear spatially invariant model of the HVS as a weighting function. Due to their implementation complexity, search-based halftoning algorithms are impractical for real-time applications such as desktop printing. However, they have been used with great success in designing screens [9] and error diffusion [10], [11] parameters.

Another meaningful classification of the halftone structure produced by a given halftoning algorithm is amplitude-modulated (AM) halftones, frequency-modulated (FM) halftones, and AM–FM hybrid halftones. In AM halftoning, the dot (a dot is comprised of multiple printed pixels) size is varied depending on the gray-level value of the underlying image, while the dot frequency is held constant. The dot sizes increase to represent a darker tone and decrease to represent a lighter tone. FM halftones have a fixed dot size, but the frequency of the dots varies with the gray level of the underlying grayscale. Thus, the dots get closer together to represent a darker tone and further apart to represent a lighter tone. AM–FM halftones are hybrids that allow both dot size and dot frequency to vary in order to represent grayscale. They aim to achieve a balance that takes advantage of the desirable qualities of both AM and FM halftones. Error diffusion and iterative methods both produce FM halftone structures. Conventional screens for printing produce AM halftones, but recent research has devoted significant attention to the design of FM and AM–FM hybrid screens.

In this chapter, fundamental ideas in the design of visually pleasing halftoning structures are introduced. Our focus is on model-based color halftoning schemes, with particular attention devoted to the use of HVS models in color halftoning. For succinctness, we assume familiarity with basic color science terms and concepts throughout this chapter. Readers unfamiliar with these ideas may refer to Chapters 1 through 3. This chapter is organized as follows. Section 7.2 discusses image halftoning by screening. We briefly review classical AM (clustered-dot) and FM screening, and then develop theory for the design of optimal AM–FM screens. Section 7.3 is devoted to a detailed frequency analysis of grayscale as well as color error diffusion and to a review of recent advances in color error diffusion. Section 7.4 reviews the state-of-the-art in iterative color halftoning, and its role in color FM screen design and color error diffusion. Section 7.5 concludes the chapter by summarizing the key ideas.

## 7.2 Screening

The oldest class of halftoning algorithms is based on a point process known as *screening*. Even today, screens or halftone masks are the most commonly implemented halftoning method. Because screening involves an independent comparison of each pixel with the overlayed screen threshold, it can be executed completely in parallel. This makes it ideal for high-volume, high-resolution, real-time systems.

A screen $S$ is an $M \times N$ array of thresholds that is tiled over an input color image $\mathbf{x}(\mathbf{m})$ to be halftoned. At pixel location $\mathbf{m} = (m_1, m_2)$, the halftone value $\mathbf{b}_k(m_1, m_2)$ of the $k$th color primary is given by

$$\mathbf{b}_k(m_1, m_2) = \begin{cases} 1 \, , \, \mathbf{x}_k(m_1, m_2) \geq S_k(mod(m_1, M), mod(m_2, N)) \\ 0 \, , \, \mathbf{x}_k(m_1, m_2) < S_k(mod(m_1, M), mod(m_2, N)) \end{cases} \tag{7.1}$$

where $\mathbf{b}_k(m_1, m_2) = 1$ denotes a printer pixel of primary color $k$ at location $(m_1, m_2)$ and $\mathbf{b}_k(m_1, m_2) = 0$ denotes the absence of a printed colorant pixel. The objective of color screen design is to find the values $S_k(m_1, m_2)$ so that the resulting image closely approximates the original continuous image when printed and viewed.

### 7.2.1 Classification of Screening Methods

Screening methods in the literature may be classified into four categories — periodic dispersed dot screens, clustered-dot or AM screening, aperiodic or FM screening, and hybrid AM–FM screening.

In the early 1970s, Bayer [12] designed a periodic dispersed screen that was optimized to reduce the visibility of the halftone structure. Dispersed textured patterns are useful for low resolution and low bit-depth displays, because display dots (unlike those of printers) are invariably stable. AM screens (aka, clustered-dot ordered dither screens) organize the threshold matrix or screen to promote the formation of printed pixel clusters that make the printed halftone robust to printer imperfections, such as dot placement error and unstable isolated printed pixel reproduction. AM halftones are typically used in laser printers and offset presses where fine dot reproduction and dot placements accuracy are issues. The dot centers in AM halftoning are distributed with constant frequency. This exposes conventional clustered dot screens to moire artifacts when printing textures such as fine lace. Color clustered-dot screen design may typically be decoupled into geometry design followed by dot design. Geometry design involves finding colorant screen geometries that satisfy dot frequency requirements as well as elminate/minimize the appearance of moire artifacts due to the superposition of colorant halftones. Intercolor moire occurs due to the interaction of the frequency grids of the different colorants. Much of color AM screen design is in choosing different screen geometries (typically screen angles) for the individual colorants such that the superposition moire is not visually annoying. These visually pleasing moire patterns are called *rosettes*. Colorant dot design is typically printer and application dependent.

FM halftones are used in printing processes where fine dots can be accurately and reliably reproduced. Most ink-jet printers use FM halftones. The goal of high-quality FM halftoning is to make the dot structure less visible by moving quantization error to the high frequencies where the human eye is less sensitive. Such high-frequency noise is referred to as *blue noise* [13]. FM screening methods such as the void and cluster method [3] and the blue-noise mask [2] strive to achieve a homogeneous distribution of dots at each gray level that is of the highest frequency possible to reproduce that gray level.

AM–FM halftones, are typically able to provide better tone transitions and detail rendition than clustered-dot screens, because their dot clusters are not confined to lie on a fixed frequency grid and offer a more stable printing process than FM halftoning in the presence of significant printer imperfections. FM halftones may be considered as special cases of AM–FM halftones. AM–FM screen design methods [9], [14], [15], [16], [17], [18] strive to achieve the *green-noise* property, where the dot patterns at a given gray level of a specified dot size have the highest frequency possible to reproduce that gray level. This results in increasing mid-frequency spectra as the dot cluster size is increased from a single printed pixel.

Figure 7.1a shows a grayscale ramp halftoned using a popular AM or clustered-dot screen. Note, that the dot size increases significantly in the darker region of the ramp. Figure 7.1b shows the halftone output of a typical blue-noise FM screen. Unlike the AM case, the dot size remains the same throughout the ramp, but the frequency or arrangement of dots is adapted (modulated) based on the gray level. Finally, the halftone generated via a hybrid or AM–FM screen is shown in Figure 7.1c.

The latter two categories of halftone screens (i.e., FM and AM–FM) are often referred to as stochastic screens and have been the focus of much recent research activity [19]. Stochastic screens hold the promise of providing much greater image detail, because they are free of the periodic artifacts or patterns introduced by AM or clustered dot halftones. However, they must be very carefully designed, because ill-designed stochastic screens add visible noise to an image and have poor robustness to printer dot gain. In this chapter, we survey

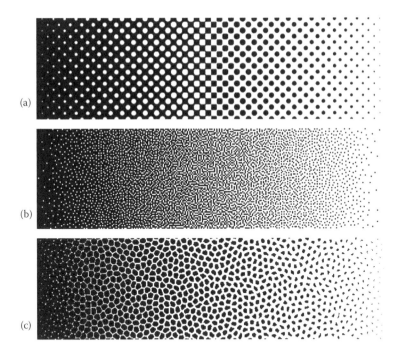

**FIGURE 7.1**
Halftones of a grayscale ramp generated using different screening methods: (a) clustered-dot or AM screen, (b) blue-noise FM screen, and (c) hybrid AM–FM screen.

the design of general stochastic screens. Kang [20] reviews well-established practices for conventional clustered dot or AM screen design.

### 7.2.2 Heuristic Stochastic Screen Design

The construction of an $L$ level, $M \times N$ screen $S(m_1, m_2)$, using a void and cluster approach with a radial filter $D(r)$ is a simple process:

1. Set starting level $l = l_0$.
2. Set $n = 0, g = l/L$. Generate donut filter $D_g(m_1, m_2)$ for gray-level $g$.
3. Filter minority pixel pattern $\phi(m_1, m_2)$ (locations where minority pixels exist are set to 1 and majority pixel locations are set to 0) for gray-level $g$ using the donut filter $D_g(m_1, m_2)$ to produce an output $O_g^{(n)}(m_1, m_2)$.
4. Find location $(m_1^*, m_2^*)$ where $O_g^{(n)}(m_1, m_2)$ is minimum (maximum) subject to the constraint that $O_g^{(n)}(m_1, m_2)$ is a majority (minority) pixel when $g \leq 0.5$ ($g \geq 0.5$). Set $S(m_1^*, m_2^*) = l$.
5. If $g \leq 0.5$ the majority pixel at $(m_1^*, m_2^*)$ is selected, and that majority pixel is converted to a minority pixel $\phi_g(m_1^*, m_2^*) = 1$.
6. If $g > 0.5$ the minority pixel at $(m_1^*, m_2^*)$ is selected, and that minority pixel is converted to a majority pixel $\phi_g(m_1^*, m_2^*) = 0$.
7. If the desired concentration of minority pixels is achieved, that is, if $n = n_{desired}$, update $l \leftarrow l + 1$ and go to step 2. If not, go to the next step. If all gray levels are processed, we are done.

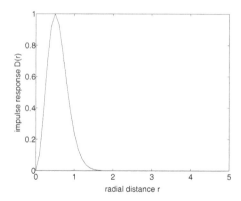

**FIGURE 7.2**
Radial impulse response of a donut filter using difference of Gaussians $D(r) = 4[e^{-5.5\frac{r^2}{2}} - e^{-5.5\,r^2}]$.

8. Update filter output as

$$O_g^{(n+1)}(m_1, m_2) \leftarrow \begin{cases} O_g^{(n)}(m_1, m_2) + D_g(mod(m_1^* - m_1, M), mod(m_2^* - m_2, N)) \,, \ g \le 0.5 \\ O_g^{(n)}(m_1, m_2) - D_g(mod(m_1^* - m_1, M), mod(m_2^* - m_2, N)) \,, \ g > 0.5 \end{cases}$$

9. Increment $n$ as $n \leftarrow n + 1$.

10. Go to step 4.

Because the filtering is linear, instead of performing step 3 every time a pixel is added, we may update the past filter output using one addition per pixel. This is encapsulated in step 8. For every new gray level, the filtering could be performed by a different donut filter using fast Fourier transform (FFT)s. The use of the FFTs implies that a circular convolution is used to perform the filtering; hence, screen tiles are designed smoothly without boundary artifacts. Typically, the pattern up to the level $l_0$ is produced using *blue-noise* methods, such as described in Reference [3]. FM halftones may be produced by choosing a Gaussian filter profile [3] $D(r) = \gamma e^{-r^2}$, and AM–FM halftones may be produced by choosing a donut-shaped filter [16] $D(r) = \gamma \left[ e^{-\lambda \frac{r^2}{2}} - e^{-\lambda\,r^2} \right]$, where $r$ is the average interminority pixel distance, and parameter $\gamma$ scales the filter to have a peak response of unity. The parameter $\lambda$ controls the size of dot clusters. A Gaussian filter produces FM halftones, because it inhibits minority pixels from forming close to existing minority pixels. Hence, the algorithm is able to break up clusters and fill voids for a homogeneous FM halftone pattern. The motivation for using a donut-shaped impulse response is that it encourages dot clusters to form close to dot centers, while inhibiting dot clusters, especially strongly midway between dot clusters. This results in the formation of stochastic dot clusters. Figure 7.2 shows a typical donut filter profile.

### 7.2.3 Halftone Statistics and Optimum AM–FM Screens

Lau, Arce, and Gallagher [15], [21] analyzed the spatial patterns produced by AM–FM halftones in the spatial and frequency domains. They found that the pattern power spectra exhibited a strong mid-frequency component; hence, they coined the term "green-noise" halftoning as opposed to conventional "blue-noise" [13] halftone patterns that had pattern spectra with strong high-frequency components. Lau, Arce, and Gallagher [15], [21] also formulated criteria for "optimum green-noise" patterns by extending Ulichney's optimum homogeneous packing argument for isolated dots to dot clusters [13]. An optimum

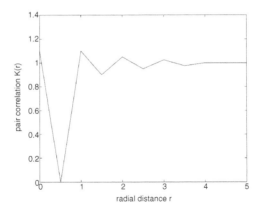

**FIGURE 7.3**
Ideal pair correlation function for a green-noise halftone pattern. The radial distance is in units of principle wavelength $\lambda_g$.

green-noise pattern for a gray-level $g$ is characterized by the average distance between the dot centers of minority pixel clusters, also called the *principle wavelength* $\lambda_g$:

$$\lambda_g = \begin{cases} 1/\sqrt{g/\overline{M}}, & 0 < g \leq 1/2 \\ 1/\sqrt{1-g/\overline{M}}, & 1/2 < g \leq 1 \end{cases} \qquad (7.2)$$

where $\overline{M}$ is the average number of minority pixels per cluster. Note that blue-noise is the special case when $\overline{M} = 1$. Following up on their work, Lau, Arce, and Gallagher presented a method to construct green-noise masks having this property [14]. Lau et al. used spatial statistics such as the pair correlation function commonly employed in stochastic geometry [22] to characterize green-noise halftones. The pair correlation function $K(r)$ is defined as the ratio of the expected number of minority pixels at distance $r$ given that the distance is measured from a minority pixel to the expected number of minority pixels at a distance $r$ from an arbitrary pixel. Figure 7.3 shows the pair correlation function for an optimum green-noise pattern. The pair correlation function for an optimum green-noise pattern exhibits a peak near the origin and has multiple peaks at positive integer multiples of $\lambda_g$ with valleys in between. As the distance from a dot cluster increases, the pair correlation function asymptotically equals 1. Note that for blue-noise, the pair correlation function is identical to the pair correlation for green noise except for the region $r < 0.5$, where the pair correlation is zero, representing the low probability of finding a minority pixel close to another minority pixel.

### 7.2.4 Optimum Donut Filters

In this section, we show that given spatial halftone statistics, we may use appropriately designed donut filters to construct halftone patterns possessing that statistic in the maximum likelihood sense [18]. The optimum screen design problem reduces to the design of the optimum donut filter to be used at each gray level. In Section 7.2.4.1, we consider the case of monochrome screen design using optimum donut filters. Section 7.2.4.2 generalizes this result to joint color screen design using optimized donut filters.

#### 7.2.4.1 Optimum AM–FM Monochrome Screen Design

We use a modification of the pair correlation function to specify the desired statistics. We define a related function called the *spatial probability profile* that encodes the probability of seeing a minority pixel at a radial distance $r$ from the center of any dot cluster of minority pixels. It is essentially a scaled version of the pair correlation function defined by

$$Z_g(r) = \begin{cases} g\,K(r), & 0 < g \leq 1/2 \\ (1-g)\,K(r), & 1/2 < g \leq 1 \end{cases} \tag{7.3}$$

According to the spatial probability profile, the probability of seeing a minority pixel at given distance $r$ from a minority pixel becomes equal to the unconditional probability of seeing a minority pixel as $r$ gets large.

Consider the situation in which a minority pixel is to be added to an existing pattern of minority pixels for a gray level $g \leq 0.5$. If the positions of all existing minority pixels are given by the set $\mathcal{Y} = \{\mathbf{y}_1, \mathbf{y}_2, \ldots, \mathbf{y}_t\}$, then the optimum majority pixel location $\mathbf{m}^* \in \mathcal{M}$ at which to add the next minority pixel is the location that maximizes the probability of observing minority pixels at $\mathcal{Y}$ given that a minority pixel is added at $\mathbf{m}$.

$$\mathbf{m}^* = \operatorname*{argmax}_{\mathbf{m} \in \mathcal{M}} P(\mathcal{Y}|\mathbf{m}) = \operatorname*{argmax}_{\mathbf{m} \in \mathcal{M}} \prod_{k=1}^{t} P(\mathbf{y}_k|\mathbf{m}) \tag{7.4}$$

where we have assumed that, given a minority pixel at $\mathbf{m}$, seeing a minority pixel at a location $\mathbf{y}_i \in \mathcal{Y}$ is independent of seeing a minority pixel at a location $\mathbf{y}_j \in \mathcal{Y}$ for $i \neq j$. This assumption is implied by the optimal spatial probability profile that assigns a probability to a minority pixel $\mathbf{y}_k \in \mathcal{Y}$ that only depends on its distance to $\mathbf{m}$. Taking the negative logarithm converts Equation 7.4 to a minimization problem:

$$\mathbf{m}^* = \operatorname*{argmin}_{\mathbf{m} \in \mathcal{M}} \sum_{k=1}^{t} -\log\left(P(\mathbf{y}_k|\mathbf{m})\right) = \operatorname*{argmin}_{\mathbf{m} \in \mathcal{M}} \sum_{k=1}^{t} -\log\left(Z_g(||\mathbf{y}_k - \mathbf{m}||)\right) \tag{7.5}$$

Because the minority pixel pattern consists of ones and zeros, the above summation may be regarded as a linear filtering operation. Thus, the maximum likelihood solution to the minority pixel placement problem is obtained by filtering the existing minority pixel pattern using a radial linear filter with a radial impulse response $-\log(Z_g(r))$ and adding a minority pixel to the majority pixel location where the filter output is minimum. When $g > 0.5$, we need to convert minority pixels to majority pixels in order to satisfy the stacking constraint. In this case, we need to find the minority pixel with the lowest likelihood of being a minority pixel and convert it to a majority pixel. The optimal minority pixel location is given by

$$\mathbf{y}^* = \operatorname*{argmax}_{\mathbf{y} \in \mathcal{Y}} \sum_{k=1}^{t} -\log\left(P(\mathbf{y}_k|\mathbf{y})\right) = \operatorname*{argmax}_{\mathbf{y} \in \mathcal{Y}} \sum_{k=1}^{t} -\log\left(Z_g(||\mathbf{y}_k - \mathbf{y}||)\right) \tag{7.6}$$

Using the maximum likelihood solution as described above does not constrain the dot growth to be homogeneous. This solution does not necessarily encourage pixels to form in regions where there are large voids. The optimal donut filter may be constructed according to the following formula:

$$D_g(r) = (1-\alpha)\frac{\log\left(\delta + Z_g(r)\right)}{\log\left(\delta + Z_g(0)\right)} + \alpha e^{-r^2} \tag{7.7}$$

The parameter $\delta$ is a small constant used to avoid the log(0) situation (we use $\delta = 10^{-15}$). The parameter $\alpha \in [0, 1]$ provides a compromise between satisfying the optimal spatial statistics and achieving homogeneous dot growth, both of which are important. At locations where the minority pixel density is large, the additional term provides a large response, while it provides a low response when a void is encountered.

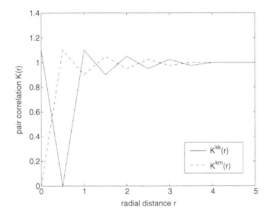

**FIGURE 7.4**

Ideal pair correlation functions $K^{kk}(r)$ and $K^{km}(r)$, $k \neq m$ for a color green-noise halftone pattern. The radial distance is in units of principle wavelength $\lambda_g$.

### 7.2.4.2 Optimum AM–FM Color Screen Design

The approach of Section 7.2.4.1 may be extended to the joint design of color screens. Joint color statistics may be defined by joint pair correlation functions [14]. Figure 7.4 shows the joint pair correlation function used by Lau et al. to generate joint colorant screens where overlap between different colorants is discouraged. Spatial probability profiles may be derived from these pair correlation functions using Equation 7.3. The spatial probability profile functions $Z_g^{kk}(r)$ represent the probability of seeing a minority pixel in the $k$th colorant plane at a distance $r$ from another minority pixel in the $k$th colorant plane. The spatial probability profile functions $Z_g^{km}(r)$, $k \neq m$ represent the probability of seeing a minority pixel in the $m$th colorant plane at a distance $r$ from another minority pixel in the $k$th colorant plane. The optimal donut filters in this case are given by the following equation:

$$
D_g^{km}(r) = \begin{cases} \gamma_{kk} \left[ (1-\alpha) \dfrac{\log \left( \delta + Z_g^{kk}(r) \right)}{\log \left( \delta + Z_g^{kk}(0) \right)} + \alpha e^{-r^2} \right], & k = m \\[2em] \gamma_{km} \left[ \log \left( \delta + Z_g^{km}(r) \right) \right], & k \neq m \end{cases}
\tag{7.8}
$$

where the homogeneity term is omitted when $k \neq m$, because it is already taken into account while designing the individual colorant planes. The constants $\gamma_{kk}$ and $\gamma_{km}$ scale the filter responses to achieve a peak value of unity.

Let us consider the joint design of an $L$ level, $M \times N$ screen $\mathbf{S}(m_1, m_2)$ with $C$ colorants. The filtering operations may be expressed as linear filtering using $1 \times C$ multifilters (i.e., filters with matrix-valued coefficients):

$$
\mathbf{D}_g^k(m_1, m_2) = \left[ \beta_g^{k1} D_g^{k1}(m_1, m_2), \ \beta_g^{k2} D_g^{k2}(m_1, m_2), \ \ldots, \ \beta_g^{kC} D_g^{kC}(m_1, m_2) \right]
\tag{7.9}
$$

where $\beta_g^{km}$ is a gray-level-dependent relative weighting factor that weights the influence of the $m$th colorant plane on the statistics of the $k$th colorant plane. The weighting constants satisfy the following equations:

$$
\sum_{m=1}^{C} \beta_{km} = 1, \quad \forall k
\tag{7.10}
$$

$$
\beta_{km} \geq 0, \quad \forall k, m
\tag{7.11}
$$

A filtering of the minority pixel color patterns $\Phi(m_1, m_2) = [\phi_g^1(m_1, m_2), \phi_g^2(m_1, m_2), \ldots, \phi_g^C(m_1, m_2)]^T$ using this multifilter is performed according to

$$O_g^k(m_1, m_2) = (\mathbf{D}_g^k \star \Phi)(m_1, m_2) = \sum_{m=1}^{C} \beta_g^{km} \left(D_g^{km} * \phi_g^m\right)(m_1, m_2) \qquad (7.12)$$

where the matrix–vector convolution operator $\star$ is represented using the scalar convolution operator $*$. As with monochrome screen design, the color screens are designed one gray level at a time:

1. Set starting level $l = l_0$.
2. Set $k = 1$, $g = l/L$, $n = 1$. Generate donut multifilters $\mathbf{D}_g^k(m_1, m_2)$ for gray-level $g$, $\forall k$.
3. Filter minority pixel pattern $\Phi(m_1, m_2)$ for gray-level $g$ using the donut multifilter $\tilde{\mathbf{D}}_g^k(m_1, m_2)$ to produce an output $O_g^{k(n)}(m_1, m_2)$.
4. Find location $(m_1^*, m_2^*)$ in colorant plane $k$ where $O_g^{k(n)}(m_1, m_2)$ is minimum (maximum) subject to the constraint that $O_g^{k(n)}(m_1, m_2)$ is a majority (minority) pixel when $g \leq 0.5$ ($g \geq 0.5$). Set $S_k(m_1^*, m_2^*) = l$.
5. If $g \leq 0.5$, the majority pixel in colorant plane $k$ at $(m_1^*, m_2^*)$ is selected, and that majority pixel is converted to a minority pixel $\phi_g^k(m_1^*, m_2^*) = 1$.
6. If $g > 0.5$, the minority pixel at $(m_1^*, m_2^*)$ in colorant plane $k$ is selected, and that minority pixel is converted to a majority pixel $\phi_g^k(m_1^*, m_2^*) = 0$.
7. Update filter output $O_g^{k(n+1)}(m_1, m_2)$ for colorant plane $k$ as

$$
\begin{cases}
O_g^{k(n)}(m_1, m_2) + \sum_{m=1}^{C} \beta_g^{km} \, D_g^{km}(mod(m_1^* - m_1, M), mod(m_2^* - m_2, N)) \, , \ g \leq 0.5 \\[2ex]
O_g^{k(n)}(m_1, m_2) - \sum_{m=1}^{C} \beta_g^{km} \, D_g(mod(m_1^* - m_1, M), mod(m_2^* - m_2, N)) \, , \ g > 0.5
\end{cases}
$$

8. If $k = C$ go to the next step, or else increment $k$ as $k \leftarrow k + 1$ and go to step 3 if $n = 1$ or step 4 if $n > 1$.
9. If the desired concentration of minority pixels in all the colorant planes is achieved, if $n = n_{desired}$, update $l \leftarrow l + 1$ and go to step 2. If not, go to the next step. If all gray levels are processed, we are done.
10. Increment $n$ as $n \leftarrow n + 1$.
11. Go to step 4.

Figure 7.5a and Figure 7.5b show the results of halftoning constant cyan–magenta gray levels of 10% and 50%, respectively, using a screen designed using the optimum donut multifilters along with their respective spatial probability profiles. We used $\beta_g^{kk} = 0.7$ and $\beta_g^{km} = 0.3$, $k \neq m$. Note that the strongest peak of $Z_g^{kk}(r)$ and the corresponding strongest valley of $Z_g^{km}(r)$ occur at the principle wavelength $\lambda_g$. The corresponding pattern for the darker tone is similar.

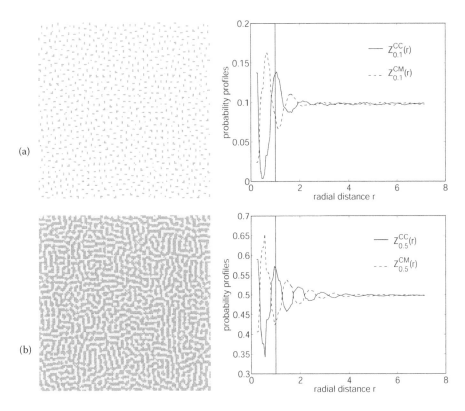

**FIGURE 7.5 (See color insert.)**
Performance of optimum color donut multifilters for (a) $g = 10\%$ and (b) $g = 50\%$; (left) cyan-magenta halftones, and (right) computed spatial probability profiles for the cyan color plane. The vertical line indicates the location of $\lambda_g$.

## 7.3 Error Diffusion

### 7.3.1 Grayscale Error Diffusion

The major 1976 advance in digital halftoning by Floyd and Steinberg [4] diffuses the quantization error over the neighboring continuous-tone pixels. As a grayscale image is raster scanned, the current pixel is thresholded against mid-gray to 1 (black) or 0 (paper white). The quantization error $e$ is scaled and added to the nearest four grayscale (unhalftoned) pixels. The scaling factors are shown below, where $\times$ represents the current pixel:

$$
\begin{array}{ccc}
 & \times & \dfrac{7}{16} \\[2ex]
\dfrac{3}{16} & \dfrac{5}{16} & \dfrac{1}{16}
\end{array}
$$

An alternate but equivalent implementation of error diffusion feeds back a filtered version of the quantization error to the input. This form, which is shown in Figure 7.6, is also known as a noise-shaping feedback coder. In Figure 7.6, $x(\mathbf{m})$ denotes the gray level of the input image at pixel location $\mathbf{m}$, such that $x(\mathbf{m}) \in [0, 1]$. The output halftone pixel is $b(\mathbf{m})$, where $b(\mathbf{m}) \in \{0, 1\}$. Here, 0 is interpreted as the absence of a printer dot, and 1 is interpreted as

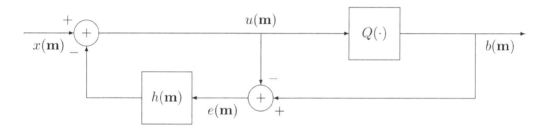

**FIGURE 7.6**
System block diagram for error diffusion halftoning where **m** represents a two-dimensional spatial index $(m_1, m_2)$, and $h(\mathbf{m})$ is the impulse response of a fixed two-dimensional nonseparable finite impulse response (FIR) error filter having scalar-valued coefficients.

the presence of a printer dot. The term $Q(\cdot)$ denotes the thresholding quantizer function given by

$$Q(x) = \begin{cases} 1 & x \geq 0 \\ 0 & x < 0 \end{cases} \tag{7.13}$$

The error filter $h(\mathbf{m})$ filters the previous quantization errors $e(\mathbf{m})$:

$$h(\mathbf{m}) * e(\mathbf{m}) = \sum_{\mathbf{k} \in \mathcal{S}} h(\mathbf{k}) \, e(\mathbf{m} - \mathbf{k}) \tag{7.14}$$

Here, $*$ means linear convolution, and the set $\mathcal{S}$ defines the extent of the error filter coefficient mask. The error filter output is feedback and is added to the input. Note that $(0,0) \notin \mathcal{S}$. The mask is causal with respect to the image scan.

To ensure that all of the quantization error is diffused, $h(\mathbf{m})$ must satisfy the constraint

$$\sum_{\mathbf{k} \in \mathcal{S}} h(\mathbf{m}) = 1 \tag{7.15}$$

This ensures that the error filter eliminates quantization noise at DC, where the HVS is most sensitive [23]. The quantizer input $u(\mathbf{m})$ and output $b(\mathbf{m})$ are given by

$$u(\mathbf{m}) = x(\mathbf{m}) - h(\mathbf{m}) * e(\mathbf{m}) \tag{7.16}$$
$$b(\mathbf{m}) = Q(u(\mathbf{m})) \tag{7.17}$$

Error diffusion halftones have significantly better quality than clustered and dispersed dot dither halftones, because they are free from periodic artifacts and shape the quantization noise into the high frequencies where the human eye is less sensitive. Because the halftone dots are of single pixel size, the illusion of continuous tone is created by varying the dot frequency with gray level. Thus, error diffusion is an example of FM halftoning. Figure 7.7 shows the original *Barbara* image and its halftone generated using classical Floyd–Steinberg (FS) error diffusion. Note the significantly improved rendition of detail over classical screening.

### 7.3.1.1  *Enhancements to Grayscale Error Diffusion*

Although Floyd–Steinberg (FS) error diffusion outperforms classical screens by virtue of its feedback mechanism, it introduces many new halftone artifacts. This includes linear distortions like sharpening, directional "worm" artifacts, and false textures. Many variations and enhancements have been developed to improve halftone quality for grayscale error diffusion, which includes threshold modulation [24], [25], [26], [27], [28], [29], variable error filter weights [13], [30], [31], [32], and different scan paths [13], [33].

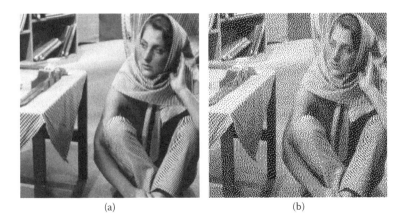

(a)                                   (b)

**FIGURE 7.7**
Classical FS error diffusion: (a) continuous-tone *Barbara* image and (b) Floyd–Steinberg error diffusion.

Because the focus of this chapter is on the color-specific aspects of halftoning, we do not discuss the aforementioned algorithms here. The interested reader is referred to Reference [34] for a detailed survey of the existing literature in grayscale error diffusion.

## 7.3.2 Color Error Diffusion

Color error diffusion is a high-quality method for color rendering continuous tone digital color images on devices with limited color palettes, such as low-cost displays and printers. For display applications, the input colorant space is a triplet of red, green, and blue (RGB) values, and the choice of output levels (i.e., the color palette) is a design parameter. For printing applications, the input colorant space is a quadruple of cyan, magenta, yellow, and black (CMYK) values, and the output levels are fixed. For example, for a bilevel CMYK printer, there are 16 possible output colors.

The application of grayscale error diffusion methods to the individual colorant planes fails to exploit the HVS response to color noise. Ideally, the quantization error must be diffused to frequencies and colors, to which the HVS is least sensitive. Further, it is desirable for the color quantization to take place in a perceptual space (such as Lab) so that the colorant vector selected as the output color is perceptually the closest to the color vector being quantized. We discuss each of the above two design principles of color error diffusion that differentiate it from grayscale error diffusion.

### 7.3.2.1 *Separable Methods*

Kolpatzik and Bouman [31] use separable error filters in a luminance–chrominance space to account for correlation among the color planes. Separate optimum scalar error filters are designed for the luminance and chrominance channels independently based on a separable model of the HVS. However, no constraints are imposed on the error filter to ensure that all of the RGB quantization error is diffused. Kolpatzik and Bouman model the error image as a white noise process and derive the optimum separable error filters to be used on the luminance and chrominance channels, respectively. Such an approach implicitly assumes that there is no correlation between the luminance and chrominance channels. This implies that the transformation matrix from RGB to the luminance–chrominance space is unitary. Damera-Venkata and Evans [35] solve for the optimum nonseparable error filter in the general case when all the error is required to be diffused, a nonseparable color vision model is used, and the linear transformation into the opponent color space is nonunitary. The luminance–chrominance separable error filters of Kolpatzik and Bouman are included in the general formulation of vector error diffusion [35].

### 7.3.2.2 Colorimetric Quantization in Error Diffusion

Haneishi et al. [36] suggested the use of the XYZ and Lab spaces to perform quantization and error diffusion. In this case, the rendering gamut is no longer a cube. The mean square error (MSE) criterion in the XYZ or Lab space is used to make a decision on the best color to output. The quantization error is a vector in the XYZ space is diffused using an error filter. Note that the Lab space is not suitable for diffusing errors due to its nonlinear variation with intensity. This method performs better than separable quantization but suffers from boundary artifacts [36], [37], such as the "smear artifact" and the "slow response artifact" at color boundaries due to accumulated errors from neighboring pixels pushing quantizer input colors outside the gamut. This causes a longer lag in canceling the errors. This effect may be reduced by clipping large color errors [36] or by using a hybrid scalar–vector quantization method called semivector quantization [37]. This method is based on the observation that when errors in colorant space are small, vector quantization does not produce the smear artifact. When large colorant space errors are detected, scalar quantization is used to avoid potential smearing. First, the colorants where the colorant space error exceeds a preset threshold are determined and quantized with scalar quantization. This restricts the possible output colors from which a color must be chosen using vector quantization in device-independent color space.

### 7.3.2.3 Vector Quantization but Separable Filtering

One suggested improvement to separable color halftoning involves limiting the number of ink colors used to render a specific pixel. Shaked et al. [38], [39] suggest a method for using error diffusion for generating color halftone patterns that carefully examines each pixel's original color values simultaneously, distinct from past error, in order to determine potential output colors. By limiting the colors used, the authors argue that a smaller range of brightness in the colors is used to create each color area, which minimizes the visibility of the halftone pattern. This criteria, which is known as the minimum brightness variation criterion (MBVC), is based on the observation that the human eye is more sensitive to changes in brightness or luminance than to changes in chrominance, as summarized next.

A given color in the RGB cube may be rendered using the eight basic colors located at the vertices of the cube. Actually, any color may be rendered using no more than four colors, where different colors require different quadruples [38]. Moreover, the quadruple corresponding to a specific color is, in general, not unique. Suppose we want to print a patch of solid color, what colors should we use? Traditional work on halftoning addresses the issue of what pattern the dots should be placed in. The issue of participating halftone color was raised in Reference [40], but it served primarily as an example of how bad things can become. MBVC gives the issue a full answer. Based on the above arguments, the authors state the criteria they arrive at as follows: "To reduce halftone noise, select from within all halftone sets by which the desired color may be rendered, the one whose brightness variation is minimal."

The method proceeds by separating the RGB color space into minimum brightness variation quadrants (MBVQs). A RGB color space can be divided into six such quadrants (see page 2 in Reference [39]). Given a pixel value RGB($\mathbf{m}$) and error $e(\mathbf{m})$, the algorithm works as follows:

1. Determine MBVQ based only on RGB($\mathbf{m}$).
2. Find the vertex $v$ MBVQ tetrahedron closest to RGB($\mathbf{m}$) + $e(\mathbf{m})$.

3. Compute the quantization error $RGB(\mathbf{m}) + v(\mathbf{m}) - v$.

4. Distribute error to the "future" pixels using standard error diffusion.

A pixel with original $R$, $G$, and $B$ values that are located within the white-cyan-magenta-yellow (WCMY) tetrahedron will end up as one of those four colors, depending on which vertex its error places it closest to. The algorithm effectively reduces the number of pixel colors visible in a given solid region. It does not modify the color appearance when viewed from a significant distance away, however, because its average color should remain the same.

### 7.3.2.4 *Vector Error Diffusion*

Separable methods for color error diffusion do not take into account the correlation among color planes. Vector error diffusion first proposed by Haneishi et al. [41] represents each pixel in a color image as a vector of values. The thresholding step would threshold each vector component separately. The vector-valued quantization error (image) would be fed back, filtered, and added to the neighboring (unhalftoned) color pixels. A matrix-valued error filter could take correlation among color planes into account. For an RGB image, each error filter coefficient would be a $3 \times 3$ matrix.

Damera-Venkata and Evans [35] generalize the linear system model of grayscale error diffusion [42] to vector color error diffusion by replacing the linear gain model with a matrix gain model and by using properties of filters with matrix-valued coefficients [35]. The proposed matrix gain model includes the earlier linear gain model by Kite et al. [42] as a special case. The matrix gain model describes vector color diffusion in the frequency domain and predicts noise shaping and linear frequency distortion produced by halftoning.

Figure 7.8 shows a model of vector color error diffusion halftoning by replacing the quantizer with a matrix gain $\tilde{\mathbf{K}}_s$ and an additive white noise image $\mathbf{n}(\mathbf{m})$. In the noise path, the gain is unity ($\tilde{\mathbf{K}}_n = \mathbf{I}$), so the quantizer appears as additive uncorrelated noise. In the signal path, the gain is a matrix $\tilde{\mathbf{K}}_s$. The matrix gain is related to the amount of sharpening, and the noise image models the quantization error. $\tilde{\mathbf{K}}_s$ is chosen to minimize the error in approximating the quantizer with a linear transformation, in the linear minimum mean squared error sense:

$$\tilde{\mathbf{K}}_s = \arg\min_{\tilde{\mathbf{A}}} E[\| \mathbf{b}(\mathbf{m}) - \tilde{\mathbf{A}}\,\mathbf{u}(\mathbf{m}) \|^2] \qquad (7.18)$$

Here, $\mathbf{b}(\mathbf{m})$ is the quantizer output process (halftone), and $\mathbf{u}(\mathbf{m})$ is the quantizer input process. When $\mathbf{b}(\mathbf{m})$ and $\mathbf{u}(\mathbf{m})$ are wide sense stationary [43], the solution for Equation 7.18 is

$$\tilde{\mathbf{K}}_s = \tilde{\mathbf{C}}_{bu}\tilde{\mathbf{C}}_{uu}^{-1} \qquad (7.19)$$

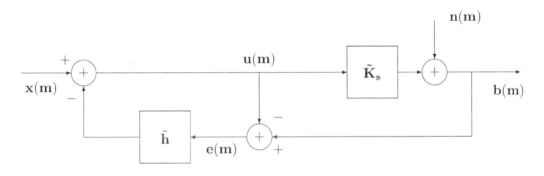

**FIGURE 7.8**

Linearized model of vector color error diffusion. The quantizer was replaced by a linear transformation by $\tilde{\mathbf{K}}_s$ plus additive noise, $\mathbf{n}(\mathbf{m})$, that is uncorrelated with $\mathbf{u}(\mathbf{m})$. The original image is $\mathbf{x}(\mathbf{m})$, and the halftone is $\mathbf{b}(\mathbf{m})$.

where $\tilde{\mathbf{C}}_{\mathbf{bu}}$ and $\tilde{\mathbf{C}}_{\mathbf{uu}}$ are covariance matrices. The linearized vector error diffusion system has two inputs (original signal $\mathbf{x}(\mathbf{m})$ and quantization noise $\mathbf{n}(\mathbf{m})$) and one output (the halftone), like its scalar counterpart. Using Equation 7.19, the signal and noise transfer functions are as follows [35]:

$$\mathbf{B}_{\mathbf{s}}(z) = \tilde{\mathbf{K}}_s \left[ \tilde{\mathbf{I}} + \tilde{\mathbf{H}}(z)(\tilde{\mathbf{K}}_s - \tilde{\mathbf{I}}) \right]^{-1} \mathbf{X}(z) \qquad (7.20)$$

$$\mathbf{B}_{\mathbf{n}}(z) = \left[ \tilde{\mathbf{I}} - \tilde{\mathbf{H}}(z) \right] \mathbf{N}(z) \qquad (7.21)$$

The overall system response is given by

$$\mathbf{B}(z) = \mathbf{B}_{\mathbf{s}}(z) + \mathbf{B}_{\mathbf{n}}(z) \qquad (7.22)$$

For RGB vector error diffusion, matrix-valued error filter coefficients are adapted in Reference [44] to reduce the mean squared error between the halftone and original. However, mean squared error does not have perceptual meaning in RGB space. Damera-Venkata and Evans [35] form an objective function $J$ that measures the average visually weighted noise energy in the halftone. The output noise is computed by inverse transforming Equation 7.21:

$$\mathbf{b}_{\mathbf{n}}(m) = [\tilde{\mathbf{I}} - \tilde{\mathbf{h}}(m)] \star \mathbf{n}(\mathbf{m}) \qquad (7.23)$$

The noise energy is weighted by a linear spatially invariant matrix-valued HVS model, $\tilde{\mathbf{v}}(\mathbf{m})$, and form

$$J = E[\|\tilde{\mathbf{v}}(\mathbf{m}) \star [\tilde{\mathbf{I}} - \tilde{\mathbf{h}}(m)] \star \tilde{\mathbf{n}}(\mathbf{m})\|^2] \qquad (7.24)$$

Given a linear spatially invariant HVS model $\tilde{\mathbf{v}}(\mathbf{m})$, the problem is to design an optimal matrix-valued error filter:

$$\tilde{\mathbf{h}}_{opt}(\mathbf{m}) = \arg \min_{\tilde{\mathbf{h}}(\mathbf{m}) \in \mathcal{C}} J \qquad (7.25)$$

where the constraint $\mathcal{C}$ enforces the criterion that the error filter diffuses all quantization error [45]:

$$\mathcal{C} = \left\{ \tilde{\mathbf{h}}(\mathbf{i}), \ \mathbf{i} \in \mathcal{S} \ \Big| \ \sum_{\mathbf{i}} \tilde{\mathbf{h}}(\mathbf{i})\mathbf{1} = \mathbf{1} \right\} \qquad (7.26)$$

The term $\mathcal{S}$ denotes the set of coordinates for the error filter support, that is, $\mathcal{S} = \{(1, 0), (1, 1), (0, 1), (-1, 1)\}$ for Floyd–Steinberg.

We now explain the design of the linear human visual system model $\tilde{\mathbf{v}}(\mathbf{m})$. The linear color model employed by Damera-Venkata and Evans [35] is based on the pattern color separable model by Wandell et al. [46], [47] They transfer device-dependent RGB values into an opponent representation [47], [48]. The three opponent visual pathways are white–black (luminance pathway) and red–green and blue–yellow (chrominance pathways). By $x - y$, we mean that in value, $x$ is at one extreme and $y$ is at the other.

Monga et al. [49] generalize this linear color model as a linear transformation $\tilde{\mathbf{T}}$ to a desired color space, which is not necessarily the opponent representation [46] but any one that satisfies pattern color separability, followed by appropriate spatial filtering in each channel. A complete HVS model is uniquely determined by the color space transformation and associated spatial filters. This generalization provides a platform for evaluation of different models in perceptual meaning and error filter quality obtained by minimizing Equation 7.24. The linear color model consists of a linear transformation $\tilde{\mathbf{T}}$ and separable spatial filtering on each channel. Each channel uses a different spatial filter. The filtering in the $z$-domain is a matrix multiplication by a diagonal matrix $\mathbf{D}(\mathbf{z})$. In the spatial domain, the linear HVS model $\tilde{\mathbf{v}}(\mathbf{m})$ is computed as

$$\tilde{\mathbf{v}}(\mathbf{m}) = \tilde{\mathbf{d}}(\mathbf{m})\tilde{\mathbf{T}} \qquad (7.27)$$

Based on this framework, they evaluate four color spaces [49] in which to optimize matrix-valued error filters: linearized CIELab [50], opponent [51], YUV, and YIQ. These color spaces are chosen because they all score well in perceptual uniformity [52] and approximately satisfy the requirements for pattern color separability [53]. Because RGB values are device dependent, they perform the color transformations based on characterizing an sRGB monitor.

The transformation to opponent color space is given by

$$\text{sRGB} \longrightarrow \text{CIEXYZ} \longrightarrow \text{opponent representation}$$

The standard transformations from sRGB to CIEXYZ and from CIEXYZ to opponent representation are taken from the S-CIELab [51] code at http://white.stanford.edu/~brian/scielab/scielab1-1, which is also the source for transformations to the YUV and YIQ representations. The linearized CIELab color space is obtained by linearizing the CIELab space about the D65 white point [50] in the following manner:

$$Y_y = 116 \frac{Y}{Y_n} - 16 \tag{7.28}$$

$$C_x = 500 \left[ \frac{X}{X_n} - \frac{Y}{Y_n} \right] \tag{7.29}$$

$$C_z = 200 \left[ \frac{Y}{Y_n} - \frac{Z}{Z_n} \right] \tag{7.30}$$

Hence, $\tilde{\mathbf{T}}$ is sRGB $\longrightarrow$ CIEXYZ $\longrightarrow$ Linearized CIELab. The $Y_y$ component is similar to the luminance, and the $C_x$ and $C_z$ components are similar to the R–G and B–Y opponent color components. The original transformation to the CIELab from CIEXYZ is nonlinear:

$$L^* = 116 f \left( \frac{Y}{Y_n} \right) - 16 \tag{7.31}$$

$$a^* = 500 \left[ f \left( \frac{X}{X_n} \right) - f \left( \frac{Y}{Y_n} \right) \right] \tag{7.32}$$

$$b^* = 200 \left[ f \left( \frac{Y}{Y_n} \right) - f \left( \frac{Z}{Z_n} \right) \right] \tag{7.33}$$

where

$$f(x) = \begin{cases} 7.787x + \dfrac{16}{116} & \text{if } 0 \le x \le 0.008856 \\ x^{1/3} & \text{if } 0.008856 < x \le 1 \end{cases}$$

The values for $X_n$, $Y_n$, and $Z_n$ are as per the D65 white point [54].

The nonlinearity in the transformation from CIELab distorts the spatially averaged tone of the images, which yields halftones that have incorrect average values [50]. The linearized color space overcomes this, and has the added benefit that it decouples the effect of incremental changes in $(Y_y, C_x, C_z)$ at the white point on $(L, a, b)$ values:

$$\nabla_{(Y_y, C_x, C_z)} (L^*, a^*, b^*)|_{D_{65}} = \frac{1}{3} \mathbf{I} \tag{7.34}$$

In the opponent color representation, data in each plane are filtered [51] by two-dimensional (2-D) separable spatial kernels:

$$f = k \sum_i \omega_i E_i \tag{7.35}$$

where $E_i = k_i \exp(-\frac{(x^2+y^2)}{\sigma_i^2})$. The parameters $\omega_i$ and $\sigma_i$ are based on psychophysical testing and are available in Reference [51]. The spatial filters for linearized CIELab and the YUV and YIQ color spaces are based on analytical models of the eye's luminance and chrominance frequency response.

Nasanen and Sullivan [55] chose an exponential function to model the luminance frequency response:

$$W_{(Y_y)}(\tilde{\rho}) = K(L)e^{-\alpha(L)\tilde{\rho}} \qquad (7.36)$$

where $L$ is the average luminance of display, $\tilde{\rho}$ is the radial spatial frequency, $K(L) = a\, L^b$, and

$$\alpha(L) = \frac{1}{c \ln(L) + d} \qquad (7.37)$$

The frequency variable $\tilde{\rho}$ is defined [50] as a weighted magnitude of the frequency vector $\mathbf{u} = (u, v)^T$, where the weighting depends on the angular spatial frequency $\phi$ [55]. Thus,

$$\tilde{\rho} = \frac{\rho}{s(\phi)} \qquad (7.38)$$

where $\rho = \sqrt{u^2 + v^2}$ and

$$s(\phi) = \frac{1-\omega}{2} \cos(4\phi) + \frac{1+\omega}{2} \qquad (7.39)$$

The symmetry parameter $\omega$ is 0.7, and $\phi = \arctan\left(\frac{v}{u}\right)$. The weighting function $s(\phi)$ effectively reduces the contrast sensitivity to spatial frequency components at odd multiples of $45°$. The contrast sensitivity of the human viewer to spatial variations in chrominance falls off faster as a function of increasing spatial frequency than does the response to spatial variations in luminance [56]. The chrominance model reflects this [31]:

$$W_{(C_x, C_z)}(\rho) = Ae^{-\alpha\rho} \qquad (7.40)$$

In the above equation, $\alpha$ is determined to be 0.419, and $A = 100$ [31]. Both the luminance and chrominance responses are low-pass in nature, but only the luminance response is reduced at odd multiples of $45°$ (Figure 7.9a and Figure 7.9b). This will place more luminance error across the diagonals in the frequency domain where the eye is less sensitive. Using this chrominance response as opposed to identical responses for both luminance and chrominance will allow for more low-frequency chromatic error, which will not be perceived by the human viewer.

The four HVS models (each specified by the corresponding color transformation followed by spatial filtering) may then be employed in Equation 7.24 to design matrix-valued error filters for color vector error diffusion. Monga et al. performed a subjective assessment procedure that evaluates halftones generated using the four different HVS models based on a paired comparison task as described in Reference [49]. They observe that the color spaces in order of increasing quality are YIQ space, YUV space, opponent color space [46], [47], and linearized CIELab or $Y_yC_xC_z$ color space [50].

Their findings on the best HVS model for measuring color reproduction errors in error diffusion halftoning match those made by Kim and Allebach [57] for color direct binary search (DBS). The HVS model based on a color transformation to the linearized CIELAB or $Y_yC_xC_z$ color space has since been used extensively by several researchers for color halftone design. Because the model was initially proposed by Flohr et al. [50], for the rest of the chapter, we refer to it as the Flohr HVS model.

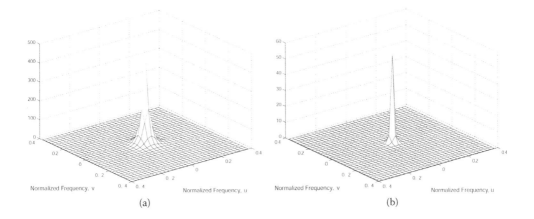

**FIGURE 7.9**
Spatial frequency responses: (a) luminance $W_{(Y_y)}(\mathbf{u})$ and (b) chrominance $W_{(C_x,C_z)}(\mathbf{u})$.

### 7.3.2.5 Illustrations

Figure 7.10a shows the original *toucan* image. Figure 7.10b shows a halftone generated by applying the Floyd–Steinberg error diffusion separably. The green color impulses on the red toucan in Figure 7.10b are easily visible on a color monitor. Figure 7.10c shows a halftone generated by applying an optimum matrix-valued error filter as given by Equation 7.25. The green color impulses in Figure 7.10b are eliminated in Figure 7.10c.

Figure 7.10d shows a halftone image generated using vector error diffusion in the device-independent XYZ space [36]. Artifacts are noticeable at color boundaries, especially on the yellow toucan. Figure 7.10e shows a halftone image generated using vector error diffusion in the device-independent XYZ space with artifact reduction by semivector quantization [37]. The boundary artifacts are significantly reduced. Figure 7.10f shows a halftone generated using the MBVC quantization as described in Reference [39]. Figure 7.10g and Figure 7.10h show magnified views of the MBVC halftone and the Floyd–Steinberg halftone, respectively. The MBVC halftone exhibits much smoother color with significantly reduced objectionable color variation.

## 7.4 Iterative Approaches to Color Halftoning

In iterative color halftoning algorithms, several passes over the halftone are made to minimize an error metric or satisfy certain constraints before the halftoning process is complete. The general approach is to start with an initial halftone and sequentially visit the individual halftone pixels to modify the halftone such that a visually meaningful error metric is reduced.

Iterative color halftoning algorithms are generally capable of creating halftones resulting with noticeably superior visual quality than the previously discussed two groups of color halftoning algorithms (i.e., point processes such as screening and neighborhood algorithms such as error diffusion). Iterative schemes, however, are computationally significantly more expensive than screening or error diffusion. For this reason, iterative algorithms cannot be implemented in current printers or displays for real-time halftoning of documents. Their value then lies in the fact that a well-designed iterative scheme serves as a practical upper bound on achievable halftone quality given any set of colorant and device constraints.

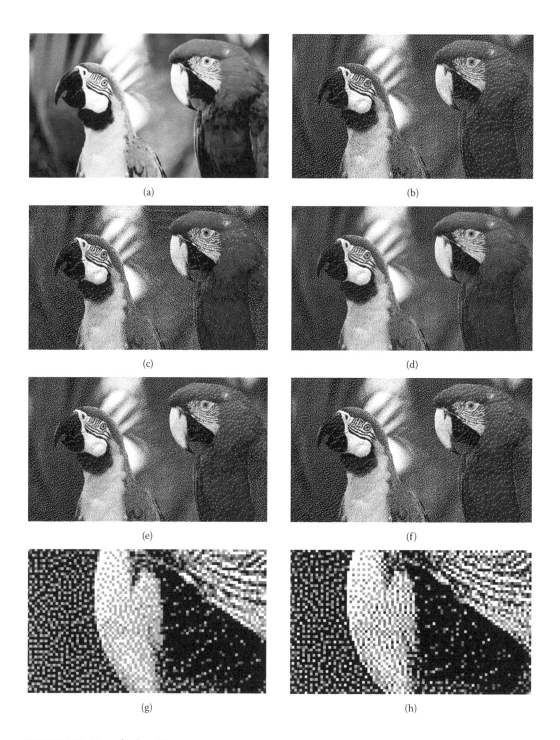

**FIGURE 7.10 (See color insert.)**

Comparison of various color error diffusion algorithms: (a) continuous tone *toucan* color image, (b) separable Floyd–Steinberg error diffusion, (c) optimum matrix-valued error filter, (d) vector error diffusion in XYZ space, (e) boundary artifact reduction of (d), (f) MBVC error diffusion, (g) detail of MBVC halftone, and (h) detail of Floyd–Steinberg error diffusion. Note the significant reduction in color halftone noise in parts (c) through (f) over separable FS error diffusion in part (b).

Hence, they can be used in training the more practical halftoning schemes (i.e., screening [9] and error diffusion [10], [11]). Such applications are reviewed in Section 7.4.2.

Because computation time is not a constraint, iterative schemes also afford the luxury of incorporating elaborate models of colorant characteristics, complex dot and media interactions, and the response of the human visual system to a color stimulus. Next, we describe color direct binary search (DBS), the most popular algorithm that is representative of the general philosophy of iterative halftoning schemes.

### 7.4.1 Color Direct Binary Search

The color direct binary search (CDBS) halftoning method [8] is an iterative search-based algorithm that minimizes a measure of the perceived error by starting from an initial halftone and modifying the error locally. Figure 7.11 shows a block diagram representation of the algorithm.

The initial halftone in color DBS is obtained by halftoning the R, G, and B components of the continuous tone color image separately by using the same screening algorithm, and then superimposing these three halftones under the assumption that $C = 1 - R$, $M = 1 - G$, $Y = 1 - B$.

For the initial halftone, the perceived error in the device-independent color space of $Y_y C_x C_z$ is computed. Then, the pixels of the halftone are processed in raster scan order. At each pixel, the effect on the error metric of toggling (changing the colorant combination) of the pixel and swapping it with its eight nearest neighbor (NN) pixels is examined. The trial change, if any, that reduces the error metric the most is accepted. The iteration continues until there are no more accepted trial changes (i.e., until the error metric reaches a local minimum).

To compute the perceived error, the original continuous tone image $\mathbf{x(m)}$, and the halftone bitmap $\mathbf{b(m)}$, need to be transformed from the device-dependent color space of RGB to the device-independent color space of $Y_y C_x C_z$ using transformations calibrated for a given

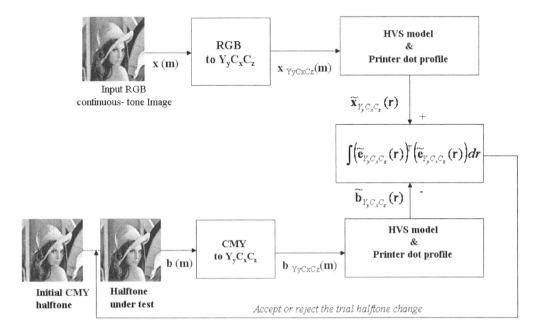

**FIGURE 7.11**
Block diagram representation of the iterative color direct binary search algorithm.

color imaging system. To transform $\mathbf{b(m)}$ into $Y_yC_xC_z$, the authors [8] use an eight-entry $CMY \longrightarrow Y_yC_xC_z$ lookup table (LUT). This LUT contains the $Y_yC_xC_z$ values of the eight possible colorant combinations known as the Neugebauer primaries ($C, M, Y, R, G, B, K, W$), measured with a spectrophotometer, for a given printer and paper substrate. The transformation from $\mathbf{x(m)}$ (specified in device RGB coordinates) to $Y_yC_xC_z$ can be made as described in Section 7.3.2.4 by an appropriate characterization of an sRGB monitor.

Then, let $\mathbf{x(m)}$ denote the $Y_yC_xC_z$ continuous tone color image and $\mathbf{b}_{Y_yC_xC_z}(\mathbf{m})$ the rendered (or halftoned) $Y_yC_xC_z$ color image. Their components are represented as $x_i(\mathbf{m})$, $b_i(\mathbf{m})$, $i = Y_y, C_x, C_z$. The error image in the $Y_yC_xC_z$ color space and its components is defined as

$$\mathbf{e}_{Y_yC_xC_z}(\mathbf{m}) \equiv \mathbf{x}_{Y_yC_xC_z}(\mathbf{m}) - \mathbf{b}_{Y_yC_xC_z}(\mathbf{m}) \tag{7.41}$$

and

$$e_i(\mathbf{m}) \equiv x_i(\mathbf{m}) - b_i(\mathbf{m}), \quad i = Y_y, C_x, C_z \tag{7.42}$$

Using the Flohr HVS model described in Section 7.3.2, and assuming additive interaction between neighboring dots, the perceived error $\tilde{\mathbf{e}}_{Y_yC_xC_z}(\mathbf{r})$ in the $Y_yC_xC_z$ color space may be modeled as

$$\tilde{\mathbf{e}}_{Y_yC_xC_z}(\mathbf{r}) = \sum_{\mathbf{m}} diag\left(\tilde{p}_{dotY_y}(\mathbf{r} - \mathbf{Rm}), \tilde{p}_{dotC_x}(\mathbf{r} - \mathbf{Rm}), \tilde{p}_{dotC_z}(\mathbf{r} - \mathbf{Rm})\right) \mathbf{e}_{Y_yC_xC_z}(\mathbf{m}) \tag{7.43}$$

where $\tilde{p}_{dot_i}(\mathbf{r}) = \tilde{p}_i(\mathbf{r}) * p_{dot}(\mathbf{r})$ is the HVS point spread function for the $i$th component of the $Y_yC_xC_z$ color space $\tilde{p}_i(\mathbf{r})$ convolved with the printer dot profile $p_{dot}(\mathbf{r})$, $\mathbf{R}$ is a periodicity matrix with columns that form the basis for the lattice of printer addressable dots, and $diag(\cdot)$ is a diagonal matrix with the diagonal elements within the parentheses. With a printer for which the lattice of addressable dots is rectangular with horizontal and vertical spacing $R$, $\mathbf{R} = diag(R, R)$. Because the printer dot profile has much more limited support than the HVS point spread function, and under the assumption that the printer dot profile has unit volume, it holds that $\tilde{p}_{dot_i}(\mathbf{r}) \approx \tilde{p}_i(\mathbf{r})$. Therefore, Equation 7.43 can be rewritten as

$$\tilde{\mathbf{e}}_{Y_yC_xC_z}(\mathbf{r}) = \sum_{\mathbf{m}} \tilde{\mathbf{P}}(\mathbf{r} - \mathbf{Rm})\mathbf{e}_{Y_yC_xC_z}(\mathbf{m}) \tag{7.44}$$

where

$$\tilde{\mathbf{P}}(\mathbf{r}) \equiv diag\left(\tilde{p}_{Y_y}(\mathbf{r}), \tilde{p}_{C_x}(\mathbf{r}), \tilde{p}_{C_z}(\mathbf{r})\right) \tag{7.45}$$

The error metric for halftone design $E$ is defined to be the sum of the total squared perceived errors in all three components of the $Y_yC_xC_z$ color space:

$$E = \int \tilde{\mathbf{e}}_{Y_y,C_x,C_z}(\mathbf{r})^T \tilde{\mathbf{e}}_{Y_y,C_x,C_z}(\mathbf{r}) \, dr \tag{7.46}$$

Substituting Equation 7.44 into Equation 7.46, we get

$$E = \sum_{\mathbf{m}} \sum_{\mathbf{n}} \mathbf{e}_{Y_y,C_x,C_z}(\mathbf{m}) \left( \int \tilde{\mathbf{P}}(\mathbf{r} - \mathbf{Rm}) \tilde{\mathbf{P}}(\mathbf{r} - \mathbf{Rn}) dr \right) \mathbf{e}_{Y_y,C_x,C_z}(\mathbf{n}) \tag{7.47}$$

The effect of trial halftone changes (i.e., toggles and swaps) on $E$ may then be found by traversing the image one pixel at a time, and evaluating Equation 7.47 for each considered toggle and swap. Efficient procedures for the same may be found in References [6], [8].

### 7.4.2 Training-Based Halftone Structures via Iterative Methods

#### 7.4.2.1 Color FM Screen Design Using DBS

Lin et al. proposed a training-based FM screen design method [9] to address the problem of dot-on-dot printing. Their design goal was to achieve a uniform rendition of any printable color using cyan, magenta, yellow, and black printer dots. In particular, Lin et al.

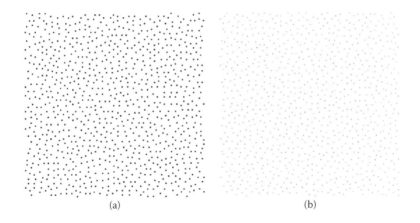

(a)                                    (b)

**FIGURE 7.12**
Magnified halftone images: (a) rendition of light gray with composite three-color black dots, and (b) rendition by a color FM screen trained using DBS. Note that halftone graininess is significantly reduced in part (b). Both the images are courtesy of Dr. Qian Lin at Hewlett-Packard labs.

use the DBS algorithm to design the dither matrix for each of the primary colors of the printer. To obtain the binary halftone pattern for any CMYK combination, they start with a random arrangement of a given number of cyan, magenta, yellow, and black dots. The design procedure then refines the initial random pattern by minimizing a color fluctuation metric [9] in a manner similar to color DBS.

Figure 7.12a and Figure 7.12b allow for comparison of two magnified halftone images of a 6.25% light gray patch (i.e., 6.25% each of cyan, magenta, and yellow dots and no black dots). The halftone output in Figure 7.12a is generated using a traditional overlay of the individual outputs of a FM halftone screen applied to each of the C, M, and Y colorant channels. The covered area contains composite black dots (made of the three inks), while the rest of the area is white paper. Because the printed dot contrasts heavily against the substrate (paper) white, this results in a grainy pattern. The halftone output of Lin's color FM screen in Figure 7.12b however, renders spatially dispersed colored dots that average to gray. In particular, the covered area in Figure 7.12b is composed of individual cyan, magenta, or yellow dots, and the uncovered area is white paper. This reduces the contrast between covered and uncovered areas, resulting in a smoother pattern.

### 7.4.2.2 Tone-Dependent Error Diffusion

Grayscale tone-dependent error diffusion (TDED) methods use error filters $h(\mathbf{m})$ with different sizes and coefficients for different gray levels [10]. The TDED algorithm [10] searches for error filter weights and thresholds to minimize a visual cost function for each input gray level. For the error filter design, the objective spectrum is the spectrum of the gray-level patch for highlights and shadows (gray levels 0 to 20 and 235 to 255). For input gray-level values in the midtones (gray levels 21 to 234), the spectrum of the direct binary search (DBS) pattern is used instead. The authors argue that using such a design procedure, error filters can be trained to produce halftone quality approaching that of DBS.

Monga et al. [11], [58] perform an extension of the grayscale TDED algorithm to color. The notion of "tone" in the case of color, however, is far more involved. To optimize over the entire color gamut, one needs to design error filters for all possible input CMY combinations. This number easily grows to be prohibitively large, for example, for 24-bit color images with eight bits per color plane, there are $(256)^3$ different combinations. To address this problem, Monga et al. design error filters for CMY combinations that correspond to the true neutrals in the device-independent gamut, that is, the locus $(L^*, 0, 0)$ in the CIELab space). Their

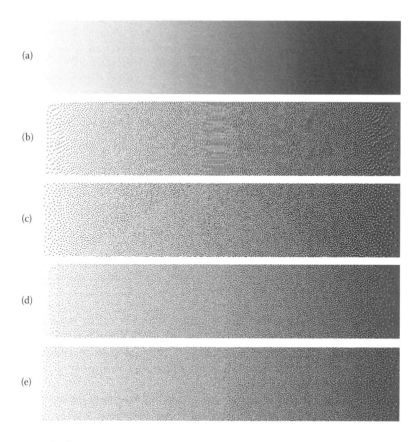

**FIGURE 7.13** (See color insert.)
A color ramp and its halftone images: (a) original color ramp image, (b) Floyd–Steinberg error diffusion, (c) separable application of grayscale TDED, (d) color TDED, and (e) colorant-based direct binary search. The halftone in part (c) is courtesy of Prof. Jan P. Allebach and Mr. Ti-Chiun Chang at Purdue University. The halftone in part (e) is courtesy of Dr. Je-Ho Lee at Hewlett-Packard and Prof. Jan P. Allebach at Purdue University.

design procedure employs a Neugebauer printer model and a color HVS model that takes into account spatial considerations in color reproduction [58].

Figure 7.13a to Figure 7.13e present halftone images of a color ramp using different error diffusion methods. It may be seen that the choice of color to render is significantly better for the color TDED halftone in Figure 7.13d over classical FS error diffusion in Figure 7.13b, as well as a separable application of the grayscale TDED [10] in Figure 7.13c. Figure 7.13e shows a halftone image generated using the CMYK color direct binary search (DBS) halftoning algorithm by Lee and Allebach [59]. The CMYK color DBS algorithm is essentially a variant of the basic color DBS algorithm reviewed in Section 7.4.1. In particular, Lee's work [59] enhances the color DBS algorithm described in Section 7.4.1 by controlling the quality of each colorant texture separately along with the total dot distribution. In order to achieve this, the authors first set the total dot arrangement and then color the dots optimally without altering the total dot arrangement. Due to the computational complexity in the search for optimal dot arrangements and subsequent color selection, the algorithm in Reference [59] cannot be directly used in real-time color printing paths. Hence, the color halftone generated via this method may be viewed as a benchmark. In fact, it may be seen that the color TDED and color DBS halftones shown, respectively, in Figure 7.13d and Figure 7.13e are virtually indistinguishable. In particular, the choice of color to render over the length of the ramp is near identical for the two halftoning methods.

## 7.5 Conclusion

Digital color halftoning is the process of transforming continuous-tone color images into images with a limited number of colors. The importance of this process arises from the fact that many color imaging systems use output devices such as color printers and low-bit depth displays that are bilevel or multilevel with a few levels. The goal is to create the perception of a continuous-tone color image using the limited spatiochromatic discrimination capability of the HVS. In decreasing order of how locally algorithms transform a given image into a halftone and, therefore, in increasing order of computational complexity and halftone quality, monochrome digital halftoning algorithms can be placed in one of three categories: point processes (screening or dithering), neighborhood algorithms (error diffusion), and iterative methods.

The naive digital color halftoning approach is to apply these monochrome halftoning techniques scalarly and independently to the color (RGB: red, green, and blue) or colorant (CMYK: cyan, magenta, yellow, and black) planes. As expected, this scalar approach leads to color artifacts and poor color rendition, because it does not exploit the correlation between color or colorant planes, which is a key element in our color perception and appreciation of the halftone quality.

Screening-based color halftoning algorithms account for colorant interaction by minimizing the occurrence of dot-on-dot printing. For instance, if the colorants are printed on top of each other, this will result in dots that contrast undesirably with the paper in the highlights. In color error diffusion, the correlation among color planes is taken into account by using color HVS models in the design of error filters, colorimetric or perceptual quantization, and employing matrix-valued filters as in vector error diffusion. For color printing, it is important for the underlying halftoning algorithm to account for nonideal characteristics of colorants and complicated dot interactions. This is accomplished by using a color hard-copy or printer model in conjunction with a color HVS model. Iterative algorithms are best suited for this purpose, because they are not limited by computation time. Halftone structures generated using iterative approaches may then be used to train screening- and error-diffusion-based color halftoning algorithms.

## References

[1] R. Ulichney, Dithering with blue noise, *Proceedings of the IEEE*, 76, 56–79, January 1988.

[2] T. Mitsa and K. Parker, Digital halftoning using a blue noise mask, *J. Opt. Soc. Am. A*, 9, 1920–1929, November 1992.

[3] R. Ulichney, The void-and-cluster method for dither array generation, in *Proceedings of SPIE Human Vision, Visual Process., and Digital Display IV*, J.P. Allebach, B.E. Rogowitz, Eds., San Jose, CA, USA, Vol. 1913, February 1993, pp. 332–343.

[4] R. Floyd and L. Steinberg, An adaptive algorithm for spatial grayscale, *Proceedings of the Society of Image Display*, Vol. 17, 1976, 75–77.

[5] T.D. Kite, Design and Quality Assessment of Forward and Inverse Error-Diffusion Halftoning Algorithms. Ph.D. thesis, Department of ECE, The University of Texas at Austin, TX, August 1998.

[6] M. Analoui and J.P. Allebach, Model based halftoning using direct binary search, *Proceedings of SPIE Human Vision, Visual Processing, and Digital Display III*, February 1992, 96–108.

[7] T. Pappas, Model-based halftoning of color images, *IEEE Trans. on Image Process.*, 6, 1014–1024, July 1997.

[8]   U.A. Agar and J.P. Allebach, Model based color halftoning using direct binary search, *Proceedings of SPIE Color Imaging: Processing, Hardcopy and Applications VI*, 2000, 521–535.

[9]   Q. Lin and J.P. Allebach, Color FM screen design using the DBS algorithm, *Proceedings of SPIE Annual Symposium on Electronic Imaging*, January 1998, 353–361.

[10]  P. Li and J.P. Allebach, Tone dependent error diffusion, in *SPIE Color Imaging: Device Independent Color, Color Hardcopy, and Applications VII*, Vol. 4663, January 2002, pp. 310–321.

[11]  V. Monga, N. Damera-Venkata, and B.L. Evans, An input-level dependent approach to color error diffusion, in *Proceedings of SPIE Color Imaging: Processing, Hardcopy and Applications IX*, Vol. 5009, January 2004, pp. 333–343.

[12]  B.E. Bayer, An optimal threshold for two-level rendition of continuous tone pictures, *Proc. IEEE Int. Conf. on Commun.*, 1, 11–15, 1973.

[13]  R. Ulichney, *Digital Halftoning*, MIT Press, Cambridge, MA, 1987.

[14]  D.L. Lau, G.R. Arce, and N.C. Gallagher, Digital color halftoning with generalized error-diffusion and green-noise masks, *IEEE Trans. on Image Process.*, 9, 923–935, May 2000.

[15]  D.L. Lau and G.R. Arce, *Modern Digital Halftoning*, Marcel Dekker, New York, 2001.

[16]  Q. Lin, Halftone Printing with Donut Filters, U.S. Patent, Vol. 6335989, January 2002.

[17]  Y. Abe, A new method of designing a dither matrix, *IEICE Transactions on Fundamentals of Electronics, Communications, and Computer Sciences, E85A*, 7, 1702–1709, July 2002.

[18]  N. Damera-Venkata and Q. Lin, *Proceedings of SPIE Annual Symposium on Electronic Imaging, Color Imaging IX: Processing, Hardcopy, and Applications*, R. Eschbach, G. G. Marcu, Eds., San Jose, CA, USA, AM-FM screen design using donut filters, January 2004, 469–480.

[19]  S.G. Wang, Stochastic halftone screen design, in *Proceedings of IS&T NIP13*, 1997, pp. 516–521.

[20]  H. Kang, *Digital Color Halftoning*, Society of Photo-Optical Instrumentation Engineers (SPIE), Bellingham, WA, 1999.

[21]  D.L. Lau, G.R. Arce, and N.C. Gallagher, Green-noise digital halftoning, *Proceedings of the IEEE*, 86, 2424–2442, December 1998.

[22]  D. Stoyan, W.S. Kendall, and J. Mecke, *Stochastic Geometry and Its Applications*, Wiley, New York, 1987.

[23]  J. Mannos and D. Sakrison, The effects of a visual fidelity criterion on the encoding of images, *IEEE Trans. on Inf. Theory*, 20, 525–536, July 1974.

[24]  C. Billotet-Hoffman and O. Brynghdahl, On the error diffusion technique for electronic halftoning, *Proceedings of the Society of Information Display*, 24, 3, 253–258, 1983.

[25]  R.L. Miller and C.M. Smith, Image processor with error diffusion modulated threshold matrix, U.S. Patent 5150429.

[26]  R. Levien, Output dependent feedback in error diffusion halftoning, *IS&T Imaging Sci. and Technol.*, 1, 115–118, May 1993.

[27]  J. Sullivan, R. Miller, and G. Pios, Image halftoning using a visual model in error diffusion, *J. Opt. Soc. Am. A*, 10, 1714–1724, August 1993.

[28]  R. Eschbach, Error-diffusion algorithm with homogeneous response in highlight and shadow areas, *J. Electron. Imaging*, 6, 1844–1850, July 1997.

[29]  N. Damera-Venkata and B.L. Evans, Adaptive threshold modulation for error diffusion halftoning, *IEEE Trans. on Image Process.*, 10, 104–116, January 2001.

[30]  P. Wong, Adaptive error diffusion and its application in multiresolution rendering, *IEEE Trans. on Image Process.*, 5, 1184–1196, July 1996.

[31]  B. Kolpatzik and C. Bouman, Optimized error diffusion for high quality image display, *J. Electron. Imaging*, 1, 277–292, January 1992.

[32]  P.W. Wong and J.P. Allebach, Optimum error diffusion kernel design, in *Proceedings of SPIE/IS&T Symposium on Electronic Imaging*, January 1997. Invited paper, 236–242.

[33]  I. Witten and R. Neal, Using Peano curves for bilevel display of continuous-tone images, *IEEE Comput. Graphics and Appl.*, 47–51, May 1982.

[34]  B.L. Evans, V. Monga, and N. Damera-Venkata, Variations on error diffusion: Retrospectives and future trends, in *Proceedings of SPIE Color Imaging: Processing, Hardcopy and Applications VIII*, Vol. 5008, January 2003, pp. 371–389.

[35]  N. Damera-Venkata and B.L. Evans, Design and analysis of vector color error diffusion halftoning systems, *IEEE Trans. on Image Process.*, 10, 1552–1565, October 2001.

[36] H. Haneishi, T. Suzuki, N. Shimonyama, and Y. Miyake, Color digital halftoning taking colorimetric color reproduction into account, *J. Electron. Imaging*, 5, 97–106, January 1996.

[37] Z. Fan and S. Harrington, Improved quantization methods in color error diffusion, *J. Electron. Imaging*, 8, 430–437, October 1999.

[38] D. Shaked, N. Arad, A. Fitzhugh, and I. Sobel, Ink Relocation for Color Halftones, HP Labs Technical Report, HPL-96-127R1, 1996.

[39] D. Shaked, N. Arad, A. Fitzhugh, and I. Sobel, Color Diffusion: Error-Diffusion for Color Halftones, HP Labs Technical Report, HPL-96-128R1, 1996.

[40] R.V. Klassen and R. Eschbach, Vector error diffusion in a distorted color spaceing, *Proceedings of IS&T 47th Annual Conference*, Rochester, NY, USA, May 1994, 489–491.

[41] H. Haneishi, H. Yaguchi, and Y. Miyake, A new method of color reproduction in digital halftone image, in *Proceedings of IS&T 47th Annual Conference*, Cambridge, MA, May 1993.

[42] T.D. Kite, B.L. Evans, and A.C. Bovik, Modeling and quality assessment of halftoning by error diffusion, *IEEE Trans. on Image Process.*, 9, 909–922, May 2000.

[43] H. Stark and J.W. Woods, *Probability, Random Processes and Estimation Theory for Engineers*, Prentice Hall, Englewood Cliffs, NJ, 1986.

[44] L. Akarun, Y. Yardimci, and A.E. Cetin, Adaptive methods for dithering color images, *IEEE Trans. on Image Process.*, 6, 950–955, July 1997.

[45] N. Damera-Venkata, Analysis and Design of Vector Error Diffusion Systems for Image Halftoning. Ph.D. thesis, Department of ECE, The University of Texas at Austin (www.ece.utexas.edu/~bevans/students/phd/niranjan/), December 2000.

[46] A.B. Poirson and B.A. Wandell, Appearance of colored patterns: Pattern-color separability, *J. Opt. Soc. Am. A*, 10, 2458–2470, December 1993.

[47] X. Zhang and B.A. Wandell, A spatial extension of CIELAB for digital color image reproduction, in *SID Digest of Technical Papers*, 1996, pp. 731–734.

[48] M.D. Fairchild, *Color Appearance Models*, Addison-Wesley, Reading, MA, 1998.

[49] V. Monga, W.S. Geisler, and B.L. Evans, Linear, color separable, human visual system models for vector error diffusion halftoning, *IEEE Signal Process. Lett.*, 10, 93–97, April 2003.

[50] T.J. Flohr, B.W. Kolpatzik, R. Balasubramanian, D.A. Carrara, C.A. Bouman, and J.P. Allebach, Model based color image quantization, in *Proceedings of SPIE Human Vision, Visual Processing and Digital Display IV*, 1993, 270–281.

[51] X. Zhang and B.A. Wandell, A spatial extension of CIELab for digital color image reproduction, *SID Tech. Dig.*, 731–734, 1996.

[52] C.A. Poynton, Frequently Asked Questions about Colour, available at www.inforamp.net/~poynton/ColorFAQ.html, 1999.

[53] A.B. Poirson and B.A. Wandell, Appearance of colored patterns: Pattern-color separability, *J. Opt. Soc. Am. A*, 10, 2458–2470, December 1993.

[54] What is sRGB? — Introduction to the Standard Default RGB Color Space Developed by Hewlett-Packard and Microsoft, available at www.srgb.com/aboutsrgb.html, 1999.

[55] J.R. Sullivan, L.A. Ray, and R. Miller, Design of minimum visual modulation halftone patterns, *IEEE Trans. Sys. Man. Cyb.*, 21, 33–38, January 1991.

[56] D.H. Kelly, Spatiotemporal variation of chromatic and achromatic contrast thresholds, *J. Opt. Soc. Am. A*, 73, 742–750, June 1983.

[57] S.H. Kim and J.P. Allebach, Impact of human visual system models on model based halftoning, *IEEE Trans. on Image Process.*, 11, 258–269, March 2002.

[58] V. Monga, N. Damera-Venkata, and B.L. Evans, Design of tone dependent color error diffusion halftoning systems, *IEEE Trans. on Image Process.*, accepted for publication.

[59] J.-H. Lee and J.P. Allebach, Colorant based direct binary search halftoning, *J. Electron. Imaging*, 11, 517–527, October 2002.

# 8

## *Secure Color Imaging*

**Rastislav Lukac and Konstantinos N. Plataniotis**

## CONTENTS

## 8.1   Introduction

In digital imaging, visual data are massively accessed, distributed, manipulated, and stored using communication and multimedia technology. To prevent unauthorized access and illegal copying and distribution, modern communication and multimedia systems utilize digital rights management (DRM) solutions to ensure media integrity, secure its transmission over untrusted communication channels, and protect intellectual property rights [1], [2], [3]. Two fundamental DRM frameworks (i.e., watermarking [4] and encryption [5]) have been suggested for protecting and enforcing the rights associated with the use of digital content [6].

Watermarking technologies are used for tasks such as identification of the content origin, copy protection, tracing illegal copies, fingerprinting, and disabling unauthorized access to content [7]. The image watermarking process embeds data, the so-called watermark, into the host image. Basically, watermarking can be performed in the spatial or frequency domain of the host image, and the visual content can be protected by embedding visible or imperceptible watermarks [1]. Examples of color watermarking solutions that operate on different principles can be found in References [8], [9], [10], [11]. Essential secure characteristics can be obtained by additive, multiplicative, or quantization embedding. The watermark should be robust to various attacks and attempts for its removal, damage, or unauthorized detection. After the transmission of watermarked images, the watermark is extracted using the secret key or blind extraction techniques. Note that most watermarking techniques are symmetric (i.e., the embedding and detection key are identical).

Encryption technologies ensure protection by scrambling the visual data into unrecognizable and meaningless variants [7], [12], [13]. In general, this transformation should be reversible in order to allow for the perfect recovery of the original content using the secret key. Thus, the security of the encryption solution depends on the secrecy of the encryption and decryption keys. Once the encrypted data are decrypted, encryption techniques do not offer any protection. To reduce computational overhead, popular image encryption solutions usually perform partial or selective encryption to protect the most important parts of the visual material [14], [15]. Most partial encryption solutions are secure coders that combine encryption and image coding to overcome the redundancy in the visual data and secure the confidentiality of compressed data by encrypting only a fraction of the total image data. The most significant portion of the data, as dictated by a compression algorithm, is encrypted to disallow decoding without the knowledge of the decryption key. Similar to the watermarking paradigm, secure characteristics can be obtained by encrypting the visual data in the spatial or frequency domain [16]. Efficient solutions for secure coding of color images can be found in References [17], [18], [19], [20].

Apart from the above DRM paradigms, secret sharing schemes have been shown to be sufficiently secure in order to facilitate distributed trust and shared control in various communication applications, such as key management, conditional access, message authentication, and content encryption [21], [22], [23], [24]. Due to the proliferation of imaging-enabled consumer electronic devices and the extensive use of digital imaging technologies in networked solutions and services, secret sharing concepts have a great potential to accomplish DRM features for securing the transmission and distribution of personal digital photographs and digital document images in public environments. This makes the secret sharing framework an excellent candidate for filling the gap between watermarking and encryption paradigms in secure imaging applications.

This chapter focuses on visual data protection using secret sharing concepts. Two main frameworks that use either the human visual system or simple logical operations to recover the secret image from the available shares are surveyed in a systematic and comprehensive manner. The presented methods can encrypt the secret image using an array of the existing threshold configurations, thus offering different design and application characteristics.

Section 8.2 starts by surveying the fundamentals of cryptographic solutions based on visual secret sharing or visual cryptography. Encryption and decryption functions are introduced and commented upon, and encryption of natural color images using halftoning and color mixing concepts is discussed. The implication of cost-effective decryption on the visual quality of the decrypted images is demonstrated.

Section 8.3 is devoted to image secret sharing with perfect reconstruction of the original visual data. The framework encrypts the decomposed bit levels of the secret color image. In the input-agnostic processing mode, the framework produces image shares with representations identical to that of the secret image. Because in practice the end user may request an increased or reduced pixel depth representation, input-specific solutions can be used to alter the level of protection and computational efficiency. Due to the symmetry between the encryption and decryption function, when the threshold constraint is satisfied during decryption, the framework perfectly reconstructs the input image data.

Section 8.4 introduces a cost-effective variant of the image secret sharing framework. The solution reduces the encryption and decryption operations from the block level to the pixel level, thus allowing significant computational and memory savings and efficient transmission of the shares in public networks. Reducing the number of shares to only two pieces, a private-key cryptosystem is obtained. Because of the symmetry constraint imposed on the encryption and decryption process, the solution satisfies the perfect reconstruction property. This section also includes a discussion of selective encryption, in terms of both bit levels or color channels of the secret color image.

The chapter concludes with Section 8.5 in which the ideas behind secret sharing of visual data are summarized. The definitions and some properties of the most popular secret sharing configurations are listed in the Appendix.

## 8.2 Visual Secret Sharing of Color Images

Secret sharing is considered a cost-effective solution that can be used to secure transmission and distribution of visual digital material over untrusted public networks. Most of the existing secret sharing schemes are generalized within the so-called $\{k, n\}$-threshold framework that confidentially divides the content of a secret message into $n$ shares in the way that requires the presence of at least $k$, for $k \leq n$, shares for the secret message reconstruction [21], [22]. Thus, the framework can use any of $n!/(k!(n-k)!)$ possible combinations of $k$ shares to recover the secret message, whereas the use of $k-1$ shares should not reveal the secret message. Among numerous possible $\{k, n\}$ configurations, the simplest case is constituted by $\{2, 2\}$ schemes that are commonly used as a private-key cryptosystem solution [25], [26].

The $\{k, n\}$-threshold framework has been popularized in the image processing community through visual secret sharing (VSS) or visual cryptography [27], [28], [29]. VSS schemes (Figure 8.1) encrypt the binary or binarized visual data — the so-called secret image — into the shares with the same data representation and use properties of the human visual system (HVS) to force the recognition of a secret image from available shares. Because binary data can be displayed either as frosted (for 0 values) or transparent (for 1 values) when printed on transparencies or viewed on the screen, overlapping shares that contain seemingly random information can reveal the secret image without additional computations or any knowledge of cryptographic keys. This makes the approach attractive for various applications. For instance, visual cryptography concepts were recently extended to enhance image watermarking solutions [30], [31], [32].

### 8.2.1 Visual Cryptography Fundamentals

In the conventional VSS framework (Figure 8.1a), the secret image is a $K_1 \times K_2$ binary image $I : Z^2 \to \{0, 1\}$ with values $I_{(r,s)}$ occupying the pixel locations $(r, s)$, for $r = 1, 2, \ldots, K_1$ and $s = 1, 2, \ldots, K_2$. Using a $\{k, n\}$ scheme operating on $I$, each binary pixel $I_{(r,s)}$ is encrypted via an encryption function [27]:

$$f_e(I_{(r,s)}) = \begin{cases} [s^{(1)}, s^{(2)}, \ldots, s^{(n)}]^T \in C_0 \text{ for } I_{(r,s)} = 0 \\ [s^{(1)}, s^{(2)}, \ldots, s^{(n)}]^T \in C_1 \text{ for } I_{(r,s)} = 1 \end{cases} \tag{8.1}$$

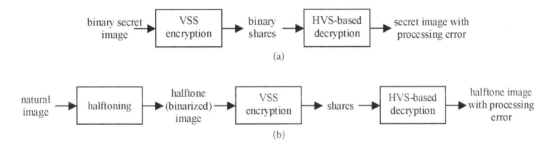

**FIGURE 8.1**
Visual secret sharing for (a) binary images and (b) natural continuous-tone images.

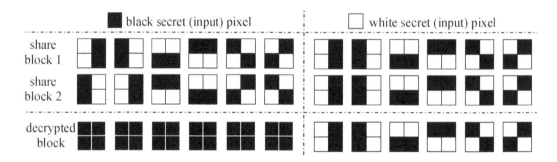

**FIGURE 8.2**
VSS concept demonstrated using a {2, 2}-threshold scheme.

to produce a $m_1 \times m_2$ block $s^{(l)} = \{s_{(m_1(r-1)+1,m_2(s-1)+1)}, s_{(m_1(r-1)+1,m_2(s-1)+2)}, \ldots, s_{(m_1r,m_2s)}\} \in S^{(l)}$, for $l = 1, 2, \ldots, n$, of binary values in each of $n$ binary shares $S^{(1)}, S^{(2)}, \ldots, S^{(n)}$. The spatial arrangement of bits in $s^{(l)}$ varies from block to block depending on the value of $I_{(r,s)}$ to be encrypted and the choice (usually guided by a random number generator) of the matrix $[s^{(1)}, s^{(2)}, \ldots, s^{(n)}]^T$ from the matrices' set $C_0$ or $C_1$. The sets $C_0$ or $C_1$ include all matrices obtained by permuting the columns of $n \times m_1m_2$ basis binary matrices $A_0$ or $A_1$, respectively. The value $m_1m_2$ is the so-called expansion factor, and therefore, the basis matrices are constructed in such a way as to minimize the expansion factor as much as possible. For example, in {2, 2}-VSS configurations, the use of $2 \times 2$ basis matrices

$$A_0 = \begin{bmatrix} 0, 1, 0, 1 \\ 1, 0, 1, 0 \end{bmatrix}, \quad A_1 = \begin{bmatrix} 0, 1, 0, 1 \\ 0, 1, 0, 1 \end{bmatrix} \tag{8.2}$$

implies the following (Figure 8.2):

$$C_0 = \left\{ \begin{bmatrix} 1, 0, 1, 0 \\ 0, 1, 0, 1 \end{bmatrix}, \begin{bmatrix} 0, 1, 0, 1 \\ 1, 0, 1, 0 \end{bmatrix}, \begin{bmatrix} 1, 1, 0, 0 \\ 0, 0, 1, 1 \end{bmatrix}, \begin{bmatrix} 0, 0, 1, 1 \\ 1, 1, 0, 0 \end{bmatrix}, \begin{bmatrix} 0, 1, 1, 0 \\ 1, 0, 0, 1 \end{bmatrix}, \begin{bmatrix} 1, 0, 0, 1 \\ 0, 1, 1, 0 \end{bmatrix} \right\} \tag{8.3}$$

$$C_1 = \left\{ \begin{bmatrix} 1, 0, 1, 0 \\ 1, 0, 1, 0 \end{bmatrix}, \begin{bmatrix} 0, 1, 0, 1 \\ 0, 1, 0, 1 \end{bmatrix}, \begin{bmatrix} 1, 1, 0, 0 \\ 1, 1, 0, 0 \end{bmatrix}, \begin{bmatrix} 0, 0, 1, 1 \\ 0, 0, 1, 1 \end{bmatrix}, \begin{bmatrix} 0, 1, 1, 0 \\ 0, 1, 1, 0 \end{bmatrix}, \begin{bmatrix} 1, 0, 0, 1 \\ 1, 0, 0, 1 \end{bmatrix} \right\} \tag{8.4}$$

Repeating Equation 8.1 for $\forall(r, s)$ encrypts the secret image $I$ into the shares $S^{(1)}, S^{(2)}, \ldots, S^{(n)}$ with dimensions of $m_1K_1 \times m_2K_2$ pixels. The reader can find the definition of basis matrices for other most commonly used $\{k, n\}$ configurations in the Appendix.

In standard practice, VSS allows for visual recovery of the encrypted images by simply stacking the shares and visually inspecting the resulting message, a feature that makes the operation cost-effective [27], [33], [34]. To understand the reconstruction of the secret image from the shares, VSS decryption can be modeled through the following decryption function [35]:

$$I'_{(u,v)} = f_d(\{s^{(l)}_{(u,v)}; l = 1, 2, \ldots, \zeta\}) = \begin{cases} 1 \text{ if } \forall s^l_{(u,v)} = 1 \\ 0 \text{ if } \exists s^l_{(u,v)} = 0 \end{cases} \tag{8.5}$$

where $u = 1, 2, \ldots, m_1K_1$, and $v = 1, 2, \ldots, m_2K_2$. The parameter $\zeta$ denotes the number of available shares, $\zeta \leq n$. Due to the utilization of the transparent/frosted concept in Equation 8.1, the VSS decryption process (Equation 8.5) recovers the decrypted pixel $I'_{(u,v)}$ as:

- black ($I'_{(u,v)} = 0$) if any of the share pixels $\{s^{(l)}_{(u,v)}, l = 1, 2, \ldots, \zeta\}$ corresponding to the same spatial location $(u, v)$ is frosted; or
- white ($I'_{(u,v)} = 1$) if all the share pixels $\{s^{(l)}_{(u,v)}, l = 1, 2, \ldots, \zeta\}$ corresponding to $(u, v)$ in the available shares are transparent.

Due to the expansion properties of VSS schemes, the original pixel $I_{(r,s)}$ is transformed by the VSS encryption/decryption process to a $m_1 \times m_2$ block of decrypted pixels:

$$f_d(f_e(I_{(r,s)})) = \{I'_{(m_1(r-1)+1,m_2(s-1)+1)}, I'_{(m_1(r-1)+1,m_2(s-1)+2)}, \ldots, I'_{(m_1r,m_2s)}\} \tag{8.6}$$

Through the construction of basis matrices, $\{k, n\}$-VSS schemes obtain the essential secure characteristics via the contrast properties of decrypted blocks. Because pixels in small spatial neighborhoods are perceived by HVS as a single pixel with the intensity averaged over its neighbors [36], [37], the contrast of the decrypted block $f_d(f_e(I_{(r,s)}))$ can be modeled as $\sum f_d(f_e(I_{(r,s)}))/(m_1m_2)$. If $\zeta < k$, then the contrast properties of decrypted blocks corresponding to $I_{(r,s)} = 0$ and $I_{(r,s)} = 1$ should be identical. The meaningful information — modeled via the different spatial contrast — can be visually revealed only if $\zeta \geq k$. This forms the following constraint:

$$\begin{aligned} \sum f_d(f_e(0)) = \sum f_d(f_e(1)) \quad &\text{if } \zeta < k \\ \sum f_d(f_e(0)) \neq \sum f_d(f_e(1)) \quad &\text{if } \zeta \geq k \end{aligned} \tag{8.7}$$

The graphical interpretation of the matrices listed in Equation 8.3 and Equation 8.4 is given in Figure 8.2. The figure also depicts the decrypted blocks obtained by stacking the share blocks. If only one arbitrary share block is used for the decryption, the spatial contrast of $f_d(f_e(I_{(r,s)}))$ is equal to $1/2$ for both $I_{(r,s)} = 0$ and $I_{(r,s)} = 1$. However, if both shares — as required by the $\{2, 2\}$-threshold scheme — are available, then the decrypted block $f_d(f_e(I_{(r,s)}))$ has the spatial contrast equal to 0 for $I_{(r,s)} = 0$ and $1/2$ for $I_{(r,s)} = 1$. Note that similar observations can be made for all $\{k, n\}$-threshold configurations listed in the Appendix. Due to the construction of basis matrices, the blocks corresponding to white secret pixels ($I_{(r,s)} = 1$) are recognized as some level of gray, but never white. Similarly, many $\{k, n\}$-threshold configurations with $k < n$ do not restore the decrypted blocks corresponding to black secret pixels ($I_{(r,s)} = 0$) as purely black. Therefore, a visually decrypted image has shifted intensity (typically darker) compared to the secret input image. An example generated using the $\{2, 2\}$-VSS scheme is shown in Figure 8.3.

### 8.2.2 Color Visual Cryptography

Given the binary nature of VSS encryption, the application of a conventional $\{k, n\}$-VSS solution to $K_1 \times K_2$ natural, continuous-tone, grayscale, and color images requires their binarization using halftoning [36], [38], [39]. As described in Chapter 7, the halftoning process transforms the input image into a $K_1 \times K_2$ halftone image by using the density of the net dots to simulate the gray or color levels. Note that there are many ways to obtain halftone images, and $\{k, n\}$-VSS solutions can work with all of them. In this work,

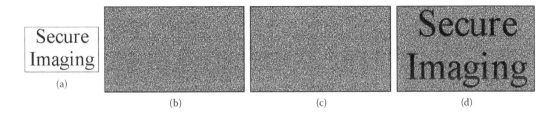

(a)  (b)  (c)  (d)

**FIGURE 8.3**
Secure binary imaging using $\{2, 2\}$-VSS scheme: (a) $111 \times 187$ binary secret image, (b,c) $222 \times 374$ binary shares, and (d) $222 \times 374$ binary decrypted image.

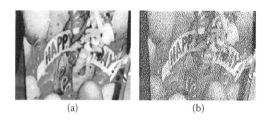

(a)                                    (b)

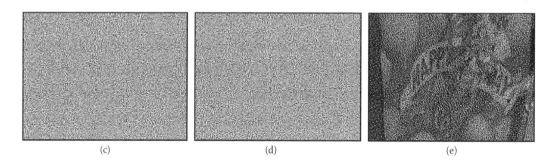

(c)                          (d)                          (e)

**FIGURE 8.4** (See color insert.)
Secure color imaging using {2, 2}-VSS scheme: (a) 120 × 160 color secret image, (b) 120 × 160 halftone image produced using Floyd–Steinberg filter, (c,d) 240 × 320 binarized color shares, and (e) 240 × 320 decrypted color image.

a simple error-diffusion procedure based on the Floyd–Steinberg filter with the following weights [40]:

$$
\begin{bmatrix}
w_{(r-1,s-1)} & w_{(r-1,s)} & w_{(r-1,s+1)} \\
w_{(r,s-1)} & w_{(r,s)} & w_{(r,s+1)} \\
w_{(r+1,s-1)} & w_{(r+1,s)} & w_{(r+1,s+1)}
\end{bmatrix}
= \frac{1}{16}
\begin{bmatrix}
0 & 0 & 0 \\
0 & 0 & 7 \\
3 & 5 & 1
\end{bmatrix}
\tag{8.8}
$$

is used to demonstrate the concept and produce the $I_{(r,s)}$ data suitable for VSS encryption.

Following the application scenario shown in Figure 8.1b, the input color image (Figure 8.4a) is halftoned to reduce the depth of the image representation. Applying the VSS encryption procedure of Equation 8.1 in a component-wise manner to the color halftone image (Figure 8.4b), shares — such as those shown in Figure 8.4c and Figure 8.4d for the {2, 2}-VSS configuration — can be produced. Figure 8.4e depicts the result of stacking two shares together using Equation 8.5. The decrypted color image has reduced visual quality due to color shifts and modified contrast. Not surprisingly, the produced outcome has the familiar form of a halftone image.

Apart from the component-wise solutions, the color {k, n}-VSS schemes can be constructed using additive or subtractive color mixing principles [36], [37], [41], [42], [43]. In the additive model (Figure 8.5a), each color is modeled using red (R), green (G), and blue (B) primaries. This concept is used in most computer monitors. On the other hand, color printers typically use the subtractive model (Figure 8.5b) with complementary cyan (C), magenta (M), and yellow (Y) colors to obtain spectrally shifted colors. Additional information on the issue can be found in Chapter 1. By decomposing the color halftone image into its RGB or CMY channels and using either the additive or subtractive model to produce the share blocks, decrypted halftone color pixels are recognizable by HVS for $\zeta \geq k$ as an average color of the corresponding stacked color share blocks of $m_1 \times m_2$ pixels. Similar to the component-wise VSS solutions, the decryption process deteriorates the visual quality of the output.

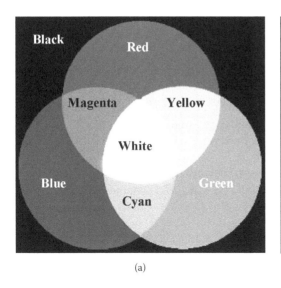
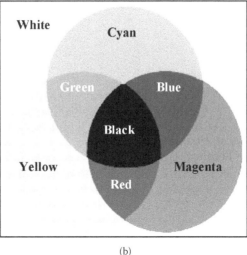

(a)                                          (b)

**FIGURE 8.5  (See color insert.)**
Two of the most common color models: (a) additive model and (b) subtractive model.

## 8.3   Perfect Reconstruction-Based Image Secret Sharing

To prevent the introduction of visual impairments into the decrypted image, a bit-level processing-based image secret sharing (ISS) framework was introduced (Figure 8.6) [35], [44]. Similar to the VSS schemes, the ISS framework operates in any $\{k, n\}$-threshold configuration (see Appendix) to encrypt the secret image into $n$ shares. By operating on the bit levels of the image array, the ISS framework: generates the shares with enhanced protection, allows for selective encryption of the decomposed bit levels, and recovers the original secret image when the required amount of shares is available for decryption.

### 8.3.1   Color Image Secret Sharing

A $K_1 \times K_2$ color image $\mathbf{x} : Z^2 \to Z^3$ represents a two-dimensional array of three-component vectorial inputs $\mathbf{x}_{(r,s)} = [x_{(r,s)1}, x_{(r,s)2}, x_{(r,s)3}]$ that occupy the spatial position $(r, s)$ with coordinates $r = 1, 2, \ldots, K_1$ and $s = 1, 2, \ldots, K_2$. Components $x_{(r,s)c}$, for $c = 1, 2, 3$, represent the $c$th elements of the color vector $\mathbf{x}_{(r,s)}$. In the case of a red, green, blue (RGB) color image, $c = 1$ denotes the R component, whereas $c = 2$ and $c = 3$ correspond to G and B components, respectively. Each color component $x_{(r,s)c}$ is coded with $B$ bits allowing $x_{(r,s)c}$ to take an integer value between 0 and $2^B - 1$. In the case of RGB color images, $x_{(r,s)c}$ is coded by eight bits ($B = 8$) ranging in the value of $x_{(r,s)c}$ from 0 to 255. Using a bit-level representation

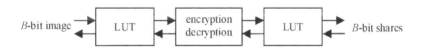

**FIGURE 8.6**
Bit-level processing-based image secret sharing. Both bit-level decomposition and stacking can be realized using lookup tables (LUTs).

[45], the color vector $\mathbf{x}_{(r,s)}$ can be equivalently expressed in a binary form as follows [44]:

$$\mathbf{x}_{(r,s)} = \sum_{b=1}^{B} \mathbf{x}_{(r,s)}^{b} 2^{B-b} \tag{8.9}$$

where $\mathbf{x}_{(r,s)}^{b} = [x_{(r,s)1}^{b}, x_{(r,s)2}^{b}, x_{(r,s)3}^{b}] \in \{0, 1\}^{3}$ denotes the binary vector at the bit level $b$, with $b = 1$ denoting the most significant bit (MSB). Thus, each binary component $x_{(r,s)c}^{b} \in \{0, 1\}$, for $c = 1, 2, 3$, is equal to 1 or 0, corresponding, respectively, to white and black in the binary representation.

Because components $x_{(r,s)c}^{b}$ represent binary data, they are ideal for VSS-like encryption. Using the basis matrices of the conventional $\{k, n\}$-VSS threshold schemes, each $x_{(r,s)c}^{b}$ can be encrypted as follows:

$$f_{e}\left(x_{(r,s)c}^{b}\right) = \begin{cases} \left[s_{c}^{(1)b}, s_{c}^{(2)b}, \ldots, s_{c}^{(n)b}\right]^{T} \in C_{0} \text{ for } x_{(r,s)c}^{b} = 0 \\ \left[s_{c}^{(1)b}, s_{c}^{(2)b}, \ldots, s_{c}^{(n)b}\right]^{T} \in C_{1} \text{ for } x_{(r,s)c}^{b} = 1 \end{cases} \tag{8.10}$$

The set $s_{c}^{(l)b} = \{s_{(m_1(r-1)+1,m_2(s-1)+1)c}^{b}, s_{(m_1(r-1)+1,m_2(s-1)+2)c}^{b}, \ldots, s_{(m_1 r, m_2 s)c}^{b}\} \in S_{c}^{(l)b}$, for $l = 1, 2, \ldots, n$, denotes a $m_1 \times m_2$ block of binary values in each of $n$ binary shares $S_{c}^{(1)b}, S_{c}^{(2)b}, \ldots, S_{c}^{(n)b}$, which are generated for the particular bit-level $b$ and the color-channel $c$.

Due to the use of random selection of $[s_{c}^{(1)b}, s_{c}^{(2)b}, \ldots, s_{c}^{(n)b}]^{T}$ from the matrices' set $C_0$ or $C_1$, component-wise bit levels $S_{c}^{(l)b}$ exhibit randomness. Thus, the process modifies both the spatial and spectral correlation between spatially neighboring binary share vectors $\mathbf{s}_{(u,v)}^{(l)b} = [s_{(u,v)1}^{(l)b}, s_{(u,v)2}^{(l)b}, s_{(u,v)3}^{(l)b}] \in S^{(l)b}$, for $u = 1, 2, \ldots, m_1 K_1$ and $v = 1, 2, \ldots, m_2 K_2$. By repeating the operation in Equation 8.10 for all values of $b$ and $c$, the generated share bits $s_{(u,v)c}^{(l)b}$ are used to obtain the full-color share vector:

$$\mathbf{s}_{(u,v)}^{(l)} = \sum_{b=1}^{B} \mathbf{s}_{(u,v)}^{(l)b} 2^{B-b} \tag{8.11}$$

where $\mathbf{s}_{(u,v)}^{(l)} = [s_{(u,v)1}^{(l)}, s_{(u,v)2}^{(l)}, s_{(u,v)3}^{(l)}]$ consists of $B$-bit color components $s_{(u,v)1}^{(l)}, s_{(u,v)2}^{(l)}, s_{(u,v)3}^{(l)}$. Thus, the ISS encryption process splits the full-color secret image $\mathbf{x}$ into seemingly random, full-color shares $\mathbf{S}^{(1)}, \mathbf{S}^{(2)}, \ldots, \mathbf{S}^{(n)}$ with an $m_1 K_1 \times m_2 K_2$ spatial resolution.

Unlike previously proposed VSS solutions, the ISS framework aims to restore the secret image in its original quality. Thus, the framework satisfies the so-called perfect reconstruction property, which is considered essential in modern visual communication systems and imaging pipelines [35]. To recover the secret image with perfect reconstruction, encryption and decryption should be symmetric (Figure 8.6). The decryption process first decomposes the color vectors $\mathbf{s}_{(u,v)}^{(1)}, \mathbf{s}_{(u,v)}^{(2)}, \ldots, \mathbf{s}_{(u,v)}^{(\varsigma)}$ from $\varsigma$ shares $\mathbf{S}^{(1)}, \mathbf{S}^{(2)}, \ldots, \mathbf{S}^{(\varsigma)}$ which are available for decryption. Then, the decryption function [46]

$$x_{(r,s)c}^{b} = f_{d}\left(\{s_{c}^{(l)b}; l = 1, 2, \ldots, \varsigma\}\right) = \begin{cases} 1 & \text{for } \left[s_{c}^{(1)b}, s_{c}^{(2)b}, \ldots, s_{c}^{(\varsigma)b}\right]^{T} \in C_{1} \\ 0 & \text{for } \left[s_{c}^{(1)b}, s_{c}^{(2)b}, \ldots, s_{c}^{(\varsigma)b}\right]^{T} \in C_{0} \end{cases} \tag{8.12}$$

is applied in the component-wise manner to the set of decomposed share blocks:

$$s_{c}^{(l)b} = \{s_{(u,v)c}^{(l)b}, s_{(u,v+1)c}^{(l)b}, \ldots, s_{(u+m_1-1, v+m_2-1)c}^{(l)b}\} \in S_{c}^{(l)b} \tag{8.13}$$

to recover the individual bits. The determination of the relationship between $\{s_{c}^{(1)b}, s_{c}^{(2)b}, \ldots, s_{c}^{(\varsigma)b}\} \subseteq \{s_{c}^{(1)b}, s_{c}^{(2)b}, \ldots, s_{c}^{(n)b}\}$ for $\varsigma \leq n$ and the matrices' sets $C_0$ and $C_1$ can be done using the contrast properties of the share blocks $s_{c}^{(1)b}, s_{c}^{(2)b}, \ldots, s_{c}^{(\varsigma)b}$ stacked together (Figure 8.2).

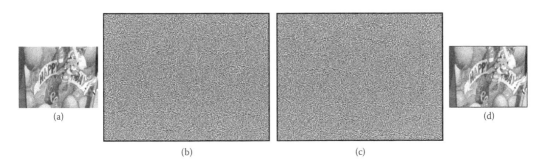

**FIGURE 8.7**
Secure color imaging using {2, 2}-ISS scheme: (a) $120 \times 160$ color secret image, (b, c) $240 \times 320$ full-color shares, and (d) $120 \times 160$ decrypted color image.

Similar to the $\{k, n\}$-VSS schemes, the difference between the stacked blocks $[s_c^{(1)b}, s_c^{(2)b}, \ldots, s_c^{(\zeta)b}]^T \in C_0$ and $[s_c^{(1)b}, s_c^{(2)b}, \ldots, s_c^{(\zeta)b}]^T \in C_1$ in Equation 8.12 reveals only if $\zeta \geq k$. In this case, the decryption process recovers the corresponding original bit $x_{(r,s)c}^b$ that can be equivalently expressed via the symmetry constraint of ISS encryption/decryption as follows:

$$f_d \left( f_e(x_{(r,s)c}^b) \right) = x_{(r,s)c}^b \tag{8.14}$$

By repeating Equation 8.12 with Equation 8.13 for all color channels $c = 1, 2, 3$, bit levels $b = 1, 2, \ldots, B$, and spatial locations $u = 1, 1 + m_1, 1 + 2m_1, \ldots, 1 + (K_1 - 1)m_1$ and $v = 1, 1 + m_2, 1 + 2m_2, \ldots, 1 + (K_2 - 1)m_2$, the procedure recovers the complete set of bits $x_{(r,s)c}^b$ in binary vectors $\mathbf{x}_{(r,s)} = [x_{(r,s)1}^b, x_{(r,s)2}^b, x_{(r,s)3}^b]$ used to represent the original color vector $\mathbf{x}_{(r,s)}$ in Equation 8.9. Completing the bit-level stacking in Equation 8.9 for $r = 1, 2, \ldots, K_1$ and $s = 1, 2, \ldots, K_2$ recovers the original full-color secret image $\mathbf{x}$ with perfect reconstruction.

Figure 8.7a to Figure 8.7d show images recorded at different stages of the ISS processing chain. The ISS shares (Figure 8.7b and Figure 8.7c) follow the full-color representation of the original image (Figure 8.7a), thus offering better protection compared to the VSS shares shown in Figure 8.4c and Figure 8.4d. Moreover, unlike the VSS output shown in Figure 8.4e, the ISS decrypted output shown in Figure 8.7d is perfectly restored in terms of both resolution and color and structural content.

## 8.3.2 Secret Sharing Solutions for Various Image Formats

Following the nature of the visual data to be encrypted, the ISS framework constitutes an input-agnostic solution [46] that produces shares with the bit representation identical to that of the secret image. In this case, the ISS solution encrypts [35] the binary secret image into the binary shares, the grayscale secret image into the grayscale shares, or the color secret image into the color shares. In all the above cases, the decryption process recovers the secret image with perfect reconstruction.

Because the input-agnostic ISS framework can be directly applied to any $B$-bit image, it can also be used to process the binary image shown in Figure 8.8a. Visual inspection of the results shown in Figure 8.8b and Figure 8.8c and Figure 8.3b and Figure 8.3c reveals that for the binary data, both VSS and ISS frameworks produce equivalent shares. However, due to the different decryption concept, the ISS decrypted output (Figure 8.8d) is identical to the original image, whereas the VSS output (Figure 8.3d) has an expanded size and suffers from various visual impairments.

The randomness of the encryption operations in Equation 8.10 fortified by the depth of the $B$-bit representation of the secret image introduces significant variations between the

(a)  (b)  (c)  (d)

**FIGURE 8.8**
Secure binary imaging using {2, 2}-ISS scheme: (a) 111 × 187 binary secret image, (b, c) 222 × 374 binary shares, and (d) 111 × 187 binary decrypted image.

original and share pixels. The degree of protection, obtained here through the depth of cryptographic noise generated by the ISS framework, increases with the number of bits used to represent the image pixel (Figure 8.9a to Figure 8.9c). Assuming that $N$ denotes the number of unique matrices either in $C_0$ or $C_1$, the $B$-bit color component $x_{(r,s)c}$ is encrypted using one of $N^B$ unique share blocks of $B$-bit values instead of one of only $N$ unique share blocks of binary values used in the traditional and halftoning-based VSS. It is not difficult to see that even for a simple {2, 2}-ISS scheme with six ($N = 6$) matrices listed in Equation 8.3 or Equation 8.4, there exist $6^{24}$ unique full-color share blocks that can be used for encryption of color RGB vectors $x_{(r,s)}$ with $B = 3 \times 8$. This suggests that the ISS framework can offer the higher protection of the visual data compared to the conventional VSS solutions.

In many practical applications, the user can request different protection levels during the encryption process or encrypt the visual data in the predetermined format. This can be done using the input-specific ISS solutions [46]. As part of the processing pipeline, the input-specific solution can require conversion of the binary or grayscale input image into the color image when the solution is color image specific to produce color shares, the binary or color input image into the grayscale image when the solution is grayscale image specific to produce grayscale shares, and the color or grayscale input image into the binary image when the solution is binary image specific to produce binary shares.

The input-specific paradigm requires format conversion, such as the replication of the input (for binary-to-grayscale, binary-to-color, and grayscale-to-color) or reduction of image representation (for color-to-grayscale, color-to-binary, and grayscale-to-binary) in order to meet the requirements for the input. Depending on the format conversion, the procedure requires the transmission of more or less share information compared to the shares produced by the input-agnostic ISS solution. Note that inverse format conversion is necessary to recover the secret image. In the data-replication encryption mode, the decryption recovers the original image. In the data-reduction encryption mode, the procedure results in the approximated secret image due to the loss in input format conversion. The reader can

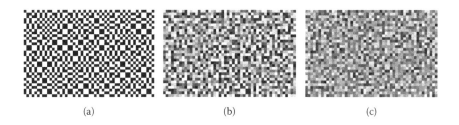

(a)  (b)  (c)

**FIGURE 8.9**
ISS share formats generated for (a) binary secret image, (b) grayscale secret image, and (c) full-color secret image.

find additional information on input-agnostic and input-specific solutions in References [46], [47].

Finally, it should be noted that both input-agnostic and input-specific ISS solutions can be used to process the secret image using an arbitrary $\{k, n\}$-threshold configuration and expansion factor. Because expanded dimensionality of the shares suggests increased requirements for their transmission, the next section will discuss the design of a nonexpansive ISS solution.

## 8.4 Cost-Effective Private-Key Solution

In practice, $\{2, 2\}$-threshold configurations are often used as the private-key cryptosystem solution [25]. In this application scenario, each of the two generated shares serves to the other as the decryption key. However, encrypting the color image using basis matrices defined in Equation 8.2 expands the spatial resolution of shares fourfold (i.e., the expansion factor is $m_1 m_2 = 4$). To reduce the complexity and allow for cost-effective transmission of the shares via public networks, the ISS solution (Figure 8.6) proposed in Reference [26] encrypts each binary component of the decomposed original vectors with a single output bit instead of the usual block of $m_1 m_2$ bits (for $m_1 \geq 2$ and $m_2 \geq 2$). Because the solution admits the nonexpansion factor $m_1 m_2 = 1$, the produced shares have the same spatial resolution as that of the original image (see Figure 8.10a to Figure 8.10d). This suggests that the encrypted visual information can be transmitted over untrusted channels at a reasonable cost (overhead).

Based on decomposed binary vectors $\mathbf{x}^b_{(r,s)} = [x^b_{(r,s)1}, x^b_{(r,s)2}, x^b_{(r,s)3}]$ obtained from the original color vector $\mathbf{x}_{(r,s)}$ in Equation 8.9, the solution generates two binary share vectors $\mathbf{s}^{(l)b}_{(r,s)} = [s^{(l)b}_{(r,s)1}, s^{(l)b}_{(r,s)2}, s^{(l)b}_{(r,s)3}]$, for $l = 1, 2$, as follows [26]:

$$f_e\left(x^b_{(r,s)c}\right) = \left[s^{(1)b}_{(r,s)c}\ s^{(2)b}_{(r,s)c}\right]^T \in \begin{cases} \{[0\ 1]^T, [1\ 0]^T\} & \text{for } x^b_{(r,s)c} = 1 \\ \{[0\ 0]^T, [1\ 1]^T\} & \text{for } x^b_{(r,s)c} = 0 \end{cases} \tag{8.15}$$

where the binary sets $[s^{(1)b}_{(r,s)c}\ s^{(2)b}_{(r,s)c}]^T$ are obtained from the basis elements 0 and 1. For simulation purposes, any conventional "rand" programming routine, which implements a random number generator seeded using the computer system clock state, can be used in Equation 8.15 to guide the encryption. However, solutions implemented in hardware may use electronic noise sources or radioactive decay [48]. The generated share bits are used in

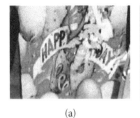
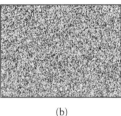
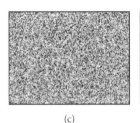
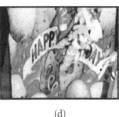

(a)  (b)  (c)  (d)

**FIGURE 8.10 (See color insert.)**
Secure color imaging using $\{2, 2\}$-ISS scheme: (a) $120 \times 160$ color secret image; (b, c) $120 \times 160$ full-color shares; and (d) $120 \times 160$ decrypted color image.

Equation 8.11 to produce the full-color share vectors $\mathbf{s}_{(r,s)}^{(1)}$ and $\mathbf{s}_{(r,s)}^{(2)}$ located at spatial position $(r, s)$ of the $K_1 \times K_2$ color shares $\mathbf{S}^{(1)}$ and $\mathbf{S}^{(2)}$, respectively.

Although each binary component $x_{(r,s)c}^b$ is encrypted by one of only two different configurations, the formation of the binary vectors $\mathbf{s}_{(r,s)}^{(l)b}$ increases the degree of protection to $2^3$. Moreover, due to bit-level stacking in Equation 8.11, the encryption process can generate the full-color shares from the set of $2^{3B}$ possible vectors. It is evident that the maximum confidentiality of the encrypted information can be obtained by repeating the encryption process in Equation 8.15 for $b = 1, 2, ..., B$ and $c = 1, 2, 3$.

During decryption, the original color and structural information is recovered by processing the share vectors at the decomposed bit level. The decryption procedure classifies the original binary components $x_{(r,s)c}^b$ under the constraint in Equation 8.14 as follows [26]:

$$x_{(r,s)c}^b = \begin{cases} 0 & \text{for } s_{(r,s)c}^{(1)b} = s_{(r,s)c}^{(2)b} \\ 1 & \text{for } s_{(r,s)c}^{(1)b} \neq s_{(r,s)c}^{(2)b} \end{cases} \tag{8.16}$$

and recovers the original color vector $\mathbf{x}_{(r,s)}$ using Equation 8.9. Due to the symmetry between Equation 8.15 and Equation 8.16, as indicated in Equation 8.14, the solution satisfies the perfect reconstruction property (Figure 8.10).

Because the above approach holds the perfect reconstruction property and is nonexpansive and easy to implement, it was recently used to encrypt the metadata information in digital camera images [49]. In this way, the acquired images can be indexed directly in the capturing device by embedding metadata information using the simple {2, 2} scheme. The concept described in this section was also extended in the JPEG domain to enable shared key image encryption for a variety of applications. The scheme proposed in Reference [50] directly works on the quantized DCT coefficients, and the shares are stored in the JPEG format. Following the symmetry of Equation 8.15 and Equation 8.16, the decryption process preserves the generated JPEG data.

To understand the importance of bit-level encryption of color images, Figure 8.11a to Figure 8.11c allow for the visual comparison of the color shares when cryptographic processing is applied to a subset of binary levels. Applying the cryptographic operations for the MSB (Figure 8.11a) or the two most significant bits (Figure 8.11b) only, fine details are

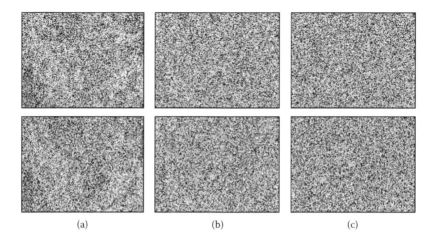

(a)                    (b)                    (c)

**FIGURE 8.11 (See color insert.)**
Color shares obtained using the nonexpansive ISS solution when cryptographic processing is performed for a reduced set of binary levels: (a) $b = 1$, (b) $b = 1, 2$, and (c) $b = 1, 2, 3$.

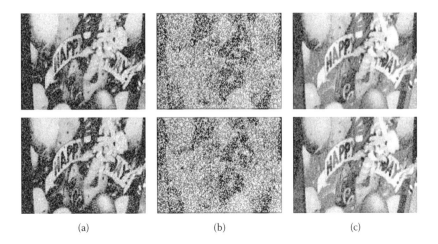

(a)                    (b)                    (c)

**FIGURE 8.12 (See color insert.)**
Color shares obtained using the nonexpansive ISS solution when cryptographic processing is performed for a single color channel: (a) R channel with $c = 1$, (b) G channel with $c = 2$, and (c) B channel with $c = 3$.

sufficiently encrypted; however, large flat regions can be partially visually revealed. As shown in Figure 8.11c, a sufficient level of protection of the whole visual information is achieved by applying Equation 8.15 to the first three most significant bits ($b = 1, 2, 3$). The remaining bits of the original image vectors can simply be copied into the shares unchanged.

Another important factor in color image encryption is the color information. Figure 8.12a to Figure 8.12c and Figure 8.13a to Figure 8.13c depict share images generated when the encryption operations are selectively applied to the particular color channels. As can be seen from the presented examples, encrypting either one (Figure 8.12a to Figure 8.12c) or two color channels (Figure 8.13a to Figure 8.13c) does not completely obscure the actual input. This suggests that for secure ISS encryption, all the channels of the color RGB image should be encrypted.

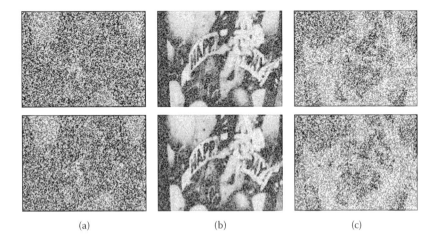

(a)                    (b)                    (c)

**FIGURE 8.13 (See color insert.)**
Color shares obtained using the nonexpansive ISS solution when cryptographic processing is performed for two color channels: (a) RG channels with $c = 1$ and $c = 2$, (b) RB channels with $c = 1$ and $c = 3$, and (c) GB channels with $c = 2$ and $c = 3$.

## 8.5  Conclusion

Secret sharing technology was used in this chapter as the means of ensuring the protection of color images intended for distribution over untrusted public networks. Using the popular $\{k, n\}$-threshold framework, secret sharing solutions encrypt color images into $n$ seemingly random, noise-like shares and recover the input image when at least $k$ shares are available for decryption. An overview was provided of the $\{k, n\}$-threshold solutions that decrypt the visual data using either the properties of the human visual system or simple logical operations.

In the first application scenario, the nature of visual secret sharing solutions requires that the color image to be encrypted should be transformed to a halftone image prior to its encryption. The generated shares are commonly printed on transparencies or viewed on the special screen. Due to the ability of the HVS to sense small image neighborhoods by averaging color information over spatially neighboring pixels, overlapping $k$ or more shares readily reveals the secret image without the need for additional computations or knowledge of cryptographic keys. However, the simplicity of decryption is obtained at the expense of reduced visual quality of the decrypted color image.

The availability of decrypted images in quality and representation identical to that of the original are essential in modern visual communication and multimedia systems. For that reason, $\{k, n\}$-threshold configurations were combined with bit-level processing and simple logical operations to provide perfect reconstruction of the original color input. Building on the bit representation of the secret image, the framework can be used to design various input-agnostic and input-specific image encryption tools. These $\{k, n\}$ image secret sharing solutions differ in their design characteristics and complexity and may secure the visual content at different protection levels and with different expansion or data reduction modes.

This overview suggests that secret sharing of color images constitutes a modern and powerful cryptographic tool that complements existing watermarking and encryption technology. It can be used to efficiently protect visual communication over untrusted public networks, and it is well suited to support value-additive services for the next generation of applications, such as secure wireless videoconferencing, online collaboration, and secure distribution and sharing of digital image materials.

## Appendix: Basis Matrices of Some Popular Threshold Configurations

Apart from the most popular $\{2, 2\}$-threshold scheme with the basis matrices defined in Equation 8.2, other popular $\{k, n\}$-threshold configurations are used to encrypt the secret image into three, four, or more shares. For example, the basis matrices

$$A_0 = \begin{bmatrix} 1, 0, 0, 0 \\ 0, 1, 0, 0 \\ 0, 0, 1, 0 \end{bmatrix}, \quad A_1 = \begin{bmatrix} 1, 0, 0, 0 \\ 1, 0, 0, 0 \\ 1, 0, 0, 0 \end{bmatrix} \tag{8.17}$$

of the $\{2, 3\}$ scheme achieve the required secure characteristics by splitting the content of the input image into three shares. The use of any two $(k = 2)$ of three $(n = 3)$ generated shares produces the spatial contrast equal to 0 for secret zero bits and $1/4$ for secret unit bits. The same spatial contrast of the stacked share blocks is obtained when the decryption is performed over all three shares generated using the following {3, 3}-threshold configuration:

$$A_0 = \begin{bmatrix} 0,0,1,1 \\ 0,1,0,1 \\ 0,1,1,0 \end{bmatrix}, \quad A_1 = \begin{bmatrix} 1,1,0,0 \\ 1,0,1,0 \\ 1,0,0,1 \end{bmatrix} \tag{8.18}$$

If the secret image is to be encrypted into four shares, three different {k, 4} configurations (for k = 2, 3, 4) are possible. The {2, 4}-threshold scheme:

$$A_0 = \begin{bmatrix} 1,0,0,0 \\ 0,1,0,0 \\ 0,0,1,0 \\ 0,0,0,1 \end{bmatrix}, \quad A_1 = \begin{bmatrix} 1,0,0,0 \\ 1,0,0,0 \\ 1,0,0,0 \\ 1,0,0,0 \end{bmatrix} \tag{8.19}$$

operates on $2 \times 2$ blocks and for two stacked shares has the spatial contrast properties similar to the configurations in Equation 8.17 and Equation 8.18. However, the construction of {3, 4} and {4, 4} basis matrices is more complex, necessitating $3 \times 3$ blocks to preserve the ratios $m_1 K_1/(m_2 K_2)$ and $K_1/K_2$ identical. Thus, the {3, 4}-threshold scheme is defined using

$$A_0 = \begin{bmatrix} 0,1,1,1,1,1,0,0 \\ 0,1,1,1,1,0,0,1,1 \\ 0,1,1,0,0,1,1,1,1 \\ 0,0,0,1,1,1,1,1,1 \end{bmatrix}, \quad A_1 = \begin{bmatrix} 1,1,1,1,1,0,0,0 \\ 1,1,1,1,0,0,1,1,0 \\ 1,1,1,0,1,0,1,0,1 \\ 1,1,1,0,0,1,0,1,1 \end{bmatrix} \tag{8.20}$$

which implies that three stacked shares produce the spatial contrast equal to 2/9 for secret zero bits and 1/3 for secret unit bits. By stacking four shares in the {4, 4}-scheme given by

$$A_0 = \begin{bmatrix} 1,0,0,1,0,0,1,0,1 \\ 1,0,1,0,0,0,1,1,0 \\ 1,0,1,0,0,1,0,0,1 \\ 0,1,1,0,0,0,1,0,1 \end{bmatrix}, \quad A_1 = \begin{bmatrix} 1,0,0,0,0,0,1,1,1 \\ 1,0,1,0,0,1,1,0,0 \\ 1,1,0,0,0,1,0,1,0 \\ 1,1,1,0,0,0,0,0,1 \end{bmatrix} \tag{8.21}$$

the secret zero and unity bits are, respectively, represented in the stacked shares by spatial contrast values 0 and 1/9.

Finally, the basis matrices of the {2, 6}-threshold scheme:

$$A_0 = \begin{bmatrix} 0,1,0,1 \\ 1,0,1,0 \\ 1,1,0,0 \\ 0,0,1,1 \\ 1,0,0,1 \\ 0,1,1,0 \end{bmatrix}, \quad A_1 = \begin{bmatrix} 0,1,0,1 \\ 0,1,0,1 \\ 0,1,0,1 \\ 0,1,0,1 \\ 0,1,0,1 \\ 0,1,0,1 \end{bmatrix} \tag{8.22}$$

are defined using $2 \times 2$ blocks. The decrypted block is recognized with the spatial contrast value 1/2 for secret unity bits, while decryption of secret zero bits can result in the contrast value 0 or 1/4 depending on which two of six generated shares are available for decryption.

The interested reader can find the guidelines for the construction of basis matrices corresponding to higher-order {k, n}-threshold configurations in References [25], [34]. However, it should be noted that expanding share dimensions may be a limiting factor in practical applications. Therefore, some recent research effort has been devoted to reduction or min-imization of share blocks used for encryption and decryption [26], [51], [52].

# References

[1] F. Bartolini, M. Barni, A. Tefas, and I. Pitas, Image authentication techniques for surveillance applications, *Proceedings of the IEEE*, 89(10), 1403–1418, October 2001.

[2] M. Wu, W. Trappe, Z.J. Wang, and K.J.R. Liu, Collusion-resistant fingerprinting for multimedia, *IEEE Signal Process. Mag.*, 21(2), 15–27, March 2004.

[3] D.C. Lou and J.L. Liu, Steganographic method for secure communications, *Comput. and Security*, 21(5), 449–460, October 2002.

[4] I. Cox, M. Miller, and J. Bloom, *Digital Watermarking*, Morgan Kaufmann, San Francisco, 2001.

[5] A. Menezes, P.V. Oorschot, and S. Vanstone, *Handbook of Applied Cryptography*, CRC Press, Boca Raton, FL, 1996.

[6] E.T. Lin, A.M. Eskicioglu, R.L. Lagendijk, and E.J. Delp, Advances in digital video content protection, *Proceedings of the IEEE*, 93(1), 171–183, January 2005.

[7] A.M. Eskicioglu and E.J. Delp, An overview of multimedia content protection in consumer electronics devices, *Signal Process.: Image Commun.*, 16(7), 681–699, April 2001.

[8] G.W. Braudaway, K.A. Magerlein, and F. Mintzer, Protecting publicly-available images with a visible image watermark, in *Proceedings of SPIE*, Vol. 2659, February 1996, pp. 126–133.

[9] M. Barni, F. Bartolini, and A. Piva, Multichannel watermarking of color images, *IEEE Trans. on Circuits and Syst. for Video Technol.*, 12(3), 142–156, March 2000.

[10] C.H. Tzeng, Z.F. Yang, and W.H. Tsai, Adaptive data hiding in palette images by color ordering and mapping with security protection, *IEEE Trans. on Commun.*, 52(5), 791–800, May 2004.

[11] C.S. Chan, C.C. Chang, and Y.C. Hu, Color image hiding scheme using image differencing, *Opt. Eng.*, 44(1), 017003, January 2005.

[12] J. Wen, M. Severa, W.J. Zeng, M. Luttrell, and W. Jin, A format-compliant configurable encryption framework for access control of video, *IEEE Trans. on Circuits and Syst. for Video Technol.*, 12(6), 545–557, June 2002.

[13] C.P. Wu and C.C.J. Kuo, Design of integrated multimedia compression and encryption systems, *IEEE Trans. on Multimedia*, 7(5), 828–839, October 2005.

[14] H. Cheng and X. Li, Partial encryption of compressed images and videos, *IEEE Trans. on Signal Process.*, 48(8), 2439–2451, August 2000.

[15] T. Lookabaugh and D.C. Sicker, Selective encryption for consumer applications, *IEEE Commun. Mag.*, 124–129, May 2004.

[16] W. Zeng and S. Lei, Efficient frequency domain selective scrambling of digital video, *IEEE Trans. on Multimedia*, 5(1), 118–129, March 2003.

[17] K. Martin, R. Lukac, and K.N. Plataniotis, Efficient encryption of wavelet-based coded color images, *Patt. Recognition*, 38(7), 1111–1115, July 2005.

[18] S. Lian, J. Sun, D. Zhang, and Z. Wang, A selective image encryption scheme based on JPEG2000 codec, *Lecture Notes in Comput. Sci.*, 3332, 65–72, 2004.

[19] A. Sinha and K. Singh, Image encryption by using fractional Fourier transform and jigsaw transform in image bit planes," *Opt. Eng.*, 44(5), 057001, May 2005.

[20] Y. Sadourny and V. Conan, A proposal for supporting selective encryption in JPSEC, *IEEE Trans. on Consumer Electron.*, 49(4), 846–849, November 2003.

[21] A.M. Eskicioglu, E.J. Delp, and M.R. Eskicioglu, New channels for carrying copyright and usage rights data in digital multimedia distribution, in *Proceedings of the International Conference on Information Technology: Research and Education (ITRE'03)*, Newark, New Jersey, USA, Vol. 16(7), August 2003, pp. 94–98.

[22] W. Lou, W. Liu, and Y. Fang, A simulation study of security performance using multipath routing in ad hoc networks, in *Proceedings of the IEEE Vehicular Technology Conference (VTC'03)*, Orlando, Florida, USA, Vol. 3, October 2003, pp. 2142–2146.

[23] D.C. Lou, J.M. Shieh, and H.K. Shieh, Copyright protection scheme based on chaos and secret sharing techniques, *Opt. Eng.*, 44(11), 117004, November 2005.

[24] C. Padró and G. Sáez, Lower bounds on the information rate of secret sharing schemes with homogeneous access structure, *Inf. Process. Lett.*, 83(6), 345–351, September 2002.

[25] G. Ateniese, C. Blundo, A. de Santis, and D.R. Stinson, Visual cryptography for general access structures, *Inf. and Comput.*, 129(2), 86–106, September 1996.

[26] R. Lukac and K.N. Plataniotis, A cost-effective encryption scheme for color images, *Real-Time Imaging, Spec. Issue on Multi-Dimensional Image Process.*, 11(5–6), 454–464, October–December 2005.

[27] M. Naor and A. Shamir, Visual cryptography, *Lect. Notes in Comput. Sci.*, 950, 1–12, 1994.

[28] C.C. Chang and J.C. Chuang, An image intellectual property protection scheme for gray-level images using visual secret sharing strategy, *Patt. Recognition Lett.*, 23(8), 931–941, June 2002.

[29] C.N. Yang, New visual secret sharing schemes using probabilistic method, *Patt. Recognition Lett.*, 25(4), 481–494, March 2004.

[30] G.C. Tai and L.W. Chang, Visual cryptography for digital watermarking in still images, *Lect. Notes in Comput. Sci.*, 3332, 50–57, December 2004.

[31] C.S. Tsai and C.C. Chang, A new repeating color watermarking scheme based on human visual model, *EURASIP J. on Appl. Signal Process.*, 2004(13), 1965–1972, October 2004.

[32] H. Guo and N.D. Georganas, A novel approach to digital image watermarking based on a generalized secret sharing schemes, *Multimedia Syst.*, 9(3), 249–260, September 2003.

[33] T. Hofmeister, M. Krause, and H. Simon, Contrast optimal $k$ out of $n$ secret sharing schemes in visual cryptography, *Theor. Comput. Sci.*, 240(2), 471–485, June 2000.

[34] P.A. Eisen and D.R. Stinson, Threshold visual cryptography schemes with specified levels of reconstructed pixels, *Design, Codes and Cryptography*, 25(1), 15–61, January 2002.

[35] R. Lukac and K.N. Plataniotis, Bit-level based secret sharing for image encryption, *Patt. Recognition*, 38(5), 767–772, May 2005.

[36] J.C. Hou, Visual cryptography for color images, *Patt. Recognition*, 36(7), 1619–1629, July 2003.

[37] T. Ishihara and H. Koga, A visual secret sharing scheme for color images based on meanvalue-color mixing, *IEICE Trans. on Fundam.*, E86-A(1), 194–197, January 2003.

[38] C.C. Lin and W.H. Tsai, Visual cryptography for gray-level images by dithering techniques, *Patt. Recognition Lett.*, 24(1–3), 349–358, January 2003.

[39] P.W. Wong and N.S. Memon, Image processing for halftones, *IEEE Signal Process. Mag.*, 20(4), 59–70, July 2003.

[40] R.A. Ulichney, Dithering with blue noise, *Proceedings of the IEEE*, 76, 56–79, January 1988.

[41] T. Ishihara and H. Koga, New constructions of the lattice-based visual secret sharing scheme using mixture of colors, *IEICE Trans. on Fundam. of Electron., Commun. and Comput. Sci.*, E85-A(1), 158–166, January 2002.

[42] H. Koga, M. Iwamoto, and H. Yamamoto, An analytic construction of the visual secret sharing scheme for color images, *IEICE Trans. on Fundam. of Electron., Commun. and Comput. Sci.*, 51(E84-A), 262–272, January 2001.

[43] A. Adhikari and S. Sikdar, A new (2, $n$) visual threshold scheme for color images, *Lect. Notes in Comput. Sci.*, 2904, 148–161, December 2003.

[44] R. Lukac and K.N. Plataniotis, Colour image secret sharing, *IEE Electron. Lett.*, 40(9), 529–530, April 2004.

[45] S. Ramprasad, N.R. Shanbha, and I.N. Hajj, Analytical estimation of signal transition activity from word-level statistics, *IEEE Trans. on Comput.-Aided Design of Integrated Circuits and Syst.*, 16(7), 718–733, July 1997.

[46] R. Lukac and K.N. Plataniotis, Image representation based secret sharing, *Commun. CCISA (Chinese Cryptology Information Security Association), Spec. Issue on Visual Secret Sharing*, 11(2), 103–114, April 2005.

[47] R. Lukac, K.N. Plataniotis, and C.N. Yang, *Encyclopedia of Multimedia*, ch. Image secret sharing. Springer, New York, 2005.

[48] C.S. Petrie and J.A. Connelly, A noise-based ic random number generator for applications in cryptography," *IEEE Trans. on Circuits and Syst. I*, 47(5), 615–621, May 2000.

[49] R. Lukac and K.N. Plataniotis, Digital image indexing using secret sharing schemes: A unified framework for single-sensor consumer electronics, *IEEE Trans. on Consumer Electron.*, 51(3), 908–916, August 2005.

[50] S. Sudharsan, Shared key encryption of JPEG color images, *IEEE Trans. on Consumer Electron.*, 51(4), 1204–1211, November 2005.

[51] C.N. Yang and T.S. Chen, Aspect ratio invariant visual secret sharing schemes with minimum pixel expansion, *Patt. Recognition Lett.*, 26(2), 193–206, January 2005.

[52] C.C. Lin and W.H. Tsai, Secret image sharing with capability of share data reduction, *Opt. Eng.*, 42(8), 2340–2345, August 2005.

# 9

## Color Feature Detection

Theo Gevers, Joost van de Weijer, and Harro Stokman

## CONTENTS

## 9.1 Introduction

The detection and classification of local structures (i.e., edges, corners, and T-junctions) in color images is important for many applications, such as image segmentation, image matching, object recognition, and visual tracking in the fields of image processing and computer vision [1], [2], [3]. In general, those local image structures are detected by differential operators that are commonly restricted to luminance information. However, most of the images recorded today are in color. Therefore, in this chapter, the focus is on the use of color information to detect and classify local image features.

The basic approach to compute color image derivatives is to calculate separately the derivatives of the channels and add them to produce the final color gradient. However, the derivatives of a color edge can be in opposing directions for the separate color channels. Therefore, a summation of the derivatives per channel will discard the correlation between color channels [4]. As a solution to the opposing vector problem, DiZenzo [4] proposes the color tensor, derived from the structure tensor, for the computation of the color gradient. Adaptations of the tensor lead to a variety of local image features, such as circle detectors and curvature estimation [5], [6], [7], [8]. In this chapter, we study the methods and techniques to combine derivatives of the different color channels to compute local image structures.

To better understand the formation of color images, the dichromatic reflection model was introduced by Shafer [9]. The model describes how photometric changes, such as shadows and specularities, influence the red, green, blue (RGB) values in an image. On the basis of this model, algorithms have been proposed that are invariant to different photometric phenomena such as shadows, illumination, and specularities [10], [11], [12]. The extension to differential photometric invariance was proposed by Geusebroek et al. [13]. Van de Weijer et al. [14] proposed photometric quasi-invariants that have better noise and stability characteristics compared to existing photometric invariants. Combining photometric quasi-invariants with derivative-based feature detectors leads to features that can identify various physical causes (e.g., shadow corners and object corners). In this chapter, the theory and practice is reviewed to obtain color invariance such as shading/shadow and illumination invariance incorporated into the color feature detectors.

Two important criteria for color feature detectors are *repeatability*, meaning that they should be *invariant* (stable) under varying viewing conditions, such as illumination, shading, and highlights; and *distinctiveness*, meaning that they should have high *discriminative power*. It was shown that there exists a trade-off between color invariant models and their discriminative power [10]. For example, color constant derivatives were proposed [11] that are invariant to all possible light sources, assuming a diagonal model for illumination changes. However, such a strong assumption will significantly reduce the discriminative power. For a particular computer vision task that assumes only a few different light sources, color models should be selected that are invariant (only) to these few light sources, resulting in an augmentation of the discriminative power of the algorithm. Therefore, in this chapter, we outline an approach to the selection and weighting of color (invariant) models for discriminatory and robust image feature detection.

Further, although color is important to express saliency [15], the explicit incorporation of color distinctiveness into the design of salient points detectors has been largely ignored. To this end, in this chapter, we review how color distinctiveness can be explicitly incorporated in the design of image feature detectors [16], [17]. The method is based upon the analysis of the statistics of color derivatives. It will be shown that isosalient derivatives generate ellipsoids in the color derivative histograms. This fact is exploited to adapt derivatives in such a way that equal saliency implies equal impact on the saliency map.

Classifying image features (e.g., edges, corners, and T-junctions) is useful for a large number of applications where corresponding feature types (e.g., material edges) from distinct images are selected for image matching, while other accidental feature types (e.g. shadow and highlight edges) are discounted. Therefore, in this chapter, a classification framework is discussed to combine the local differential structure (i.e., geometrical information such as edges, corners, and T-junctions) and color invariance (i.e., photometrical information, such as shadows, shading, illumination, and highlights) in a multidimensional feature space [18]. This feature space is used to yield proper rule-based and training-based classifiers to label salient image structures on the basis of their physical nature [19].

In summary, in this chapter, we will review methods and techniques solving the following important issues in the field of color feature detection: to obtain color invariance, such as with shading and shadows, and illumination invariance; to combine derivatives of the different color channels to compute local image structures, such as edges, corners, circles, and so forth; to select and weight color (invariant) models for discriminatory and robust image feature detection; to improve color saliency to arrive at color distinctiveness (focus-of-attention); and to classify the physical nature of image structures, such as shadow, highlight, and material edges and corners.

This chapter is organized as follows. First, in Section 9.2, a brief review is given on the various color models and their invariant properties based on the dichromatic reflection model. Further, color derivatives are introduced. In Section 9.3, color feature detection is proposed based on the color tensor. Information on color feature detection and its application to color feature learning, color boosting, and color feature classification is given in Sections 9.4, 9.5, and 9.6.

## 9.2 Color Invariance

In this section, the dichromatic reflection model [9] is explained. The dichromatic reflection model explains the image formation process and, therefore, models the photometric changes, such as shadows and specularities. On the basis of this model, methods are discussed containing invariance. In Section 9.2.1, the dichromatic reflection model is introduced. Then, in Sections 9.2.2 and 9.2.3, color invariants and color (invariant) derivatives will be explained.

### 9.2.1 Dichromatic Reflection Model

The dichromatic reflection model [9] divides the light that falls upon a surface into two distinct components: specular reflection and body reflection. Specular reflection is when a ray of light hits a smooth surface at some angle. The reflection of that ray will reflect at the same angle as the incident ray of light. This kind of reflection causes highlights. Diffuse reflection is when a ray of light hits the surface and is then reflected back in every direction.

Suppose we have an infinitesimally small surface patch of some object, and three sensors are used for red, green, and blue (with spectral sensitivities $f_R(\lambda)$, $f_G(\lambda)$ and $f_B(\lambda)$) to obtain an image of the surface patch. Then, the sensor values are [9]

$$C = m_b(\mathbf{n}, \mathbf{s}) \int_\lambda f_C(\lambda)e(\lambda)c_b(\lambda)d\lambda + m_s(\mathbf{n}, \mathbf{s}, \mathbf{v}) \int_\lambda f_C(\lambda)e(\lambda)c_s(\lambda)d\lambda \qquad (9.1)$$

for $C \in \{R, G, B\}$, and where $e(\lambda)$ is the incident light. Further, $c_b(\lambda)$ and $c_s(\lambda)$ are the surface albedo and Fresnel reflectance, respectively. The geometric terms $m_b$ and $m_s$ are the geometric dependencies on the body and surface reflection component, $\lambda$ is the wavelength, $\mathbf{n}$ is the surface patch normal, $\mathbf{s}$ is the direction of the illumination source, and $\mathbf{v}$ is the direction of the viewer. The first term in the equation is the diffuse reflection term. The second term is the specular reflection term.

Let us assume that white illumination is when all wavelengths within the visible spectrum have similar energy: $e(\lambda) = e$. Further assume that the neutral interface reflection model holds, so that $c_s(\lambda)$ has a constant value independent of the wavelength ($c_s(\lambda) = c_s$). First, we construct a variable that depends only on the sensors and the surface albedo:

$$k_C = \int_\lambda f_c(\lambda)c_b(\lambda)d\lambda \qquad (9.2)$$

Finally, we assume that the following holds:

$$\int_\lambda f_R(\lambda)d\lambda = \int_\lambda f_G(\lambda)d\lambda = \int_\lambda f_B(\lambda)d\lambda = f \tag{9.3}$$

With these assumptions, we have the following equation for the sensor values from an object under white light [11]:

$$C_w = e m_b(\mathbf{n}, \mathbf{s})k_C + e m_s(\mathbf{n}, \mathbf{s}, \mathbf{v})c_s f \tag{9.4}$$

with $C_w \in \{R_w, G_w, B_w\}$.

### 9.2.2   Color Invariants

To derive that normalized color, given by,

$$r = \frac{R}{R + G + B} \tag{9.5}$$

$$g = \frac{G}{R + G + B} \tag{9.6}$$

$$b = \frac{B}{R + G + B} \tag{9.7}$$

is insensitive to surface orientation, illumination direction, and illumination intensity, the diffuse reflection term

$$C_b = e m_b(\mathbf{n}, \mathbf{s})k_C \tag{9.8}$$

is used.

By substituting Equation 9.8 in the equations of $r$, $g$, and $b$, we obtain

$$r(R_b, G_b, B_b) = \frac{k_R}{k_R + k_G + k_B} \tag{9.9}$$

$$g(R_b, G_b, B_b) = \frac{k_G}{k_R + k_G + k_B} \tag{9.10}$$

$$b(R_b, G_b, B_b) = \frac{k_B}{k_R + k_G + k_B} \tag{9.11}$$

and hence, $rgb$ is only dependent on the sensor characteristics and surface albedo. Note that $rgb$ is dependent on highlights (i.e., dependent on the specular reflection term of Equation 9.4).

The same argument holds for the $c_1c_2c_3$ color space:

$$c_1(R_b, G_b, B_b) = \arctan\left(\frac{k_R}{\max\{k_G, k_B\}}\right) \tag{9.12}$$

$$c_2(R_b, G_b, B_b) = \arctan\left(\frac{k_G}{\max\{k_R, k_B\}}\right) \tag{9.13}$$

$$c_1(R_b, G_b, B_b) = \arctan\left(\frac{k_B}{\max\{k_G, k_R\}}\right) \tag{9.14}$$

Invariant properties for saturation

$$S(R, G, B) = 1 - \frac{\min(R, G, B)}{R + G + B} \tag{9.15}$$

**TABLE 9.1**

Invariance for Different Color Spaces for Varying Image Properties

| System | Viewpoint | Geometry | Illumination Color | Illumination Intensity | Highlights |
|--------|-----------|----------|--------------------|-----------------------|-----------|
| $RGB$ | − | − | − | − | − |
| $rgb$ | + | + | − | + | − |
| $Hue$ | + | + | − | + | + |
| $S$ | + | + | − | + | − |
| $I$ | − | − | − | − | − |
| $c_1c_2c_3$ | + | + | − | + | − |

*Note*: A "+" means that the color space is not sensitive to the property; a "−" means that it is.

are obtained by substituting the diffuse reflection term into the equation of saturation:

$$S(R_b, G_b, B_b) = 1 - \frac{\min\{k_R, k_G, k_B\}}{(k_R + k_G + k_B)} \tag{9.16}$$

where $S$ is only dependent on the sensors and the surface albedo.

Further, hue

$$H(R, G, B) = \arctan\left(\frac{\sqrt{3}(G - B)}{((R - G) + (R - B))}\right) \tag{9.17}$$

is also invariant to surface orientation, illumination direction, and intensity:

$$H(R_b, G_b, B_b) = \arctan\left(\frac{\sqrt{3}em_b(\mathbf{n}, \mathbf{s})(k_G - k_B)}{em_b(\mathbf{n}, \mathbf{s})((k_R - k_g) + (k_R - k_B))}\right)$$

$$= \arctan\left(\frac{\sqrt{3}(k_G - k_B)}{(k_R - k_G) + (k_R - k_B)}\right) \tag{9.18}$$

In addition, hue is invariant to highlights:

$$H(R_w, G_w, B_w) = \arctan\left(\frac{\sqrt{3}(G_w - B_w)}{(R_w - G_w) + (R_w - B_w)}\right)$$

$$= \arctan\left(\frac{\sqrt{3}em_b(\mathbf{n}, \mathbf{s})(k_G - k_B)}{em_b(\mathbf{n}, \mathbf{s})((k_R - k_G) + (k_R - k_B))}\right)$$

$$= \arctan\left(\frac{\sqrt{3}(k_G - k_B)}{(k_R - k_G) + (k_R - k_B)}\right) \tag{9.19}$$

A taxonomy of color invariant models is shown in Table 9.1.

### 9.2.3 Color Derivatives

Here we describe three color coordinate transformations from which derivatives are taken [20]. The transformations are derived from photometric invariance theory, as discussed in the previous section.

For an image $\mathbf{f} = (R, G, B)^T$, the spherical color transformation is given by

$$\begin{pmatrix} \theta \\ \varphi \\ r \end{pmatrix} = \begin{pmatrix} \arctan\left(\dfrac{G}{R}\right) \\ \arcsin\left(\dfrac{\sqrt{R^2 + G^2}}{\sqrt{R^2 + G^2 + B^2}}\right) \\ r = \sqrt{R^2 + G^2 + B^2} \end{pmatrix} \tag{9.20}$$

The spatial derivatives are transformed to the spherical coordinate system by

$$S(\mathbf{f}_x) = \mathbf{f}_x^s = \begin{pmatrix} r \sin \varphi \, \theta_x \\ r\varphi_x \\ r_x \end{pmatrix} = \begin{pmatrix} \dfrac{G_x R - R_x G}{\sqrt{R^2 + G^2}} \\ \dfrac{R_x RB + G_x GB - B_x(R^2 + G^2)}{\sqrt{R^2 + G^2}\sqrt{R^2 + G^2 + B^2}} \\ \dfrac{R_x R + G_x G + B_x B}{\sqrt{R^2 + G^2 + B^2}} \end{pmatrix} \tag{9.21}$$

The scale factors follow from the Jacobian of the transformation. They ensure that the norm of the derivative remains constant under the transformation, hence $|\mathbf{f}_x| = |\mathbf{f}_x^s|$. In the spherical coordinate system, the derivative vector is a summation of a shadow–shading variant part, $\mathbf{S}_x = (0, 0, r_x)^T$ and a shadow–shading quasi-invariant part, given by $\mathbf{S}_x^c = (r \sin \varphi \theta_x, r\varphi_x, 0)^T$ [20].

The opponent color space is given by

$$\begin{pmatrix} o1 \\ o2 \\ o3 \end{pmatrix} = \begin{pmatrix} \dfrac{R - G}{\sqrt{2}} \\ \dfrac{R + G - 2B}{\sqrt{6}} \\ \dfrac{R + G + B}{\sqrt{3}} \end{pmatrix} \tag{9.22}$$

For this, the following transformation of the derivatives is obtained:

$$O(\mathbf{f}_x) = \mathbf{f}_x^o = \begin{pmatrix} o1_x \\ o2_x \\ o3_x \end{pmatrix} = \begin{pmatrix} \dfrac{1}{\sqrt{2}}(R_x - G_x) \\ \dfrac{1}{\sqrt{6}}(R_x + G_x - 2B_x) \\ \dfrac{1}{\sqrt{3}}(R_x + G_x + B_x) \end{pmatrix} \tag{9.23}$$

The opponent color space decorrelates the derivative with respect to specular changes. The derivative is divided into a specular variant part, $\mathbf{O}_x = (0, 0, o3_x)^T$, and a specular quasi-invariant part $\mathbf{O}_x^c = (o1_x, o2_x, 0)^T$.

The hue–saturation–intensity is given by

$$\begin{pmatrix} h \\ s \\ i \end{pmatrix} = \begin{pmatrix} \arctan\left(\dfrac{o1}{o2}\right) \\ \sqrt{o1^2 + o2^2} \\ o3 \end{pmatrix} \tag{9.24}$$

The transformation of the spatial derivatives into the *hsi* space decorrelates the derivative with respect to specular, shadow, and shading variations,

$$H(\mathbf{f}_x) = \mathbf{f}_x^h = \begin{pmatrix} s\,h_x \\ s_x \\ i_x \end{pmatrix} = \begin{pmatrix} \dfrac{(R\,(B_x - G_x) + G\,(R_x - B_x) + B\,(G_x - R_x))}{\sqrt{2(R^2 + G^2 + B^2 - RG - RB - GB)}} \\ \dfrac{R\,(2R_x - G_x - B_x) + G\,(2G_x - R_x - B_x) + B\,(2B_x - R_x - G_x)}{\sqrt{6(R^2 + G^2 + B^2 - RG - RB - GB)}} \\ \dfrac{(R_x + G_x + B_x)}{\sqrt{3}} \end{pmatrix}$$

(9.25)

The shadow–shading–specular variant is given by $\mathbf{H}_x = (0, 0, i_x)^T$, and the shadow–shading–specular quasi-invariant is given by $\mathbf{H}_x^c = (sh_x, s_x, 0)^T$.

Because the length of a vector is not changed by orthonormal coordinate transformations, the norm of the derivative remains the same in all three representations $|\mathbf{f}_x| = |\mathbf{f}_x^c| = |\mathbf{f}_x^o| = |\mathbf{f}_x^h|$. For both the opponent color space and the hue–saturation–intensity color space, the photometrically variant direction is given by the $L1$ norm of the intensity. For the spherical coordinate system, the variant is equal to the $L2$ norm of the intensity.

## 9.3 Combining Derivatives

In the previous section, color (invariant) derivatives were discussed. The question is how to combine these derivatives into a single outcome. A default method to combine edges is to use equal weights for the different color features. This naive approach is used by many feature detectors. For example, to achieve color edge detection, intensity-based edge detection techniques are extended by taking the sum or Euclidean distance from the individual gradient maps [21], [22]. However, the summation of the derivatives computed for the different color channels may result in the cancellation of local image structures [4]. A more principled way is to sum the orientation information (defined on $[0, \pi)$) of the channels instead of adding the direction information (defined on $[0, 2\pi)$). Tensor mathematics provide a convenient representation in which vectors in opposite directions will reinforce one another. Tensors describe the local orientation rather than the direction (i.e., the tensor of a vector and its 180° rotated counterpart vector are equal). Therefore, tensors are convenient for describing color derivative vectors and will be used as a basis for color feature detection.

### 9.3.1 The Color Tensor

Given a luminance image $f$, the structure tensor is given by [6]

$$G = \begin{pmatrix} \overline{f_x^2} & \overline{f_x f_y} \\ \overline{f_x f_y} & \overline{f_y^2} \end{pmatrix}$$

(9.26)

where the subscripts indicate spatial derivatives, and the bar (¯) indicates convolution with a Gaussian filter. The structure tensor describes the local differential structure of images and is suited to find features such as edges and corners [4], [5], [7]. For a multichannel image $\mathbf{f} = (f^1, f^2, ..., f^n)^T$, the structure tensor is given by

$$G = \begin{pmatrix} \overline{\mathbf{f}_x \cdot \mathbf{f}_x} & \overline{\mathbf{f}_x \cdot \mathbf{f}_y} \\ \overline{\mathbf{f}_y \cdot \mathbf{f}_x} & \overline{\mathbf{f}_y \cdot \mathbf{f}_y} \end{pmatrix}$$

(9.27)

In the case that $\mathbf{f} = (R, G, B)$, Equation 9.27 is the color tensor. For derivatives that are accompanied by a weighting function, $w_x$ and $w_y$, which appoint a weight to every measurement in $\mathbf{f}_x$ and $\mathbf{f}_y$, the structure tensor is defined by

$$G = \begin{pmatrix} \dfrac{\overline{w_x^2 \mathbf{f}_x \cdot \mathbf{f}_x}}{\overline{w_x^2}} & \dfrac{\overline{w_x w_y \mathbf{f}_x \cdot \mathbf{f}_y}}{\overline{w_x w_y}} \\[4mm] \dfrac{\overline{w_y w_x \mathbf{f}_y \cdot \mathbf{f}_x}}{\overline{w_y w_x}} & \dfrac{\overline{w_y^2 \mathbf{f}_y \cdot \mathbf{f}_y}}{\overline{w_y^2}} \end{pmatrix} \tag{9.28}$$

### 9.3.2 Color Tensor-Based Features

In this section, a number of detectors are discussed that can be derived from the weighted color tensor. In the previous section, we described how to compute (quasi) invariant derivatives. In fact, dependent on the task at hand, either quasi-invariants are selected for detection or full invariants. For feature detection tasks quasi-invariants have been shown to perform best, while for feature description and extraction tasks, full invariants are required [20]. The features in this chapter will be derived for a general derivative $\mathbf{g}_x$. To obtain the desired photometric invariance for the color feature detector, the inner product of $\mathbf{g}_x$, see Equation 9.27, is replaced by one of the following:

$$\overline{\mathbf{g}_x \cdot \mathbf{g}_x} = \begin{cases} \overline{\mathbf{f}_x \cdot \mathbf{f}_x} & \text{if no invariance is required} \\[2mm] \overline{\mathbf{S}_x^c \cdot \mathbf{S}_x^c} \quad \text{or} \quad \overline{\mathbf{H}_x^c \cdot \mathbf{H}_x^c} & \text{for invariant feature detection} \\[2mm] \dfrac{\overline{\mathbf{S}_x^c \cdot \mathbf{S}_x^c}}{|\mathbf{f}|^2} \quad \text{or} \quad \dfrac{\overline{\mathbf{H}_x^c \cdot \mathbf{H}_x^c}}{|\mathbf{s}|^2} & \text{for invariant feature extraction} \end{cases} \tag{9.29}$$

where $\mathbf{s}$ is the saturation.

In Section 9.3.2.1, we describe features derived from the eigenvalues of the tensor. Further, more features are derived from an adapted version of the structure tensor, such as the Canny edge detection, in Section 9.3.2.2, and the detection of circular objects in Section 9.3.2.3.

#### 9.3.2.1 Eigenvalue-Based Features

Two eigenvalues are derived from the eigenvalue analysis defined by

$$\lambda_1 = \frac{1}{2} \left( \overline{\mathbf{g}_x \cdot \mathbf{g}_x} + \overline{\mathbf{g}_y \cdot \mathbf{g}_y} + \sqrt{(\overline{\mathbf{g}_x \cdot \mathbf{g}_x} - \overline{\mathbf{g}_y \cdot \mathbf{g}_y})^2 + (2\overline{\mathbf{g}_x \cdot \mathbf{g}_y})^2} \right)$$

$$\lambda_2 = \frac{1}{2} \left( \overline{\mathbf{g}_x \cdot \mathbf{g}_x} + \overline{\mathbf{g}_y \cdot \mathbf{g}_y} - \sqrt{(\overline{\mathbf{g}_x \cdot \mathbf{g}_x} - \overline{\mathbf{g}_y \cdot \mathbf{g}_y})^2 + (2\overline{\mathbf{g}_x \cdot \mathbf{g}_y})^2} \right) \tag{9.30}$$

The direction of $\lambda_1$ points in the direction of the most prominent local orientation:

$$\theta = \frac{1}{2} \arctan \left( \frac{2\overline{\mathbf{g}_x \cdot \mathbf{g}_y}}{\overline{\mathbf{g}_x \cdot \mathbf{g}_x} - \overline{\mathbf{g}_y \cdot \mathbf{g}_y}} \right) \tag{9.31}$$

The $\lambda$ terms can be combined to give the following local descriptors:

- $\lambda_1 + \lambda_2$ describes the total local derivative energy.
- $\lambda_1$ is the derivative energy in the most prominent direction.
- $\lambda_1 - \lambda_2$ describes the line energy (see Reference [23]). The derivative energy in the prominent orientation is corrected for the energy contributed by the noise $\lambda_2$.
- $\lambda_2$ describes the amount of derivative energy perpendicular to the prominent local orientation.

The Harris corner detector [24] is often used in the literature. In fact, the color Harris operator $H$ can easily be written as a function of the eigenvalues of the structure tensor:

$$\begin{aligned} H\mathbf{f} &= \overline{\mathbf{g}_x \cdot \mathbf{g}_x}\ \overline{\mathbf{g}_y \cdot \mathbf{g}_y} - \overline{\mathbf{g}_x \cdot \mathbf{g}_y}^2 - k(\overline{\mathbf{g}_x \cdot \mathbf{g}_x} + \overline{\mathbf{g}_y \cdot \mathbf{g}_y})^2 \\ &= \lambda_1 \lambda_2 - k(\lambda_1 + \lambda_2)^2 . \end{aligned} \tag{9.32}$$

Further, the structure tensor of Equation 9.27 can also be seen as a local projection of the derivative energy on two perpendicular axes [5], [7], [8], namely, $\mathbf{u}_1 = (1\ 0)^T$ and $\mathbf{u}_2 = (0\ 1)^T$,

$$\mathbf{G}^{\mathbf{u}_1, \mathbf{u}_2} = \begin{pmatrix} \overline{(\mathbf{G}_{x,y}\mathbf{u}_1)\cdot(\mathbf{G}_{x,y}\mathbf{u}_1)} & \overline{(\mathbf{G}_{x,y}\mathbf{u}_1)\cdot(\mathbf{G}_{x,y}\mathbf{u}_2)} \\ \overline{(\mathbf{G}_{x,y}\mathbf{u}_1)\cdot(\mathbf{G}_{x,y}\mathbf{u}_2)} & \overline{(\mathbf{G}_{x,y}\mathbf{u}_2)\cdot(\mathbf{G}_{x,y}\mathbf{u}_2)} \end{pmatrix} \tag{9.33}$$

in which $\mathbf{G}_{x,y} = (\mathbf{g}_x\ \mathbf{g}_y)$. From the Lie group of transformation, several other choices of perpendicular projections can be derived [5], [7]. They include feature extraction for circle, spiral, and star-like structures.

The star and circle detector is given as an example. It is based on $\mathbf{u}_1 = \frac{1}{\sqrt{x^2+y^2}}(x\ y)^T$, which coincides with the derivative pattern of a circular patterns and $\mathbf{u}_2 = \frac{1}{\sqrt{x^2+y^2}}(-y\ x)^T$, which denotes the perpendicular vector field that coincides with the derivative pattern of star-like patterns. These vectors can be used to compute the adapted structure tensor with Equation 9.33. Only the elements on the diagonal have nonzero entries and are equal to

$$\mathbf{H} = \begin{pmatrix} \overline{\frac{x^2}{x^2+y^2}\mathbf{g}_x\cdot\mathbf{g}_x} + \overline{\frac{2xy}{x^2+y^2}\mathbf{g}_x\cdot\mathbf{g}_y} + \overline{\frac{y^2}{x^2+y^2}\mathbf{g}_y\cdot\mathbf{g}_y} & 0 \\ 0 & \overline{\frac{x^2}{x^2+y^2}\mathbf{g}_y\cdot\mathbf{g}_y} - \overline{\frac{2xy}{x^2+y^2}\mathbf{g}_x\cdot\mathbf{g}_y} + \overline{\frac{y^2}{x^2+y^2}\mathbf{g}_x\cdot\mathbf{g}_x} \end{pmatrix} \tag{9.34}$$

where $\lambda_1$ describes the amount of derivative energy contributing to circular structures and $\lambda_2$ the derivative energy that describes a star-like structure.

Curvature is another feature that can be derived from an adaption of the structure tensor. For vector data, the equation for the curvature is given by

$$\kappa = \frac{\overline{w^2\mathbf{g}_v\cdot\mathbf{g}_v} - \overline{w^2\cdot\mathbf{g}_w\cdot\mathbf{g}_w} - \sqrt{(\overline{w^2\cdot\mathbf{g}_w\cdot\mathbf{g}_w} - \overline{w^2\mathbf{g}_v\cdot\mathbf{g}_v})^2 + 4\overline{w^2\cdot\overline{w}\mathbf{g}_v\cdot\mathbf{g}_w}^2}}{2\overline{w^2\cdot\overline{w}\mathbf{g}_v\cdot\mathbf{g}_w}} \tag{9.35}$$

in which $\mathbf{g}_v$ and $\mathbf{g}_w$ are the derivatives in gauge coordinates.

### 9.3.2.2  Color Canny Edge Detection

We now introduce the Canny color edge detector based on eigenvalues. The algorithm consists of the following steps:

1. Compute the spatial derivatives, $\mathbf{f}_x$, and combine them if desired into a quasi-invariant, as discussed in Section 9.2.3.

2. Compute the maximum eigenvalue using Equation 9.30 and its orientation using Equation 9.31.

3. Apply nonmaximum suppression on $\lambda_1$ in the prominent direction.

To illustrate the performance, the results of Canny color edge detection for several photometric quasi-invariants is shown in Figure 9.1a to Figure 9.1e. The image is recorded in three RGB colors with the aid of the SONY XC-003P CCD color camera (three chips) and the

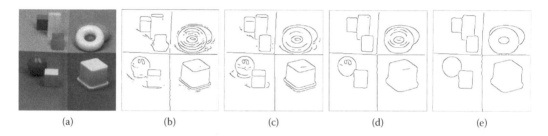

**FIGURE 9.1**
(a) Input image with Canny edge detection based on, successively, (b) luminance derivative, (c) *RGB* derivatives, (d) the shadow–shading quasi-invariant, and (e) the shadow–shading–specular quasi-invariant.

Matrox Magic Color frame grabber. Two light sources of average daylight color are used to illuminate the objects in the scene. The digitization was done in 8 bits per color. The results show that the luminance-based Canny (Figure 9.1b) misses several edges that are correctly found by the RGB-based method (Figure 9.1c). Also, the removal of spurious edges by photometric invariance is demonstrated. In Figure 9.1d, the edge detection is robust to shadow and shading changes and only detects material and specular edges. In Figure 9.1e, only the material edges are depicted.

### 9.3.2.3  Circular Object Detection

In this section, the combination of photometric invariant orientation and curvature estimation is used to detect circles robust against varying imaging conditions such as shadows and illumination changes.

The following algorithm is introduced for the invariant detection of color circles [20]:

1. Compute the spatial derivatives, $\mathbf{f}_x$, and combine them if desired into a quasi-invariant as discussed in Section 9.2.3.

2. Compute the local orientation using Equation 9.31 and curvature using Equation 9.35.

3. Compute the Hough space [25], $H\left(R, x^0, y^0\right)$, where $R$ is the radius of the circle, and $x^0$ and $y^0$ indicate the center of the circle. The computation of the orientation and curvature reduces the number of votes per pixel to one. Namely, for a pixel at position $\mathbf{x} = (x^1, y^1)$,

$$R = \frac{1}{\kappa}$$
$$x^0 = x^1 + \frac{1}{\kappa}\cos\theta \qquad (9.36)$$
$$y^0 = y^1 + \frac{1}{\kappa}\sin\theta$$

Each pixel will vote by means of its derivative energy $\sqrt{\mathbf{f}_x \cdot \mathbf{f}_x}$.

4. Compute the maxima in the hough space. These maxima indicate the circle centers and the radii of the circle.

To illustrate the performance, the results of the circle detection are given in Figure 9.2a to Figure 9.2c. Images have been recorded by the Nikon Coolpix 950, a commercial digital camera of average quality. The images have size $267 \times 200$ pixels with JPEG compression. The digitization was done in 8 bits per color. It is shown that the luminance-based circle

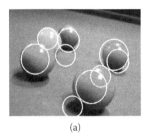 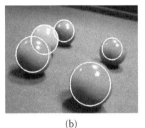 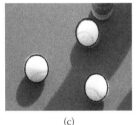

(a)              (b)              (c)

**FIGURE 9.2**
(a) Detected circles based on luminance, (b) detected circles based on shadow–shading–specular quasi-invariant, and (c) detected circles based on shadow–shading–specular quasi-invariant.

detection is sensitive to photometric variations, as nine circles are detected before the five balls were extracted. For the circle detector based on the (shadow–shading–specular) quasi-invariant, the five most prominent peaks in the hough space (not shown here) correspond to the radii and center points of the circles found. In Figure 9.2c, an outdoor example with a shadow partially covering the objects (tennis balls) is given. The detector finds the right circular objects and, hence, performs well, even under severe varying imaging conditions, such as shading and shadow, and geometrical changes of the tennis balls.

## 9.4 Color Feature Detection: Fusion of Color Derivatives

In the previous section, various image feature detection methods to extract locale image structures such as edges, corners, and circles were discussed. As there are many color invariant models available, the inherent difficulty is how to automatically select the weighted subset of color models producing the best result for a particular task. In this section, we outline how to select and weight color (invariant) models for discriminatory and robust image feature detection.

To achieve proper color model selection and fusion, we discuss a method that exploits nonperfect correlation between color models or feature detection algorithms derived from the principles of diversification. As a consequence, an optimal balance is obtained between repeatability and distinctiveness. The result is a weighting scheme that yields maximal feature discrimination [18], [19].

### 9.4.1 Problem Formulation

The measuring of a quantity $u$ can be stated as

$$u = E(u) \pm \sigma_u \tag{9.37}$$

where $E(u)$ is the best estimate for $u$ (e.g., the average value), and $\sigma_u$ represents the uncertainty or error in the measurement of $u$ (e.g., the standard deviation). Estimates of a quantity $u$, resulting from $N$ different methods, may be constructed using the following weighting scheme:

$$E(u) = \sum_i^N w_i E(u_i) \tag{9.38}$$

where $E(u_i)$ is the best estimate of a particular method $i$. Simply taking the weighted average of the different methods allows features from very different domains to be combined.

For a function $u(u_1, u_2, \cdots, u_N)$ depending on $N$ correlated variables, the propagated error $\sigma_u$ is

$$\sigma_u(u_1, u_2, \cdots, u_N) = \sum_{i=1}^{N} \sum_{j=1}^{N} \frac{\partial u}{\partial u_i} \frac{\partial u}{\partial u_j} \text{cov}(u_i, u_j) \tag{9.39}$$

where $\text{cov}(u_i, u_j)$ denotes the covariance between two variables. From this equation, it can be seen that if the function $u$ is nonlinear, the resulting error, $\sigma_u$, depends strongly on the values of the variables $u_1, u_2, \cdots, u_N$. Because Equation 9.38 involves a linear combination of estimates, the error of the combined estimate is only dependent on the covariances of the individual estimates. So, through Equation 9.39, we established that the proposed weighting scheme guarantees robustness, in contrast to possible, more complex, combination schemes.

Now we are left with the problem of determining the weights $w_i$ in a principled way. In the next section, we will propose such an algorithm.

### 9.4.2 Feature Fusion

When using Equation 9.38, the variance of the combined color models can be found through Equation 9.39:

$$\sigma_u^2 = \sum_{i=1}^{N} \sum_{j=1}^{N} w_i w_j \text{cov}(u_i, u_j) \tag{9.40}$$

or, equivalently,

$$\sigma_u^2 = \sum_{j=1}^{N} w_i^2 \sigma_{u_i}^2 + \sum_{i=1}^{N} \sum_{j \neq i} w_i w_j \text{cov}(u_i, u_j) \tag{9.41}$$

where $w_i$ denotes the weight assigned to color channel $i$, $u_i$ denotes the average output for channel $i$, $\sigma_u$ denotes the standard deviation of quantity $u$ in channel $i$, and $\text{cov}(u_i, u_j)$ corresponds to the covariance between channels $i$ and $j$.

From Equation 9.41, it can be seen how diversification over various channels can reduce the overall variance due to the covariance that may exist between channels. The Markowitz selection model [26] is a mathematical method for finding weights that achieve an optimal diversification. The model will minimize the variance for a given expected estimate for quantity $u$ or will maximize the expected estimate for a given variance $\sigma_u$. The model defines a set of optimal $u$ and $\sigma_u$ pairs. The constraints of this selection model are given as follows:

$$\textit{minimize } \sigma_u \tag{9.42}$$

for the formula described in Equation 9.38. The weights are constrained by the following conditions:

$$\sum_{i=1}^{N} w_i = 1 \tag{9.43a}$$

$$-1 <= w_i <= 1, i = 1, \cdots, N \tag{9.43b}$$

The constraint in Equations 9.43a ensures that all channels are fully allocated, and the constraint in Equation 9.43b limits the search space for $w_i$.

This model is quadratic with linear constraints and can be solved by linear programming [27]. When $\sigma_u$ is varied parametrically, the solutions for this system will result in mean–variance pairs representing different weightings of the feature channels. The pairs that maximize the expected $u$ versus $\sigma_u$ or minimize the $\sigma_u$ versus expected $u$, define the optimal frontier. They form a curve in the mean–variance plane, and the corresponding weights are optimal.

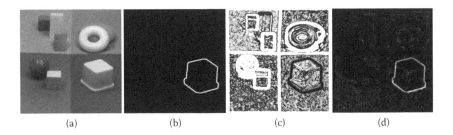

|  (a) | (b) | (c) | (d) |

**FIGURE 9.3**

(a) Lab image and (b) ground-truth for learning edges. Input image for the edge and corner detection: on the left, the edge is indicated for the learning algorithm. (c) The $\chi$-squared error of the transformed image and the predicted expected value: here the edges have a very low intensity. (d) The local signal-to-noise ratio for the transformed image. The edges have a higher ratio.

A point of particular interest on this curve is the point that has the maximal ratio between the expected combined output $E(u)$ and the expected variance $\sigma_u^2$. This point has the weights for which the combined feature space offers the best trade-off between repeatability and distinctiveness.

In summary, the discussed selection model is used to arrive at a set of weights to combine different color models into one feature. The expected value of this feature $E(u)$ is the weighted average of its component expected values. The standard deviation of this combined feature will be less than or equal to the weighted average of the component standard deviations. When the component colors or features are not perfectly correlated, the weighted average of the features will have a better variance-to-output ratio than the individual components on their own. New features or colors can always be safely added, and the ratio will never deteriorate, because zero weights can be assigned to components that will not improve the ratio.

### 9.4.3 Corner Detection

The purpose is to detect corners by learning. Our aim is to arrive at an optimal balance between color invariance (repeatability) and discriminative power (distinctiveness). In the context of combining feature detectors, in particular, in the case of color (invariant) edge detection, a default method to combine edges is to use equal weights for the different color features. This naive approach is used by many feature detectors. Instead of experimenting with different ways to combine algorithms, in this section, we use the principled method, outlined in the previous section, on the basis of the benefits of diversification. Because our method is based on learning, we need a set of training examples. The problem of corners is, however, that there are always a few pixels at a corner, making it hard to create a training set. We circumvent this problem by training on the edges, the first-order derivatives, where many more pixels are located.

Because the structure tensor (Equation 9.28) and the derived Harris operator (Equation 9.32) are based on spatial derivatives, we will train the weighting vector **w** on edges. This will allow for a much simpler collection of training points. So, the weights are trained with the spatial derivatives of the color channels as input. The resulting weights are then put in the **w** weights vector of the Harris operator.

To illustrate the performance of the corner detector based on learning, the first experiment was done on the image of Section 9.3, recorded in three RGB colors with the aid of the SONY XC-003P CCD color camera. The weights were trained on the edges of the green cube — see Figure 9.3a and Figure 9.3b. The edges were trained on the first-order derivatives in

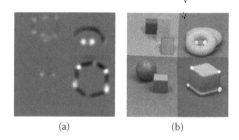

(a)                          (b)

**FIGURE 9.4**
(a) Results of the Harris corner detector. (b) Corners projected on the input image. The results of the Harris corner detector, trained on the lower right cube.

all color spaces. The results of applying these weights to the same image are shown in Figure 9.3c and Figure 9.3d. The edge is especially visible in the signal-to-noise image. Using the weights learned on the edges with the Harris operator, according to Equation 9.32, the corners of the green cube particularly stand out (see Figure 9.4a and Figure 9.4b).

Another experiment is done on images taken from an outdoor object — a traffic sign (see Figure 9.5a and Figure 9.5b). The weights were trained on one image and tested on images of the same object while varying the viewpoint. Again, the edges were defined by the first-order derivative in gauge coordinates. The results of the Harris operator are shown in Figure 9.6. The corner detector performs well even under varying viewpoints and illumination changes. Note that the learning method results in an optimal balance between repeatability and distinctiveness.

## 9.5   Color Feature Detection: Boosting Color Saliency

So far, we have outlined how to obtain color invariant derivatives for image feature detection. Further, we discussed how to learn a proper set of weights to yield proper color model selection and fusion of feature detection algorithms.

In addition, it is known that color is important to express saliency [15], [17]. To this end, in this section, we review how color distinctiveness can be explicitly incorporated in the design of image feature detectors [16], [17]. The method is based upon the analysis of the statistics of color derivatives. When studying the statistics of color image derivatives, points of equal frequency form regular structures [17]. Van de Weijer et al. [17] propose a color saliency boosting function based on transforming the color coordinates and using

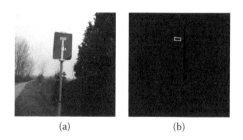

(a)                          (b)

**FIGURE 9.5**
The input image for the edge and corner detection: (a) the training image and (b) the trained edges.

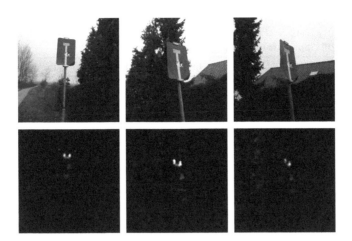

**FIGURE 9.6**
Original images (top) and output (bottom) of the Harris corner detector trained on red–blue edges.

the statistical properties of the image derivatives. The RGB color derivatives are correlated. By transforming the RGB color coordinates to other systems, photometric events in images can be ignored as discussed in Section 9.2, where it was shown that the spatial derivatives are separated into photometrical variant and invariant parts. For the purpose of color saliency, the three different color spaces are evaluated — the spherical color space in Equation 9.21, the opponent color space in Equation 9.23, and the *hsi* color space in Equation 9.25. In these decorrelated color spaces, only the photometric axes are influenced by these common photometric variations.

The statistics of color images are shown for the Corel database [28], which consists of 40,000 images (black and white images were excluded). In Figure 9.7a to Figure 9.7c, the distributions (histograms) of the first-order derivatives, $f_x$, are given for the various color coordinate systems.

When the distributions of the transformed image derivatives are observed from Figure 9.7, regular structures are generated by points of equal frequency (i.e., isosalient surfaces). These surfaces are formed by connecting the points in the histogram that occur the same number

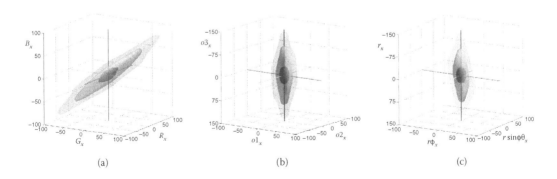

**FIGURE 9.7**
The histograms of the distribution of the transformed derivatives of the Corel image database in, respectively, (a) the RGB coordinates, (b) the opponent coordinates, and (c) the spherical coordinates. The three planes correspond with the isosalient surfaces that contain (from dark to light), respectively, 90%, 99%, and 99.9% of the total number of pixels.

**TABLE 9.2**

The Diagonal Entries of $\Lambda$ for the Corel Data Set Computed for Gaussian Derivatives With $\sigma = 1$

| Parameter | $\mathbf{f}_x$ | $|\mathbf{f}_x|_1$ | $\mathbf{f}_x^s$ | $\tilde{\mathbf{S}}_x^c$ | $\mathbf{f}_x^{\tilde{o}}$ | $\tilde{\mathbf{O}}_x^c$ | $\mathbf{f}_x^h$ | $\mathbf{H}_x^c$ |
|---|---|---|---|---|---|---|---|---|
| $\Lambda_{11}$ | 0.577 | 1 | 0.851 | 0.856 | 0.850 | 0.851 | 0.858 | 1 |
| $\Lambda_{22}$ | 0.577 | — | 0.515 | 0.518 | 0.524 | 0.525 | 0.509 | 0 |
| $\Lambda_{33}$ | 0.577 | — | 0.099 | 0 | 0.065 | 0 | 0.066 | 0 |

of times. The shapes of the isosalient surfaces correspond to ellipses. The major axis of the ellipsoid coincides with the axis of maximum variation in the histogram (i.e., the intensity axes). Based on the observed statistics, a saliency measure can be derived in which vectors with an equal information content have an equal effect on the saliency. This is called the "color saliency boosting function." It is obtained by deriving a function that describes the isosalient surfaces.

More precisely, the ellipsoids are equal to

$$\left(\alpha h_x^1\right)^2 + \left(\beta h_x^2\right)^2 + \left(\gamma h_x^3\right)^2 = |\Lambda h(\mathbf{f}_x)|^2 \tag{9.44}$$

and then the following holds:

$$p\left(\mathbf{f}_x\right) = p(\mathbf{f}_x') \leftrightarrow |\Lambda h(\mathbf{f}_x)| = \left|\Lambda^T h(\mathbf{f}_x')\right| \tag{9.45}$$

where $\Lambda$ is a $3 \times 3$ diagonal matrix with $\Lambda_{11} = \alpha$, $\Lambda_{22} = \beta$, and $\Lambda_{33} = \gamma$. $\Lambda$ is restricted to $\Lambda_{11}^2 + \Lambda_{22}^2 + \Lambda_{33}^2 = 1$. The desired saliency boosting function is obtained by

$$g\left(\mathbf{f}_x\right) = \Lambda h\left(\mathbf{f}_x\right) \tag{9.46}$$

By a rotation of the color axes followed by a rescaling of the axis, the oriented isosalient ellipsoids are transformed into spheres, and thus, vectors of equal saliency are transformed into vectors of equal length.

Before color saliency boosting can be applied, the $\Lambda$-parameters have to be initialized by fitting ellipses to the histogram of the data set. The results for the various transformations are summarized in Table 9.2. The relation between the axes in the various color spaces clearly confirms the dominance of the luminance axis in the RGB cube, because $\Lambda_{33}$, the multiplication factor of the luminance axis, is much smaller than the color-axes multiplication factors, $\Lambda_{11}$ and $\Lambda_{22}$. After color saliency boosting, there is an increase in information context, see Reference [17] for more details.

To illustrate the performance of the color-boosting method, Figure 9.8a to Figure 9.8d show the results before and after saliency boosting. Although focus point detection is already an extension from luminance to color, black-and-white transition still dominates the result. Only after boosting the color saliency are the less interesting black-and-white structures in the image ignored and most of the red Chinese signs are found.

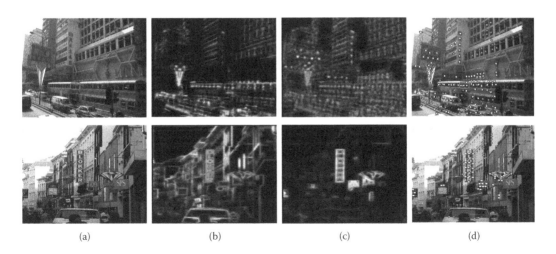

(a)           (b)           (c)           (d)

**FIGURE 9.8 (See color insert.)**
In columns, respectively, (a) input image, (b) RGB-gradient-based saliency map, (c) color-boosted saliency map, and (d) the results with red dots (lines) for gradient-based method and yellow dots (lines) for salient points after color saliency boosting.

## 9.6 Color Feature Detection: Classification of Color Structures

In Section 9.2, we showed that color models may contain a certain amount of invariance to the imaging process. From the taxonomy of color invariant models, shown in Table 9.1, we now discuss a classification framework to detect and classify local image structures based on photometrical and geometrical information [18]. The classification of local image structures (e.g., shadow versus material edges) is important for many image processing and computer vision tasks (e.g., object recognition, stereo vision, three-dimensional reconstruction).

By combining the differential structure and reflectance invariance of color images, local image structures are extracted and classified into one of the following types: shadow–geometry edges, corners, and T-junctions; highlight edges, corners, and T-junctions; and material edges, corners, and T-junctions. First, for detection, the differential nature of the local image structures is derived. Then, color invariant properties are taken into account to determine the reflectance characteristics of the detected local image structures. The geometrical and photometrical properties of these salient points (structures) are represented as vectors in a multidimensional feature space. Finally, a classifier is built to learn the specific characteristics of each class of image structures.

### 9.6.1 Combining Shape and Color

By combining geometrical and photometrical information, we are able to specify the physical nature of salient points. For example, to detect highlights, we need to use both a highlight invariant color space, and one or more highlight variant spaces. It was already shown in Table 9.1 that hue is invariant to highlights. Intensity $I$ and saturation $S$ are not invariant. Further, a highlight will yield a certain image shape: a local maximum ($I$) and a local minimum ($S$). These local structures are detected by differential operators as discussed in Section 9.2. Therefore, in the brightness image, we are looking for a local maximum.

The saturation at a highlight is lower than its surroundings, yielding a local minimum. Finally, for hue, the values will be near zero at that location. In this way, a five-dimensional feature vector is formed by combining the color space $HSI$ and the differential information on each location in an image.

The same procedure holds for the detection of shadow–geometry/highlight/material edges, corners, and T-junctions. The features used to detect shadow–geometry edges are first-order derivate applied on both the RGB and the $c_1c_2c_3$ color channels. Further, the second-order derivative is only applied on the RGB color image. To be precise, in this section, we use the curvature gauge to characterize local structures that are only characterized by their second-order structure. It is a coordinate system on which the Hessian becomes diagonal, yielding the $(p, q)$-coordinate system. The two eigenvectors of the Hessian are $\kappa_1$ and $\kappa_2$ and are defined by

$$\kappa_1 = f_{xx} + f_{yy} - \sqrt{(f_{xx} + f_{yy})^2 + 4f_{xy}^2} \tag{9.47}$$

$$\kappa_2 = f_{xx} + f_{yy} + \sqrt{(f_{xx} + f_{yy})^2 + 4f_{xy}^2} \tag{9.48}$$

To obtain the appropriate density distribution of feature values in feature space, classifiers are built to learn the density functions for shadow–geometry/highlight/material edges, corners, and T-junctions.

In this section, the learning-based classification approach is taken as proposed by Gevers and Aldershoff [19]. This approach is adaptive, as the underlying characteristics of image feature classes are determined by training. In fact, the probability density functions of the local image structures are learned by determining the probability that an image patch under consideration is of a particular class (e.g., edge, corner, or T-junctions). If two image patches share similar characteristics (not only the same color, but also the same gradient size, and curvature), both patches are represented by the same point in feature space. These points are represented by a $(n \times d)$-matrix, in which $d$ depends on the number of feature dimensions and $n$ on the number of training samples.

Then, the density function $p(\mathbf{x}|\omega)$ is computed, where $\mathbf{x}$ represents the data of the pixel under consideration, and $\omega$ is the class to be determined. From the data and training points, the parameters of the density function $p(\mathbf{x}|\omega)$ are estimated. We use a single Gaussian and multiple Gaussians (mixture of Gaussians [MoG]). Besides this, the $k$-nearest neighbor method is used.

### 9.6.2  Experimental Results

In this section, the results are given to classify the physical nature of salient points by learning. A separate set of tests is computed for each classifier (i.e., Gaussian, mixture of Gaussians, and $k$-nearest neighbor).

The images are recorded in three RGB colors with the aid of the SONY XC-003P CCD color camera (three chips) and the Matrox Magic Color frame grabber. Two light sources of average daylight color are used to illuminate the objects in the scene. The digitization was done in 8 bits per color. Three examples of the five images are shown in Figure 9.9a to Figure 9.9c. For all experiments, $\sigma = 2$ is used for the Gaussian smoothing parameter of the differential operators.

The classifiers are trained using all but one image. This last image is used as a test image. In this way, the test image is not used in the training set. In all experiments, a total of three Gaussian components is used for the MoG classifier, and $k = 3$ for the $k$-NN classifier.

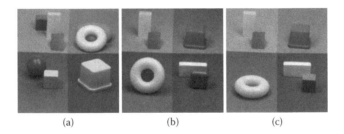

**FIGURE 9.9**
(a) Example image 1 (b) example image 2, and (c) example image 3. The images are recorded in three RGB-colors with the aid of the SONY XC-003P CCD color camera (three chips) and the Matrox Magic Color frame grabber. Two light sources of average daylight color are used to illuminate the objects in the scene.

### 9.6.3   Detection of Highlights

The features used for highlight detection are $\kappa_1$ and $\kappa_2$ applied on the *HSB* color channels yielding a five-dimensional space for each image point:

- **Gaussian:** The Gaussian method performs well to detect highlights, see Figure 9.10b. Most of the highlights are detected. However, only a few false positives are found (e.g., bar-shaped structures). This is because the reflectances at these structures are composed of a portion of specular reflection.

- **Mixture of Gaussians:** The MoG method gives slightly better results than the Gaussian method (see Figure 9.10c). For this method, the highlighted bars, found by the Gaussian method, are discarded.

- *k*-**Nearest neighbor:** This method performs slightly worse as opposed to the detection method based on a single Gaussian (see Figure 9.10d). The problem with the highlighted bars is still present.

- **Summary:** The detection methods based on a single Gaussian as well as on the MoG are well suited for highlight detection.

### 9.6.4   Detection of Geometry/Shadow Edges

The features that are used to detect geometry/shadow edges are the first-order derivatives applied on both the RGB and the $c_1c_2c_3$ color models. Further, the second-order derivative is applied on the RGB color images:

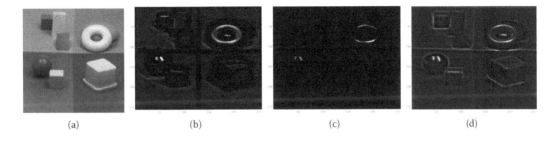

**FIGURE 9.10**
(a) Test image, (b) Gaussian classifier, (c) mixture of Gaussians, and (d) *k*-nearest neighbor. Based on the (training) efficiency and accuracy of the results, the Gaussian or MoG are most appropriate for highlight detection.

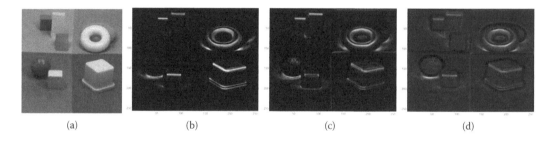

(a)                          (b)                          (c)                          (d)

**FIGURE 9.11**
(a) Test image, (b) Gaussian classifier, (c) mixture of Gaussians, and (d) *k*-nearest neighbor. For geometry–shadow detection, the best results are obtained by the Gaussian method. MoG and *k*-nearest neighbor perform a bit less.

- **Gaussian:** The detection method, based on a single Gaussian, performs well (see Figure 9.11b). Most of the geometry–shadow edges were detected. Further, there are nearly no false positives present. Besides that, the recall is very high.

- **Mixture of Gaussians:** The method based on a mixture of gaussians has similar performance as the Gaussian method (see Figure 9.11c). For a few instances, however, material edges are detected.

- *k*-**Nearest neighbor:** The accuracy of the method is somewhat lower than the other two classifiers (see Figure 9.11d). Still, most of the geometry and shadow edges are detected correctly.

- **Summary**: For geometry–shadow detection, the best results are obtained by the Gaussian method. MoG and *k*-nearest neighbor perform a bit less.

### 9.6.5   Detection of Corners

The first-order derivative ($f_w$) and second-order derivative ($f_{vv}$) of the RGB color space are used for corner learning and classification. To determine the thresholds for corner detection,

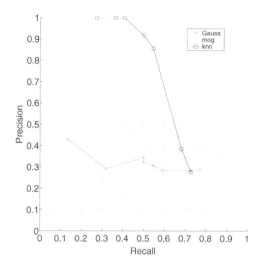

**FIGURE 9.12**
Precision/recall graph for the classifiers of corners.

**TABLE 9.3**

Classifiers and Their Performance for
Corner Detection

| Classifier | Precision | Recall |
|---|---|---|
| Gaussian | 34.9% | 56.6% |
| Mixture of Gaussians | 77.8% | 52.8% |
| $k$-Nearest neighbor | 83.9% | 58.5% |

various settings have been examined. The results are shown in Figure 9.12. The threshold providing the highest accuracy, and subsequently used in our experiments, is 0.75.

From Table 9.3, it is observed that the $k$-nearest neighbor classifier provides the highest performance. Examining the precision/recall graphs for the three classifiers reveals that this method provides good performance. Further, the MoG performs slightly better than the single Gaussian method.

The $k$-nearest neighbor classifier provides the best performance to detect corners. Although the recall of all three methods is similar, the precision of the $k$-NN classifier is higher.

## 9.7 Conclusion

In this chapter, we discussed methods and techniques in the field of color feature detection. In particular, the focus was on the following important issues: color invariance, combining derivatives, fusion of color models, color saliency boosting, and classifying image structures.

To this end, the dichromatic reflection model was outlined first. The dichromatic reflection model explains the RGB values variations due to the image formation process. From the model, various color models are obtained showing a certain amount of invariance. Then, color (invariant) derivatives were discussed. These derivatives include quasi-invariants that have proper noise and stability characteristics. To combine color derivatives into a single outcome, the color tensor was used instead of taking the sum or Euclidean distance. Tensors are convenient to describe color derivative vectors. Based on the color tensor, various image feature detection methods were introduced to extract locale image structures such as edges, corners, and circles. The experimental results of Canny color edge detection for several photometric quasi-invariants showed stable and accurate edge detection. Further, a proper model was discussed to select and weight color (invariant) models for discriminatory and robust image feature detection. The use of the fusion model is important, as there are many color invariant models available. In addition, we used color to express saliency. It was shown that after color saliency boosting, (less interesting) black-and-white structures in the image are ignored and more interesting color structures are detected. Finally, a classification framework was outlined to detect and classify local image structures based on photometrical and geometrical information. High classification accuracy is obtained by simple learning strategies.

In conclusion, this chapter provides a survey on methods solving important issues in the field of color feature detection. We hope that these solutions on low-level image feature detection will aid the continuing challenging task of handling higher-level computer vision tasks, such as object recognition and tracking.

## References

[1] R. Haralick and L. Shapiro, *Computer and Robot Vision*, Vol. II, Addison-Wesley, Reading, MA, 1992.

[2] C. Schmid, R. Mohr, and C. Bauckhage, Evaluation of interest point detectors, *Int. J. Comput. Vision*, 37, 2, 151–172, 2000.

[3] J. Shi and C. Tomasi, Good features to track, in *Proceedings of IEEE Conference on Computer Vision and Pattern Recognition*, Seattle, pp. 819–825, 1994.

[4] S. Di Zenzo, Note: A note on the gradient of a multi-image, *Comput. Vision, Graphics, and Image Process.*, 33, 1, 116–125, 1986.

[5] J. Bigun, Pattern recognition in images by symmetry and coordinate transformations, *Comput. Vision and Image Understanding*, 68, 3, 290–307, 1997.

[6] J. Bigun, G. Granlund, and J. Wiklund, Multidimensional orientation estimation with applications to texture analysis and optical flow, *IEEE Trans. on Patt. Anal. and Machine Intelligence*, 13, 8, 775–790, 1991.

[7] O. Hansen and J. Bigun, Local symmetry modeling in multi-dimensional images, *Patt. Recognition Lett.*, 13, 253–262, 1992.

[8] J. van de Weijer, L. van Vliet, P. Verbeek, and M. van Ginkel, Curvature estimation in oriented patterns using curvilinear models applied to gradient vector fields, *IEEE Trans. Patt. Anal. and Machine Intelligence*, 23, 9, 1035–1042, 2001.

[9] S. Shafer, Using color to seperate reflection components, *COLOR Res. Appl.*, 10, 210–218, Winter 1985.

[10] T. Gevers and H. Stokman, Robust histogram construction from color invariants for object recognition, *IEEE Trans. on Patt. Anal. and Machine Intelligence (PAMI)*, 26, 1, 113–118, 2004.

[11] T. Gevers and A. W. M. Smeulders, Color based object recognition, *Patt. Recognition*, 32, 453–464, March 1999.

[12] G. Klinker and S. Shafer, A physical approach to color image understanding, *Int. J. Comput. Vision*, 4, 7–38, 1990.

[13] J. Geusebroek, R. van den Boomgaard, A. Smeulders, and H. Geerts, Color invariance, *IEEE Trans. Patt. Anal. Machine Intelligence*, 23, 12, 1338–1350, 2001.

[14] J. van de Weijer, T. Gevers, and J. Geusebroek, Edge and corner detection by photometric quasi-invariants, *IEEE Trans. Patt. Anal. and Machine Intelligence*, 27, 4, 625–630, 2005.

[15] L. Itti, C. Koch, and E. Niebur, Computation modeling of visual attention, *Nat. Rev. Neuroscience*, 2, 194–203, March 2001, 365–372.

[16] J. van de Weijer and T. Gevers, Boosting color saliency in image feature detection, in *International Conference on Computer Vision and Pattern Recognition*, San Diego, CA, USA, pp. 365–372, 2005.

[17] J. van de Weijer, T. Gevers, and A. Bagdanov, Boosting color saliency in image feature detection, *IEEE Trans. Patt. Anal. and Machine Intelligence*, 28, 1, 150–156, 2006.

[18] T. Gevers and H. Stokman, Classification of color edges in video into shadow-geometry, highlight, or material transitions, *IEEE Trans. on Multimedia*, 5, 2, 237–243, 2003.

[19] T. Gevers and F. Aldershoff, Color feature detection and classification by learning, in *Proceedings IEEE International Conference on Image Processing (ICIP)*, Vol. II, pp. 714–717, 2005.

[20] J. van de Weijer, T. Gevers, and A. Smeulders, Robust photometric invariant features from the color tensor, *IEEE Trans. Image Process.*, 15, 1, 118–127, 2006.

[21] S.D. Zenzo, A note on the gradient of a multi-image, *Comput. Vision, Graphics, and Image Process.*, 33, 116–125, 1986.

[22] G. Sapiro and D.L. Ringach, Anisotropic diffusion of multivalued images with applications to color filtering, *IEEE Trans. Patt. Anal. and Machine Intelligence*, 5, 1582–1586, 1996.

[23] G. Sapiro and D. Ringach, Anisotropic diffusion of multivalued images with applications to color filtering, *IEEE Trans. Image Process.*, 5, 1582–1586, October 1996.

[24] C. Harris and M. Stephens, A combined corner and Manchester, UK edge detector, in *Proceedings of the Fourth Alvey Vision Conference*, Manchester, UK, Vol. 15, 1988, pp. 147–151.

[25] D.H. Ballard, Generalizing the Hough transform to detect arbitrary shapes, *Patt. Recognition*, 12, 111–122, 1981.

[26] H. Markowitz, Portfolio selection, *J. Finance*, 7, 1952.

[27] P. Wolfe, The simplex method for quadratic programming, *Econometrica*, 27, 1959.

[28] C. Gallery, www.corel.com.

# 10

# Color Spatial Arrangement for Image Retrieval by Visual Similarity

Stefano Berretti and Alberto Del Bimbo

## CONTENTS

## 10.1 Introduction

The rapid advancements in multimedia technology have increased the relevance that repositories of digital images are assuming in a wide range of information systems. Effective access to such archives requires that conventional searching techniques based on external textual keywords be complemented by content-based queries addressing appearing visual features of searched data [1], [2]. To this end, a number of models were experimented with that permit the representation and comparison of images in terms of quantitative indexes of visual features [3], [4], [5]. In particular, different techniques were identified and experimented with to represent the content of single images according to low-level features, such as color [6], [7], [8], texture [9], [10], shape [11], [12], [13], and structure [14], [15];

intermediate-level features of saliency [16], [17], [18] and spatial relationships [19], [20], [21], [22], [23]; or high-level traits modeling the semantics of image content [24], [25], [26]. In doing so, extracted features may either refer to the overall image (e.g., a color histogram), or to any subset of pixels constituting a spatial entity with some apparent visual cohesion in the user's perception. This can be the set of pixels constituting any object with high-level semantics, such as a character, a face, or a geographic landmark. Or it can be a set of pixels with low-level visual cohesion, induced by a common chrominance or texture, or by a common position within a predefined area of the image. As a limit case, the overall image can be regarded as a particular spatial entity.

Selecting the entities on which content representation should be based entails a trade-off between the significance of the model and the complexity of its creation: models containing high-level entities permit a closer fit to the users' expressive habits, but they also require some assistance in the archiving stage for the identification and the classification of significant entities.

Information associated with each entity generally combines a set of salient entity features, along with additional indexes that can be measured once the entity has been extracted: a high-level object is usually associated with a symbolic type [19], [27], an image region derived through a color-based segmentation is associated with a chromatic descriptor [28], and both of them can be associated with a measure of size, or with any other shape index [29], [30], [31]. When multiple entities are identified, the model may also capture information about their mutual spatial relationships. This can improve the effectiveness of retrieval by registering perceived differences and similarities that depend on the arrangement of entities rather than on their individual features. Relational information associated with multiple entities can capture high-level concepts, such as an action involving represented objects or spatial relationships between the pixel sets representing different entities. Relationships of the latter kind are most commonly employed in content-based image retrieval (CBIR) due to the possibility of deriving them automatically and to their capability of conveying a significant semantics.

In particular, image representations based on chromatic indexes have been widely experimented and comprise the basic backbone of most commercial and research retrieval engines, such as QBIC [32], Virage [33], VisualSeek [20], PickToSeek [34], BlobWorld [35], and SIMPLIcity [36], [37], to mention a few. This apparently depends on the capability of color-based models to combine robustness of automatic construction with a relative perceptual significance of the models.

However, despite the increased descriptive capability enabled by relational models that identify separate spatial entities, in the early and basic approaches, the chromatic content of the overall image has been represented by a global histogram. This is obtained by tessellating the (three-dimensional) space of colors into a finite set of reference parts, each associated with a bin representing the quantity of pixels with color that belongs to the part itself [38]. The similarity between two images is thus evaluated by comparing bins and their distribution [39]. In doing so, the evaluation of similarity does not account for the spatial arrangement and coupling of colors over the image. This plays a twofold role in the user's perception, serving to distinguish images with common colors and to perceive similarities between images with different colors but similar arrangements. To account for both these aspects, chromatic information must be associated with individual spatial entities identified over the image. According to this, integration of spatial descriptors and color has been addressed to extend the significance of color histograms with some index of spatial locality.

In early work [40], the image is partitioned into blocks along a fixed grid, and each block is associated with an individual local histogram. In this case, similarity matching also considers adjacency conditions among blocks with similar histograms. However, because blocks are created according to a static partitioning of the image, representation of spatial arrangement does not reflect the user-perceived patching of colors. In Reference [41], the spatial arrangement of the components of a color histogram is represented through color correlograms, capturing the distribution of distances between pixels belonging to different bins. In Reference [28], a picture is segmented into color sets and partitioned into a finite number of equally spaced slices. The spatial relationship between two color sets is modeled by the number of slices in which one color set is above the other. In Reference [31], the spatial distribution of a set of pixel blocks with common chromatic features is indexed by the two largest angles obtained in a Delaunay triangulation over the set of block centroids. Though quantitative, these methods still do not consider the actual extensions of spatial entities.

To overcome the limit, the image can be partitioned into entities collecting pixels with homogeneous chromatic content [42]. This can be accomplished through an automated segmentation process [43], [44], which clusters color histograms around dominating components, and then determines entities as image segments collecting connected pixels under common dominating colors [45], [46], [47], [48]. In general, few colors are sufficient to partition the histogram in cohesive clusters, which can be represented as a single average color without significant loss for the evaluation of similarity. However, color clusters may be split into several nonconnected image segments when they are back-projected from the color space to the image. This produces an exceedingly complex model, which clashes with the human capability to merge regions with common chromatic attributes. An effective solution to this problem was proposed in References [21], and [49], where weighted walkthroughs are proposed to quantitatively model spatial relationships between nonconnected clusters of color in the image plane. Following a different approach, in Reference [50], spatial color distribution is represented using local principal component analysis (PCA). The representation is based on image windows that are selected by a symmetry-based saliency map and an edge and corner detector. The eigenvectors obtained from local PCA of the selected windows form color patterns that capture both low and high spatial frequencies, so they are well suited for shape as well as texture representation.

To unify efforts aiming to define descriptors that effectively and efficiently capture the image content, the International Standards Organization (ISO) has developed the MPEG-7 standard, specifically designed for the description of multimedia content [51], [52], [53]. The standard focuses on the representation of descriptions and their encoding, so as to enable retrieval and browsing applications without specific ties to a single content provider. According to this, descriptors are standardized for different audiovisual features, such as dominant color, texture, object's contour shape, camera motion, and so forth. (All MPEG-7 descriptors are outlined in Reference [54].) This has permitted research efforts to focus mainly on optimization mechanisms rather than on the definition and extraction of the descriptors. In particular, CBIR applications have usefully exploited the features provided by the standard. For example, solutions like those proposed in References [55] and [56] have tried to combine MPEG-7 descriptors with relevance feedback mechanisms [57] in order to improve the performances of retrieval systems. In other works, because the MPEG-7 does not standardize ways whereby content descriptions should be compared, effective models for evaluating similarities among descriptors have been investigated [58].

In these approaches, chromatic descriptors are widely used. Specifically, MPEG-7 provides seven color descriptors, namely, *Color space, Color Quantization, Dominant Colors, Scalable Color, Color Layout, Color-Structure*, and *Group of Frames/Group of Pictures Color*. Among these, the color layout descriptor (CLD) and the color-structure descriptor (CSD) are capable of conveying spatial information of the image color distribution. The CSD provides information regarding color distribution as well as localized spatial color structure in the image. This is obtained by taking into account all colors in a structuring element of $8 \times 8$ pixels that slides over the image, instead of considering each pixel separately. Unlike the color histogram, this descriptor can distinguish between two images in which a given color is present in identical amounts, but where the structure of the groups of pixels having that color is different. Information carried out by the CSD are complemented using the CLD, which provides information about the color spatial distributions by dividing images into 64 blocks and extracting a representative color from each of the blocks to generate an $8 \times 8$ icon image. When regions are concerned, the region locator descriptor (RLD) can be used to enable region localization within images by specifying them with a brief and scalable representation of a box or a polygon.

However, these kinds of descriptors permit some information to be embedded on the spatial localization of color content into color histograms but may not be appropriate for capturing binary spatial relationships between complex spatial entities. For example, this is the case in which users are interested in retrieving images where several entities, identified either by high-level types or low-level descriptors, are mutually positioned according to a given pattern of spatial arrangement. Moreover, this difficulty is particularly evident in expressing spatial relationships between nonconnected entities.

In this chapter, we propose an original representation of the spatial arrangement of chromatic content that contributes to the state-of-the-art in two main respects. First, the color information is captured by partitioning the image space in color clusters collecting pixels with common chromatic attributes, regardless of their spatial distribution in separate segments. This improves perceptual robustness and facilitates matching and indexing. In particular, this avoids the excessive complexity of descriptions arising in segmenting images based on connected regions of homogeneous color. However, it also poses some major difficulties related to the spatial complexity of the projection of color clusters and to the consequent difficulty in representing their arrangement. To this end, as a second contribution of this work, we propose and expound a descriptor, called *weighted walkthroughs*, that is able to capture the binary directional relationship between two complex sets of pixels, and we embed it into a graph theoretical model. In fact, weighted walkthroughs enable a quantitative representation of the joint distribution of masses in two extended spatial entities. This relationship is quantified over the dense set of pixels that comprise the two entities, without reducing them to a minimum embedding rectangle or to a finite set of representative points. This improves the capability to discriminate perceptually different relationships and makes the representation applicable for complex and irregular-shaped entities. Matching a natural trait of vagueness in spatial perception, the relationship between extended entities is represented as the union of the primitive directions (the walkthroughs) which connect their individual pixels. The mutual relevance of different directions is accounted for by quantitative values (the weights) that enable the establishment of a quantitative metric of similarity. Breaking the limits of Boolean classification of symbolic models, this prevents classification discontinuities and improves the capability to assimilate perceptually similar cases. Weights are computed through an integral form that satisfies a main property of compositionality. This permits efficient computation of the relationships between two entities by linear combination of the relationships between their parts, which is not possible for models based on symbolic classification. This is the actual basis that permits us to ensure consistency in the quantitative weighting of spatial relationships and to deal with extended entities beyond the limits of the minimum embedding rectangle approximation.

A prototype retrieval engine is described, and experimental results are reported that indicate the performance of the proposed model with respect to a representation based on a global color histogram, and to a representation that uses centroids orientation to model spatial relationships between color clusters.

The rest of the chapter is organized into five sections and a conclusion. First, to evidence the innovative aspects of weighted walkthroughs, in the remainder of this section, we discuss previous work on modeling techniques for representation and comparison of spatial relationships as developed in the context of image databases (Section 10.1.1).

In Section 10.2, we introduce the representation of chromatic spatial arrangement based on color clusters and their mutual spatial relationships. In particular, we define weighted walkthroughs as original techniques for modeling spatial relationships and discuss their theoretical foundations and properties. Efficient derivation of weighted walkthroughs is expounded in Section 10.3. In Section 10.4, the image representation is cast to a graph theoretical model, and a graph matching approach for the efficient computation of image similarity is prospected. A retrieval engine based on this model is briefly described in Section 10.5. In Section 10.6, we report a two-stage evaluation of the effectiveness of the proposed model, focusing first on a benchmark of basic synthetic arrangements of three colors, and then on a database of real images. Finally, conclusions are drawn in Section 10.7.

### 10.1.1 Related Work on Modeling Techniques for Representing Spatial Relationships

Several different solutions have been practiced to model spatial relationships in image databases. In particular, at the higher level, representation structures for spatial relationships can be distinguished into object-based and relation-based structures.

The first group comprises those structures that treat spatial relationships and visual information as one inseparable entity. In these approaches, spatial relationships are not explicitly stored, but visual information is included in the representation. As a consequence, spatial relationships are retrieved examining objects coordinates. Object-based structures are based on space partitioning techniques that allow a spatial entity to be located in the space that it occupies. In that some of the data structures used for the indexing of $n$-dimensional points can also handle, in addition to points, spatial objects such as rectangles, polygons, or other geometric bodies, they are particularly suited to being employed as spatial access methods to localize spatial entities in an image. According to this, object-based representations rely on $R$-trees [59], $R^+$ [60], $R^*$ [61], and their variations [62], [63]. $R$-trees are commonly used to represent the spatial arrangement of rectangular regions and are probably the most popular spatial representation, due to their easy implementation. $R$-trees are particularly effective for searching points or regions. $R^+$ and $R^*$ trees are improvements of the $R$-tree based on different philosophies. Applications exploiting the spatial properties of these representations have been used mainly in the context of geographical information systems (GISs).

Structures in the second category do not include visual information and preserve only a set of spatial relationships, discarding all uninteresting relationships. Objects are represented symbolically, and spatial relationships explicitly. These approaches may address topological set-theoretical concepts (e.g., inclusion, adjacency, or distance) [64], [65] or directional constructs (e.g., above or below) [19], [66], [67], [68]. In both cases, relationships can be interpreted over a finite set of predefined (symbolic) classes [65], [66], or they can be associated with numeric descriptors taking values in dense spaces [19], [64]. The latter approach enables the use of distance functions that change with continuity and avoid classification thresholds, thus making them better able to cope with the requirements of retrieval by visual similarity [21], [69].

In Reference [64], the topological relationship between pixel sets is encoded by the emptiness/nonemptiness of the intersections between their inner, border, and outer parts. In Reference [65], this approach is extended to the nine-intersection model, so as to allow the representation of topological relationships between regions, lines, and points. Each object is represented as a point set with an interior region, a boundary, and an exterior region. The topological relationship between two objects is described considering the nine possible intersections of their interior, boundary, and exterior.

In References [67], [68], and [70], the directional relationship between point-like objects is encoded in terms of the relative quadrants in which the two points are lying. Directional relationships are usually the strict relationships north, south, east, and west. To these are often added the mixed directional relationships northeast, northwest, southeast, and southwest. Other solutions consider the positional directional relationships: left, right, above, and below. Developing on this model, directional spatial relationships are extended to the case of points and lines in Reference [71], while in Reference [72], direction relations for crisp regions are proposed. Generalization of the directional model to regions with broad boundaries is considered in Reference [73].

In the theory of symbolic projection, which underlies a large part of the literature on image retrieval by spatial similarity, both directional and topological relationships between the entities in a two-dimensional (2-D) scene are reduced to the composition of the qualitative ordering relationships among their projections on two reference axes [27], [66]. In the original formulation [66], spatial entities are assimilated to points (usually the centroids) to avoid overlapping and to ensure a total and transitive ordering of the projections on each axis. This permits the encoding of the bidimensional arrangement of a set of entities into a sequential structure, the 2-D-string, which reduces matching from quadratic to linear complexity. However, this point-like representation loses soundness when entities have a complex shape or when their mutual distances are small with respect to individual dimensions. Much work has been done around this model to account for the extent of spatial entities, trading the efficiency of match for the sake of representation soundness. In the 2-DG-string and the 2-DC-string, entities are cut into subparts with disjoint convex hulls [74], [75]. In the 2-D-B string [76], [77], the mutual arrangement of spatial entities is represented in terms of the interval ordering of the projections on two reference axes. Because projections on different axes are independent, the representation subtends the assimilation of objects to their minimum embedding rectangles, which largely reduces the capability to discriminate perceptually distant arrangements. In References [78] and [79], this limit is partially smoothed by replacing extended objects through a finite set of representative points. In particular, in Reference [78], the directional relationship between two entities is interpreted as the union of the primitive directions (up, up-right, right, down-right, down, down-left, left, up-left, coincident), capturing the displacement between any of their respective representative points.

In general, the effectiveness of qualitative models is basically limited by inherent Boolean classification thresholds that determine discontinuities between perceived spatial arrangements and their representation. This hurdles the establishment of quantitative metrics of similarity and basically limits the robustness of comparison. These limits of Boolean matching are faced in quantitative models by associating spatial relationships with numeric values, which enables the evaluation of a continuous distance between nonexact matching arrangements. In the most common approach, directional information is represented through the orientation of the line connecting object centroids [19], [80]. This type of representation inherently requires that extended entities be replaced by a single representative point used to take the measure of orientation. This still limits the capability to distinguish perceptually dissimilar configurations. Representations based on directional histograms have partially solved this limit [81], [82], [83]. The approach in Reference [81] avoids assimilating an object to representative points, like the centroid, or to the minimum bounding rectangle, by computing the histogram of angles between any two points in both the objects. This histogram, normalized by the maximum frequency, represents the directional relationship between the two objects. In Reference [82], histograms are extended to consider pairs of longitudinal sections instead of pairs of points. In this way, it is possible to exploit the power of integral calculus to ensure the processing of raster data as well as of vector data, explicitly considering both angular and metric information. Instead, in Reference [83], the histogram of angles is modified by incorporating both angles and labeled distances. The set of angles from any pixel on the boundaries of two spatial entities expresses their directional relationships. In summary, these angle histogram approaches provide quantitative representation of directional relationships, but they do not provide explicit metric (distance) information and do not support the extraction of topological spatial relationships like "inside" or "overlap."

## 10.2   Modeling Spatial Arrangements of Color

Using a clustering process [84], the color histogram of an image can be partitioned into a few cohesive clusters, which can be effectively represented by their average color without significant loss of information for the evaluation of similarity. In general, using the CIE $L^*u^*v^*$ color space for color representation, we found that a number of clusters not higher than 8, at most 16, is definitely sufficient to maintain a nonambiguous association between an image and its reduced representation, in which colors are replaced by the average value of their cluster. However, in the backprojection from the color space to the image, each color cluster may be split into several nonmutually connected image segments. This produces an exceedingly complex model, that does not reflect the human capability to merge multiple regions with common chromatic attributes (see Figure 10.1a).

  To overcome the limitation, we consider the pixels of each color cluster as a single spatial entity, regardless of their spatial distribution and of their connection in the image space (see Figure 10.1b). The entity is associated with the triple of $L^*u^*v^*$ normalized coordinates of the average color in the cluster. Clusters are also associated with their number of pixels, even if this has only a limited significance due to the capability of the clustering algorithm to produce sets with an approximately equal number of pixels.

### 10.2.1   Representing Spatial Relationships between Color Clusters

The spatial layout of color clusters is usually complex: color clusters are usually not connected; their mutual distances may be small with respect to their dimensions; and they may be tangled in a complex arrangement evading any crisp classification. These

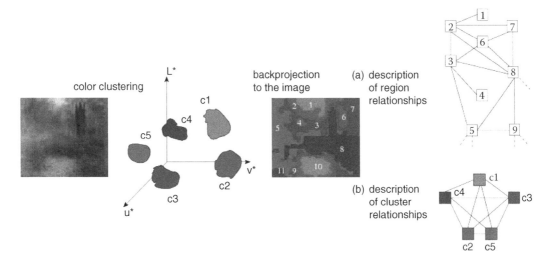

**FIGURE 10.1**

Pixels are grouped in the color space by using chromatic similarity, so that image content is effectively partitioned into a few clusters. (a) Backprojection in the image space results in a high number of separated segments, yielding an exceedingly complex model for the image. (b) All the pixels obtained from the backprojection of a common cluster are collected within a single entity in the image space.

complexities cannot be effectively managed using conventional spatial descriptors based on centroids or embedding rectangles. To overcome the limit, spatial relationships between color clusters are represented with weighted walkthroughs [21]. In the rest of this subsection, we further develop the original model of weighted walkthroughs to fit the requirements of retrieval by color similarity.

### 10.2.1.1 Weighted Walkthroughs

In a Cartesian reference system, a point $a$ partitions the plane into four quadrants: upper-left, upper-right, lower-left, and lower-right. These quadrants can be encoded by an index pair $< i, j >$, with $i$ and $j$ taking values $\pm 1$. In this perspective, the directional relationship between the point $a$ and an extended set $B$, can be represented by the number of points of $B$ that are located in each of the four quadrants. This results in four weights $w_{\pm 1, \pm 1}(a, B)$ that can be computed with an integral measure on the set of points of $B$:

$$w_{i,j}(a, B) = \frac{1}{|B|} \int_B C_i(x_b - x_a) C_j(y_b - y_a) \, dx_b dy_b \tag{10.1}$$

where $|B|$ denotes the area of $B$ and acts as dimensional normalization factor $\langle x_a, y_a \rangle$ and $\langle x_b, y_b \rangle$, respectively, denote the coordinates of the point $a$, and of points $b \in B$ (see Figure 10.2). The terms $C_{\pm 1}(\cdot)$ denote the characteristic functions of the positive and negative real semi-axes $(0, +\infty)$ and $(-\infty, 0)$, respectively. In particular, $C_{\pm 1}(t)$ are defined in the following way:

$$C_{-1}(t) = \begin{cases} 1 & \text{if } t < 0 \\ 0 & \text{otherwise} \end{cases} \qquad C_1(t) = \begin{cases} 1 & \text{if } t > 0 \\ 0 & \text{otherwise} \end{cases} \tag{10.2}$$

where, according to Equation 10.1, $t = x_b - x_a$ for $C_i(\cdot)$, and $t = y_b - y_a$ for $C_j(\cdot)$.

The model can be directly extended to represent the directional relationship between two extended sets of points $A$ and $B$, by averaging the relationships between the individual points of $A$ and $B$:

$$w_{i,j}(A, B) = \frac{1}{|A||B|} \int_A \int_B C_i(x_b - x_a) C_j(y_b - y_a) \, dx_b dy_b dx_a dy_a \tag{10.3}$$

In doing so, the four-tuple $w(A, B)$ provides a measure of the number of pairs of points in $A$ and $B$ that have a displacement that falls within each of the four directional relationships: $w_{1,1}$ evaluates the number of point pairs $a \in A$ and $b \in B$ such that $b$ is upper-right from $a$;

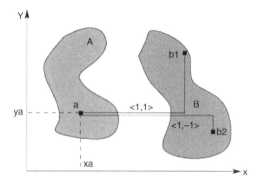

**FIGURE 10.2**
Walkthroughs connecting the point $a \in A$, to two points $b_1, b_2 \in B$. Because $b_1$ is in the upper-right quadrant of $a$, it contributes to the weight $w_{1,1}$. Being $b_2$ in the lower-right quadrant of $a$, it contributes to the weight $w_{1,-1}$.

in a similar manner, $w_{-1,1}$ evaluates the number of point pairs such that $b$ is upper-left from $a$; $w_{1,-1}$ evaluates the number of point pairs such that $b$ is lower-right from $a$; and $w_{-1,-1}$ evaluates the number of point pairs such that $b$ is lower-left from $a$.

### 10.2.1.2  Properties of Weighted Walkthroughs

Because the functions $C_{\pm1}(\cdot)$ are positive defined, and due to the normalization factor in Equation 10.3, the four weights $w_{i,j}$ are adimensional positive numbers. They are also antisymmetric, that is, $w_{i,j}(A, B) = w_{-i,-j}(B, A)$:

$$\int_A \int_B C_i(x_b - x_a)C_j(y_b - y_a)\, dx_b dy_b\, dx_a dy_a = \int_A \int_B C_{-i}(x_a - x_b)C_{-j}(y_a - y_b)\, dx_b dy_b\, dx_a dy_a$$

as a direct consequence of Equation 10.3, and the antisymmetric property of characteristic functions (i.e., $C_{\pm1}(t) = C_{\mp1}(-t)$).

In addition, weighted walkthroughs between two sets $A$ and $B$ are invariant with respect to shifting and zooming of the two sets:

$$w_{i,j}(\alpha A + \beta, \alpha B + \beta) = w_{i,j}(A, B)$$

Shift invariance descends from the fact that $w_{i,j}(A, B)$ is a relative measure (i.e., it depends on the displacement between points in $A$ and $B$ rather than on their absolute position). Scale invariance derives from integration linearity and from the scale invariance of characteristic functions $C_{\pm1}(\cdot)$.

More importantly, weights inherit from the integral operator of Equation 10.3 a major property of compositionality, by which the weights between $A$ and the union $B_1 \cup B_2$ can be derived by linear combination of the weights between $A$ and $B_1$, and between $A$ and $B_2$:

*THEOREM 10.2.1*
For any point set $A$, and for any two disjoint point sets $B_1$ and $B_2$ (i.e., $B_1 \cap B_2 = \varnothing$, and $B_1 \cup B_2 = B$):

$$w_{i,j}(A, B) = w_{i,j}(A, B_1 \cup B_2) = \frac{|B_1|}{|B_1 \cup B_2|}w_{i,j}(A, B_1) + \frac{|B_2|}{|B_1 \cup B_2|}w_{i,j}(A, B_2) \qquad (10.4)$$

**PROOF**  From Equation 10.3 directly descends

$$w_{i,j}(A, B_1 \cup B_2) \cdot |A| \cdot |B_1 \cup B_2| = \int_A \int_{B_1 \cup B_2} C_i(x_b - x_a)C_j(y_b - y_a)dx_b dy_b dx_a dy_a$$

$$= \int_A \int_{B_1} C_i(x_b - x_a)C_j(y_b - y_a)dx_b dy_b dx_a dy_a$$

$$+ \int_A \int_{B_2} C_i(x_b - x_a)C_j(y_b - y_a)dx_b dy_b dx_a dy_a$$

$$= w_{i,j}(A, B_1) \cdot |A| \cdot |B_1| + w_{i,j}(A, B_2) \cdot |A| \cdot |B_2|$$

and dividing both sides by the term $|A| \cdot |B_1 \cup B_2|$, the thesis of the theorem follows.  ∎

The property of compositionality permits the derivation of the four-dimensional integral of Equation 10.3 through the linear combination of a number of terms corresponding to subintegrals taken over elementary domains for which the weights can be easily computed in closed form. In particular, the four-tuple of weighted walkthroughs can be easily computed over rectangular domains. For example, the weight $w_{1,1}$ between two rectangular

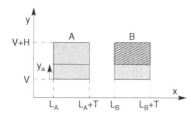

**FIGURE 10.3**
Determination of $w_{1,1}(A, B)$.

entities with projections that are disjoint along the $X$ axis and perfectly aligned along the $Y$ axis, is computed as follows:

$$w_{11}(A, B) = \frac{1}{T^2 H^2} \int_A \int_B C_1(x_b - x_a) C_1(y_b - y_a) dx_b dy_b dx_a dy_a$$

$$= \frac{1}{T^2 H^2} \int_{L_A}^{L_A+T} dx_a \int_{L_B}^{L_B+T} dx_b \int_V^{V+H} \int_{y_a}^{V+H} dy_b dy_a$$

$$= \frac{T^2}{T^2 H^2} \int_V^{V+H} [V + H - y_a] dy_a = \frac{1}{H^2} \left[ (V + H) y_a - \frac{y_a^2}{2} \right]_V^{V+H} = \frac{1}{2}$$

where, as shown in Figure 10.3, the integration domain along the $y$ dimension of $B$ is limited to the set of points such that $yb > ya$, $\forall y_a \in A$. Similar computations permit the derivation of the weights $w_{i,j}$ among rectangular domains arranged in the nine basic cases (Figure 10.4a and Figure 10.4b) that represent the possible relationships occurring between two elementary rectangles. This has particular relevance in the context of a digital image with a discrete domain, constituted by individual pixels, that can be regarded as a grid of elementary rectangular elements. In this way, the discrete case can be managed by using the results derived in the continuous domain for the basic elements.

Based on the property of compositionality, and the existence of a restricted set of arrangements between basic elements, if $A$ and $B$ are approximated by any multirectangular shape (see Figure 10.5a), their relationship can be computed by exploiting Equation 10.4 on rectangular domains. According to this, the property of compositionality is used in the computation of weighted walkthroughs between two color regions $A$ and $B$ (see

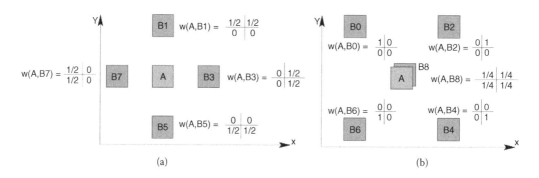

**FIGURE 10.4**
The tuples of weights for the nine basic arrangements between rectangular entities. The weights are represented as elements of a two-by-two matrix. (a) Projections of two rectangular entities are aligned along one of the coordinate axes; and (b) disjoint projections and perfect overlap of rectangular entities.

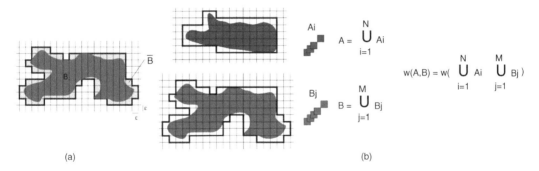

(a)                                                              (b)

**FIGURE 10.5**
(a) Entity $B$ is approximated by the minimum embedding multirectangle $\bar{B}$ made up of elements of size $\epsilon \times \epsilon$; and (b) Computation of weighted walkthroughs between $A$ and $B$ is reduced to that of a set of rectangular parts arranged in the nine reference positions.

Figure 10.5b), as well as in the composition of relationships between multiple regions within the same color cluster (Figure 10.6).

Finally, it can be observed that the sum of the four weights is equal to one in each of the nine basic cases. As a consequence, the four weights undergo to the following bound:

*THEOREM 10.2.2*
For any two multirectangular pixel sets $A$ and $B$, the sum of the four weights is equal to 1:

$$\sum_{i=\pm 1}\sum_{j=\pm 1} w_{i,j}(A, B) = 1 \tag{10.5}$$

**PROOF** Demonstration runs by induction on the set of rectangles that composes $A$ and $B$. By the property of compositionality (Theorem 10.2.1), for any partition of $B$ in two disjoint subparts $B_1$ and $B_2$, the coefficients of $w(A, B)$ can be expressed as

$$w_{i,j}(A, B) = \frac{|B_1|}{|B_1 \cup B_2|} w_{i,j}(A, B_1) + \frac{|B_2|}{|B_1 \cup B_2|} w_{i,j}(A, B_2)$$

Because this is a convex combination, that is,

$$\frac{|B_1|}{|B_1 \cup B_2|} + \frac{|B_2|}{|B_1 \cup B_2|} = 1$$

coefficients of $w(A, B)$ are a convex combination of coefficients of $w(A, B_1)$ and $w(A, B_2)$, respectively, and so is also the sum of the coefficients themselves. This implies that, by

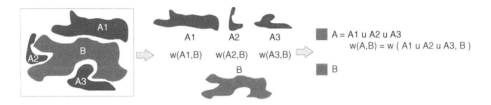

**FIGURE 10.6**
Property of compositionality applied to the relationship between the nonconnected color cluster $A$ (composed of segments A1, A2 and A3) and the color cluster $B$ (composed of one segment).

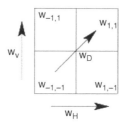

**FIGURE 10.7**
Directional indices.

recursive decomposition of $A$ and $B$, the sum of the coefficients of $w(A, B)$ is a convex combination of the sum of the coefficients of the weighted walkthroughs between elementary rectangles mutually arranged in the basic cases.

In all the basic cases of Figure 10.4a and Figure 10.4b, the sum of weights is equal to 1. This implies that any convex combination of the sum of the coefficients of the weighted walkthroughs among any set of elementary rectangles mutually arranged in the basic cases is equal to 1.  ■

### 10.2.1.3  Distance between Weighted Walkthroughs

Because the four weights have a sum equal to 1, they can be replaced, without loss of information, with three directional indexes, taking values within 0 and 1 (Figure 10.7):

$$
\begin{aligned}
w_H(A, B) &= w_{1,1}(A, B) + w_{1,-1}(A, B) \\
w_V(A, B) &= w_{-1,1}(A, B) + w_{1,1}(A, B) \\
w_D(A, B) &= w_{-1,-1}(A, B) + w_{1,1}(A, B)
\end{aligned}
\tag{10.6}
$$

In doing so, $w_H(A, B)$ and $w_V(A, B)$ account for the degree by which $B$ is on the right, and up of $A$, respectively; $w_D(A, B)$ accounts for the degree by which $A$ and $B$ are aligned along the diagonal direction of the Cartesian reference system.

In order to compare spatial arrangements occurring between two pairs of spatial entities, the three directional indexes are used. In particular, we experimentally found that a city-block distance constructed on the indices provides effective results in terms of discrimination accuracy between different arrangements. According to this, composition of differences in homologous directional indexes is used as the metric of dissimilarity $\mathcal{D}_S$ for the relationships between two pairs of entities $\langle A, B \rangle$, and $\langle \bar{A}, \bar{B} \rangle$ represented by weights tuples $w$ and $\bar{w}$:

$$
\begin{aligned}
\mathcal{D}_S(w, \bar{w}) &= \alpha_H \cdot |w_H - \bar{w}_H| + \alpha_V \cdot |w_V - \bar{w}_V| + \alpha_D \cdot |w_D - \bar{w}_D| \\
&= \alpha_H \cdot d_H(w, \bar{w}) + \alpha_V \cdot d_V(w, \bar{w}) + \alpha_D \cdot d_D(w, \bar{w})
\end{aligned}
\tag{10.7}
$$

where $\alpha_H$, $\alpha_V$, and $\alpha_D$ are a convex combination (i.e., they are nonnegative numbers with sum equal to 1), and $d_H$, $d_V$, and $d_D$ are the distance components evaluated on the three directional indexes of Equation 10.6. In our framework, we experimentally found that better results are achieved by equally weighting the three distance components ($\alpha_H = \alpha_V = \alpha_D = 1/3$). Due to the city-block structure, $\mathcal{D}_S$ is nonnegative ($\mathcal{D}_S \geq 0$), autosimilar ($\mathcal{D}_S(w, \bar{w}) = 0$ iff $w = \bar{w}$), symmetric ($\mathcal{D}_S(w, \bar{w}) = \mathcal{D}_S(\bar{w}, w)$) and triangular (for any three weights tuples $w, \bar{w}, \hat{w}$: $\mathcal{D}_S(w, \bar{w}) \leq \mathcal{D}_S(w, \hat{w}) + \mathcal{D}_S(\hat{w}, \bar{w})$). In addition, $\mathcal{D}_S$ is normal (i.e., $\mathcal{D}_S \in [0, 1]$) as a consequence of the bound existing on the sum of the weights (Theorem 10.2.2). As an example, Figure 10.8 shows the distance computation between two spatial arrangements.

Weights also satisfy a basic property of continuity by which small changes in the shape or arrangement of entities result in small changes of their relationships. This results in the following theorem for the distance between spatial arrangements:

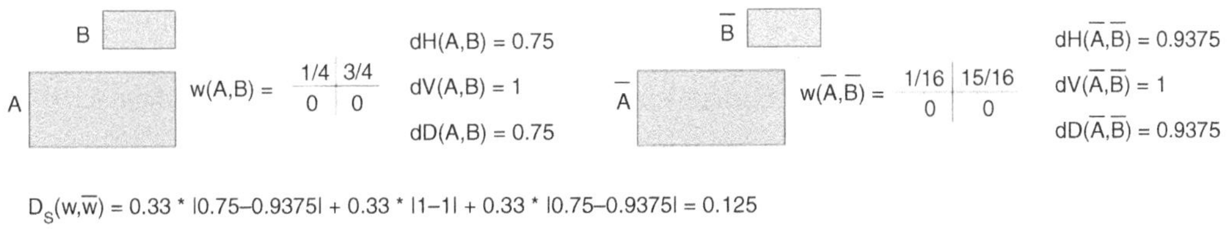

B
A
w(A,B) =
1/4 3/4
0 0
dH(A,B) = 0.75
dV(A,B) = 1
dD(A,B) = 0.75
B̄
Ā
w(Ā,B̄) =
1/16 15/16
0 0
dH(Ā,B̄) = 0.9375
dV(Ā,B̄) = 1
dD(Ā,B̄) = 0.9375
Ds(w,w̄) = 0.33 * |0.75–0.9375| + 0.33 * |1–1| + 0.33 * |0.75–0.9375| = 0.125


**FIGURE 10.8**
Spatial distance $\mathcal{D}_S$ between two pairs of entities $\langle A, B\rangle$ and $\langle \bar{A}, \bar{B}\rangle$.

*THEOREM 10.2.3*
Let $A$ and $B$ be a pair of pixel sets, and let $\bar{B}$ be the minimum multirectangular extension of $B$ on a grid of size $\epsilon$ (see Figure 10.5a). Let $B_\epsilon$ denote the difference between $\bar{B}$ and $B$ (i.e., $\bar{B} = B \cup B_\epsilon$ and $B \cap B_\epsilon = \oslash$). The distance $\mathcal{D}_S(w(A, B), w(A, \bar{B}))$ between the walkthroughs capturing the relationships between $A$ and $B$, and between $A$ and $\bar{B}$ undergoes the following bound:

$$\mathcal{D}_S(w(A, B), w(A, \bar{B})) \leq \frac{B_\epsilon}{\bar{B}} \tag{10.8}$$

**PROOF** Separate bounds are derived for the three distance components $d_H$, $d_V$, and $d_D$. By the property of compositionality (Theorem 10.2.1), $d_H(w(A, B), w(A, \bar{B}))$ can be decomposed as

$$\begin{aligned} d_H(w(A, B), w(A, \bar{B})) &= |(w_{1,1}(A, B) + w_{1,-1}(A, B)) - (w_{1,1}(A, \bar{B}) + w_{1,-1}(A, \bar{B}))| \\ &= |(w_{1,1}(A, B) + w_{1,-1}(A, B)) - \left(\frac{B}{\bar{B}}(w_{1,1}(A, B) + w_{1,-1}(A, B) \right. \\ &\quad \left. + \frac{B_\epsilon}{\bar{B}}(w_{1,1}(A, B_\epsilon) + w_{1,-1}(A, B_\epsilon))\right)| \\ &= \frac{B_\epsilon}{\bar{B}}|(w_{1,1}(A, B) + w_{1,-1}(A, B)) - (w_{1,1}(A, B_\epsilon) + w_{1,-1}(A, B_\epsilon))| \\ &= \frac{B_\epsilon}{\bar{B}} d_H(w(A, B), w(A, B_\epsilon)) \end{aligned}$$

which, by the normality of $d_H(\cdot)$, yields

$$d_H(w(A, B), w(A, \bar{B})) \leq \frac{B_\epsilon}{\bar{B}}$$

The same estimate can be applied to $d_V(w(A, B), w(A, \bar{B}))$ and $d_D(w(A, B), w(A, \bar{B}))$, from which the thesis of the theorem follows. ■

## 10.3 Efficient Computation of Weights

In the straightforward approach, if $A$ and $B$ are decomposed in $N$ and $M$ rectangles, respectively, the four weights of their directional relationship can be computed by repetitive composition of the relationships between the $N$ parts of $A$ and the $M$ parts of $B$:

$$w(A, B) = w\left(\bigcup_{n=1}^{N} A_n, \bigcup_{m=1}^{M} B_m\right) = \frac{1}{|A||B|}\sum_{n=1}^{N}|A_n|\sum_{m=1}^{M}|B_m| \cdot w(A_n, B_m) \tag{10.9}$$

If component rectangles of $A$ and $B$ are cells of a regular grid partitioning the entire picture, each elementary term $w(A_n, B_m)$ is one of the four-tuples associated with the nine basic arrangements of Figure 10.4a and Figure 10.4b. This permits the computation of $w(A, B)$ in time $O(N \cdot M)$.

A more elaborate strategy permits the derivation of the relationship with a complexity that is linear in the number of cells contained in the intersection of the bounding rectangles of the two entities. This is expounded in the rest of this section.

### 10.3.1 Representation of Spatial Entities

We assume that each entity is approximated as a set of rectangular cells taken over a regular grid partitioning the entire picture along the horizontal and vertical directions of the Cartesian reference system. The set of cells comprising each entity is partitioned in any number of segments. Each of these segments is assumed to be connected, but not necessarily maximal with respect to the property of the connection (as an example, in Figure 10.6, the nonconnected entity $A$ is decomposed into the three connected segments $A_1$, $A_2$, and $A_3$). Here, we expound the representation of segments and the computation of their mutual relationships. Relationships between the union of multiple segments are derived by direct application of the property of compositionality (Equation 10.4). The following clauses illustrate the derivation:

$$
\begin{aligned}
WW_{i,j}^{0,0} &= 1 \quad \text{if the cell } \langle i, j \rangle \text{ is part of } A \\
&\quad\ 0 \quad \text{otherwise} \\
WW_{i,j}^{-1,0} &= 0 \quad \text{if } j = 0 \text{ (i.e., } j \text{ is the leftmost column of } A) \\
&\quad\ WW_{i,j-1}^{-1,0} + WW_{i,j}^{0,0} \quad \text{otherwise} \\
WW_{i,j}^{1,0} &= \text{is derived by scanning the row } i \text{ if } j = 0 \\
&\quad\ WW_{i,j-1}^{1,0} - WW_{i,j}^{0,0} \quad \text{otherwise} \\
WW_{i,j}^{0,-1} &= 0 \quad \text{if } i = 0 \text{ (i.e., } i \text{ is the lowermost row of } A) \\
&\quad\ WW_{i-1,j}^{0,-1} + WW_{i-1,j}^{0,0} \quad \text{otherwise} \\
WW_{i,j}^{0,1} &= \text{is derived by scanning the column } j \text{ if } i = 0 \\
&\quad\ WW_{i-1,j}^{0,1} - WW_{i,j}^{0,0} \quad \text{otherwise} \\
WW_{i,j}^{-1,1} &= 0 \quad \text{if } j = 0 \\
&\quad\ WW_{i,j-1}^{-1,1} + WW_{i,j-1}^{0,1} \quad \text{otherwise} \\
WW_{i,j}^{-1,-1} &= 0 \quad \text{if } i = 0 \text{ or } j = 0 \\
&\quad\ WW_{i,j-1}^{-1,-1} + WW_{i,j-1}^{0-1} \quad \text{otherwise} \\
WW_{i,j}^{1,-1} &= 0 \quad \text{if } i = 0 \\
&\quad\ WW_{i-1,j}^{1,-1} + WW_{i-1,j}^{1,0} \quad \text{otherwise} \\
WW_{i,j}^{1,1} &= N - WW_{i,j}^{0,0} - WW_{i,j}^{0,1} - WW_{i,j}^{1,0} \quad \text{if } j = 0 \text{ and } i = 0 \\
&\quad\ WW_{i,j-1}^{1,1} - WW_{i,j}^{0,0} - WW_{i,j}^{0,1} \quad \text{if } j = 0 \text{ and } i > 0 \\
&\quad\ WW_{i-1,j}^{1,1} - WW_{i,j}^{0,0} - WW_{i,j}^{1,0} \quad \text{if } j > 0
\end{aligned}
\tag{10.10}
$$

Each segment $A$ is represented by a data structure that encompasses the following information: the number of cells of $A$, and the indexes $\langle i_l, j_l \rangle$ and $\langle i_u, j_r \rangle$ of the cells of the lower-left and of the upper-right corners of the bounding rectangle of $A$. The segment $A$ is also associated with a matrix $WW$ with size equal to the number of cells in the bounding rectangle of $A$, which associates each cell $\langle i, j \rangle$ in the bounding rectangle of A with a nine-tuple $WW_{i,j}$ that encodes the number of cells of $A$ in each of the nine directions centered in the cell $\langle i, j \rangle$: $WW_{i,j}^{0,0}$ is equal to 1 if the cell $\langle i, j \rangle$ is part of A, and it is equal to zero otherwise; $WW_{i,j}^{1,0}$ is the number of cells of $A$ that are on the right of cell $\langle i, j \rangle$ (i.e., the number of cells of $A$ with indexes $\langle i, k \rangle$ such that $k > j$); in a similar manner, $WW_{i,j}^{-1,0}$ is the number of cells of $A$

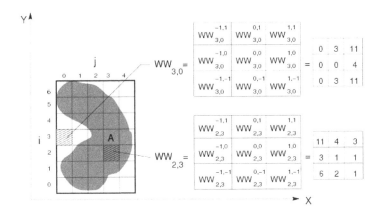

**FIGURE 10.9**
Examples of the data structure $WW$, computed for the cells $\langle 3, 0 \rangle$ and $\langle 2, 3 \rangle$ of the bounding rectangle enclosing the entity $A$.

that are on the left of $\langle i, j \rangle$, while $WW_{i,j}^{0,1}$ and $WW_{i,j}^{0,-1}$ are the number of cells of $A$ over and below cell $\langle i, j \rangle$, respectively; finally, $WW_{i,j}^{1,1}$ is the number of cells of $A$ that are upper-right from $\langle i, j \rangle$ (i.e., the cells of $A$ with indexes $\langle h, k \rangle$ such that $h > i$ and $k > j$). In a similar manner, $WW_{i,j}^{1,-1}$, $WW_{i,j}^{-1,-1}$ and $WW_{i,j}^{-1,1}$ are the numbers of cells of $A$ that are lower-right, lower-left, and upper-left from the cell $\langle i, j \rangle$, respectively. Figure 10.9 shows the $WW$ matrix computed for two cells of the bounding rectangle of an entity $A$.

The matrix $WW$ of the segment $A$ is derived in linear time with respect to the number of cells in the bounding rectangle of $A$. To this end, the elements of the matrix are computed starting from the lower-left corner, covering the matrix by rows and columns. In doing so, the nine coefficients associated with any cell $\langle i, j \rangle$ can be derived by relying on the coefficients of the cells $\langle i - 1, j \rangle$ (lower adjacent), and $\langle i, j - 1 \rangle$ (left adjacent).

In the overall derivation, a constant time $O(1)$ is spent for evaluating coefficients of each cell; thus requiring a total cost $O(L_A \cdot H_A)$, where $L_A$ and $H_A$ are the numbers of columns and rows of the bounding box of $A$, respectively. In addition, the entire column of each cell in the first row, and the entire row of each cell in the first column must be scanned, with a total cost $O(2 \cdot L_A \cdot H_A)$. According to this, the total complexity for the derivation of the overall matrix $WW$ is linear in the number of cells in the bounding rectangle of $A$.

## 10.3.2 Computation of the Four Weights

Given two segments $A$ and $B$, the four weights of their relationship are computed from the respective descriptions, in a way that depends on the intersection between the projections of $A$ and $B$ on the Cartesian reference axes:

- If the projections of $A$ and $B$ have null intersections on both the axes, then the descriptor has only a nonnull weight (and this weight is equal to 1) that is derived in constant time (see Figure 10.4b).

- If the projections of $A$ and $B$ on the $Y$ axis have a nonnull intersection, but the projections on the $X$ axis are disjoints (see, for example, Figure 10.10), then the descriptor has two null elements and is determined with complexity $O(H_{AB})$, where $H_{AB}$ is the number of cells by which the projections intersect along the $Y$ axis. Of course, the complementary case that the projections of $A$ and $B$ have nonnull intersection along the $X$ axis is managed in the same manner.

    We expound here the method for the case in which $B$ is on the right of $A$ (see Figure 10.10). In the complementary case ($B$ on the left of $A$), the same algorithm

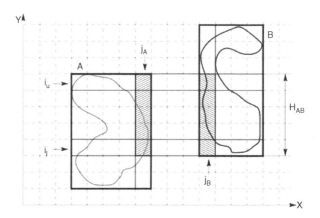

**FIGURE 10.10**
Projections of bounding rectangles $A$ and $B$ intersect along the $Y$ axis. The gray patterns indicate cells that are scanned in the evaluation of coefficient $w_{1,1}(A, B)$. This is sufficient to evaluate the complete relationship between entities represented by segments $A$ and $B$.

serves to derive the relationship $w(B, A)$, which can then be transformed into $w(A, B)$ by applying the property of antisymmetry of weighted walkthroughs. Because all the cells of $A$ are on the left of $B$, the two upper-left and lower-left weights $w_{-1,1}(A, B)$ and $w_{-1,-1}(A, B)$ are equal to 0. In addition, because the sum of the four weights is equal to 1, the derivation of the upper-right weight $w_{1,1}(A, B)$ is sufficient to fully determine the descriptor (as $w_{1,-1}(A, B) = 1 - w_{1,1}(A, B)$).

The upper-right weight $w_{1,1}(A, B)$ is computed by summing up the number of cells of $A$ that are lower-left or left from cells of $B$. According to the forms computed in the nine basic cases of Figure 10.4a and Figure 10.4b, for any cell $\langle i, j \rangle$ in $A$, the contribution to $w_{1,1}(A, B)$ is equal to 1 for each cell of $B$ having indexes $\langle h, k \rangle$ with $h > i$ and $k > j$, and it is equal to 1/2 for each cell of $B$ having indexes $\langle h, k \rangle$ with $h = i$ and $k > j$. In the end of the computation, the total sum is normalized by dividing it by the product of the number of cells in $A$ and $B$.

By relaying on matrixes $WW$ in the representation of segments $A$ and $B$, the computation can be accomplished by scanning only once a part of the rightmost column of the bounding box of $A$ and of the leftmost column of the bounding box of $B$, without covering the entire set of cells in $A$ and $B$. The algorithm is reported in Figure 10.11. $UR$ denotes the weight $w_{1,1}(A, B)$ being computed. For the simplicity of notation, matrixes $WW$ of segments $A$ and $B$ are denoted by $A$ and $B$. Notations $j_A$ and $j_B$ denote the indexes of the right column of the bounding box of $A$ and of the left column of the bounding box of $B$, respectively. Finally, $i_l$ and $i_u$ indicate the indexes of the lowest and topmost rows that contain cells of both $A$ and $B$, respectively (see Figure 10.10).

In the statement on line 1, the term $(A_{i_l, j_A}^{-1, -1} + A_{i_l, j_A}^{0, -1})$ evaluates the number of cells of $A$ that are lower-left, or lower-aligned with respect to $i_l, j_A$; for each of these cells, there are no cells of B that are aligned on the right-hand side, and the number of cells of $B$ that are in the upper-right position is equal to the term $(B_{i_l, j_B}^{0,0} + B_{i_l, j_B}^{0,1} + B_{i_l, j_B}^{1,0} + B_{i_l, j_B}^{1,1})$. According to this, statement 1 initializes $UR$ by accounting for the contribution of all the (possibly existing) rows of $A$ that are below row $i_l$. The statement in line 2 controls a loop that scans the cells in the right column of A and in the left column of $B$, throughout the height of the intersection of the projections of $A$ and $B$ on the vertical axis. Note that, because $i_u$ is the topmost row of $A$ or of $B$, there cannot be any other cell of $A$ that is over row

1. $UR = (A_{i_l,j_A}^{-1,-1} + A_{i_l,j_A}^{0,-1}) \cdot (B_{i_l,j_B}^{0,0} + B_{i_l,j_B}^{0,1} + B_{i_l,j_B}^{1,0} + B_{i_l,j_B}^{1,1}) \cdot 1;$
2. for $i = i_l : i_u$
3. $\quad UR = UR + (A_{i,j_A}^{-1,0} + A_{i,j_A}^{0,0}) \cdot ((B_{i,j_B}^{0,0} + B_{i,j_B}^{1,0}) \cdot 1/2 + (B_{i,j_B}^{0,1} + B_{i,j_B}^{1,1}) \cdot 1);$
4. $UR = UR/(N \cdot M);$

**FIGURE 10.11**
Algorithm for the case in which $A$ and $B$ have a null intersection along the $X$ axis.

$i_u$, and that has any cell of $B$ up-right or aligned-right. The statement 3, in the body of the loop, adds to $UR$ the contribution of all the cells of $A$ belonging to row $i$: $(A_{i,j_A}^{-1,0} + A_{i,j_A}^{0,0})$ is the number of cells of $A$ in row $i$; each of these cells has $(B_{i,j_B}^{0,0} + B_{i,j_B}^{1,0})$ cells of $B$ aligned on the right-hand side (contributing the weight $1/2$), and $(B_{i,j_B}^{0,1} + B_{i,j_B}^{1,1})$ cells of $B$ that are up-right (each contributing the weight $1$). The statement in line 4 normalizes the weight.

- When projections of $A$ and $B$ have a nonnull intersection on both the axes (i.e., when the bounding boxes of $A$ and $B$ overlap [see Figure 10.12], all four weights can be different than 0, and three of them must be computed (the fourth can be determined as the complement to 1). The derivation of each of the three weights is accomplished in time linear with respect to the number of cells falling within the intersection of bounding boxes of $A$ and $B$.

We expound here the derivation of $w_{1,1}(A, B)$. Of course, any of the other three weights can be derived in a similar manner, with the same complexity.

The derivation of $w_{1,1}(A, B)$ consists of evaluating how many cells of $A$ have how many cells of $B$ in the upper-right quadrant, in the upper column, in the right row, or coincident. According to the forms computed in the nine basic arrangements of Figure 10.4a and Figure 10.4b, each cell in the upper-right quadrant provides a contribution equal to 1, each cell in the upper column or in the right row provides a contribution equal to 1/2, and each cell coincident provides a contribution equal to 1/4.

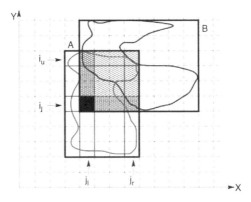

**FIGURE 10.12**
Projections of bounding rectangles of $A$ and $B$ have a nonnull intersection on both the axes. During the evaluation of relationships, the cells filled with the less dense pattern are scanned once, those with a more dense pattern are scanned twice, and the black cell is scanned three times.

1. $UR = (A_{i_l, j_l}^{-1, -1}) \cdot (B_{i_l, j_l}^{0,0} + B_{i_l, j_l}^{0,1} + B_{i_l, j_l}^{1,0} + B_{i_l, j_l}^{1,1}) \cdot 1;$
2. for $i = i_l : i_u$
3.     $UR = UR + (A_{i, j_l}^{-1,0}) \cdot ((B_{i, j_l}^{0,1} + B_{i, j_l}^{1,1}) \cdot 1 + (B_{i, j_l}^{0,0} + B_{i, j_l}^{1,0}) \cdot 1/2);$
4. for $j = j_l : j_r$
5.     $UR = UR + (A_{i_l, j}^{0,-1}) \cdot ((B_{i_l, j}^{1,0} + B_{i_l, j}^{1,1}) \cdot 1 + (B_{i_l, j}^{0,0} + B_{i_l, j}^{0,1}) \cdot 1/2);$
6. for $i = i_l : i_u$
7.     for $j = j_l : j_r$
8.         $UR = UR + (A_{i, j}^{0,0}) \cdot ((B_{i, j}^{1,1}) \cdot 1 + (B_{i, j}^{1,0} + B_{i, j}^{0,1}) \cdot 1/2 + (B_{i, j}^{0,0}) \cdot 1/4);$
9. $UR = UR/(N \cdot M);$

**FIGURE 10.13**
Algorithm for the case in which $A$ and $B$ have a nonnull intersection on both the $X$ and $Y$ axes.

Also, in this case, matrices $WW$ associated with $A$ and $B$ permit the evaluation by scanning only once a limited set of cells of $A$ and $B$. The algorithm is reported in Figure 10.13. In this case, indexes $i_l$, $i_u$, $j_l$, and $j_r$ indicate the lower and upper row, and the left and right column of the intersection of bounding boxes of $A$ and $B$, respectively (see Figure 10.12).

Statement 1 initializes the weight $w_{1,1}(A, B)$, denoted as $UR$, by summing up the contribution of the $(A_{i_l, j_l}^{-1, -1})$ cells of $A$ that are in the lower-left quadrant of the cell $\langle i_l, j_l \rangle$. The loop in statements 2 and 3 adds to $UR$ the contribution of all the cells of $A$ that are on the left of the intersection area of the bounding boxes of $A$ and $B$. These cells yield a different contribution on each row $i$ in the range between $i_l$ and $i_u$. In a similar manner, the loop in statements 4 and 5 adds to $UR$ the contribution of all the cells that are below the intersection area of the bounding boxes of $A$ and $B$. Finally, the double loop in statements 6, 7, and 8 adds the contribution of the cells of $A$ that fall within the intersection of the bounding boxes of $A$ and $B$. Statement 9 normalizes the weight.

## 10.4   Graph Representation and Comparison of Spatial Arrangements

Color clusters and their binary spatial relationships can be suitably represented and compared in a graph–theoretical framework. In this case, an image is represented as an attributed relational graph (ARG):

$$\text{image model} \overset{def}{=} < E, a, w >, \quad \begin{aligned} &E = \text{set of spatial entities} \\ &a : E \to A \cup \{\text{any}_a\} \\ &w : E \times E \to W \cup \{\text{any}_s\} \end{aligned} \quad (10.11)$$

where spatial entities are represented by vertices in $E$, and their chromatic features are captured by the attribute label $a$; spatial relationships are the complete set of pairs in $E \times E$, each labeled by the spatial descriptor $w$. To accommodate partial knowledge and intentional detail concealment, we also assume that both edges and vertices can take a neutral label any, yielding an exact match in every comparison (i.e., $\forall w \in W$, $\mathcal{D}_S(w, \text{any}_s) = 0$, and $\forall a \in A$, $\mathcal{D}_A(a, \text{any}_a) = 0$).

In so doing, $\mathcal{D}_S$ is the spatial distance defined in Section 10.2.1, while $\mathcal{D}_A$ is the metric of chromatic distance defined in the $L^* u^* v^*$ color space. In particular, the $L^* u^* v^*$ color space has been specifically designed to be "perceptual," this meaning that the distance between two colors with coordinates that are not far apart in the space, can be evaluated by using the Euclidean distance. According to this, attributes $a_1$ and $a_2$ of two entities are compared by using an Euclidean metric distance:

$$\mathcal{D}_A(a_1, a_2) \overset{def}{=} \sqrt{\alpha_L \cdot (L^*_{a_1} - L^*_{a_2})^2 + \alpha_u \cdot (u^*_{a_1} - u^*_{a_2})^2 + \alpha_v \cdot (v^*_{a_1} - v^*_{a_2})^2} \qquad (10.12)$$

where $\alpha_L$, $\alpha_u$, and $\alpha_v$ is a convex combination (i.e., $\alpha_L$, $\alpha_u$, and $\alpha_v$ are nonnegative numbers with sum equal to 1). Because there is not a preferred coordinate in the space, we set $\alpha_L, \alpha_u, \alpha_v = 1/3$. Distance $\mathcal{D}_A$ is nonnegative, autosimilar, symmetric, and normal, and satisfies the triangular inequality.

The comparison of the graph models of a query specification $< Q, a^q, w^q >$ and an archive image description $< D, a^d, w^d >$ involves the association of the entities in the query with a subset of the entities in the description. This is represented by an injective function $\Gamma$ that we call *interpretation*.

The distance between two image models $Q$ and $D$, under an interpretation $\Gamma$ can be defined by combining the metrics of chromatic distance $\mathcal{D}_A$, and spatial distance $\mathcal{D}_S$, associated with entity attributes (vertices) and relationship descriptors (edges), respectively. Using an additive composition, this is expressed as follows:

$$\mu^\Gamma(Q, D) \overset{def}{=} \lambda \sum_{k=1}^{N_q} \mathcal{D}_A(q_k, \Gamma(q_k)) + (1 - \lambda) \sum_{k=1}^{N_q} \sum_{h=1}^{k-1} \mathcal{D}_S([q_k, q_h], [\Gamma(q_k), \Gamma(q_h)]) \qquad (10.13)$$

where $N_q$ is the number of entities in the query graph $Q$, and $\lambda \in [0, 1]$ balances the mutual relevance of spatial and chromatic distance: for $\lambda = 1$, distance accounts only for the chromatic component.

In general, given the image models $Q$ and $D$, a combinatorial number of different interpretations $\Gamma$ are possible, each scoring a different value of distance. The distance is thus defined as the minimum distance under any possible interpretation:

$$\mu(Q, D) \overset{def}{=} \min_\Gamma \mu^\Gamma(Q, D) \qquad (10.14)$$

In doing so, computation of the distance between two image models becomes an optimal error-correcting (sub)graph isomorphism problem [85], which is a NP-complete problem with exponential time solution algorithms.

In the proposed application, the problem of matching a query graph $Q$ against a description graph $D$ is faced following the approach proposed in Reference [86]. To avoid exhaustive inspection of all possible interpretations $\Gamma$ of $Q$ on $D$, the search is organized in an incremental approach by repeatedly growing a partial assignment of the vertices of the query to the vertices of the description. In doing so, the space of solutions is organized as a tree, where the $k$th level contains all the partial assignments of the first $k$ entities of the query. Because the function of distance is monotonically growing with the level, any partial interpretation scoring a distance over a predefined threshold of maximum acceptable dissimilarity $\mu_{max}$ can be safely discarded without risk of false dismissal. While preserving the exactness of results, this reduces the complexity of enumeration. Following the approach of the $A^*$ algorithm [87], a search is developed in depth-first order by always extending the partial interpretation toward the local optimum, and by backtracking when the scored distance of the current assignment runs over a maximum acceptable threshold. When the inspection reaches a complete interpretation, a match under the threshold is found. This is not guaranteed to be the global optimum, but its scored distance comprises a stricter threshold for acceptable distance that is used to efficiently extend the search until the global optimum is found.

In Reference [86], a look-ahead strategy is proposed that extends the basic $A^*$ schema using an admissible heuristic to augment the cost of the current partial interpretation with a lower estimate of the future cost that will be spent in its extension to a complete match. This permits a more "informed" direction of search and enables the early discard of partial assignments that cannot lead to a final match with acceptable similarity. This reduces the complexity of the search while preserving the optimality of results. The approach results were compatible with the dimension encountered in the application context of retrieval by spatial arrangement.

## 10.5 A Retrieval System

The metric of similarity in Equation 10.13 and Equation 10.14, based on the joint combination of color clusters and weighted walkthroughs, was employed within a prototype retrieval engine.

In the archiving stage, all images are segmented into eight clusters and are represented by eight-vertices complete graphs. This resulted as a trade-off between the accuracy of representation and the efficiency of the graph matching process. The usage of graphs with fixed size permits the exploitation of the metric properties of the graph distance, thus enabling the exploitation of a metric indexing scheme [86]. The system supports two different query modalities: global similarity and *sketch*.

In a query by *global similarity*, the user provides an example by directly selecting an image from the database (see Figure 10.14), and the retrieval engine compares the query

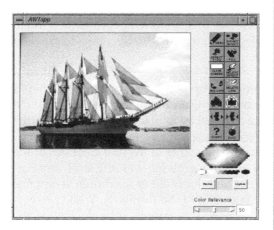
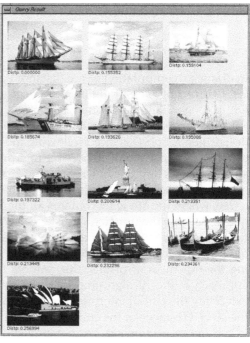

**FIGURE 10.14 (See color insert.)**
A query by image example (left), and the corresponding retrieval set (right).

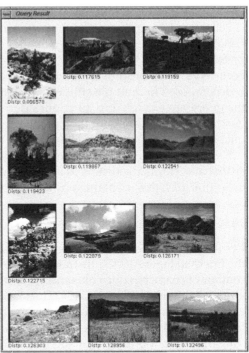

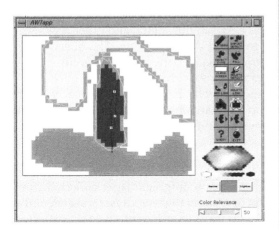

**FIGURE 10.15  (See color insert.)**
A query by sketch (left), and the corresponding retrieval set (right).

graph with database descriptions. In a query by *sketch*, the user expresses the query by drawing, coloring, and positioning a set of regions that capture only the color patches and relationships that are relevant to the user (see Figure 10.15 and Figure 10.16). From this representation, a query graph is automatically derived following a decomposition approach. Each region corresponds to a variable number of color clusters, depending on its size normalized with respect to that of the drawing area. This has a twofold effect.

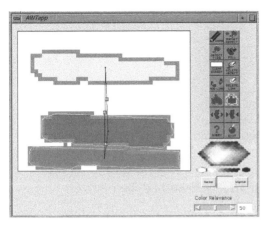

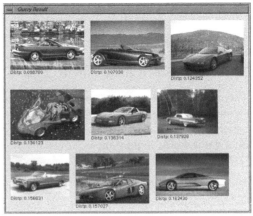

**FIGURE 10.16**
A query by sketch (left), and the corresponding retrieval set for $\lambda = 0.5$ (color relevance set to 50) (right).

On the one hand, the different relevance of regions, implicitly associated with their size, is considered by splitting them into a different number of graph entities. On the other hand, this partially replicates the behavior of the clustering algorithms, which splits sets of pixels according to their size, thus providing multiple clusters for colors with a predominant occurrence. Relationships between entities are those explicitly drawn by the user. If a region is decomposed in multiple entities, relationships between this region and other regions in the query are extended to all entities derived from the decomposition. The query graph derived from this representation involves a restricted match between the $N_q$ entities in the query against the $N_d$ entities in the database descriptions (with $N_q \leq N_d$).

For both queries, the user is allowed to dynamically set the balance of relevance by which spatial and chromatic distances are combined in the searching process. In the framework of Section 10.4, this is obtained by setting parameter $\lambda$ in Equation 10.13.

### 10.5.1 Retrieval Examples

Results are reported for a database of about 10,000 photographic images collected from the Internet. Figure 10.15 illustrates the querying operation: the user draws a sketch of the contour of characterizing color entities and positions them so as to reproduce the expected arrangement in searched images. The sketch is interpreted by the system as a set of color clusters and their spatial relationships and is checked against the descriptions stored in the archive. Matching images are displayed in a separate window, sorted by decreasing similarity from top to bottom and from left to right (see Figure 10.15). The user can tune, with the slide bar *color relevance*, the balance of color and spatial distances to the overall measure.

In Figure 10.16, a query for a different sketch is shown; the interpretation of the sketch takes into account only those spatial relationships that are marked by the user (made explicit by lines on the screen). In this case, the color relevance is set equal to 50, corresponding to $\lambda = 0.5$, so that color and spatial similarities are given equal weight.

Figure 10.14 shows the expression of a query by example. In this case, one of the database images is used as a query example, and the system searches for the most similar images, using all the color entities and relationships that appear in the query representation. In the particular example, the system retrieves the query image in the first position, and other images with a similar arrangement. Some of the retrieved images show a lower consistency in the semantics of the imaged scenes but still have a high relevance in terms of chromatic content and spatial arrangement.

## 10.6 User-Based Assessment

The perceptual significance of the metric of dissimilarity derived through the joint representation of color and spatial content was evaluated in a two-stage test, focusing first on a benchmark of images representing basic synthetic arrangements of three colors, and then on a database of real images.

### 10.6.1 A Benchmark Database of Basic Spatial Arrangements of Color

The first stage of the evaluation was oriented to investigate the capability of the proposed model to capture differences and similarities in basic spatial arrangements of colors, by abstracting from other relevant features, such as color distribution and size and shape of color patches.

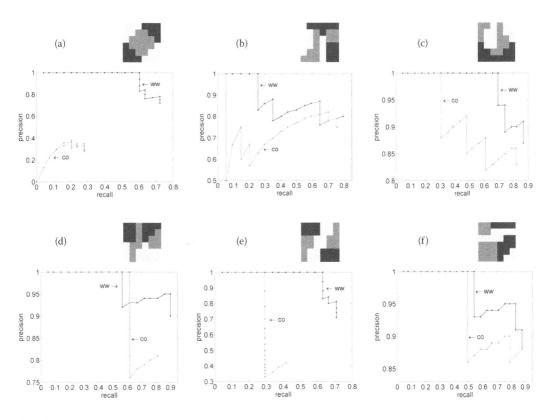

**FIGURE 10.17**
The six query images used in the test, and their corresponding plots of precision/recall. Plotted values correspond to those obtained by resolving the query using both the weighted walkthroughs (WW), and the centroid orientation (CO).

To this end, the evaluation was carried out on a benchmark based on an archive with $6 \times 3 \times 9$ synthetic pictures. The archive was derived from six reference pictures, obtained by different compositions of an equal number of red, yellow, and blue squares within a six-by-six grid. Reference pictures (displayed on the top of the plots of Figure 10.17) were created so as to contain five or six separate regions each. Preliminary pilot tests indicated that this number results in a complexity that is sufficient to prevent the user from acquiring an exact memory of the arrangement. Though these images are completely synthetic and not occurring in real application contexts, they are useful in testing the effectiveness of spatial descriptors independently from chromatic components. In fact, their structure allows for an easier evaluation by the users which can focus on spatial arrangements rather than on the semantics or other image features that could bias the results of the evaluation in the case of real images.

For each reference picture, three sets of mutations were derived automatically by a random engine changing the arrangement of blocks through shift operations on randomly selected rows or columns. Each set includes nine variations of the reference picture, which attain different levels of mutation by applying a number of shift operations ranging from one to nine. (Figure 10.18 indicates the level of mutation for the nine variations in each of the three sets of a reference picture.) In order to avoid the introduction of a perceivable ordering, mutations were derived independently (i.e., the mutation at level $n$ was obtained through $n$ shifts on the reference picture rather than through one shift on the mutation at level $n-1$). By construction, the mutation algorithm maintains the overall picture histogram and the multirectangular shape of segments, but it largely increases the fragmentation of

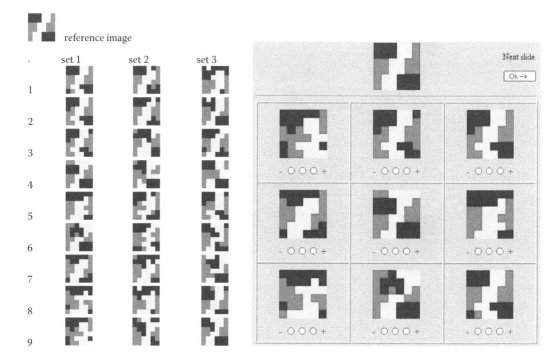

**FIGURE 10.18**
The columns on the left are the images, listed from top to bottom in increasing order of variation, comprised in the three sets of mutations of the reference image on the top left. A page of the user test for the reference image and the mutation set 1 is shown on the right.

regions. Preliminary pilot tests with variations including more than eight regions resulted in major complexity for the user in comparing images and ranking their similarity. The algorithm was thus forced to accept only arrangements resulting in less than eight regions.

The six reference pictures were employed as queries against the $6 \times 3 \times 9$ pictures of the archive, and queries were resolved using the metric of dissimilarity defined in Equation 10.13.

### 10.6.2 Ground Truth

Evaluation of the effectiveness of retrieval obtained on the benchmark requires a ground-truth about the similarity $V_{qd}$ between each reference picture $q$ and each archive image $d$. With six queries against an archive of 162 images, this makes 972 values of similarity, which cannot be realistically obtained with a fully user-based rank. To overcome the problem, user rankings have been complemented with inference [88].

Each user was shown a sequence of $3 \times 6$ html pages, each showing a reference picture and a set of nine variations. (Figure 10.18 reports a test page, while the overall testing session is available online at http://viplab.dsi.unifi.it/color/test). Pages presenting variations of the same reference picture were presented subsequently, so as to maximize the correlation in the ranking of variations included in different sets. On each page, the user was asked to provide a three-level rank of the similarity between the reference picture and each of the nine variations. To reduce the stress of the test, users were suggested to first search for the most similar images and then extend the rank toward low similarities, thus emphasizing the relevance of high ranks.

The testing session was administered to a sample of 22 volunteers and took an average time ranging between 10 and 21 min, with an average of 14.6 min. This appeared to be a realistic limit for the user capability and willingness in maintaining attention throughout the test. The overall sizing of the evaluation, and, in particular, the number of reference pictures and queries considered, was based on preliminary evaluation of this limit.

User ranks were employed to evaluate a ground value of similarity between each reference picture and its compared variations. In order to reflect the major relevance of higher ranks, a score of three was attributed for each high rank received; a score of 1 was attributed for each intermediate rank. No score was attributed for low ranks, as in the testing protocol, these correspond to cases that are not relevant to the user. The average number of scores obtained by each variation $d$ was assumed as the value of similarity with the reference picture $q$ of its set.

The ground truth acquired in the comparison of each query against three sets of variations was extended to cover the comparison of each query against the overall archive through two complementary assumptions. On the one hand, we assume that the ranking obtained for variations of the same reference pictures belonging to different sets can be combined. Concretely, this means that for each reference picture, the user implicitly sets an absolute level of similarity that is maintained throughout the three subsequent sets of variations. The assumption is supported by the statistical equivalence of different sets (which are generated by a uniform random algorithm), and by the fact that different variations of the same reference picture are presented sequentially without interruption. On the other hand, we assume that any picture $d_1$ deriving from mutation of a reference picture $q_1$ has a null value of similarity with respect to any other reference picture $q_2$. This is to say that if $d_1$ would be included in a set of the reference picture $q_2$, then the user would rank the similarity at the lowest level. To verify the assumption, a sample of $6 \times 9$ images collecting a variation set for each reference picture was created and displayed on a page. Three pilot users were then asked to identify which variations derived from each of the six reference pictures. All the users identified a variable number of variations, ranging between four and six, with no false classifications. None of the selected images turned out to have an average rank higher than 1.2.

Based on the two assumptions, the average user-based ranking was extended to complete the array $V_{qd}$ capturing the value of any archive picture $d$ as a member of the retrieval set for any query $q$.

## 10.6.3 Results

Summarized in Figure 10.17 are the results of the evaluation. Reference pictures employed as queries are reported on the top, while the plots on the bottom are the curves of *precision/recall* obtained by resolving the query on the archive according to the joint metric of similarity based on color and weighted walkthroughs (WW), and color and centroids orientation (CO). Defining as *relevant* those images in the archive which are similar to the query in the users' perception, and as *retrieval set* the set of images retrieved in each retrieval session, the *recall* is defined as the ratio between the number of relevant retrieved images and the overall number of relevant images in the archive; instead, the *precision* is the ratio between the number of relevant retrieved images and the size of the current retrieval set.

In the plots, each point represents the values of precision and recall computed for the retrieval set which extends up to comprise the image represented by the point itself. In this way, points are added to each plot from left to right, representing retrieval sets of size varying from one image up to a maximum that depends on the specific query. In fact, the maximum size of the retrieval set for a query is determined as the number of images in the three mutation sets of the query that users recognize as similar to the query (values are 24, 24, 21, 25, 20, 23 for the six queries, respectively). In this representation, a perfect accordance of retrieval with the user ranking would result in a flat curve of precision 1 at every recall, which is possible if the retrieval set is constituted only by relevant pictures. Instead, any misclassification is highlighted by a negative slope of the curve that derives from the "anticipated" retrieval of nonrelevant pictures. For all six queries, WW closely fit the ideal user-based curve in the ranking of the first, and most relevant, variations. A significant divergence is observed only on the second query for the ranking of variations taking the positions between six and nine.

In all the cases tested, WW outperformed CO. In particular, CO evidenced a main limit in the processing of the first and the fifth queries. In particular, the long sequences with constant recall (in the case (a), the top-ranked images in the retrieval set scored a null value of recall and precision) indicate that this problem of CO derives from a misclassification that confuses variations of the query with those of different reference pictures. Analysis of the specific results of retrieval indicates that CO are not able to discriminate the first and fifth reference pictures, which are definitely different in the user perception but share an almost equal representation in terms of the centroids of color sets. Finally, note that, because all the images share a common proportion of colors, a representation based on a global histogram cannot discriminate any two images in the benchmark. As a consequence, in all the cases tested, WW outperformed the color histogram, which ranks, by construction, all the images in the same position.

### 10.6.4   A Benchmark Database of Real Images

The second stage of the evaluation was aimed at extending the experimental results to the case of images with realistic complexity. To this end, the weighted walkthroughs and the centroids orientation were experimented within the prototype system introduced in Section 10.5 and compared against a solution based on the sole use of a global color histogram. For the experiments, the system was applied to an archive of about 1000 reference paintings featured by the library of WebMuseum [89]. The test was administered to a set of 10 volunteers, all with university educations. Only two of them had experience in using systems for image retrieval by content.

Before the start of the testing phase, users were trained with two preliminary examples, in order to ensure their understanding of the system. During the test, users were asked to retrieve a given set of eight target images (shown in Figure 10.19a, from $T_1$ to $T_8$), representing the aim of the search, by expressing queries by sketch (see Figure 10.19b in which the query images for a particular user are shown). To this end, users were shown each target image, and they were requested to express a query with three regions to retrieve it (see Figure 10.15). Only one trial was allowed for each target image.

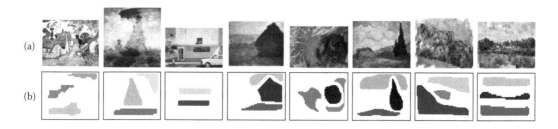

**FIGURE 10.19  (See color insert.)**
(a) The target images used in the test; and (b) a user's query sketches for the eight images.

**FIGURE 10.20**
Different users' queries for the same target image (leftmost image).

The overall time to express queries for all eight target images was about 20 min, and this permitted the users to maintain attention. The time spent for each query, about 2 min, appeared to mainly derive from the difficulty in selecting an appropriate color capable of representing the visual appearance of the image. This is basically a limit of the interface, which is not presently engineered with respect to usability quality factors. Figure 10.20 shows some of the queries drawn from users during the search of the sixth target image. It is worth noting that different users employed noticeably different sketches to find the same target image.

For each query, the ranking of similarity on the overall set of 1000 pictures was evaluated using the joint modeling of color and spatial relationships (weighted walkthroughs and centroid orientation have been used separately to model spatial relationships), and the global color histogram. Results were summarized within two indexes of *recall* and *precision*. For each target image, the *recall* is 1 if the target image appears within the set of the first 20 retrieved images, 0 otherwise. Thus, recall expresses with a true/false condition, the presence of the target image within the retrieval set. *Precision* considers the rank scored by the target image in the retrieval set: it is 1 if the target image is ranked in the first position, and gradually decreases to 0 when the target is ranked from the first toward the 20th position (i.e., precision is assumed zero when the target is ranked out of the first 20 retrieved images). In this way, precision measures the system capability in classifying images according to the implicit ordering given by the target image. System recall and precision for each of the eight target images are derived by averaging the individual values scored for a target image on the set of users' queries.

Results are reported in Figure 10.21a and Figure 10.21b. Figure 10.21a compares values of recall for the proposed model (here indicated as *WW*), for the centroid orientation (*CO*),

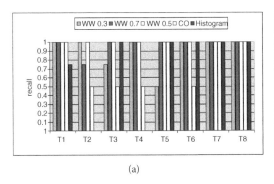 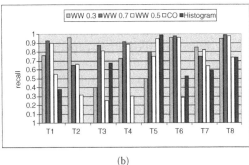

(a)                                            (b)

**FIGURE 10.21**
Values of recall (a) and precision (b) are compared for the proposed model (*WW*), for centroid orientation (*CO*), and for global color histogram (*Histogram*). Results for *WW* are reported for $\lambda = 0.5$, which corresponds to an equal weight for the contribution of color and spatial distance; $\lambda = 0.3$ and $\lambda = 0.7$ correspond to a reduced or increased contribution for the color distance, respectively. It can be noticed as the global histogram definitely fails in ranking the second and fourth target images, whose recall and precision values are both null.

and for the color histogram (*Histogram*). For *WW*, results are reported for different values of the parameter $\lambda$, which weights the contribution of color and spatial distance in Equation 10.13. Though *Histogram* provides an average acceptable result, it becomes completely inappropriate in two of the eight cases ($T_2$ and $T_4$), where the recall becomes zero. Color used jointly with centroid orientation shows a recall even greater than 0.5 and performs better than *Histogram* in six of the eight cases ($T_3$ and $T_6$ are the exceptions). Differently, search based on the *WW* model provides optimal results for each of the eight tested cases. In particular, it can be observed that better results are scored for $\lambda$ set equal to 0.5, while for unbalanced combinations, there are cases that both penalize a major weight for color ($T_2$, and this directly descends from the fact that the color histogram failed, thus evidencing the inadequacy of the sole color in obtaining the correct response for this image), and cases that penalize a major weight for spatial contribution ($T_3$ and $T_5$).

*Histogram* is clearly disadvantaged when the system effectiveness is measured as rank of the target image in the retrieval set, as evidenced in plots of precision of Figure 10.21b. By considering a spatial coordinate, ranking provided from the system is much closer to the user expectation, than that given by global histogram. In almost all the tested cases ($T_1$, $T_3$, $T_4$, and $T_5$), a solution that privileges the contribution of color distance scores better results than that favoring the spatial component ($T_2$ and $T_7$). In the remaining two cases ($T_6$ and $T_8$), there is no substantial difference for the three values of $\lambda$. Finally, for the target image $T_5$, the histogram outperforms *WW*, basically due to the low spatial characterization of this image.

## 10.7 Conclusions

In image search based on chromatic similarity, the effectiveness of retrieval can be improved by taking into account the spatial arrangement of colors. This can serve both to distinguish images with the same colors in different arrangements and to capture the similarity between images with different colors but similar arrangements.

In this chapter, we proposed a model of representation and comparison that attains this goal by partitioning the image in separate entities and by associating them with individual chromatic attributes and with mutual spatial relationships. Entities are identified with the sets of image pixels belonging to color clusters derived by a clustering process in the $L^*u^*v^*$ color space. In doing so, a spatial entity may be composed of multiple nonconnected segments, mirroring the human capability to merge regions with common chromatic attributes. To support this modeling approach, a suitable spatial descriptor was proposed which is able to capture the complexity of directional relationships between the image projections of color clusters.

The effectiveness of the proposed model was assessed in a two-stage experimental evaluation. In the first stage, basic chromatic arrangements were considered to evaluate the capability of the model to rank the similarity of images with equal histograms but different spatial arrangements (which cannot be distinguished using a global histogram). In the second stage, the model was experimented with to evaluate the capability to reflect perceived similarity between user sketches and images of realistic complexity. In both cases, experimental results showed the capability of the model to combine and balance account for chromatic and spatial similarity, thus improving the effectiveness of retrieval with respect to a representation based on a global histogram and a representation using centroids orientation to model spatial relationships between color clusters.

# References

[1] A. Gupta and R. Jain, Visual information retrieval, *Commun. ACM*, 40, 70–79, May 1997.

[2] A. Del Bimbo, *Visual Information Retrieval*, Academic Press, San Francisco, CA, 1999.

[3] R. Veltkamp and M. Tanase, Content-Based Image Retrieval Systems: A Survey, Technical Report UU-CS-2000-34, Utrecht University, Utrecht, the Netherlands, 2002.

[4] A. Smeulders, M. Worring, S. Santini, A. Gupta, and R. Jain, Content based image retrieval at the end of the early years, *IEEE Trans. on Patt. Anal. and Machine Intelligence*, 22, 1349–1380, December 2000.

[5] T. Gevers, A. Smeulders, *Emerging Topics in Computer Vision*, S.B. Kang, and G. Medioni (Eds.), ch. Content-based image retrieval: An overview. Prentice Hall, New York, 2004.

[6] T. Gevers, *Principles of Visual Information Retrieval*, M. Lew, Ed., ch. Color in image search engines. Springer-Verlag, Heidelberg, February 2001, 11–48.

[7] R. Schettini, G. Ciocca, and S. Zuffi, *A Survey of Methods for Color Image Indexing and Retrieval in Image Databases*, ch. Color imaging science: Exploiting digital media, R. Luo and L. Mac Donald, Eds., John Wiley & Sons, New York, 2001.

[8] C. Theoharatos, N. Laskaris, G. Economou, and S. Fotopoulos, A generic scheme for color image retrieval based on the multivariate wald-wolfowitz test, *IEEE Trans. on Knowledge and Data Eng.*, 17, 808–819, June 2005.

[9] N. Sebe and M. Lew, *Texture Features for Content-Based Retrieval*, ch. Principles of visual information Retrieval. Springer-Verlag, Heidelberg, 2001.

[10] J. Zhang and T. Tan, Brief review of invariant texture analysis methods, *Patt. Recognition*, 35, 735–747, March 2002.

[11] B. Günsel and M. Tekalp, Shape similarity matching for query-by-example, *Patt. Recognition*, 31, 931–944, July 1998.

[12] S. Loncaric, A survey of shape analysis techniques, *Patt. Recognition*, 34, 983–1001, August 1998.

[13] D. Zhang and G. Lu, Review of shape representation and description techniques, *Patt. Recognition*, 37, 1–19, January 2004.

[14] D. Hoiem, R. Sukthankar, H. Schneiderman, and L. Huston, Object-based image retrieval using the statistical structure of images, in *Proceedings of the IEEE Conference on Computer Vision and Pattern Recognition*, Washington, DC, IEEE Computer Society, Vol. 2, June 2004, pp. 490–497.

[15] S. Maybank, Detection of image structures using the fisher information and the rao metric, *IEEE Trans. on Patt. Anal. and Machine Intelligence*, 26, 1579–1589, December 2004.

[16] C. Schmid, R. Mohr, and C. Bauckhage, Evaluation of interest point detectors, *Int. J. Comput. Vision*, 37, 151–172, June 2000.

[17] D. Lowe, Distinctive image features from scale-invariant keypoints, *Int. J. Comput. Vision*, 60, 91–110, February 2004.

[18] J.V. de Weijer and T. Gevers, Boosting saliency in color image features, in *Proceedings of the IEEE International Conference on Computer Vision and Pattern Recognition*, IEEE Computer Society, San Diego, CA, Vol. 1, June 2005, pp. 365–372.

[19] V. Gudivada and V. Raghavan, Design and evaluation of algorithms for image retrieval by spatial similarity, *ACM Trans. on Inf. Syst.*, 13, 115–144, April 1995.

[20] J. Smith and S. Chang, Visualseek: A fully automated content-based image query system, in *Proceedings of the ACM Conference on Multimedia*, Boston, MA, February 1996, ACM Press, pp. 87–98.

[21] S. Berretti, A. Del Bimbo, and E. Vicario, Weighted walkthroughs between extended entities for retrieval by spatial arrangement, *IEEE Trans. on Multimedia*, 5, 52–70, March 2003.

[22] J. Amores, N. Sebe, and P. Radeva, Fast spatial pattern discovery integrating boosting with constellations of contextual descriptors, in *Proceedings of the IEEE Conference on Computer Vision and Pattern Recognition*, San Diego, CA, Vol. 2, June 2005, pp. 769–774.

[23] M. Rodríguez and M. Jarur, A genetic algorithm for searching spatial configurations, *IEEE Trans. on Evol. Computation*, 9, 252–270, June 2005.

[24] C. Colombo, A. Del Bimbo, and P. Pala, Semantics in visual information retrieval, *IEEE Multimedia*, 6, 38–53, July–September 1999.

[25] B. Bradshaw, Semantic based image retrieval: A probabilistic approach, in *Proceedings of the ACM Multimedia*, Marina del Rey, Los Angeles, CA, October 2000, ACM Press, pp. 167–176.

[26] Y. Marchenco, T.-S. Chua, and I. Aristarkhova, Analysis and retrieval of paintings using artistic color concepts, in *Proceedings of the IEEE International Conference on Multimedia and Expo*, Amsterdam, the Netherlands, July 2005, IEEE Computer Society, pp. 1246–1249.

[27] S. Chang and E. Jungert, Pictorial data management based upon the theory of symbolic projections, *J. Visual Languages and Computing*, 2, 195–215, June 1991.

[28] J. Smith and C.-S. Li, Decoding image semantics using composite region templates, in *Proceedings of the IEEE Workshop on Content-Based Access of Image and Video Libraries*, Santa Barbara, CA, June 1998, IEEE Computer Society, pp. 9–13.

[29] R. Mehrotra and J. Gary, Similar-shape retrieval in shape data management, *IEEE Comput.*, 28, 57–62, September 1995.

[30] K. Siddiqi and B. Kimia, Parts of visual form: Computational aspects, *IEEE Trans. on Patt. Anal. and Machine Intelligence*, 17, 239–251, March 1995.

[31] Y. Tao and W. Grosky, Spatial color indexing: A novel approach for content-based image retrieval, in *Proceedings of the IEEE International Conference on Multimedia Computing and Systems*, Florence, Italy, Vol. 1, June 1999, pp. 530–535.

[32] M. Flickner, W. Niblack, H. Sawhney, J. Ashley, Q. Huang, B. Dom, M. Gorkani, J. Hafner, D. Lee, D. Petkovic, D. Steele, and P. Yanker, Query by image and video content: The qbic system, *IEEE Comput.*, 28, 23–32, September 1995.

[33] J. Bach, C. Fuler, A. Gupta, A. Hampapur, B. Horowitz, R. Humphrey, R. Jain, and C. Shu, The virage image search engine: An open framework for image management, in *Proceedings of the SPIE Conference on Storage and Retrieval for Image and Video Databases IV*, San Jose, CA, Vol. 2670, March 1996, I.K. Sethi and R. Jain, Eds., SPIE, pp. 76–87.

[34] T. Gevers and A. Smeulders, Pictoseek: Combining color and shape invariant features for image retrieval, *IEEE Trans. on Image Process.*, 9, 102–119, January 2000.

[35] C. Carson, S. Belongie, H. Greenspan, and J. Malik, Blobworld: Image segmentation using expectation maximization and its application to image querying, *IEEE Trans. on Patt. Anal. and Machine Intelligence*, 24, 1026–1038, August 2002.

[36] J. Wang, J. Li, and G. Wiederhold, Simplicity: Semantics-sensitive integrated matching for picture libraries, *IEEE Trans. on Patt. Anal. and Machine Intelligence*, 23, 947–963, September 2001.

[37] J. Li and J. Wang, Automatic linguistic indexing of pictures by a statistical modeling approach, *IEEE Trans. on Patt. Anal. and Machine Intelligence*, 25, 1075–1088, September 2003.

[38] M. Swain and D. Ballard, Color indexing, *Int. J. Comput. Vision*, 7, 11–32, March 1991.

[39] Y. Rubner, C. Tomasi, and L. Guibas, A metric for distributions with applications to image databases, in *Proceedings of the IEEE International Conference on Computer Vision*, Bombay, India, January 1998, Narosa Publishing House, pp. 59–66.

[40] A. Nagasaka and Y. Tanaka, Automatic video indexing and full video search for object appearances, in *Proceedings of the IFIP Transactions, Working Conference on Visual Database Systems II*, 1992, pp. 113–127.

[41] J. Huang, S. Kumar, M. Mitra, W.-J. Zhu, and R. Zabih, Image indexing using color correlograms, in *Proceedings of the IEEE Conference on Computer Vision and Pattern Recognition*, San Juan, Puerto Rico, June 1997, IEEE Computer Society, pp. 762–768.

[42] J. Smith and S. Chang, Integrated spatial and feature image query, *Multimedia Syst.*, 7, 129–140, March 1999.

[43] J. Chen, T. Pappas, A. Mojsilovic, and B. Rogowitz, Adaptive perceptual color-texture image segmentation, *IEEE Trans. on Image Process.*, 14, 1524–1536, October 2005.

[44] S. Makrogiannis, G. Economou, S. Fotopoulos, and N. Bourbakis, Segmentation of color images using multiscale clustering and graph theoretic region synthesis, *IEEE Trans. on Syst., Man and Cybernetics, Part A*, 35, 224–238, March 2005.

[45] A. Del Bimbo, M. Mugnaini, P. Pala, and F. Turco, Visual querying by color perceptive regions, *Patt. Recognition*, 31, 1241–1253, September 1998.

[46] R. Haralick and L. Shapiro, Image segmentation techniques, *Comput. Vision Graphics and Image Process.*, 29, 100–132, 1985.

[47] M. Arbib and T. Uchiyama, Color image segmentation using competitive learning, *IEEE Trans. on Patt. Anal. and Machine Intelligence*, 16, 1197–1206, December 1994.

[48] D. Androutsos, K. Plataniotis, and A. Venetsanopoulos, A novel vector-based approach to color image retrieval using vector angular based distance measure, *Comput. Vision and Image Understanding*, 75, 46–58, July 1999.

[49] S. Berretti, A. Del Bimbo, and E. Vicario, Spatial arrangement of color in retrieval by visual similarity, *Patt. Recognition*, 35, 1661–1674, August 2002.

[50] G. Heidemann, Combining spatial and colour information for content based image retrieval, *Comput. Vision and Image Understanding*, 94, 234–270, April–June 2004.

[51] Multimedia Content Description Interface — part 3: Visual, Final Commitee Draft, Technical Report 15938-3, Doc. N4062, ISO/IEC, Singapore, 2001.

[52] J. Martinez, R. Koenen, and F. Pereira, Mpeg-7: The generic multimedia content description standard, part 1, *IEEE Trans. on Multimedia*, 9, 78–87, April/June 2002.

[53] M. Abdel-Mottaleb and S. Krishnamachari, Multimedia descriptions based on mpeg-7: Extraction and applications, *IEEE Trans. on Multimedia*, 6, 459–468, June 2004.

[54] B. Manjunath, J.-R. Ohm, V. Vasudevan, and A. Yamada, Color and texture descriptors, *IEEE Trans. on Circuits and Syst. for Video Technol.*, 11, 703–715, June 2001.

[55] A. Doulamis and N. Doulamis, Generalized nonlinear relevance feedback for interactive content-based retrieval and organization, *IEEE Trans. on Circuits and Syst. for Video Technol.*, 14, 656–671, May 2004.

[56] J. Laaksonen, M. Koskela, and E. Oja, Picsom — self-organizing image retrieval with mpeg-7 content descriptors, *IEEE Trans. on Neural Networks*, 13, 841–853, July 2002.

[57] Y. Rui, T. Huang, M. Ortega, and S. Mehrotra, Relevance feedback: A power tool for interactive content-based image retrieval, *IEEE Trans. on Circuits and Syst. for Video Technol.*, 8, 644–655, September 1998.

[58] A. Kushki, P. Androutsos, K. Plataniotis, and A. Venetsanopoulos, Retrieval of images from artistic repositories using a decision fusion framework, *IEEE Trans. on Image Process.*, 13, 277–292, March 2004.

[59] A. Guttmann, R-trees: A dynamic index structure for spatial searching, in *Proceedings of the ACM International Conference on Management of Data*, Boston, MA, June 1984, ACM Press, pp. 47–57.

[60] T. Sellis, N. Roussopoulos, and C. Faloustos, The r+ tre: A dynamic index for multidimensional objects, in *Proceedings of the International Conference on Very Large Databases*, P. M. Stocker, W. Kent, and P. Hammersley, Eds., Brighton, U.K., September 1987, Morgan Kaufmann, pp. 507–518.

[61] N. Beckmann, H. Kriegel, R. Schneider, and B. Seeger, The r* tree: An efficient and robust access method for points and rectangles, in *Proceedings of the ACM International Conference on Management of Data*, Atlantic City, NJ, May 1990, ACM Press, pp. 322–331.

[62] D. White and R. Jain, Similarity indexing with the ss-tree, in *Proceedings of the IEEE International Conference on Data Engineering*, New Orleans, LA, February 1996, pp. 516–523.

[63] N. Katayama and S. Satoh, The sr-tree: An index structure for high-dimensional nearest neighbor queries, in *Proceedings of the ACM International Conference on Management of Data*, Tucson, AZ, ACM Press, May 1997, pp. 369–380.

[64] M. Egenhofer and R. Franzosa, Point-set topological spatial relations, *Int. J. Geogr. Inf. Syst.*, 5, 2, 161–174, 1991.

[65] M. Egenhofer and R. Franzosa, On the equivalence of topological relations, *Int. J. Geogr. Inf. Syst.*, 9, 2, 133–152, 1995.

[66] S. Chang, Q. Shi, and C. Yan, Iconic indexing by 2-d strings, *IEEE Trans. on Patt. Anal. and Machine Intelligence*, 9, 413–427, July 1987.

[67] A. Frank, Qualitative spatial reasoning about distances and directions in geographic space, *J. Visual Languages and Computing*, 3, 343–371, September 1992.

[68] C. Freksa, Using orientation information for qualitative spatial reasoning, in *Proceedings of the International Conference on Theories and Methods of Spatio-Temporal Reasoning in Geographic Space, Lecture Notes in Computer Science*, Pisa, Italy, Vol. 639, Springer-Verlag, 1992, pp. 162–178.

[69] S. Berretti, A. Del Bimbo, and E. Vicario, Modeling spatial relationships between color sets, in *Proceedings of the IEEE International Workshop on Content Based Access of Image and Video Libraries*, Hilton Head, SC, June 2000, IEEE Computer Society, pp. 73–77.

[70] D. Papadias and T. Sellis, The semantics of relations in 2d space using representative points: Spatial indexes, *J. Visual Languages and Computing*, 6, 53–72, March 1995.

[71] R. Goyal and M. Egenhofer, Consistent queries over cardinal directions across different levels of detail, in *Proceedings of the International Workshop on Database and Expert Systems Applications*, A.M. Tjoa, R. Wagner, and A. Al Zobaidie, Eds., September 2000, Greenwich, U.K., IEEE Press, pp. 876–880.

[72] R. Goyal and M. Egenhofer, Cardinal directions between extended spatial objects, *IEEE Trans. on Knowledge and Data Engineering* (in press).

[73] S. Cicerone and P. Di Felice, Cardinal relations between regions with a broad boundary, in *Proceedings of the ACM Symposium on Geographical Information Systems*, K. -J. Li, K. Makki, N. Pissinou, S. Ravada, Eds., Washington, DC, November 2000, ACM Press, pp. 15–20.

[74] S. Chang, E. Jungert, and T. Li, Representation and retrieval of symbolic pictures using generalized 2d strings, in *SPIE Proceedings of Visual Communications and Image Processing IV*, Philadelphia, Vol. 1199, November 1989, pp. 1360–1372.

[75] S. Lee and F. Hsu, Spatial reasoning and similarity retrieval of images using 2d c-strings knowledge representation, *Patt. Recognition*, 25, 305–318, March 1992.

[76] S. Lee, M. Yang, and J. Cheng, Signature file as spatial filter for iconic image database, *J. Visual Languages and Computing*, 3, 373–397, December 1992.

[77] E. Jungert, Qualitative spatial reasoning for determination of object relations using symbolic interval projections, in *Proceedings of the IEEE International Workshop on Visual Languages*, Bergen, Norway, August 1993, IEEE Computer Society, pp. 83–87.

[78] A. Del Bimbo and E. Vicario, Specification by-example of virtual agents behavior, *IEEE Trans. on Visualization and Comput. Graphics*, 1, 350–360, December 1995.

[79] D. Papadias, Spatial relation-based representation systems, in *Proceedings of the European Conference on Spatial Information Theory*, Marciana Marina, Italy, September 1993, pp. 234–247.

[80] V. Gudivada, Spatial knowledge representation and retrieval in 3-d image databases, in *Proceedings of the International Conference on Multimedia and Computing Systems*, Washington DC, IEEE Computer Society, May 1995, pp. 90–97.

[81] K. Miyajima and A. Ralescu, Spatial organization in 2d segmented images: Representation and recognition of primitive spatial relations, *Int. J. Fuzzy Sets and Systems*, 65, 225–236, July 1994.

[82] P. Matsakis and L. Wendling, A new way to represent the relative position between areal objects, *IEEE Trans. on Patt. Anal. and Machine Intelligence*, 21, 634–643, July 1999.

[83] Y. Wang and F. Makedon, R-histogram: Qualitative representation of spatial relations for similarity-based image retrieval, in *Proceedings of the ACM Multimedia*, Berkeley, CA, November 2003, pp. 323–326.

[84] G. Dong and M. Xie, Color clustering and learning for image segmentation based on neural networks, *IEEE Trans. on Neural Networks*, 16, 925–936, July 2005.

[85] M. Eshera and K.-S. Fu, A graph distance measure for image analysis, *IEEE Trans. on Syst., Man, Cybernetics*, 14, 398–407, May/June 1984.

[86] S. Berretti, A. Del Bimbo, and E. Vicario, Efficient matching and indexing of graph models in content based retrieval, *IEEE Trans. on Patt. Anal. and Machine Intelligence*, 23, 1089–1105, October 2001.

[87] J. Ullman, An algorithm for subgraph isomorphism, *J. ACM*, 23, 31–42, January 1976.

[88] J. Smith, Image retrieval evaluation, in *Proceedings of the IEEE Workshop of Content-Based Access of Image and Video Libraries*, Santa Barbara, CA, June 1998, IEEE Computer Society, pp. 112–113.

[89] N. Pioch, WebMuseum, www.ibiblio.org/wm/, 2003.

# 11

# *Semantic Processing of Color Images*

Stamatia Dasiopoulou, Evaggelos Spyrou, Yiannis Kompatsiaris,
Yannis Avrithis, and Michael G. Strintzis

## CONTENTS

## 11.1 Introduction

Image understanding continues to be one of the most exciting and fastest-growing research areas in the field of computer vision. The recent advances in hardware and telecommunication technologies, in combination with the Web proliferation witnessed, have boosted the wide-scale creation and dissemination of digital visual content. However, this rate of growth has not been matched by concurrent emergence of technologies to support efficient image analysis and retrieval. As a result, this ever-increasing flow of available visual content has resulted in overwhelming users with large volumes of information, thus hindering access to appropriate content. Moreover, the number of diverse, emerging application areas, which rely increasingly on image understanding systems, has further revealed the tremendous potential of the effective use of visual content through semantic analysis. Better access to image databases, enhanced surveillance and authentication support, content filtering, summarization, adaptation and transcoding services, and improved human and computer interaction, are among the several application fields that can benefit from semantic image analysis.

Acknowledging the need for providing image analysis at the semantic level, research efforts focus on the automatic extraction of image descriptions in a way that matches human perception. The ultimate goal characterizing such efforts is to bridge the so-called *semantic gap* between low-level visual features that can be automatically extracted from the visual content, and the high-level concepts capturing the conveyed meaning. The emerged approaches fall into two categories — data-driven and knowledge-driven — depending on the creation processes of these high-level descriptions. The former adhere to the monolithic computational paradigm, in which the interpretation and retrieval to follow are based on some appropriately defined function computed directly from the data. No hierarchy of meaningful intermediate interpretations is created. By contrast, the latter follow the signals to symbol paradigm, in which intermediate levels of description are emphasized. They are based on the widely held belief that computational vision cannot proceed in a single step from signal-domain information to spatial and semantic understanding.

Data-driven approaches work on the basis of extracting low-level features and deriving the corresponding higher-level content representations without any prior knowledge apart from the developer's inherent one. Thus, these approaches concentrate on acquiring fully automated numeric descriptors from objective visual content properties, and the subsequent retrieval based on criteria that somehow replicate the human perception of visual similarity. The major weakness of such approaches is that they fail to interact meaningfully with the users' higher level of cognition, because the built-in associations between image semantics and its low-level quantitative descriptions are of no perceptual meaning to the users. Consequently, the underpinning linking mechanism remains a "black box" to the user, thus not allowing for efficient access or, more importantly, for the discovery of semantically related content. Systems based on the query-by-example paradigm, as well as traditional content-based image retrieval systems, are well-known application examples belonging in this category. Although they are efficient for restricted domains, such approaches lack the capability to adapt to different domains. Techniques like relevance feedback and incremental learning have been used to improve traditional content-based approaches by injecting some knowledge on user perception in the analysis and similarity matching process.

Knowledge-driven approaches, on the other hand, utilize high-level domain knowledge to produce appropriate content descriptions by guiding feature extraction, analysis and elimination of the unimportant ones, description derivation, and reasoning. These approaches form an interdisciplinary research area, trying to combine and benefit from the computer vision, signal processing, artificial intelligence, and knowledge management communities joined efforts for achieving automatic extraction of visual content semantics through the application of knowledge and intelligence. More specifically, the task of such image analysis approaches is to abstract users' visual content experience by means of computational models (i.e., reduce the volumes of multimodal data to concise representations that only capture their essence). Enabling intelligent processing of visual content requires appropriate sensors, formal frameworks for knowledge representation, and inference support. The relevant literature considers two types of approaches, depending on the knowledge acquisition and representation process — explicit, realized by formal model definitions, or implicit, realized by machine learning methods.

The main characteristic of learning-based approaches is the ability to adjust their internal structure according to input and corresponding desired output data pairs in order to approximate the associations (relations) that are implicit in the provided training data, thus elegantly simulating a reasoning process. Consequently, the use of machine learning techniques to bridge the semantic gap between image features and high-level semantic annotations provides a relatively powerful method for discovering complex and hidden relationships and mappings, and a significant number of such approaches have been proposed for a variety of applications. Neural networks, fuzzy systems, support vector machines, statistical models, and case-based reasoning are among the techniques that have been widely used in the area of object recognition and scene classification. However, due to this inherent "black box" method learning-based approaches may be difficult to develop and maintain, as their effectiveness relies upon the design and configuration of multiple variables and options. In addition, extensive and detailed training data sets are required to ensure optimum tuning and performance. The main disadvantage of machine-learning-based image analysis systems is a direct result of their implementation principle, i.e., they are built specifically for one particular domain and as a result they cannot be easily adapted to other domains or simply extended with further features for application on the same domain.

Following an alternative methodology, model-based image analysis approaches exploit prior knowledge in the form of explicitly defined facts, relations and rules about the problem under consideration. Such approaches attempt to bridge the gap between low-level descriptions and high-level interpretations by encompassing a structured representation of objects, events, relations, attributes, and so forth, of the examined domain. Thus, because the terms of the employed representation formalism (ontologies, semantic nets, etc.) carry meaning that is directly related to the visual entities, they provide a coherent semantic domain model, required to support "visual" inference in the context specified by the current set of logical statements. However, the computational complexity of such systems increases exponentially with the number of objects of interest, restricting the applicability of such approaches to settings where only a reasonable number of well-defined concepts are to be identified within a scene. Although appropriate, parameterized or generic models can be employed for improving performance, such model-based systems are computationally infeasible for unconstrained variety and complexity of supported concepts, because in such cases, the search space can become too large. As a result, in most knowledge-assisted approaches that make use of explicitly defined knowledge, objects are first detected without prior usage of such models, and recognition takes place afterwards based on contextual knowledge and fusion of the extracted facts. Controlling the variability of the scene is still a necessary condition for keeping the problem tractable.

It is worth noticing that although there is no consensus on which of these two classes of approaches is superior to the other, studies have revealed that human perception organization includes some kind of preattentive stage of visual processing. During this stage, different image features are detected, which are joined into complex objects at a second stage. Treisman [1] hypothesized that the visual system starts with extracting a set of useful properties, and then a map of locations is formed in which the presence of discontinuities is recorded. By focusing attention on this map, object hypotheses are created which are matched against stored object descriptions, for their recognition. In the latter stage, prior knowledge and expectations play an important role. Treisman further hypothesized that the preattentive visual system does not produce a single representation such as a single partitioned image. Rather, different image partitions are produced to support distinct channels in the human visual system which analyze the image along a number of different dimensions (such as color, depth, motion, etc.). Although Treisman studies do not provide a direct answer on which of the two categories best matches the semantic image analysis needs, they provide significant and useful guidelines on the individual tasks that the image interpretation process can be considered to consist of.

To conclude, automating the process of visual content semantics extraction is the final frontier in image understanding. The main challenge lies in bridging the gap between low-level visual descriptors and representations that can be automatically computed from visual content, and their associated high-level semantics as perceived by humans. In this chapter, semantic image analysis for the purpose of automatic image understanding and efficient visual content access and retrieval at the semantic level is discussed. The overview presented in Section 11.2 surveys current state-of-the-art analysis approaches aimed at bridging the "semantic gap" in image analysis and retrieval. It highlights the major achievements of the existing approaches and sheds light on the challenges still unsolved. Section 11.3 presents a generic framework for performing knowledge-assisted semantic analysis of images. Knowledge representation and modeling, content processing, and inferencing support aspects are detailed, providing further insight into requirement and specification issues for realizing automatic semantic description generation from visual content. Section 11.4 begins with a brief overview of the MPEG-7 standardized descriptors used within the presented framework and a few methods used for matching followed by the ontology infrastructure developed. It also presents the way the knowledge-assisted analysis is performed, using Semantic Web technologies. Finally, conclusions are drawn in Section 11.5, and plans for future work are presented.

## 11.2  State of the Art

Enabling efficient access to still images based on the underlying semantics presents many challenges. Image understanding includes the extraction of scene semantics in terms of global and local level conceptual entity recognition. The former may refer to general annotations, such as indoor/outdoor and city/landscape classifications, while the latter considers finer-grained descriptions addressing the presence of particular semantic entities, objects, or events (e.g., sunset, beach, airplane, etc.). The visual content of different information modalities (i.e., color, texture, shape) in combination with the inherent uncertainty render the extraction of image semantics impossible without the use of considerable amounts of *a priori* knowledge. As illustrated in the literature reviewed in the following, numerous standardized and proprietary low-level feature descriptors have been applied to capture the information conveyed by the different modalities characterizing visual information. In addition, diverse approaches have been used for knowledge representation and inference realization. Some of the most commonly used methods include neural and Bayesian networks, Markov random fields, decision trees, factor graphs, fuzzy systems, and ontologies.

Stochastic approaches include, among others, the work presented in Reference [2], where the problem of bridging the gap between low-level representation and high-level semantics is formulated as a probabilistic pattern recognition problem. A factor graph network of probabilistic multimedia objects, multijects, is defined in a probabilistic pattern recognition fashion using hidden Markov models (HMMs) and Gaussian mixture models. HMMs are combined with rules in the COBRA (COntend-Based RetrievAl) model described in Reference [3], where objects and events descriptions are formalized through appropriate grammars, and at the same time, the stochastic aspect provides the means to support visual structures that are too complex to be explicitly defined. A hierarchical model based on *Markov random fields* (MRF) was used in Reference [4] for implementing unsupervised image classification.

Histogram-based image classification is performed using a support vector machine (SVM) in Reference [5], while an object support vector machine classifier that is trained once on a small set of labeled examples is presented in Reference [6]. An SVM is applied to represent conditioned feature vector distributions within each semantic class and a Markov random field is used to model the spatial distributions of the semantic labels, for achieving semantic labelling of image regions in Reference [7]. To address cases in which more than one label fit the image data, Li, Wang, and Sung [8] propose a multilabel SVM active learning approach to address multilabel image classification problems.

In Reference [9], machine-learning techniques are used to semantically annotate images with semantic descriptions defined within ontologies, while in Reference [10], the use of the maximum entropy approach is proposed for the task of automatic image annotation. In Reference [11], a methodology for the detection of objects belonging to predefined semantic classes is presented. Semantic classes are defined in the form of a description graph, including perceptual and structural knowledge about the corresponding class objects, and are further semantically organized under a binary partition tree. Another nice example of a domain-driven semiautomated algorithm for semantic annotation is given in Reference [12], where a specific animal face tracker is formed from user-labeled examples utilizing an Adaboost classifier and a Kanade–Lucas–Tomasi tracker. The semi-automatic image annotation system proposed in Reference [13] uses hints given in natural language to prune the search space of object detection algorithms. The user can give hints like "in the upper left corner there is a L-shaped building." The system uses spatial constraints to reduce the area in which to search for an object, and other constraints to reduce the number of possible shapes or object types, supporting even complex queries describing several objects and their configurations.

Fuzziness is introduced in Reference [14], where neuro-fuzzy networks are used to locate human faces within images. An object-oriented high-resolution image classification based on fuzzy rules is described in Reference [15]. Domain experts define domain-specific rules through a graphical interface, and the system using these rules can automatically generate semantic annotations for any image of the given domain. A fuzzy rule-based inference approach is also followed in Reference [16] for building image classification. Knowledge representation is based on a fuzzy reasoning model in order to establish a bridge between visual primitives and their interpretations. A trainable system for locating clothed people in photographic images is presented in Reference [17]. Within this system, a tree is constructed with nodes that represent potentially segmentable human parts, while the edges represent distributions over the configurations of those parts. This classifier adapts automatically to an arbitrary scene by learning to use context features. A context-aware framework for the task of image interpretation is also described in Reference [18], where constraints on the image are generated by a natural language processing module performing on the text accompanying the image.

A method for classifying images based on knowledge discovered from annotated images using WordNet is described in Reference [19]. Automatic class discovery and classifier combination are performed using the extracted knowledge (i.e., the network of concepts with the associated image and text examples). This approach of automatically extracting semantic image annotation by relating words to images was reported in a number of other research efforts, such as in Reference [20] using latent semantics analysis, [21], [22], and so forth.

Following the recent Semantic Web advances, several approaches have emerged that use ontologies as the means to represent the necessary-for-the-analysis tasks domain knowledge, and take advantage of the explicit semantics representation for performing high-level inference. In Reference [23], an ontology-based cognitive vision platform for the automatic recognition of natural complex objects is presented. Three distributed knowledge-based systems drive the image processing, the mapping of numerical data into symbolical data and the semantic interpretation process. A similar approach is taken in the FUSION project [24], where ontology-based semantic descriptions of images are generated based on appropriately defined RuleML rules that associate MPEG-7 low-level features to the concepts included in the FUSION ontology. Also enhanced by rules is the user-assisted approach for automatic image annotation reported in Reference [25], while fuzzy algebra and fuzzy ontological information are exploited in Reference [26] for extracting semantic information in the form of thematic categorization. Ontology-based image classification systems are also presented in References [27] and [28]. In Reference [29], the problem of injecting semantics into visual data is addressed by introducing a data model based on description logics for describing both the form and the content of such documents, thus allowing queries on both structural and conceptual similarity.

Medical image understanding is another application field in which semantic image analysis has received particularly strong interest. Medical image interpretation is mainly required for diagnosis purposes in order to reduce repetitive work, and for providing assistance in difficult diagnoses or unfamiliar cases. Thus, the automatic acquisition of accurate interpretation is a strict requirement, and in addition, the efficient management of the huge volumes of information concentrated in medical image databases is vital. The approaches reported in the literature cover a wide variety of medical imaging cases such as tomography, mammography, ophthalmology, radiology, and so forth. Computer tomography images are analyzed in Reference [30] using two case-based reasoners, one for segment identification and another for a more holistic interpretation of the image. The system STARE (STructured Analysis of the REtina), presented in Reference [31], is a management system for medical images that supports, among others, automated retinal diagnosis using Bayesian networks to realize an inference mechanism. KBIUS (Knowledge-Based Image Understanding System) [32] is another knowledge-assisted rule-based image understanding system that supports x-ray bone images segmentation and interpretation.

Despite the sustained efforts during the last years, state of the art for semantic image understanding still cannot meet users' expectations for systems capable of performing analysis at the same level of complexity and semantics that a human would employ while analyzing the same content. Although a significant number of approaches with satisfactory results have been reported, semantic image understanding remains an unsolved problem, because most state-of-the-art techniques make no attempt to investigate generic strategies for incorporating domain knowledge and contextual information, but rather rely on ad hoc, application-targeted solutions that adopt hard-coded application-oriented analysis and interpretation approaches [33]. Consequently, due to the unrestricted potential content and the lack of temporal context that would assist in the recognition of perceptual entities, the presented technical challenges render semantic image analysis a fascinating research area awaiting new advances. Additionally, as can be seen in the presented literature, there is a significant diversity in the approaches taken for knowledge-assisted semantic image analysis. The followed knowledge representation formalisms vary from ad hoc hard-coded representations to formal logic-based ones, while the analysis and interpretation tasks include implementations ranging from probabilistic- and rule-based ones to logic inference tasks, providing or not support for uncertainty.

Furthermore, recent studies revealed that apart from the need to provide semantic-enabled image access and management, the inherent dynamic interpretation of images under different circumstances should be taken into consideration in future efforts [34]. Perceptual similarity depends upon the application, the person, and the context of usage.

Thus, machines not only need to understand the visual content and underlying meaning associations but also have to acquire and interpret them online while interacting with users. Finally, in order for image understanding to mature, understanding how to evaluate and define appropriate frameworks for benchmarking features, methods, and systems is of paramount importance.

## 11.3   Knowledge-Assisted Analysis

Building on the considerations resulting from the presented state of the art on semantic image analysis, this section presents a generic framework for performing semantics extraction from images based on explicitly defined *a priori* knowledge. The proposed semantic analysis framework does not consider global semantics extraction, at least not directly as detailed in the following, but rather focuses on the recognition of salient semantic entities at object level (e.g., sea and sand in a beach image or the presence of a mountain in an image depicting an outdoors scene). The extraction of these higher-level semantic descriptions is performed based on the available domain knowledge and appropriately defined rules that model the context on which such concepts occur (e.g., an image of a player scoring a goal presupposes a particular spatial arrangement of the ball, the goalpost, etc.). Further and more abstract annotations can be acquired based on these initially extracted annotations by further exploiting the examined domain conceptualization.

Before proceeding with the detailed description of the proposed analysis framework, the process of knowledge-assisted image analysis and understanding is briefly overviewed to better highlight the challenges and open issues involved and, thus, demonstrate how the proposed framework provides the means to address them.

The goal of knowledge-based semantic image analysis that uses explicit knowledge is to extract semantic descriptions from low-level image representations based on the facts, relations, rules, etc., provided about the domain examined. Such domain knowledge includes prototypical descriptions of the important domain concepts in terms of their visual properties and context of appearance, as well as information on their relations, and thus allows for their identification. For this reason, visual descriptions of the image data need to be extracted and matched against the corresponding definitions included in the available domain knowledge. Thereby, through a stepwise, one direction or iterative, process the extraction of semantic description is performed. Already from this very rough description, it can be seen that among the issues of particular importance are knowledge representation, the way the interpretation itself is realized, whether or not uncertainty support is provided, as well as the principle on which interpretation takes place, i.e., in an iterative or monolithic manner. As already described in the previous section, with respect to knowledge representation ad hoc solutions limit interoperability and reusability, and thus should be avoided. Providing support for uncertainty is equally crucial due to the inherent in multimedia ambiguity and the role of cues rather than evidence that visual information provides. Considering the implementation of the interpretation process, an iterative hypothesize-and-test approach seems to be more appropriate than trying to reach the final semantic interpretation in a single step. However, following such an approach requires extremely complex and sophisticated control mechanisms to tackle cases with a high number of supported concepts that moreover interrelate to each other. Thus, partitioning the involved tasks into smaller units and successively move to more refined graded annotations appears to be a reasonable tradeoff.

Complementary to the aforementioned aspects, are the challenges introduced by the limitations of the low-level processing techniques and segmentation in particular. Partitioning the image into a set of meaningful regions is prerequisite before any analysis can take place, because the analysis and interpretation tasks to follow are based on the visual features extracted from these regions. However, partitioning of an image into meaningful regions is a very challenging task [35]. The sensory data is inherently noisy and ambiguous, and the available segmentation approaches perform on a purely numerical basis, thus leading to segmentations that are unreliable and vary in an uncontrollable way (i.e., regions may result as fragmented or falsely merged). In addition, the various domain objects can be characterized by diverse visual properties requiring more than one image partitioning scheme in order to capture them. For example, objects with indicative shape properties require shape-driven segmentation approaches, while texturized objects need segmentations based on, possibly different per object, texture descriptors. Thus, the knowledge-assisted analysis and interpretation tasks need to take into account the inconsistencies introduced by erroneous segmentation and be able to recognize a single semantic entity despite being over-segmented and handle the semantics of partonomic relations between a concept and its constituent parts. Ideally handling under-segmentation cases would be desirable, however this again necessitates for particularly complex control and processing when dealing with unconstrained and ill-defined domains.

From the above mentioned, it is evident that semantic image analysis has to deal with multiple low-level representations based on the different modalities of visual information, overcome the syntactic nature of existing segmentation approaches, and exploit domain knowledge to control the complexity of the semantics extraction decision-making process. To assist in these extremely challenging tasks, the framework presented adopts a formal knowledge representation to ensure consistent inference services, and exploits the knowledge available within each stage of the analysis process.

The main knowledge structures and functional modules of the proposed generic semantic analysis framework, as well as their interactions, have been shown in Figure 11.1. As illustrated, ontologies have been used for representing the required knowledge components. This choice is justified by the recent Semantic Web technologies advances and the consequent impacts on knowledge sharing and reusability. Several ontology languages that provide support for expressing rich semantics have been proposed, providing the formal definition framework required for making these semantics explicit [36]. Furthermore, ontology alignment, merging, and modularization are receiving intense research interest, leading to methodologies that further establish and justify the use of ontologies as knowledge representation formalism. In addition, tools for providing inference support have emerged that

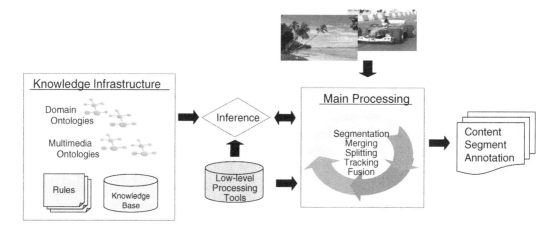

**FIGURE 11.1**
Knowledge-assisted semantic image analysis framework.

allow for reasoning about the existing facts and deriving knowledge that was previously implicit. If image content is to be fully exploited by search engines, services, and application agents within the Semantic Web context, semantic analysis should target the generation of annotations that meet the currently formulated semantics description standards. A detailed description of each of the presented framework components and its respective role and contribution in the semantic analysis process are described in the sequel.

Due to the two-layer semantics of visual content (i.e., the semantics of the actual conveyed meaning and the semantics referring to the media, different kinds of ontologies have been defined. More specifically, domain ontologies have been employed to model the conveyed content semantics with respect to specific real-world domains. They are defined in such a way as to provide a general model of the domain, with focus on the user-specific point of view. Consequently, each domain ontology includes those concepts that are of importance for the examined domain (i.e., the salient domain objects and events) and their interrelations.

On the other hand, multimedia analysis ontologies model the actual analysis process. They include knowledge specific to the media type, descriptive definitions for representing low-level visual features and attributes related to spatial topology, and in addition, the low-level processing algorithms definitions. By building this unifying model of all aspects of image analysis, all related parts can be treated as ontological concepts, thus supporting interoperability and reusability of the presented analysis framework. In addition, by associating the content-processing tools with visual properties, the analysis process gets decoupled from application-specific requirements and can be easily adapted to other domains.

Linking the domain and multimedia ontologies results in enhancing the former with qualitative and quantitative descriptions of the defined domain concepts. Thus, the domain ontologies model the examined domain in a way that, on the one hand, makes the retrieval of images more efficient for end users and, on the other hand, the defined concepts can also be automatically extracted through image analysis. In other words, the concepts are recognizable by the automatic analysis methods, while they remain comprehensible to humans. Populating the domain ontologies results in enriching the knowledge base with the appropriate models (i.e., prototypical visual and spatial descriptions) of the domain concepts that need to be detected.

To determine how the extraction of semantic concepts, their respective low-level features, and the processing algorithms execution order relate to each other, appropriate rules need to be defined. As a result, sufficiently expressive languages need to be employed for defining such rules and for allowing reasoning on top of the knowledge defined in the domain and the multimedia analysis ontologies. Naturally the need for sufficiently rich ontology languages holds also for the definition of the domain and multimedia ontologies. In particular, the latter specifically require for representing the data types and relations that are common in multimedia content. These requirements apply to the storing and querying mechanisms as well, so as to ensure effective access and retrieval to the available knowledge.

To conclude, a generic ontology-based framework for knowledge-assisted domain-specific semantic image analysis was presented that couples domain and multimedia specific ontologies to provide a coherent model that allows the automatic detection of concepts while keeping them comprehensible to humans. The considered knowledge includes qualitative object attributes, quantitative low-level features, as well as low-level processing methods. In addition, rules are employed to describe how tools for image analysis should be applied, depending on object attributes and low-level features, for the detection of objects corresponding to the semantic concepts defined in the ontology. The added value comes from the coherent architecture achieved by using an ontology to describe both the analysis process and the domain of the examined visual content. Following such an approach, the semantic image analysis process depends largely on the knowledge base of the system, and, as a result, the method can be easily applied to different domains provided that the knowledge base is enriched with the respective domain knowledge. In the following section, a specific implementation built on the aforementioned framework is presented that employs the RDFS language for knowledge representation and follows the MPEG-7 standard for the multimedia ontologies definition.

## 11.4 Knowledge-Assisted Analysis Using MPEG-7 and Semantic Web Technologies

### 11.4.1 Overview of MPEG-7 Visual Descriptors

The goal of the ISO/IEC MPEG-7 standard [37] is to allow interoperable searching, indexing, filtering, and browsing of audiovisual (AV) content. Unlike its predecessors, the focus was on nontextual description of multimedia content, aiming to provide interoperability among applications that use audiovisual content descriptions.

In order to describe AV content, the MPEG-7 standard specifies a set of various color, texture, shape, and motion standardized descriptors to represent visual, low-level, non-semantic information from images and videos and use it to create structural and detailed descriptions of AV information. A descriptor defines the syntax and the semantics of an elementary AV feature, which may be low level (e.g., color) or high level (e.g., author). For tasks like image classification or object recognition, visual MPEG-7 descriptors [38] are considered. A brief overview of the most important MPEG-7 visual descriptors that are applicable to still color images follows.

#### 11.4.1.1 Color Descriptors

Color is probably the most expressive of all the visual features. Thus, it has been extensively studied in the area of image retrieval during the last years. Apart from that, color features are robust to viewing angle, translation, and rotation of the regions of interest. The MPEG-7 color descriptors [39] comprise histogram descriptors, a dominant color descriptor, and a color layout descriptor (CLD). The presentation of the color descriptors begins with a description of the color spaces used in MPEG-7:

- *Dominant color descriptor* is probably the most useful MPEG-7 descriptor for applications like similarity retrieval, as a set of dominant colors in a region of interest or in an image provides a compact yet effective representation. Prior to the evaluation of the descriptor, the colors present are clustered in order to minimize the number of considered colors. This clustering is followed by the calculation of their percentages and optionally their variances. These colors are not fixed in the color space but are computed each time based on the given image. Each image can have up to 8 dominant colors, however experimental results have shown that 3 to 4 colors are generally sufficient to provide a satisfactory characterization.

- *Color space descriptor* is introduced, as each color descriptor uses a certain color space, and therefore, a short description of the most widely used color spaces is essential. The color spaces supported are the monochrome, RGB, HSV, YCbCr, and the new HMMD [39]. These color space descriptors are also used outside of the visual descriptors (i.e., in specifying "media properties" in suitable description schemes).

- *Color layout descriptor* (CLD) is a compact MPEG-7 visual descriptor designed to represent the spatial distribution of color in the YCbCr color space. It can be used globally in an image or in an arbitrary-shaped region of interest. The given picture or region of interest is divided into $8 \times 8 = 64$ blocks, and the average color of each block is calculated as its representative color. A discrete cosine transformation is performed in the series of the average colors, and a few low-frequency coefficients are selected using zigzag scanning. The CLD is formed after quantization of the remaining coefficients, as described in Reference [40].

- *Scalable color descriptor* (SCD) is a Haar-transform-based encoding scheme that measures color distribution over an entire image. The color space used is the HSV, quantized uniformly to 256 bins. To sufficiently reduce the large size of this representation, the histograms are encoded using a Haar transform, allowing also the desired scalability.

- *Color-structure descriptor* (CSD) captures both the global color features of an image and the local spatial structure of the color. The latter feature of the CSD provides the descriptor the ability to discriminate between images that have the same global color features but different structure; thus, a single global color histogram would fail. An $8 \times 8$ structuring element scans the image, and the number of times a certain color is found within it is counted. This way, the local color structure of an image is expressed in the form of a "color structure histogram." This histogram is identical in form to a color histogram but is semantically different. The color representation is given in the HMMD color space. The CSD is defined using four-color space quantization operating points (184, 120, 64, and 32 bins) to allow scalability, while the size of the structuring element is kept fixed.

### 11.4.1.2 Texture Descriptors

Texture refers to the visual patterns that may or may not have properties of homogeneity, which results from the presence of multiple colors or intensities in the image. It is a property of virtually any surface, and contains important structural information of surfaces and their relationship to the surrounding environment. Describing texture in images by appropriate MPEG-7 texture descriptors [39] provides a powerful means for similarity matching and retrieval for both homogeneous and non-homogeneous textures. The three texture descriptors, standardized by MPEG-7, are texture-browsing descriptor, homogeneous texture descriptor, and local edge histogram:

- *Texture-browsing descriptor* provides a qualitative characterization of a texture's regularity, directionality, and coarseness. The regularity of a texture is described by an integer ranging from 0 to 3, where 0 stands for an irregular/random texture, and 3 stands for a periodic pattern. Up to two dominant directions may be defined, and their values range from $0°$ to $150°$ in steps of $30°$. Finally, coarseness is related to image scale or resolution and is quantized to four levels, with the value 0 indicating a fine-grain texture and the value 3 indicating a coarse texture.

- *Homogeneous texture descriptor* (HTD) provides a quantitative characterization of texture and is an easy-to-compute and robust descriptor. The image is first filtered with orientation and scale-sensitive filters. The mean and standard deviations of the filtered outputs are computed in the frequency domain. The frequency space is divided in 30 channels, as described in Reference [40], and the energy and the energy deviation of each channel are computed and logarithmically scaled.

- *Local edge histogram* captures the spatial distribution of edges and represents local-edge distribution in the image. Specifically, dividing the image in $4 \times 4$ subimages, the local edge distribution for each subimage can be represented by a histogram. To generate this histogram, edges in the subimages are categorized into five types: vertical, horizontal, 45° diagonal, 135° diagonal, and nondirectional edges. Because there are 16 subimages, a total of $5 \times 16 = 80$ histogram bins are required. This descriptor is useful for image-to-image matching, even when the underlying texture is not homogeneous.

### 11.4.1.3  Shape Descriptors

Humans can often recognize objects solely from their shapes, as long as they have a characteristic one. This is a unique feature of the shape descriptors, which discriminates them from color and texture. Thus, shape usually contains semantic information for an object. It is obvious that the shape of an object may be a very expressive feature when used for similarity search and retrieval. MPEG-7 proposes three shape descriptors [41]: region-based shape descriptor, contour-based shape descriptor, and two-dimensional (2-D)/three-dimensional (3-D) shape descriptor.

- *Region-based shape descriptor* expresses the 2-D pixel distribution within an object or a region of interest. It is based both on the contour pixel and the inner pixels of the object or region of interest; therefore, it is able to describe complex objects as well as simple objects with or without holes. The shape analysis technique used is based on moments, and a complex 2-D angular radial transformation (ART) is applied. Then the descriptor is constituted by the quantized magnitudes of the ART coefficients. In conclusion, the region-based shape descriptor gives a compact, efficient, and robust way to describe both complex and simple objects.

- *Contour-based shape descriptor* captures the characteristic features of the contours of the objects. It is based on an extension of the curvature scale-space (CSS) representation of the contour and can effectively describe objects with contours that are characteristic; thus rendering the region-based shape descriptor redundant. Contour-based shape descriptor can also discriminate objects with regions that are similar but have different contours. This descriptor emulates the shape similarity perception of the human eye system and provides a compact and robust to nonrigid deformations and perspective transformations description of objects of region of interest.

- *2-D/3-D shape descriptor* combines 2-D descriptors of a visual feature of an object or region of interest, seen from various different angles, thus forming an entire 3-D representation of it. Experiments have shown that a combination of contour-based shape descriptors of a 3-D object is an effective way to obtain a multiview description of it.

### 11.4.1.4  Descriptor Matching

As described in Section 11.4, knowledge-assisted image analysis approaches exploit *a priori* knowledge about the domain under consideration to perform semantic analysis tasks, such as object recognition and image classification. As detailed above, the provided knowledge includes information about the domain conceptualization, the image in terms of its structure, and the modeled domain concepts in the form of visual descriptors and spatial relations. Among the possible representations, the information considering low-level visual features is often encoded using low-level descriptors similar to those that are proposed by the MPEG-7 standard. It is obvious that a key factor in such tasks is the measure selected for the estimation of the distance between the descriptors. When the descriptors to be considered are MPEG-7 standardized, there are certain measures to evaluate their similarities, which, in some cases, are explicit. This subsection presents a few similarity measures for some of the above described descriptors as they were defined by the MPEG-7.

For example, matching with the *dominant color* descriptor can be performed in the following way: Let

$$F_1 = \{\{c_{1i}, p_{1i}, v_{1i}\}, s_1\}, i = 1, \ldots, N_1$$
$$F_2 = \{\{c_{2i}, p_{2i}, v_{2i}\}, s_2\}, i = 1, \ldots, N_2$$

be two dominant color descriptors. Ignoring variances and spatial coherencies (which are optional), the dissimilarity between them may be defined as

$$D^2(F_1, F_2) = \sum_{i=1}^{N_1} P_1 i^2 + \sum_{j=1}^{N_2} P_2 i^2 - \sum_{i=1}^{N_1} \sum_{j=1}^{N_2} 2a_{1i,2j} p_{1i} p_{2j}$$

where $a_{ij}$ is the similarity coefficient between two colors $c_k$ and $c_l$, defined by

$$a_{k,l} = \begin{cases} 1 - d_{k,l}/d_{max} & \text{if} \quad d_{k,l} \leq T_d \\ 0 & \text{if} \quad d_{k,l} > T_d \end{cases}$$

and $d_{k,l}$ is the Euclidean distance between the two colors $c_k$ and $c_l$, $T_d$ is the maximum distance for two colors, and $d_{max} = a T_d$. More details about the determination of $T_d$ and $a$, and also for modifications that can be made to take into account the variances and the spatial coherencies, can be found in Reference [42].

MPEG-7 does not strictly standardize the distance functions to be used and sometimes does not propose a specific dissimilarity function, leaving the developers with the flexibility to develop their own dissimilarity/distance functions. A few techniques can be found in the MPEG-7 eXperimentation Model (XM) [42]. Apart from that, there are many general-purpose distances that may be applied in order to simplify some complex distance function or even to improve the performance [43]. A large number of successful distance measures from different areas (statistics, psychology, medicine, social and economic sciences, etc.) can be applied on MPEG-7 data vectors.

However, in order to achieve better performance, combining two or more low-level descriptors seems essential. This problem remains open, and there are not any standardized methods to achieve it. Apart from that, fusion of the descriptors is necessary, as they would be otherwise incompatible and inappropriate to directly include, for example, in a Euclidean distance. A classic approach to combine the results of many descriptors is to normalize the distances between images according to the different descriptors, then add these distances to obtain a unique distance for each pair (additive fusion) [44]. A drawback of this additive fusion is that it computes the average of the distances (by summing them) and, therefore, risks neglecting the good performances of a given descriptor because of the poor performances of another. Merging fusion as in Reference [45] simply consists of merging all the descriptions into a unique vector. If $D_1, D_2, \ldots, D_n$ are the $n$ descriptors to combine, then the merged descriptor is equal to

$$D_{merged} = [D_1|D_2|\ldots|D_n]$$

This fusing method requires all features to have more or less the same numerical values to avoid scale effects. An alternative is to rescale the data using for instance principal component analysis. Rescaling is not necessary in the case of the MPEG-7 descriptors because they are already scaled to integer values of equivalent magnitude. Assigning fixed weights as in Reference [46] can be an efficient method, especially when the number of the visual features is small. The assignment of the weights can be done either experimentally through a try-and-error procedure, by simply observing the results and giving more weight to the descriptors that seem to have more discriminative power, or by using a statistical method as in Reference [47], where each feature is used separately, and the matching values assigned to the first two outputs of the system are added up. Then the average of this sum over the whole query set is found and the corresponding weight for each method is defined to be inversely proportional to this average.

## 11.4.2   Ontology Structure

As noted in Section 11.4, among the possible knowledge representation formalisms, ontologies [36] present a number of advantages. They provide a formal framework for supporting explicit, machine-processable, semantics definitions, and they facilitate inference and the derivation of new knowledge based on the already existing one. Thus, ontologies appear to be ideal for expressing multimedia content semantics in a formal machine-processable representation that will allow automatic analysis and further processing of the extracted semantic descriptions. In the developed knowledge-assisted analysis framework, the RDF vocabulary description language (RDFS) has been used for expressing the considered domain and multimedia ontologies.

*Resource Description Framework Schema (RDFS)* is a simple modeling language on top of the RDF formalism[1], both being developed by the World Wide Web Consortium (W3C). *Web Ontology Language (OWL)*, a language inspired by description logics and also developed by the W3C, is designed to be used by applications that need increased expressive power compared to that supported by RDFS, by providing additional vocabulary along with formal semantics. In our framework, RDFS was chosen as the modeling language due to the fact that full usage of the increased expressiveness of OWL requires specialized and more advanced inference engines that are not yet widely available.

As shown in Figure 11.2, the developed ontology structure [48] consists of a *core ontology* whose role is to serve as a starting point for the construction of new ontologies, a *visual descriptor ontology* that contains the representations of the MPEG-7 visual descriptors, a *multimedia structure ontology* that models basic multimedia entities from the MPEG-7 Multimedia Description Scheme [49], and *domain ontologies* that model the content layer of multimedia content with respect to specific real-world domains.

### 11.4.2.1   Core Ontology

In general, core ontologies are typically conceptualizations that contain specifications of domain-independent concepts and relations based on formal principles derived from philosophy, mathematics, linguistics, and psychology. The role of the core ontology in this overall framework is to serve as a reference point for the construction of new ontologies, to provide a reference point for comparisons among different ontological approaches, and to serve as a bridge between existing ontologies. In the presented framework, the *DOLCE* [50] ontology is used for this purpose. DOLCE has been explicitly designed as a core ontology: it is minimal in the sense that it includes only the most reusable and widely applicable upper-level categories, rigorous in terms of axiomatization, and extensively researched and documented.

Although the DOLCE core ontology provides a means for representing spatiotemporal qualities, reasoning with such descriptions requires the coding of additional relations that describe the relationship between space and time regions. Based on concepts taken from the

---

[1] RDF is not a knowledge representation system but tries to improve data interoperability on the Web. This is achieved by specializing the XML data model through a graph-based data model similar to the semantic networks formalism.

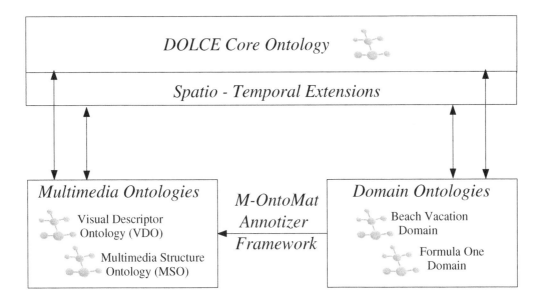

**FIGURE 11.2**
Ontology structure overview.

"Region Connecting Calculus" [51], Allen's interval calculus [52], and directional models [53], [54], the `Region` concept branch of DOLCE was extended to accommodate topological and directional relations between the spatial and temporal regions concepts of DOLCE, i.e., the `TimeRegion` and `2DRegion` ones. Directional spatial relations describe how visual segments are placed and relate to each other in 2-D or 3-D space (e.g., left and above). Topological spatial relations describe how the spatial boundaries of the segments relate (e.g., touch and overlap). In a similar way, temporal segment relations are used to represent temporal relationships among segments or events; the normative binary temporal relations correspond to Allen's temporal interval relations.

### 11.4.2.2  *Visual Descriptor Ontology*

The visual descriptor ontology (VDO) [55] represents the visual part of the MPEG-7 and thus, contains the representations of the set of visual descriptors used for knowledge-assisted analysis. Its modeled concepts and properties describe the visual characteristics of the objects. The construction of the VDO attempted to follow the specifications of the MPEG-7 Visual Part [56]. Because strict attachment to the MPEG-7 Visual Part was not possible due to the syntactic semantics underlying it, several requisite modifications were made in order to adapt the XML schema provided by MPEG-7 to an ontology and the data-type representations available in RDFS.

The tree of the VDO consists of four main concepts, which are `VDO:Region`, `VDO:Feature`, `VDO:VisualDescriptor` and `VDO:Metaconcepts`, as illustrated in Figure 11.3. None of these concepts is included in the XML schema defined by the MPEG-7 standard, but their definition was required for ensuring correct ontology engineering. The `VDO:VisualDescriptor` concept contains the visual descriptors, as these are defined by MPEG-7. The `VDO: Metaconcepts` concept, on the other hand, contains some additional concepts that were necessary for the VDO, but they are not clearly defined in the XML schema of MPEG-7. The remaining two concepts that were defined, `VDO:Region` and `VDO:Feature`, are also not included in the MPEG-7 specification, but their definition was necessary in order to enable the linking of visual descriptors to the actual image regions.

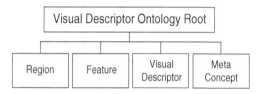

**FIGURE 11.3**
The visual descriptor ontology (VDO).

For example, consider the VDO:VisualDescriptor concept, which consists of six sub-concepts, one for each category of the MPEG-7-specified visual descriptors. These are *color, texture, shape, motion, localization,* and *basic descriptors*. Each of these subconcepts includes a number of relevant descriptors. These descriptors are defined as concepts in the VDO. Only the VDO:BasicDescriptors category was modified regarding the MPEG-7 standard and does not contain all the MPEG-7 descriptors.

### 11.4.2.3  Multimedia Structure Ontology

The multimedia structure ontology (MSO) models basic multimedia entities from the MPEG-7 Multimedia Description Scheme [49] and mutual relations like decomposition. Within MPEG-7, multimedia content is classified into five types: image, video, audio, audiovisual, and multimedia. Each of these types has its own segment subclasses that correspond to the subsegments to which they can be decomposed. MPEG-7 provides a number of tools to describe the structure of multimedia content in time and space. The Segment DS [49] describes a spatial or temporal fragment of multimedia content. A number of specialized subclasses are derived from the generic Segment DS. These subclasses describe the specific types of multimedia segments, such as video segments, moving regions, still regions, and mosaics, which result from spatial, temporal, and spatiotemporal segmentation of the different multimedia content types. Multimedia resources can be segmented or decomposed into subsegments through four types of decomposition: spatial, temporal, spatiotemporal, and media source.

### 11.4.2.4  Domain Ontologies

In the presented framework, the domain ontologies model the content layer of multimedia content, with respect to specific real-world domains, such as Formula One and beach vacations. Because the DOLCE ontology was selected as the core ontology of the ontology infrastructure, all the domain ontologies are explicitly based on or aligned to it, and thus interoperability between different domain ontologies is ensured through their linking to the DOLCE concepts.

In the context of this work, domain ontologies are defined in a way to provide a general model of the domain, with focus on the user's specific point of view. More specifically, ontology development was performed in a way that, on the one hand, the retrieval becomes more efficient for a user of a multimedia application, and on the other hand, the included concepts can also drive their automatic extraction from the multimedia layer. In other words, the defined semantic concepts are recognizable by automatic analysis methods while at the same time remaining comprehensible to users.

### 11.4.3  Domain Ontologies Population

In order to exploit the presented ontology infrastructure, the domain ontology needs to be populated with appropriate instances (i.e., visual descriptors and spatial relations of

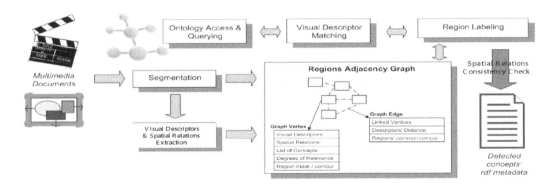

**FIGURE 11.4**
The developed knowledge-assisted semantic image analysis system architecture.

the defined domain objects), because, as described in Section 11.4, the produced semantic annotations are generated through matching against these object prototypes. To accomplish this, the low-level descriptors that are included in the definition of each domain object need to be extracted for a sufficiently large number of corresponding object samples and be associated with the domain ontology. Within the described implementation, a user-oriented tool was developed. Users are able to select regions that correspond to domain concepts and then choose the MPEG-7 Descriptor to be extracted. Triggered by the user's extraction command, the requested MPEG-7 Descriptors are extracted through calls to appropriate routines based on the MPEG-7 XM, a reference model utilizing the MPEG-7 visual descriptors [42].

### 11.4.4 Semantic Multimedia Analysis

The implemented semantic multimedia analysis architecture is presented in Figure 11.4. As illustrated, analysis starts by segmenting the input image content and extracting the low-level descriptors and the spatial relations in accordance with the domain ontology definitions. In the sequel, a first set of possible semantic concepts that might be depicted in each of the segmented regions is produced by querying the knowledge base and matching the previously extracted low-level descriptors with the ones of the objects prototype instances. To evaluate the plausibility of the produced hypotheses labels for each region and to reach the final semantic annotation, spatial context information is used. Thereby, the image semantics are extracted, and respective content description metadata are generated. The implementation details of each of these processing steps are given in the following.

#### 11.4.4.1 Image Representation

A region adjacency graph (RAG) has been selected as the means for storing internally the related to the analyzed image information. More specifically, each vertex of the graph holds the MPEG-7 visual descriptors of the image region it represents, the spatial relations between the region and its neighboring regions, and the degree of confidence to which this region matches a specific domain concept. Additionally, a list[2] of all the pixels that constitute the region and a list of all region's pixels that constitute its contour are also stored to improve performance. Finally, each edge of the graph stores the two linked regions, the

---

[2] This list is more efficient than keeping the binary mask of the region, in terms of memory usage and time required for the analysis of an image.

distance of these regions estimated based on each visual descriptor, and a list of pixels that constitute the common contour of the two linked regions. Presently, the RAG is used only for efficient representation and storage purposes and not in the actual process of the analysis (i.e., no graph matching takes place, but instead the subsequently described descriptor matching and spatial content consistency check are applied for generating semantic descriptions).

### 11.4.4.2   Image Segmentation

The first step should be to formulate a segmentation algorithm that will generate a few tens of connected regions and initialize the graph. The segmentation used is an extension of the well-known recursive shortest spanning tree (RSST) algorithm based on a new color model and so-called syntactic features [57].

### 11.4.4.3   Low-Level Visual Descriptor Extraction

The currently supported low-level descriptors, are the MPEG-7 dominant color and the region shape descriptors, and their extraction is based on the guidelines given by the MPEG-7 XM.

### 11.4.4.4   Spatial Relations Extraction

As previously mentioned, apart from low-level descriptions, it is necessary to include in the domain knowledge definitions information about the objects' spatial context as well, because this is the only way to discriminate between objects with similar visual appearance and ensure robust performance in cases of significant intraclass variability. Objects such as *Sky* and *Sea* are among the simplest and most common examples where spatial context is required to lead to correct interpretation. The information about neighboring (i.e., adjacent) regions can be found directly in the structure of the graph. However, apart from the adjacency information provided by the graph, additional topological and directional information is needed in order to further assist the analysis and improve performance. The currently supported spatial relations are *above of*, *below of*, *left of*, *right of*, and *contained in*. In addition, two absolute relations were introduced, the *bottom-most* and *top-most* relations, because during experimentation, they proved to be particularly useful in the cases of particular semantic concepts, such as the *Sky*.

### 11.4.4.5   Descriptors Matching

After having extracted all information about the visual features of the regions of the image and their spatial relations, the next step is to calculate the degree of matching between the descriptors included in the domain knowledge and the ones extracted from the segmented regions, and thus generate possible labels for each region. To accomplish this, the distances between each region descriptors and the corresponding ones of the domain concepts need to be estimated and then combined to form a single distance for each region against the defined domain concepts. Because MPEG-7 does not provide a standardized method of combining these distances or of estimating a single distance based on more than one visual descriptor, the following approaches are used:

- A *weighted sum* of the two distances, where the weight of the dominant color descriptor is greater than the one of the region shape descriptor, because dominant color has been proven to have a better discriminative performance during the descriptor evaluation process.

- A *backpropagation neural network* [45], which is trained to estimate the similarity between two regions; it has as input a vector formed by the low-level descriptions of two regions or a region and a prototype instance, and responds with their "normalized" distance.

A fundamental difference between the aforementioned techniques is that the first requires the computation of all distances (based on every available descriptor) and then combines them through a weighted sum, while the latter produces a unique distance based on all available low-level visual features. In this simple scenario of only two descriptors, both approaches exhibited satisfactory performance. A typical normalization function is used, and then the distance is inverted to acquire the *degree of confidence*, which is the similarity criterion for all matching and merging processes. From this whole procedure, a list of possible concepts along with a degree of confidence for all regions is derived and stored appropriately in the graph.

In the case that two or more neighboring regions have been assigned to only one concept, or other possible concepts have a degree less than a predefined threshold, these regions are assumed to be part of a bigger region that was not segmented correctly due to the well-known segmentation limitations. By merging the graph's vertices and updating all corresponding graph's fields (the visual descriptors are again extracted, the contour of the region is updated along with the edges of the graph, etc.), the whole process of analysis can be realized in an iterative manner, by repeating the individual processing steps until meeting a termination criterion. However, in the presented initial implementation this possibility was not investigated and the one direction approach was followed.

### 11.4.4.6 Spatial Context Consistency Check

The descriptors matching step, by only examining low-level features information, often results in more than one possible semantic labels for each region of the image. To evaluate the plausibility of each of these hypotheses and to reach the final interpretation, spatial context is used. More specifically, for each region, the system checks whether the region's extracted spatial characteristics match the spatial context associated with the possible labels assigned to it.

### 11.4.4.7 Knowledge-Base Retrieval

Whenever new multimedia content is provided as input for analysis, the existing *a priori* knowledge base is used to compare, by means of matching the MPEG-7 visual descriptors and the spatial context information, each region of the image to the prototype instances of the provided domain knowledge. For this reason, the system needs to have full access to the overall knowledge base consisting of all domain concept prototype instances. These instances are applied as references to the analysis algorithms, and with the help of appropriate rules related to the supported domains, the presented knowledge-assisted analysis system extracts semantic concepts that are linked to specific regions of the image or video shot.

For the actual retrieval of the object prototype descriptors instances, the *OntoBroker*[3] engine is used to deal with the necessary queries to the knowledge base. OntoBroker supports the loading of RDFS ontologies, so all appropriate ontology files can be easily loaded. For the analysis purposes, OntoBroker needs to load the domain ontologies where high-level concepts are defined, the VDO that contains the low-level visual descriptor

---

[3] See www.ontoprise.de/products/ontobroker_en.

**TABLE 11.1**

Formula One and Beach Vacations Domain Definitions

| Concept | Visual Descriptors | Spatial Relations |
|---------|--------------------|--------------------|
| Road | Dominant color | Road ADJ grass, sand |
| Car | Region shape, motion activity | Car INC road |
| Sand | Dominant color | Sand ADJ grass, road |
| Grass | Dominant color | Grass ADJ road, sand |
| Sky | Dominant color | Sky ABV Sea |
| Sea | Dominant color | Sea ABV, ADJ sand |
| Sand | Dominant color | Sand BEL, ADJ sea |
| Person | Region shape | Person INC sea, sand |

*Note: ADJ*: adjacency relation; *ABV*: above relation; *BEL*: below relation; *INC*: inclusion relation.

definitions, and the prototype instances files that include the knowledge base and provide the linking of domain concepts with descriptor instances. Appropriate queries are defined, which permit the retrieval of specific values from various descriptors and concepts. The OntoBroker's query language is *F-Logic*.[4] F-Logic is both a representation language that can be used to model ontologies and a query language, so it can be used to query OntoBroker's knowledge.

### 11.4.4.8 Semantic Metadata Creation

Having identified the domain concepts that correspond to the different image regions, the next step is to produce metadata in a form that can be easily communicated and shared among different applications. Taking into consideration the proliferation of the Semantic Web and the various emerging applications that use these technologies, the RDF schema was chosen for representing the extracted annotation metadata. Thereby, and due to the interoperability ensured by the linking to the DOLCE concepts, existing semantic-based retrieval systems can be utilized directly to benefit from the produced annotations. As also mentioned earlier, the produced annotations can be further enhanced and refined through further reasoning over the produced annotations with respect to the domain conceptualization itself (e.g., an image of an organized beach is one including regularly arranged umbrellas and sunbeds). It is worth noticing here, that such functionality can be supported due to the well-defined semantics that ontologies provide. Although this aspect is equally interesting and challenging, the current implementation has focused on the generation of the initial annotations.

### 11.4.5 Results

The presented knowledge-assisted semantic image analysis approach was tested in the Formula One and beach vacation domains. Analysis was performed by enriching the knowledge infrastructure with the appropriate domain ontology and by providing prototype instances for the corresponding defined domain objects. The defined semantic objects for each of the two examined domains, along with their visual descriptors and their spatial relations are given in Table 11.1. For example, the concept *Sea* in the beach vacations domain ontology is represented using the dominant color descriptor and is defined to be below the concept *Sky* and above or adjacent to the concept *Sand*. In a similar manner, the

---

[4] See www.ontoprise.de/documents/tutorial_flogic.pdf.

definitions of the other objects can be derived from Table 11.1. It must be noted that the results for the Formula One domain were obtained by analyzing image sequences and not still images. However, this does not discredit the proposed analysis framework, because each frame was processed separately following the above-described methodology, and the motion activity descriptor was employed only to further improve the attained performance for the *Car* concept. As illustrated in Figure 11.5 and Figure 11.6, respectively, the system output is a segmentation mask outlining the semantic description of the scene where different colors representing the object classes defined in the domain ontology are assigned to the segmented regions.

As previously mentioned, the use of spatial information captures part of the visual context, consequently resulting in the extraction of more meaningful descriptions, provided that the initial color-based segmentation has not segmented two objects as one region. The benefits obtained by the use of spatial information are particularly evident in the beach vacations domain results, where the semantic concepts *Sea* and *Sky*, despite sharing similar visual features, are correctly identified due to their differing spatial characteristics. The unknown label shown in the produced semantic annotations was introduced to account for the cases where a region does not match any of the semantic objects definitions included in the domain ontology.

## 11.5 Conclusions and Future Work

This chapter reported on the challenges and current state of the art in semantic image analysis and presented an integrated framework for semantic multimedia content annotation and analysis. The employed knowledge infrastructure uses ontologies for the description of low-level visual features and for linking these descriptions to concepts in domain ontologies. Despite the early stage of experimentation, the first results obtained based on the presented ontological framework are promising and show that it is possible to apply the same analysis algorithms to process different kinds of images by simply employing different domain ontologies. In addition, the generation of the visual descriptors and the linking with the domain concepts is embedded in a user-friendly tool, which hides analysis-specific details from the user. Thus, the definition of appropriate visual descriptors can be accomplished by domain experts, without the need to have a deeper understanding of ontologies or low-level multimedia representations.

However, there is still plenty of space for improvements. Because the performance of the analysis depends on the availability of sufficiently descriptive and representative concepts definitions, among the first future priorities is the investigation of additional descriptors and methodologies for their effective fusion. Related to this is the development of methodologies to efficiently handle issues regarding the prototype instances management (i.e., how many are necessary, how can they be further processed to exploit the available knowledge, etc.). Furthermore, the use of additional spatial and partonomic relations will allow for the definition of more complex semantic concepts and for the derivation of higher-level descriptions based on the already extracted ones, such as the concept of an *Island*, which can be detected as being associated to adjacent regions corresponding to the *Rock*, *Vegetation*, and so forth, concepts and which are related through the inside relation to the region corresponding to the *Sea* concept. Finally, apart from visual descriptions and relations, future focus will concentrate on the reasoning process and the creation of rules in order to detect more complex concepts. The examination of the interactive process between ontology evolution and use of ontologies for content analysis will also be the target of

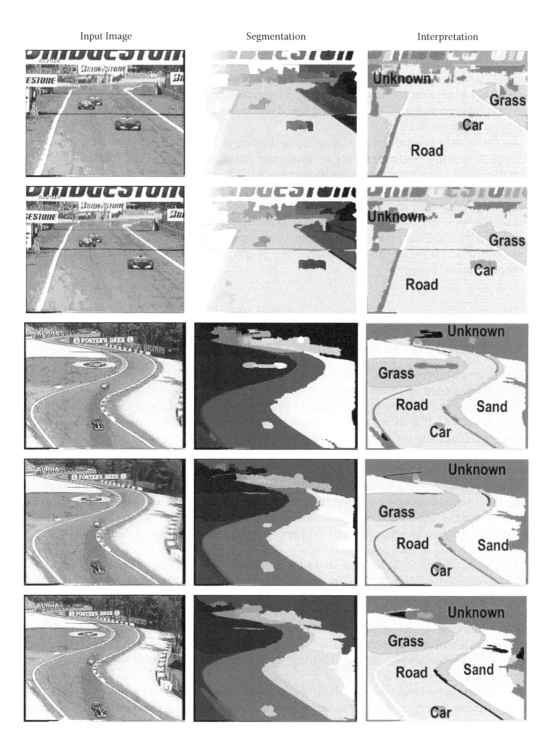

**FIGURE 11.5**
Semantic analysis results for the Formula One domain.

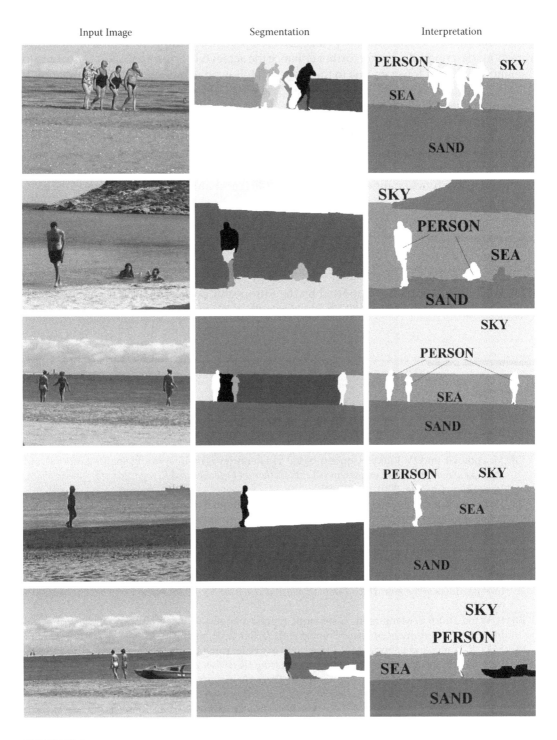

**FIGURE 11.6**
Semantic analysis results for the beach vacations domain.

our future work, in the direction of handling the semantic gap in multimedia content interpretation.

To conclude, the proposed approach presents many appealing properties and produces satisfactory results even at this early stage of development. The implementation of the future directions described above will further enhance the achieved performance and contribute to semantic analysis. However, due to the approach followed in modeling the domain knowledge (i.e., the definition of explicit models), there will be cases of semantic concepts with description that will be infeasible due to increased complexity or incomplete knowledge. To support such cases, the proposed framework can be appropriately extended to couple the domain ontology definitions with implicit representations based on the internal structure of learning-based techniques such as the specific weights values of a neural network, etc. Thereby, more accurate semantic descriptions will become available, benefiting from the complementary functionalities provided by explicit and implicit knowledge modeling.

## Acknowledgments

This research was partially supported by the European Commission under contracts FP6-001765 aceMedia and FP6-507482 KnowledgeWeb.

## References

[1] A. Treisman, Features and objects in visual processing, *Scientific American*, 255, 114–125, 1986.

[2] M.R. Naphade, I.V. Kozintsev, and T.S. Huang, A factor graph framework for semantic video indexing, *IEEE Trans. on Circuits and Syst. for Video Technol.*, 12, 40–52, 2002.

[3] M. Petkovic and W. Jonker, Content-based video retrieval by integrating spatio-temporal and stochastic recognition of events, in *IEEE Workshop on Detection and Recognition of Events in Video*, Vancouver, Canada, 2001, pp. 75–82.

[4] Z. Kato, J. Zerubia, and M. Berthod, Unsupervised parallel image classification using a hierarchical Markovian model, in *Proceedings of the Fifth International Conference on Computer Vision*, Cambridge, MA, USA, pp. 169–174, June 1995.

[5] O. Chapelle, P. Haffner, and V. Vapnik, Support vector machines for histogram-based image classification, *IEEE Trans. on Neural Networks*, 10, 1055–1064, September 1999.

[6] B. Bose and E. Grimson, Learning to use scene context for object classification in surveillance, in *Proceedings of the Joint IEEE International Workshop on VS-PETS*, Nice, France, October 2003, pp. 94–101.

[7] L. Wang and B.S. Manjunath, A semantic representation for image retrieval, in *Proceedings of International Conference on Image Processing (ICIP'02)*, 2003, pp. 523–526.

[8] X. Li, L. Wang, and E. Sung, Multi-label svm active learning for image classification, in *Proceedings of International Conference on Image Processing (ICIP'04)*, 2004, Singapore, pp. 2207–2210.

[9] O. Marques and N. Barman, Semi-automatic semantic annotation of images using machine learning techniques, in *International Semantic Web Conference*, 2003, Florida, USA, pp. 550–565.

[10] S. Jeanin and A. Divakaran, MPEG-7 visual motion descriptors, *IEEE Trans. on Circuits and Syst. for Video Technol.*, 11, 6, 720–724, 2001.

[11] X. Giro and F. Marques, Detection of semantic objects using description graphs, in *Proceedings of International Conference on Image Processing (ICIP'05)*, Genova, Italy, September 2005.

[12] T. Burghardt, J. Calic, and B. Thomas, Tracking animals in wildlife videos using face detection, in *Proceedings of the European Workshop on the Integration of Knowledge, Semantics and Digital Media Technology (EWIMT'04)*, London, UK, 2004.

[13] R.K. Srihari and Z. Zhang, Show&tell: A semi-automated image annotation system, *IEEE MultiMedia*, 7, 61–71, 2000.

[14] A.Z. Kouzani, Locating human faces within images, *Comput. Vision and Image Understanding*, 91, 247–279, September 2003.

[15] F.B.A.C. Lingnau and J.A.S. Centeno, Object oriented analysis and semantic network for high resolution image classification, *Boletim de Ciencias Geodesicas*, 9, 233–242, 2003.

[16] A. Dorado and E. Izquierdo, Exploiting problem domain knowledge for accurate building image classification, in *Proceedings of the Conference on Image and Video Retrieval (CIVR'04)*, 2004, Dublin, Ireland, pp. 199–206.

[17] N. Sprague and J. Luo, Clothed people detection in still images, in *Proceedings of the International Conference on Pattern Recognition (ICPR'02)*, 2002, Quebec, Canada, pp. 585–589.

[18] R. Chopra and R.K. Srihari, Control structures for incorporating picture-specific context in image interpretation, in *IJCAI*, 1995, pp. 50–55.

[19] A.B. Benitez and S.F. Chang, Image classification using multimedia knowledge networks, in *Proceedings of International Conference on Image Processing (ICIP'03)*, 2003, Barcelona, Spain, pp. 613–616.

[20] R. Tansley, C. Bird, W. Hall, P.H. Lewis, and M.J. Weal, Automating the linking of content and concept, in *ACM Multimedia*, Los Angeles, CA, USA, 2000, pp. 445–447.

[21] K. Barnard, P. Duygulu, D.A. Forsyth, N. Freitas, D.M. Blei, and M.I. Jordan, Matching words and pictures, *J. Machine Learning Res.*, 3, 1107–1135, 2003.

[22] V. Lavrenko, R. Manmatha, and J. Jeon, A model for learning the semantics of pictures, in *Neural Information Processing Systems (NIPS'03)*, Vancouver, Canada, 2003.

[23] C. Hudelot and M. Thonnat, A cognitive vision platform for automatic recognition of natural complex objects, in *ICTAI*, 2003, Sacramento, CA, USA, pp. 398–405.

[24] J. Hunter, J. Drennan, and S. Little, Realizing the hydrogen economy through semantic web technologies, *IEEE Intelligent Syst.*, 19, 40–47, 2004.

[25] S. Little and J. Hunter, Rules-by-example—a novel approach to semantic indexing and querying of images, in *International Semantic Web Conference*, Hiroshima, Japan, 2004, pp. 534–548.

[26] M. Wallace, G. Akrivas, and G. Stamou, Automatic thematic categorization of multimedia documents using ontological information and fuzzy algebra, in *Proceedings of the IEEE International Conference on Fuzzy Systems (FUZZ-IEEE'03)*, St. Louis, MO, 2003.

[27] L. Wang, L. Khan, and C. Breen, Object boundary detection for ontology-based image classification, in *Proceedings of Multimedia Data Mining—Mining Integrated Media and Complex Data (MDM/KDD'02)*, Edmonton, Alberta, Canada, 2002, pp. 51–61.

[28] C. Breen, L. Khan, and A. Ponnusamy, Image classification using neural networks and ontologies, in *DEXA Workshops*, Aix-en-Provence, France, 2002, pp. 98–102.

[29] C. Meghini, F. Sebastiani, and U. Straccia, Reasoning about the form and content of multimedia objects, in *Proceedings of the AAAI Spring Symposium on the Intelligent Integration and Use of Text, Image, Video and Audio Corpora*, Stanford, CA, USA, 1997.

[30] M. Grimnes and A. Aamodt, A two layer case-based reasoning architecture for medical image understanding, in *EWCBR*, 1996, Lausanne, Switzerland, pp. 164–178.

[31] M. Goldbaum, S. Moezzi, A. Taylor, S. Chatterjee, E. Hunter, and R. Jain, Automated diagnosis and image understanding with object extraction, objects classification and inferencing in retinal images, in *Proceedings of International Conference on Image Processing (ICIP'96)*, Lausanne, Switzerland, 1996.

[32] S. Linying, B. Sharp, and C.C. Chibelushi, Knowledge-based image understanding: A rule-based production system for x-ray segmentation, in *Proceedings of the International Conference on Enterprise Information Systems (ICEIS'02)*, Ciudad Real, Spain, 2002, pp. 530—533.

[33] A.W.M. Smeulders, M. Worring, S. Santini, A. Gupta, and R. Jain, Content-based image retrieval at the end of the early years, *IEEE Trans. Patt. Anal. Machine Intelligence*, 22, 1349–1380, 2000.

[34] N. Sebe, M.S. Lew, X.S. Zhou, T.S. Huang, and E.M. Bakker, The state of the art in image and video retrieval, in *Proceedings of the Conference on Image and Video Retrieval (CIVR'03)*, Urbana-Champaign, IL, USA, 2003, pp. 1–8.

[35] P. Salembier and F. Marques, Region-based representations of image and video: Segmentation tools for multimedia services, *IEEE Trans. on Circuits and Syst. for Video Technol. (CSVT)*, 9, 1147–1169, December 1999.

[36] S. Staab and R. Studer, *Handbook on Ontologies*, Springer–Verlag, Heidelberg, 2004.

[37] S.-F. Chang, T. Sikora, and A. Puri, Overview of the MPEG-7 standard, *IEEE Trans. on Circuits and Syst. for Video Technol.*, 11, 688–695, 2001.

[38] T. Sikora, The MPEG-7 visual standard for content description—an overview, *IEEE Trans. on Circuits and Syst. for Video Technol.*, 11, 696–702, 2001.

[39] B. Manjunath, J. Ohm, V. Vasudevan, and A. Yamada, Color and texture descriptors, *IEEE Trans. on Circuits and Syst. for Video Technol.*, 11, 703–715, 2001.

[40] MPEG-7, Multimedia Content Description Interface—part 3: Visual, ISO/IEC/JTC1/SC29/WG11, Document N4062, 2001.

[41] M. Bober, MPEG-7 visual shape descriptors, *IEEE Trans. on Circuits and Syst. for Video Technol.*, 11, 716—719, 2001.

[42] MPEG-7, Visual Experimentation Model (XM) Version 10.0, ISO/IEC/ JTC1/SC29/WG11, Document N4062, 2001.

[43] H. Eidenberger, Distance measures for MPEG-7-based retrieval, in *ACM MIR03*, Berkeley, CA, USA, 2003.

[44] J. Stauder, J. Sirot, H. Borgne, E. Cooke, and N. O'Connor, Relating visual and semantic image descriptors, in *European Workshop on the Integration of Knowledge, Semantics and Digital Media Technology*, London, 2004.

[45] E. Spyrou, H. LeBorgne, T. Mailis, E. Cooke, Y. Avrithis, and N. O'Connor, Fusing MPEG-7 visual descriptors for image classification, in *International Conference on Artificial Neural Networks (ICANN)*, Warsaw, Poland, 2005.

[46] B. Bustos, D. Keim, D. Saupe, T. Schreck, and D. Vranic, Automatic selection and combination of descriptors for effective 3d similarity search, in *IEEE International Workshop on Multimedia Content-Based Analysis and Retrieval*, Miami, Florida, USA, 2004.

[47] F. Mokhtarian and S. Abbasi, Robust automatic selection of optimal views in multi-view free-form object recognition, *Patt. Recognition*, 38, 7, 1021–1031, July 2005.

[48] S. Bloehdorn, K. Petridis, C. Saathoff, N. Simou, V. Tzouvaras, Y. Avrithis, S. Handschuh, I. Kompatsiaris, S. Staab, and M.G. Strintzis, Semantic annotation of images and videos for multimedia analysis, in *Proceedings of the Second European Semantic Web Conference (ESWC)*, Heraklion, Greece, May 2005, 592–607.

[49] "ISO/IEC 15938-5 FCD Information Technology—Multimedia Content Description Interface—Part 5: Multimedia Description Schemes, March 2001, Singapore.

[50] A. Gangemi, N. Guarino, C. Masolo, A. Oltramari, and L. Schneider, Sweetening ontologies with DOLCE, in *Knowledge Engineering and Knowledge Management. Ontologies and the Semantic Web, Proceedings of the 13th International Conference on Knowledge Acquisition, Modeling and Management, EKAW 2002*, Vol. 2473 of *Lecture Notes in Computer Science*, Siguenza, Spain, 2002, 166–181.

[51] A. Cohn, B. Bennett, J.M. Gooday, and N.M. Gotts, *Representing and Reasoning with Qualitative Spatial Relations about Regions*, Kluwer, Dordrecht, 1997, pp. 97–134.

[52] J. Allen, Maintaining knowledge about temporal intervals, *Commun. ACM*, 26, 832–843, 1983.

[53] D. Papadias and Y. Theodoridis, Spatial relations, minimum bounding rectangles, and spatial data structures, *Int. J. Geographical Inf. Sci.*, 11, 111–138, 1997.

[54] S. Skiadopoulos and M. Koubarakis, Composing cardinal direction relations, *Artif. Intelligence*, 152, 143–171, 2004.

[55] N. Simou, V. Tzouvaras, Y. Avrithis, G. Stamou, and S. Kollias, A visual descriptor ontology for multimedia reasoning, in *Proceedings of Workshop on Image Analysis for Multimedia Interactive Services (WIAMIS '05), Montreux, Switzerland, April 13–15, 2005*.

[56] ISO/IEC 15938-3 FCD Information Technology—Multimedia Content Description Interface—Part 3: Visual, March 2001, Singapore.

[57] T. Adamek, N. O'Connor, and N. Murphy, Region-based segmentation of images using syntactic visual features, in *Proceedings of the Workshop on Image Analysis for Multimedia Interactive Services, WIAMIS 2005*, Montreux, Switzerland, April 13–15, 2005, 5–15.

# 12

## Color Cue in Facial Image Analysis

Birgitta Martinkauppi, Abdenour Hadid, and Matti Pietikäinen

### CONTENTS

## 12.1  Introduction

Color is a low-level cue for object detection that can be implemented in a computationally fast and effective way for locating objects. It also offers robustness against geometrical changes under a stable and uniform illumination field. In some cases, it can clearly discriminate objects from a background. Therefore, its popularity in machine vision applications is most understandable. Unfortunately, color information is very sensitive to changes in illumination — which are, in practice, common. Therefore, several strategies have been developed to cope with such changes. One strategy is to use only the chromaticity coordinates of a color space which properly separate chromaticity from intensity. Although this works quite well with intensity-related light changes, it does not cancel out illumination chromaticity variations. In order to eliminate light changes due to illumination chromaticity, a mass of color constancy algorithms have been suggested, but so far they have not produced reliable enough results for machine vision purposes, except in very limited cases (see, e.g., Reference [1]). Instead of correcting colors or canceling illumination changes, some other work aims at developing approaches that can tolerate or can be adapted to changes. Such methods are yielding promising results, as will be demonstrated in this chapter.

The information about skin color can be exploited as a feature for facial image analysis. It can be utilized in two ways: as a classifier to label pixels as skin and nonskin candidates or as a verifier to determine whether a found area possibly contains skin or not. In both cases, its role is to separate skin from nonskin background. This chapter deals with the role of color in facial image analysis tasks such as face detection and recognition. First, we explain how color information is involved in the field of facial image analysis (Section 12.2). Then in Section 12.3, we give an introduction to color formation and discuss the effect of illumination on color appearance, and its consequences. We discuss skin color modeling in Section 12.4. Section 12.5 explains, through exemplification, the use of color in face detection, while the contribution of color to face recognition is covered in Section 12.6. Finally, conclusions are drawn in Section 12.7.

## 12.2 Color Cue and Facial Image Analysis

Analyzing facial images is useful in several applications, like the tracking and identification of persons, human–machine interaction, videoconferencing, and content-based image retrieval. Facial image analysis may include face detection and facial feature extraction, face tracking and pose estimation, face and facial expression recognition, and face modeling and animation.

The properties of the face pose a very difficult problem for facial image analysis: a face is a dynamic and nonrigid object that is difficult to handle. Its appearance varies due to changes in pose, expressions, illuminations, and other factors, such as age and makeup. As a consequence, most of the facial analysis tasks generally involve heavy computations due to the complexity of facial patterns. Therefore, one may need some additional cues, such as color or motion, in order to assist and accelerate the analysis. These additional cues also offer an indication of the reliability of the face analysis results: the more the cues support the analysis, the more one can be confident about the results. For instance, with appearance-based face detection, an exhaustive scan (at different locations and scales) of the images is conducted when searching the face [2]. However, when the color cue is available, one can reduce the search regions by preprocessing the images and selecting only the skin-like areas. Therefore, it is not surprising that the color of skin has been commonly used to assist face detection. Also, in face recognition, it has been argued that color plays a role under degraded conditions by facilitating low-level facial image analysis, such as better estimations of the boundaries, shapes, and sizes of facial features [3]. As mentioned above, among the advantages of using color is the computational efficiency and robustness against some geometric changes, such as scaling and rotation, when the scene is observed under a uniform illumination field. However, the main limitation with the use of color lies in its sensitivity to illumination changes (especially changes in the chromaticity of the illuminant source which are difficult to cancel out).

Let us consider the general block diagram of face analysis shown in Figure 12.1. The color cue is involved at different stages. In the first stage, the color images (or video sequences) are acquired and pre-processed. The preprocessing may include gamma correction, color space transformation, and so on. It is often preferable to get rid of the dependencies on lighting intensity as much as possible. The perfect case would be to also cancel-out the effect of the illuminant color (by defining a color representation that is only a function of

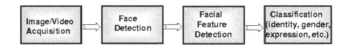

**FIGURE 12.1**
A general block diagram of face analysis that shows different phases of facial image analysis.

the surface reflectance), but so far, this has not been achieved in machine vision. The human visual system is superior in this sense, because human visual perception in which the color is perceived by the eye depends quite significantly on surface reflectance, although the light reaching the eye is a function of surface reflectance, illuminant color, and lighting intensity.

Among the different stages shown in Figure 12.1, the use of color in face detection is probably the most obvious. It is generally used to select the skin-like color regions. Then, simple refining procedures can be launched to discriminate the faces from other skin-like regions, such as hands, wood, etc. Thus, much faster face detectors are generally obtained when the color cue is considered. Section 12.5 describes a typical example of a face detector exploiting the color information.

Using the fact that some facial features, such as eyes, are darker than their surrounding regions, holes should then appear in the face area when labeling the skin pixels. Such an observation is commonly exploited when detecting facial features in color images [2], [4], [5].

Does color information contribute to face recognition? The answer to this question is not obvious, although some studies have suggested that color also plays a role in face recognition, and this contribution becomes evident when the shape cues are degraded [3]. Section 12.6 discusses this issue.

## 12.3 Color Appearance for Color Cameras

### 12.3.1 Color Image Formation and the Effect of Illumination

Color cameras represent colors using three descriptors, usually, red (R), green (G), and blue (B). An example of color camera filters is shown in Figure 12.2. The operation of a color camera can be divided into two parts: the initial response for the incoming light, and

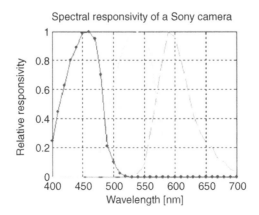

**FIGURE 12.2**
Spectral responsivity curves of a Sony camera, originally obtained from a graph provided by the manufacturer.

the gain control (or normalization) of the initial response. The initial response of an RGB camera is commonly modeled using the following expression:

$$D_{plain} = \int \eta_D(\lambda) I(\lambda) S(\lambda) d\lambda \qquad (12.1)$$

where $D$ is R,G, or B response; $\lambda$ is the wavelength; $\eta$ is the spectral responsivity of a spectral filter; $I$ is the spectral power distribution (SPD) of the light; and $S$ is the spectral reflectance of the surface. Note that the spectral power distribution of light can be expressed in an enormous number of ways due to different "normalization" methods, and the selected method may influence the end results. The normalization factor depends on the illumination SPD.

The plain RGB responses in Equation 12.1 need to be scaled to so that the responses of a certain white surface are identical under different lights. The scaling of values is also referred to as the white balancing or calibration. The first phase is the "cancellation" or "normalization" of effects of illumination, as shown in the following equation for the red channel:

$$R = \frac{\int \eta_R(\lambda) I(\lambda) S(\lambda) d\lambda}{\int \eta_R(\lambda) I(\lambda) d\lambda} \qquad (12.2)$$

where $p$ = prevailing (illumination), and $c$ = calibration (illumination).

It is a common practice in simulations to use a Planckian with corresponding color temperatures as a substitute for the actual light. The radiation spectrum of a heated blackbody or a Planckian [6] is completely determined by its (color) temperature. A high color temperature contains a more bluish component than red and vice versa for lower color temperatures. The color temperature does not directly correspond to the SPD, and this should be taken into account in the selection of an illuminant set for testing [7].

The placement differences between two adjacent chromaticity responses for adjacent Planckian illuminants in Figure 12.3 clearly demonstrate that the camera response is dissimilar for an object under different illuminants. The differences in intensity values are

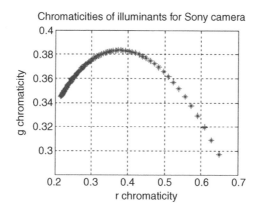

**FIGURE 12.3**
The illumination chromaticity response of the Sony camera varies widely for the Planckian illuminants. Note also that the chromaticity pairs form a curve that follows the color temperature of the illuminant. The leftmost marker corresponds to the Planckian of 10,000 K and the rightmost one to that of 2000 K. The chromaticity points between these two extreme points are formed by the Planckians with color temperatures that increase by 100 K from right to left.

even larger. The curve formed by these chromaticity pairs can be called the Planckian locus for the Sony camera. Figure 12.3 clearly indicates the need for response "normalization" by white. The normalization of plain responses is important, because they vary widely.

The second phase is a simple multiplication, the wanted output range by a constant factor, which is calculated for the canonical case. In real cameras, the process is carried out by adjusting the gains of different channels. The reference white is not ideal in practical cases, which, of course, can distort between real and theoretical results.

The relationship between illumination used in calibration and prevailing illumination is an important factor for determining the color appearance. If the prevailing illumination is the same as the illumination used in calibration, then the image is called a canonical image or calibrated case image, and correspondingly, the colors are canonical colors. Otherwise, they are uncanonical or uncalibrated ones. The effect of the relationship between calibration and prevailing illumination is discussed in more detail in Section 12.3.2. However, the modeling of uncanonical cases is problematic. The problem of normalization can be demonstrated theoretically [7]. Let us assume that the prevailing illumination is originally $I_{np}$, and its normalization factor is the constant factor $f_p$, and the calibration illumination is in the unnormalized format $I_{nc}$, which is normalized by the factor constant $f_c$. For example, if we insert these variables into Equation 12.2, we can derive the following format:

$$R = \frac{\int \eta_R(\lambda) I_p(\lambda) S(\lambda) d\lambda}{\int \eta_R(\lambda) I_c(\lambda) d\lambda} = \frac{\int \eta_R(\lambda) \frac{I_{np}(\lambda)}{f_p} S(\lambda) d\lambda}{\int \eta_R(\lambda) \frac{I_{nc}(\lambda)}{f_c} d\lambda} = \frac{f_c}{f_p} \frac{\int \eta_R(\lambda) I_{np}(\lambda) S(\lambda) d\lambda}{\int \eta_R(\lambda) I_{nc}(\lambda) d\lambda} \qquad (12.3)$$

The ratio $f_c/f_p$ is one only when the illumination conditions are the same. Different choices for normalization methods may produce different results [7]. There is no clear standard for which the currently available illumination normalization method, if any, should be used.

## 12.3.2 The Effect of White Balancing

In this section, we will examine more closely the effect of white balancing on the perceived images and colors. White balancing is a very important factor that determines the quality of the obtained images. Many digital images have been taken under canonical conditions or very near to them, because the users tend to notice color distortion as an annoying artifact. This is especially true for certain colors that humans remember very well, and thus, they are referred to as memory colors. One of these memory colors is, quite naturally, skin tone. Humans are very sensitive to any distortion in skin tones [8], [9], so it is not surprising that these have been investigated a lot. Skin tones refer here to the correct or acceptable colors for skin as perceived by a human. Skin colors refers to all those RGBs that a camera can perceive as skin under different illuminations.

It is sometimes impossible or difficult to determine when to conduct white balancing. This is especially true under varying illumination, which can cause more drastic color changes. For example, when the object is illuminated by two different light sources with different SPDs, it is not possible to conduct the correct white balancing for the whole image. This is demonstrated in Figure 12.4, in which the face is illuminated by the nonuniform illumination field, and the white balancing partially fails. The camera was calibrated to the light of fluorescent lamps on the ceiling, and the facial area under this light appears in skin tones. The incoming daylight from the window causes the bluish color shift on the right side of the face. Those facial regions between these two extremes exhibit different degrees of color shifts. Although these kinds of situations are common, they are rarely considered in most face detection and recognition systems. Therefore, we need to study more closely the factors that affect correct and incorrect white balancing.

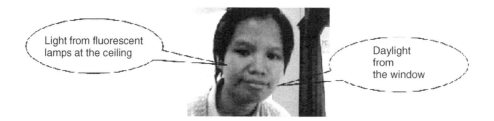

**FIGURE 12.4  (See color insert.)**
The face is illuminated by the nonuniform illumination field, and the white balancing partially fails. The color appearance of the face varies at different parts of the light field.

### 12.3.2.1  Canonical Images and Colors

In canonical images, the appearance of white is in an ideal case constant over different light sources. Real cameras present a white surface quite constantly over a range of color temperatures of light sources. Their gain control possibilities are limited due to physical limitations; therefore, at some point, the presentation of a white surface can no longer be restored.

   If the camera exhibits a linear response at a certain input signal range, then those grays that fall in this range are reproduced with values independent of the illumination of a certain color temperature range. The grays here refer to those objects with reflectance that differs only by a level from the reflectance of the white surface used in calibration. If the spectral reflectance differs also by shape, then the illumination cancellation does not work well, and the color appearance is affected to a different degree, depending on the shape difference, by the prevailing illumination. So the linearity of the camera cannot guarantee anything other than the similar appearance of grays and white over a certain color temperature range.

   This is demonstrated for three different skin complexions (shown in Figure 12.5) by calculating their theoretical RGB values for the Sony camera. Skin complexions have been roughly divided into three groups [34]: pale, yellowish, and dark. As can be seen from the

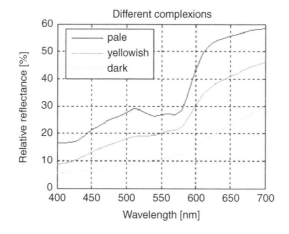

**FIGURE 12.5**
Skin complexions of three skin groups: pale, yellowish, and dark. Their reflectances are smooth and similar, mainly separated by their levels. Measured skin reflectances are available, for example, in the physics-based face database (See Marszalec, E., Martinkauppi, B., Soriano, M., and Pietikäinen, M., *J. Electron. Imaging*, 9, 32, 2000).

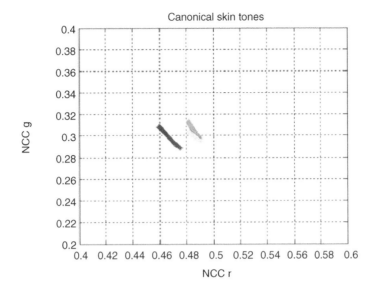

**FIGURE 12.6**
Canonical skin tones were obtained by converting the theoretical skin RGBs to normalized color coordinate (NCC) space.

figure, skin reflectances are smooth and similar, and they are mainly separated by their levels. This suggests that chromaticities of different complexions are quite near each other. The similarity of the reflectances is due to the biological factors underlying skin appearance: skin appearance arises mainly from three colorants — melanin, carotene, and hemoglobin [10]. Skin is a natural object with spectral reflectance that varies slightly from point to point.

The theoretical skin normalized color coordinate (NCC) chromaticities for the Sony camera are presented in Figure 12.6. As can be observed from the figure, the canonical skin values differ even in the ideal case, and they behave as a function of illumination. The difference is, nonetheless, small when you compare the results with real images. In Figure 12.7, we demonstrate the same phenomena for real images taken with the Sony camera. The selected light sources were four common ones encountered in many situations: horizon (light at sunset/sunrise), incandescent A, fluorescent lamp TL84, and daylight D65. The skin chromaticities from the image taken under the horizon lamp cover a bigger area than the others, maybe because the white balancing was not as successful as for the other light sources. There is a significant overlap between chromaticities values obtained under these illuminants.

### 12.3.2.2  Noncanonical Images and Colors

When the prevailing illumination mismatches the calibration one, the shift in color appearance can be bigger than in the canonical case. Figure 12.8 displays this for the case of four different light sources when only one was used in calibration. The upper image series presents what happened when the Sony camera was calibrated to the light source horizon (first image on the left), and the light was then changed to incandescent A, TL84, and daylight, respectively. The lower image series shows the opposite: first the camera was calibrated to daylight (first image on the right), and then the light was changed to TL84, A, and horizon.

The color shift in skin appearance tends to follow the direction of the color change of the light: if the prevailing illumination color is more reddish than the calibration, then the

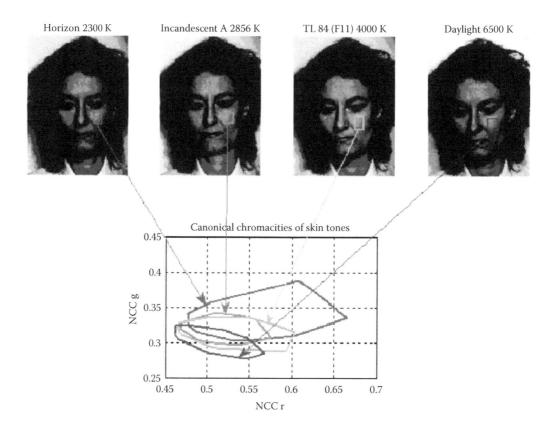

**FIGURE 12.7  (See color insert.)**
The skin tone appearance difference can be clearly observed in the four images taken with the Sony camera (see Figure 12.2). From the selected area marked with a box, the RGB values were taken and converted to NCC color space. As shown in the graph below the images, the areas of canonical chromaticities more or less overlap.

image colors shift toward red. When the prevailing illumination is more bluish, then the image colors tend to have an additional blue component. The limited dynamic response range causes distortion in color due to saturation or under-exposure. This problem can be at least partially alleviated if the camera has either a manual or an automatic brightness control. However, the manual control can be tedious and inaccurate, while the automatic control might produce false corrections.

Figure 12.9a and Figure 12.9b present theoretical chromaticities of the skin for one calibration while the illumination changes. From this figure, we can see that the chromaticity range depends on the calibration illumination and the possible color temperature range of prevailing illuminations. The number of calibrations also affects the possible range of skin colors. As we saw in Figure 12.9a and Figure 12.9b, different white balancing illuminants have dissimilar ranges of possible skin chromaticities and, therefore, produce separate skin locus. Figure 12.10 gathers all different calibration/prevailing illumination pairs. When comparing these two images, it is obvious that the skin locus with one white balancing is smaller than the one with several balancings. The size of the range of white balancing illuminants affects the locus size, too. Some settings of the camera, like gamma, contribute to the color production, and if these settings change, it may also affect the skin chromaticity range. To conclude, the size of the locus is affected by many factors that should be taken into account while creating the chromaticity constraint. Among the most important factors

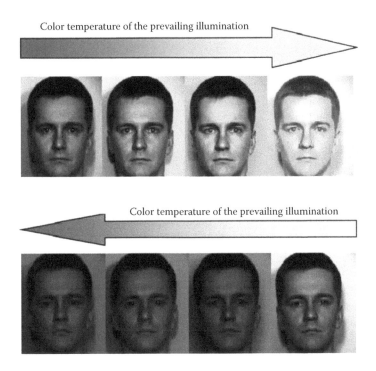

**FIGURE 12.8 (See color insert.)**
The color appearance shift. The color temperature of the light sources increases from left to right. The arrow indicates the change in the color of the light. The limited dynamic response range causes distortion in color: pixels can saturate to a maximum value (the rightmost image at the upper row) or be underexposed to zero (the leftmost image at the lower row).

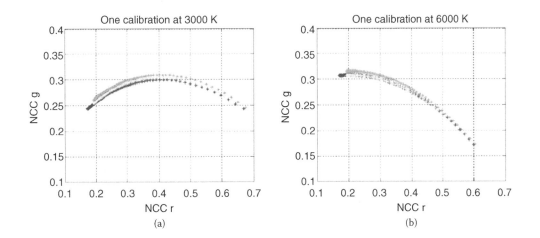

**FIGURE 12.9**
The skin NCC chromaticities were simulated using the data of the Sony camera (see Figure 12.2) and the skin reflectances from Figure 12.5: (a) possible skin chromaticities when the camera was calibrated to a Planckian of 3000 K and (b) when the calibration illumination was a Planckian of 6000 K. The chromaticity range depends on the calibration illumination and the possible color temperature range of prevailing illuminations.

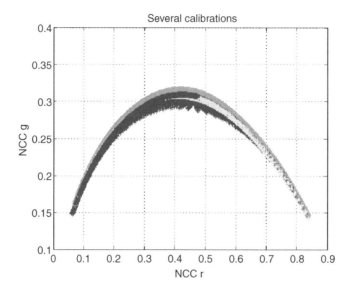

**FIGURE 12.10**
The skin locus formed with all prevailing illumination/white balancing combinations.

for the one camera case are the illumination variation range, the range of white balancing illuminants, and the camera settings.

## 12.4   Skin Color Modeling

When starting to build a skin color model, three issues should be taken into account: the first is the selection of the color spaces for modeling; the second is the illumination conditions and camera calibration; the last is the selection of a mathematical model. All these issues affect the effectiveness and optimality of the use of a skin color cue.

Several comparative studies of methods for skin detection were made for different data [11], [12]. The contradictory results obtained from the different studies are not surprising, because the optimality of the model depends on its purpose, material, and modeling parameters.

### 12.4.1   Color Spaces for Skin

Skin color modeling has been applied to several color spaces. So far, none of the color spaces has been shown to be clearly superior to the others, and it might well be that the optimal color space depends on the data. Those color spaces, that do not separate intensity properly from chromaticity are not so different from RGBs. Color spaces, that do separate intensity from chromaticity differ much more.

One popular choice for the color space is the NCC. This color space and CIE xy have been shown to be more efficient for face detection than several other color spaces and to produce more transferable skin color models between different cameras [11]. A more detailed summary of color spaces for skin detection can be found in Reference [13].

NCC effectively cancels intensity information from chromaticity information. The uniform intensity level changes in a pixel are effectively eliminated in chromaticity coordinates, because they are calculated by dividing the descriptor value of the channel by the sum of all descriptor values (intensity) at that pixel:

$$r = \frac{R}{R + G + B} \tag{12.4}$$

$$g = \frac{G}{R + G + B} \tag{12.5}$$

In NCC, a color is uniquely defined by its intensity information and two chromaticity coordinates, because $r + g + b = 1$. Therefore, one can use only the two chromaticity coordinates of NCC to cope with illumination intensity changes. The intensity changes are typically common in videos and images, because the skin areas can be located from deep shadows to bright lighting. This strategy is commonly used in skin detection, because it is easy to do. Of course, some models include intensity (like Reference [14]) but it is questionable if this information is useful, because the amount of data needed to construct a reliable model with all possible intensity levels is huge, and the third component increases the amount of computation.

## 12.4.2 Skin Color Model and Illumination

As shown in Section 12.3, the color appearance of skin depends on the illumination in two ways: by the prevailing illumination and by the illumination used in white balancing. This dependency is camera specific: the camera sensors and internal image preprocessing of the camera affect the color production and thus the end results. Therefore, creating a universal model is difficult.

Most of the research published so far concentrates on the situation in which the images have canonical or near canonical color appearance. This is not a bad approach if the image data are acquired mostly under these kinds of conditions, because the canonical skin colors overlap quite well. This kind of image data set can include personal photos, which are most likely taken under ideal conditions. However, this approach will only work on certain fixed cases.

If the illumination conditions are not fixed, the previous approaches are most likely to fail. Of course, it would be possible to use suggested color corrections, but this has been demonstrated to be even worse than no correction in some situations [12]. The color correction approach was suggested by Hsu et al. [5]. The basic idea is to correct the image colors so that the the skin would appear with skin tones and then apply the skin color model for segmentation. The color correction is based on finding pixels with high brightness value. They are assumed to belong to a white object on the image, and they are used for calculating the correction coefficient (this is a kind of white patch method). As mentioned earlier, the correction may fail, as shown in Figure 12.11.

Another approach was presented Cho et al. [15], who suggested an adaptive skin color filter. The basic idea is to first roughly select the possible skin color range and then fine-tune to find the face. The initial color range was determined from a set of images, but not so much detail was given about the selection criteria. The fine-tuning phase also makes some assumptions about the color distribution, such as the assumption that the facial skin color histogram is unimodal. It can also fail if the face is not the dominant skin-colored object on the image.

To build a better model, one should determine the possible illumination variation, white balancing of the camera, and camera settings and use this information to create the model. This is the basic idea behind the skin locus-based approach [16]: to understand the behavior under different conditions. When the behavior of skin is known, it is possible

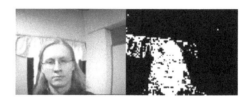

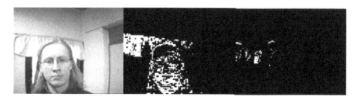

**FIGURE 12.11**
The upper row shows the color segmentation results using the model by Hsu et al. [5] without their color correction. The lower row shows the results with their color correction method. The color correction fails, because the yellow curtains have the highest brightness values.

to exclude particular nonskin tones — however, this is not the case with simple constraint. The model can be constructed either by simulations or by actually taking images under different conditions. One should note that the skin loci of different cameras may not overlap very well.

The skin locus-based models generally consist of more color tones than the canonical color models. This means that more nonskin objects will be considered skin candidates by the locus model than by the canonical model. This is the price one pays for the generality of the model. On the other hand, color is rarely enough to determine whether the target is skin or not, and canonical models tolerate illumination changes very poorly.

### 12.4.3  Mathematical Models for Skin Color

The mathematical skin color modeling can be approached from two different perspectives according to whether one can attach a probability for color tones or not. More details can be found in Reference [13]. The first approach assumes that skin is more likely to appear with certain color tones or provide higher discrimination between backgrounds and skin. The second one presumes that the probability of a certain color varies between images or that skin colors have equal appearance probability.

The challenge of the probability-based approach is to be able to reliably find the probability of color tones. This requires one to collect a representative data set of images (or then one assumes that some earlier formed statistical model is valid and can be used for the present data). So far, a statistical reliable color model for skin and nonskin Internet images was presented by Jones and Rehg [17]. They calculated the histogram and Gaussian models using over 1 billion labeled pixels. In addition to the statistical model, one has to determine the threshold limit for separating skin from nonskin areas. It is difficult to automatically find the threshold value, because the probability model found may not be valid for all images.

The second approach uses a spatial constraint in the color space to define possible skin areas. The shape of the constraint can be made up of simple thresholds like in Reference [15] or a more complex shaped function like in Reference [5]. No thresholding is needed, because there were no assumptions about the distribution of skin color in images. This can sometimes be overgenerous: all pixels within the constraint are labeled as skin.

Current frame

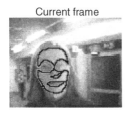

Next frame

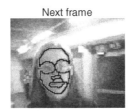

Chromacities from the two consecutive frames

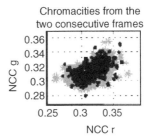

**FIGURE 12.12**
Two consecutive frames are selected from a video sequence (the first and second image from the left). The face areas of these frames are manually selected, and their RGB values are then converted to the NCC chromaticity space. The chromaticities from these two frames are marked with different colors in the right image. As can be observed from the rightmost image, the overlap between chromaticities is significant.

### 12.4.3.1 Video Sequences

Frames of a video sequence can be handled separately as if they were single, independent images. Skin detection can be made in this case by using the methods presented earlier. However, there are often sequential dependencies between frames, as shown in Figure 12.12. As can be seen, the overlap between the chromaticities from two consecutive frames is significant.

So, if skin detection is conducted for image sequences, it might be possible to use additional information to further tune the skin color model. When the illumination between images changes slowly enough (no abrupt total object color changes), the model can be made adaptive. Note that we assume also that the skin-colored target will move with a finite speed, because the illumination field over the image area can be nonuniform. To date, three different adaptive schemes were suggested: two of them use spatial constraints [18], [19] (see Figure 12.13), and the other uses skin locus [16]. The basic idea is the same: to use some constraint to select the pixels for model updating. The method presented by Raja et al. [18] updates the skin color model using pixels inside the localized face area. The pixels are selected from an area that is 1/3 of the localization area and 1/3 from the localization boundaries. Yoo and Oh [19] argued that the localization should resemble the shape of the object (face), and they used all pixels inside the elliptical face localization. The skin locus

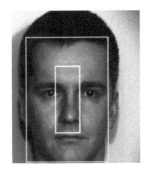
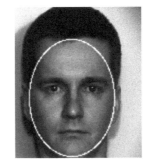

**FIGURE 12.13**
Spatial constraints suggested for adaptive skin color modeling: (left) the method suggested by Raja et al. (Raja, Y., McKenna, S., and Gong, G., *Proceedings of IEEE Third International Conference on Automatic Face and Gesture Recognition*, 1998) with the outer box indicating the localized face and the inner box determining the pixels used for model updating, (right) elliptical constraint by Yoo and Oh (Yoo, T.W., and Oh, I.S., *Patt. Recognition Lett.*, 20, 967, 1999).

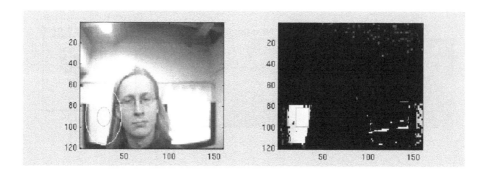

**FIGURE 12.14**
The face tracking based on Raja et al.'s method failed and adapted to nonfacial target. The left image displays the localized "face." The right image shows the pixels selected by the current skin color model. The box shows the pixels used for refreshing the model.

can be used in two ways: either the whole locus or partial locus is used to select skin-colored pixels from the localized face and its near surroundings.

There are many possible methods for updating the skin color model, but maybe a common method is the moving average, as presented in the following expression:

$$\check{M} = \frac{(1 - \alpha) * M_t + \alpha * M_{t-1}}{max((1 - \alpha) * M_t + \alpha * M_{t-1})} \tag{12.6}$$

where $\check{M}$ is a new, refreshed model; $M$ is the model; $t$ is the frame number; and $\alpha$ is a weighting factor. Quite often, the weighting factor is set to 0.5 to get equal emphasis on the skin color model of current and previous frames. The moving average method provides a smooth transition between models from different frames. It also reduces the effect of noise, which can change pixel color without any variation in external factors and thus be detrimental to the models.

However, the spatial constraint models have been shown to be very sensitive to localization errors; therefore, they can easily adapt to nonskin objects [12], [13]. The failure due to these constraints can happen even under fairly moderate illumination change. In Figure 12.14, Raja et al.'s method has failed while tracking a face on a video sequence, and the skin color model is adapted to a nonskin-colored target as shown in this image.

The constraint suggested by Raja et al. easily fails under nonuniform illumination field change as demonstrated in Figure 12.15. The model is updated using the pixel inside the

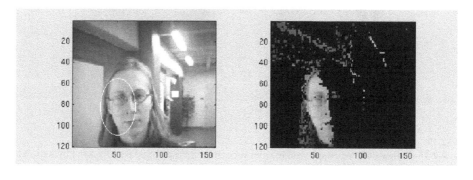

**FIGURE 12.15**
The constraint suggested by Raja et al. selects a nonpresentative set of skin pixels.

localization, and therefore, it can adapt only to global illumination changes, not to the nonuniform illumination field variation.

The localization of face for the skin-locus-based approach is not so critical, because the nonskin-colored pixels can be filtered out. Of course, there can be problem if there are large skin-colored objects connected to the face, but this would also be a problem for other methods relying only on color information.

## 12.5 Color Cue in Face Detection

As mentioned above, color is a useful cue for face detection, as it can greatly reduce the search area by selecting only the skin-like regions. However, it is obvious that the use of skin color only is not enough to distinguish between faces and other objects with a skin-like appearance (such as hands, wood, etc.). Therefore, other procedures are needed to verify whether the selected regions are (or contain) faces or not. Depending on the robustness of the skin model and changes in the illumination conditions, one can notice two cases:

- *Case #1*: The initial skin color detection step produces consistently reliable results. The skin color model is valid for the illumination conditions, the camera, and its settings. The skin color model can be designed either for stable, controlled illumination (typical case) or for variable illumination (skin locus). In such cases, it is generally enough to consider each connected resultant component from the skin detection as a face candidate. Then, one can verify the "faceness" of the candidate by simple and fast heuristics.

- *Case #2*: The initial skin color detection step produces unsatisfactory results or even fails. In this case, the skin color model does not correspond to the prevailing illumination, camera used, or settings of the camera. One may hope that the results would indicate the locations of the faces, but their size estimation is too unreliable. Therefore, a different method for face detection (either an appearance-based or feature-based one) or a different skin color model should be used when searching the faces in and around the detected skin regions.

In both cases, the use of color accelerates the detection process. In the following, we first review some methods based on color information for detecting faces and then describe in more detail an example of a color-based face detector [4].

### 12.5.1 Overview of Color-Based Face Detection Methods

Most color-based face detectors start by determining the skin pixels that are then grouped using connected component analysis. Then, for each connected component, the best fit ellipse is computed using geometric moments, for example. The skin components that verify some shape and size constraints are selected as face candidates. Finally, features (such as eyes and mouth) are searched for inside each face candidate based on the observation that holes inside the face candidate are due to these features being different from skin color.

Therefore, most of the color-based face detection methods mainly differ in the selection of the color space and the design of the skin model. In this context, as seen in Section 12.4, many methods for skin modeling in different color spaces have been proposed. For comparison studies, refer to References [11], [12], and [20].

Among the works using color for face detection is Hsu et al.'s system that consists of two major modules: face localization for finding face candidates and facial feature detection for verifying detected face candidates [5]. For finding the face candidates, the skin tone pixels are labeled using an elliptical skin model in the $YC_bC_r$ color space, after applying a lighting compensation technique. The detected skin tone pixels are iteratively segmented using local color variance into connected components that are then grouped into face candidates. Then, a facial feature detection module constructs eye, mouth, and face boundary maps to verify the face candidates. Good detection results have been reported on several test images. However, no comparative study has been made.

Garcia and Tziritas [21] presented another approach for detecting faces in color images. First, color clustering and filtering using approximations of the $YC_bC_r$ and hue, saturation and value (HSV) skin color subspaces are applied on the original image, providing quantized skin color regions. Then a merging stage is iteratively performed on the set of homogeneous skin color regions in the color quantized image, in order to provide a set of face candidates. Finally, constraints related to shape and size of faces are applied, and face intensity texture is analyzed by performing a wavelet packet decomposition on each face area candidate in order to detect human faces. The authors have reported a detection rate of 94.23% and a false dismissal rate of 5.76% on a data set of 100 images containing 104 faces. Though the method can handle nonconstrained scene conditions, such as the presence of a complex background and uncontrolled illumination, its main drawback lies in that it is computationally expensive due to its complicated segmentation algorithm and time-consuming wavelet packet analysis.

Sobottka and Pitas presented a method for face localization and facial feature extraction using shape and color [22]. First, color segmentation in the HSV space is performed to locate skin-like regions. After facial feature extraction, connected component analysis, and best-fit ellipse calculation, a set of face candidates is obtained. To verify the "faceness" of each candidate, a set of 11 lowest-order-geometric moments is computed and used as input to a neural network. The authors reported a detection rate of 85% on a test set of 100 images.

Haiyuan et al. [23] presented a different approach for detecting faces in color images. Instead of searching for facial features to verify the face candidates, the authors modeled the face pattern as a composition of a skin part and a hair part. They made two fuzzy models to describe the skin color and hair color in the CIE XYZ color space. The two models are used to extract the skin color regions, and the hair color regions, which are compared with the prebuilt head-shape models by using a fuzzy-theory-based pattern-matching method to detect the faces.

Several other approaches using color information for detecting and tracking faces and facial features in still images and video sequences were proposed [2], [24]. Most of the methods have reported their results on specific and limited data sets, and this fact does not facilitate performing a comparative analysis between the methods. In addition, most of these methods have not been tested under practical illumination changes (usually only mild changes are considered), which places them in the first category (Case #1) described above.

## 12.5.2 Case Study: Face Detection Using Skin Locus and Refining Stages

Here we present an example of a color-based face detector. It uses the skin locus model to extract skin-like region candidates and performs the selection by simple but efficient refining stages. The refining stages are organized in a cascade to achieve high accuracy and to keep the system simple and fast.

### 12.5.2.1 Skin Detection Using a Skin Locus Model

To determine the skin-like regions, we use the skin locus method, which has performed well with images under widely varying conditions [12], [16]. Skin locus is the range of skin chromaticities under varying illumination/camera calibration conditions in NCC space.

The name "skin locus" came from Störring et al. [25], who showed that the track of skin chromaticities follows the curve of Planckian radiator's chromaticities in NCC space. The main properties of the skin locus model are its robustness against changing intensity and also some relative tolerance toward varying illumination chromaticity [13].

The skin locus for a camera can be calculated based on spectral information or obtained directly from an image set. In our case (a Sony camera), we first collected several images for different camera calibrations and illumination conditions. We then manually selected the skin areas in the collected images. Finally, we converted the RGB values of the selected skin into a chromaticity space.

In NCC space, only the intensity and two chromaticity coordinates are sufficient for specifying any color uniquely (because $r + g + b = 1$). We considered $r - b$ coordinates to obtain both robustness against intensity variance and a good overlap of chromaticities of different skin colors. To define the skin locus, we used a quadratic function to define the upper bound, while the lower bound was defined by a five-degree polynomial function.

### 12.5.2.2 Verification Stages

We start by extracting skin-like regions using the skin locus. By using morphological operations (that is, a majority operator and application of dilations followed by erosions until the image no longer changes), we reduce the number of these regions. For every candidate, we verify whether it corresponds to a facial region or not. We organize the verification operations according to a cascade structure. The scheme shown in Figure 12.16 summarizes the verification steps.

To deal with faces of different orientations, we calculate that ellipse which best fits the face candidate. To find the best-fit ellipse, we can use an approach based either on regions or on edges. In our case, we computed the best-fit ellipse based on the borders of the connected component corresponding to the face candidate. For this purpose, we used the least square ellipse-fitting algorithm. Figure 12.17 shows an example of ellipse fitting.

After the best-fit ellipse operation, we only kept candidates in which the ratio of the major axis to the minor axis was within a certain range. We fixed the range to [1.11, 3.33].

Based on the observation that pixel value variations of facial regions are always more significant than those of other parts, such as hands (which is due to the fact that features

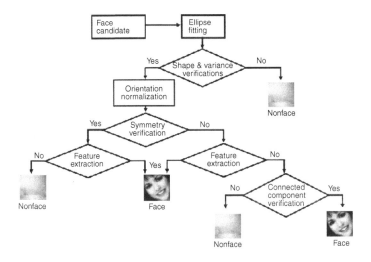

**FIGURE 12.16**
Face detection scheme.

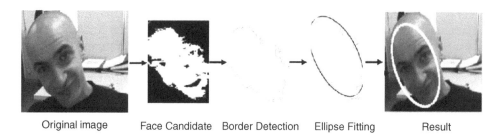

Original image        Face Candidate   Border Detection    Ellipse Fitting            Result

**FIGURE 12.17**
Example of ellipse fitting.

such as eyes, mouth, and eyebrows have different colors than skin), we removed all the candidates with a variance smaller than a threshold. Because facial features are better represented in the red channel, we only considered this channel when computing the variance. Due to illumination changes and other factors, not all hands will be removed. We also kept the threshold very small so as to not remove facial patterns.

After computing the best-fit ellipse for each candidate, we performed image rotation with the use of bilinear interpolation. Let us assume that $\theta$ denotes the angle of the ellipse that fits the face candidate. Then, the new coordinates of a pixel with coordinates $(x, y)$ are determined as follows:

$$x_{rotated} = x \cos \theta + y \sin \theta \qquad (12.7)$$

$$y_{rotated} = y \cos \theta - x \sin \theta \qquad (12.8)$$

We found in the experiments that when the symmetry of the face is verified, it is easier to detect the facial features. Thus, we implemented the idea of discarding all candidates when the symmetry is verified but no facial features have been found. After normalization for both scale and orientation, we computed a symmetry measure ($SD$) between the left and right sides of the face. We use $3 \times 3$ nonoverlapping windows to scan both sides. For every $3 \times 3$ window, we report local symmetry if the difference between the means of the pixel values corresponding to the given $3 \times 3$ windows in both parts is smaller than a threshold (we fixed this threshold at 8). The $SD$ equals the ratio of a number of local symmetries to the number of scanned windows. If more than 75% of the $3 \times 3$ windows verifies the local symmetry, then we consider that the face candidate is globally symmetric.

In relation to the face candidate after rotation, we consider the green channel in the interior of the connected component, as the experiments have shown that the green channel better discriminates the features we are looking for in the gradient images. Because the eyes and eyebrows are located in the upper half of the face, we consider only this region of the face. We calculate the gradient of the image on the $x$ dimension, then we determine the $y$-projection by computing the mean value of every row in the gradient image. By analyzing the $y$-projection, we found that the maximum corresponds to the horizontal position of the eyebrows (as shown in Figure 12.18).

Having obtained the horizontal position, the vertical position is then determined by the $x$-projection. The $x$-projection is computed by averaging the pixel values around the three-pixel neighborhoods of the horizontal position. In the case of eyes, we proceed in a similar way on the gradient image now computed on the $y$ dimension. Once we obtain the positions of the eyes and the eyebrows, we verify their spatial relationships. The horizontal position of the eyes should be below the horizontal position of the eyebrows. In addition, the ratio of the vertical eye–eyebrow distance to the face size should be within a certain range. (We fixed it to [0.1, 0.25].)

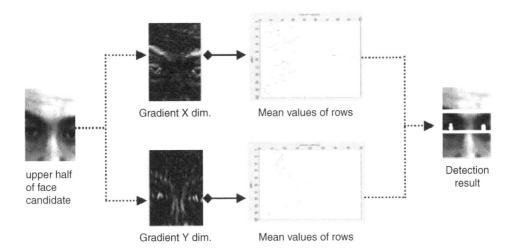

**FIGURE 12.18**
Example of eyes and eyebrow detection.

In cases where the detection of the eyes and eyebrows failed, we performed connected component analysis. Consider the example shown in Figure 12.19.

The algorithm fails to detect the features. Because a face contains eyes, a mouth, and eyebrows with darker colors than skin, empty areas should exist inside the connected components of the face. Therefore, we defined five models for connected components of skin (Figure 12.19). We determined the best representative model for the face candidate and reported the "faceness" of the candidate according to this matching value.

### 12.5.2.3  Experiments and Results

We applied the system to detect faces in different images with natural illuminations. Figure 12.20 shows an example in which the system detected two candidates (face and hand). After variance and symmetry verifications, both regions were selected. Successful detection of eyes and eyebrows was only reported for the face candidate. After failure of feature detection in the hand region, the connected component analysis step rejected the false candidate (hand).

Figure 12.21 shows some detection examples performed by the system under different conditions. After analyzing different filtering detectors and according to statistics obtained from a set of 500 detected faces, we found that in most successful cases (56%), the detections were made based on the features, not the symmetry. Only a few face candidates (18%)

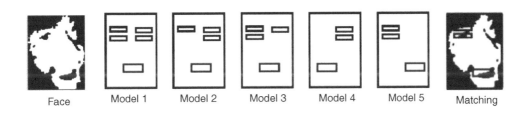

**FIGURE 12.19**
Example of connected component analysis. Five face models are defined. In this case, the face candidate is matched to the fifth model.

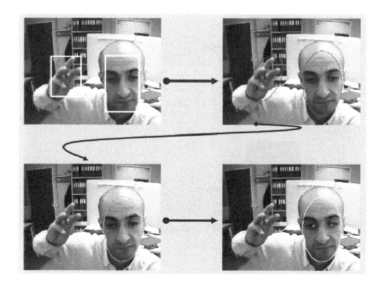

**FIGURE 12.20**
An example in which the system detected two candidates. After verification steps, only the face region is kept.

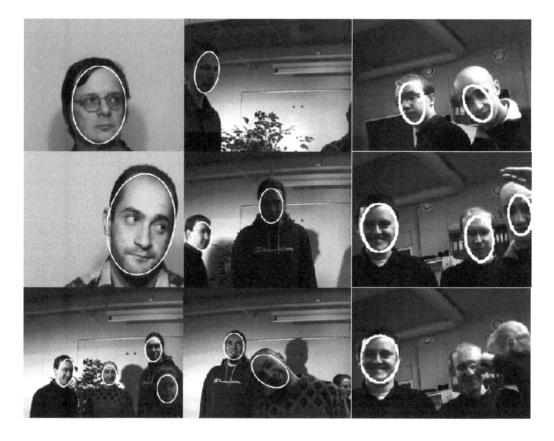

**FIGURE 12.21**
An example of detections performed by the system.

verified the face symmetry. In 26% of the cases, detection needed connected component analysis. However, the system failed to detect faces when they were broken into small pieces of skin color due to occlusions. Figure 12.21 shows failure detection, because the face skin had merged into a hand. The same failure is observed when two faces are too close. By analyzing the importance of the different steps in removing the false face candidates, and according to statistics obtained from a set of 800 rejected candidates, we found that variance verification allowed 13% of removals. In 9% of the cases, this is due to feature detection failure with successful symmetry verification. Considering these 800 cases, shape verification allowed for the removal of 79 false candidates (about 10%). In 68% of the cases, the false face candidates passed through all the possible refining stages.

The color-based face detector described here is currently in use in an experimental system for access control based on face recognition [26]. So far, it works well (detection rate over 90%) and meets the requirements of the access control system. In a preliminary analysis using common test sets, the color-based face detector is about ten times faster than another detector [27] based only on grayscale information. This is an indication of the usefulness of color cueing in face detection.

It is worth noting that the ideas behind some of the heuristics used in the refining stages are not very original. For instance, the symmetry property of the face is used by many other researchers [2]. However, the way they were used and implemented is different. Importantly, the novelty of the approach is the structure of the refining stages: it is not entirely a cascade but rather a tree scheme.

The goal of this section is not to compare the color-based face detectors but rather to describe an example of using color cue for face detection. The results showed that including color information may greatly accelerate the processing procedure. One problem of color-based face detectors lies in the fact that they are generally camera specific. Among the attempts to define a standard protocol and a common database for testing color-based face detectors is the work of Sharma and Reilly [28].

## 12.6 Color Cue in Face Recognition

The role of color information in the recognition of nonface objects has been the subject of much debate. However, there has only been a small amount of work that examines its contribution to face recognition. Most of the work has only focused on the luminance structure of the face, thus ignoring color cues, due to several reasons.

The first reason lies in the lack of evidence from human perception studies about the role of color in face recognition. A notable study in this regard was done in Reference [29], in which the authors found that the observers were able to quite normally process even those faces that had been subjected to hue reversals. Color seemed to contribute no significant recognition advantages beyond the luminance information. In another piece of work [3], it is explained that the possible reason for a lack of observed color contribution in these studies is the availability of strong shape cues that make the contribution of color not very evident. The authors then investigated the role of color by designing experiments in which the shape cues were progressively degraded. They concluded that the luminance structure of the face is undoubtedly of great significance for recognition, but that color cues are not entirely discarded by the face recognition process. They suggested that color plays a role under degraded conditions by facilitating low-level facial image analysis, such as better estimations of the boundaries, shapes, and sizes of facial features [3].

A second possible reason for a lack of work on color-based face recognition relates to the difficulties of associating illumination with white balancing of cameras. Indeed, as discussed in Section 12.3, illumination is still a challenging problem in automatic face recognition; therefore, there is no need to further complicate the task.

A third possible reason for ignoring color cues in the development of automatic recognition systems is the lack of color image databases[1] available for the testing of the proposed algorithms, in addition to the unwillingness to develop methods that cannot be used with the already existing monochrome databases and applications.

However, the few attempts to use color in automatic face recognition include the work conducted by Torres et al. [30], who extended the eigenface approach to color by computing the principal components from each color component independently in three different color spaces (RGB, YUV, and HSV). The final classification is achieved using a weighted sum of the Mahalanobis distances computed for each color component. In their experiments using one small database (59 images), the authors noticed performance improvements for the recognition rates when using YUV (88.14%) and HSV (88.14%) color spaces, while a RGB color space provided the same results (84.75%) when using R, G, or B separately and exactly the same results as using the luminance Y only. Therefore, they concluded that color is important for face recognition. However, the experiments are very limited, as only one small face database is used, and the simple eigenface approach is tested.

In another piece of work that deals with color for face recognition [31], it was argued that performance enhancement could be obtained if a suitable conversion from color images to monochromatic forms would be adopted. The authors derived a transformation from color to grayscale images using three different methods (PCA, linear regression, and genetic algorithms). They compared their results with those obtained after converting the color images to a monochromatic form by using a simple transformation $I = \frac{R+G+B}{3}$, and they noticed a performance enhancement of 4% to 14% using a database of 280 images. However, the database considered in the experiments is rather small, so one should test the generalization performance of the proposed transformation on a larger set of images from different sources.

Rajapakse et al. [32] considered an approach based on nonnegative matrix factorization (NMF) and compared the face recognition results using color and grayscale images. On a test set of 100 face images, the authors claimed a performance enhancement when also using color information for recognition.

More recently, Jones attempted to extend the Gabor-based approach for face recognition to color images by defining the concept of quaternions (four-component hypercomplex numbers) [33]. On a relatively limited set of experiments, the author reported performance enhancement on the order of 3% to 17% when using the proposed quaternion Gabor-based approach instead of the conventional monochromatic Gabor-based method.

## 12.7 Conclusion

Color is a useful cue in facial image analysis. Its use for skin segmentation and face detection is probably the most obvious, while its contribution to face recognition is not very clear. The first important issues when planning the use of color in facial image analysis are the selection of a color space and the design of a skin model. Several approaches were

---

[1] Note that recently, some color image databases have finally been collected (e.g., the color FERET database: http://www.itl.nist.gov/iad/humanid/colorferet/home.html).

proposed for these purposes, but unfortunately, there is no optimal choice. Choice depends on the requirement of the application and also on the environment (illumination conditions, camera calibration, etc.).

Once a skin model has been defined, the contribution of color to face detection, not surprisingly, plays an important role in preprocessing the images and in selecting the skin-like areas. Then, other refining stages can also be launched in order to find faces among skin-like regions. Following these lines, we presented an example for face detection in color images. The results show that color-based face detectors could be significantly much faster than other detectors based only on grayscale information.

In relation to the contribution of color to face recognition, our conclusion is that it makes sense for automatic face recognition, systems not to rely on color for recognition because its contribution is not well established.

## References

[1] B. Funt, K. Barnard, and L. Martin, Is machine colour constancy good enough?, in *Proceedings of fifth European Conference on Computer Vision*, June 1998, Springer, pp. 445–459.

[2] M.-H. Yang, D.J. Kriegman, and N. Ahuja, Detecting faces in images: A survey, *IEEE Trans. on Patt. Anal. and Machine Intelligence*, 24, 34–58, 2002.

[3] A.W. Yip and P. Sinha, Contribution of color to face recognition, *Perception*, 31, 8, 995–1003, 2002.

[4] A. Hadid, M. Pietikäinen, and B. Martinkauppi, Color-based face detection using skin locus model and hierarchical filtering," in *Proceedings of the 16th International Conference on Pattern Recognition*, Quebec, Canada, August 2002, IEEE Computer Society, pp. 196–200.

[5] R.L. Hsu, M. Abdel-Mottaleb, and A.K. Jain, Face detection in color images, *IEEE Trans. on Patt. Anal. and Machine Intelligence*, 24, 696–706, 2002.

[6] G. Wyszecki and W.S. Stiles, Eds., *Color Science Concepts and Methods, Quantitative Data and Formulae*, 2nd ed., John Wiley & Sons, New York, 2000.

[7] B. Martinkauppi and G. Finlayson, Designing a simple 3-channel camera for skin detection, in *Proceeding of the 12th Color Imaging Conference: Color Science and Engineering: Systems, Technologies, and Applications*, November 2004, The Society for Imaging Science and Technology, pp. 151–156.

[8] L. Harwood, A chrominance demodulator ic with dynamic flesh correction, *IEEE Trans. on Consumer Electron.*, CE-22, 111–117, 1976.

[9] E. Lee and Y. Ha, Automatic flesh tone reappearance for color enhancement in TV, *IEEE Trans. on Consumer Electron.*, 43, 1153–1159, 1997.

[10] E. Edwards and S. Duntley, The pigments and color of living human skin, *Am. J. Anat.*, 65, 1–33, 1939.

[11] J.C. Terrillon, M.N. Shirazi, H. Fukamachi, and S. Akamatsu, Comparative performance of different skin chrominance models and chrominance spaces for the automatic detection of human faces in color images, in *Proceedings of the Fourth IEEE International Conference on Automatic Face and Gesture Recognition*, March 2000, IEEE Computer Society, pp. 54–61.

[12] B. Martinkauppi, M. Soriano, and M. Pietikäinen, Comparison of skin color detection and tracking methods under varying illumination, *J. Electron. Imaging*, 14, 4, 043014-1–042014-19.

[13] B. Martinkauppi and M. Pietikäinen, Facial skin color modeling, in *Handbook of Face Recognition*, S.Z. Li and A.K. Jain, Eds., Springer, Berlin, 2005, pp. 109–131.

[14] R.L. Hsu, Face Detection and Modeling for Recognition, Ph.D. thesis, Michigan State University, 2002.

[15] K.M. Cho, J.H. Jang, and K.S. Hong, Adaptive skin-color filter, *Patt. Recognition*, 34, 1067–1073, 2001.

[16] M. Soriano, B. Martinkauppi, S. Huovinen, and M. Laaksonen, Adaptive skin color modeling using the skin locus for selecting training pixels, *Patt. Recognition*, 36, 3, 681–690, 2003.

[17] M. Jones and J. Rehg, Statistical color models with application to skin detection, *Int. J. Comput. Vision*, 46, 81–96, 2002.

[18] Y. Raja, S. McKenna, and G. Gong, Tracking and segmenting people in varying lighting conditions using colour, in *Proceedings of IEEE Third International Conference on Automatic Face and Gesture Recognition*, April 1998, IEEE Computer Society, pp. 228–233.

[19] T.W. Yoo and I.S. Oh, A fast algorithm for tracking human faces based on chromaticity histograms, *Patt. Recognition Lett.*, 20, 967–978, 1999.

[20] B. Martinkauppi, M. Soriano, and M. Laaksonen, Behavior of skin color under varying illumination seen by different cameras in different color spaces, in *Proceedings of the SPIE Vol. 4301 Machine Vision in Industrial Inspection IX*, 2001, pp. 102–113.

[21] C. Garcia and G. Tziritas, Face detection using quantized skin color regions merging and wavelet packet analysis, *IEEE Trans. on Multimedia*, 1, 264–277, 1999.

[22] K. Sobottka and I. Pitas, Face localization and facial feature extraction based on shape and color information, in *IEEE Conference on Image Processing*, IEEE Computer Society, Vol. 3, 1996, pp. 483–486.

[23] W. Haiyuan, C. Qian, and M. Yachida, Face detection from color images using a fuzzy pattern matching method, *IEEE Trans. on Patt. Anal. and Machine Intelligence*, 21, 557–563, 1999.

[24] E. Hjelmas and B.K. Low, Face detection: A survey, *Comput. Vision and Image Understanding*, 83, 236–274, 2001.

[25] M. Störring, H.J. Andersen, and E. Granum, Physics-based modelling of human skin colour under mixed illuminants, *J. Robotics and Autonomous Syst.*, 35, 131–142, 2001.

[26] A. Hadid, M. Heikkilä, T. Ahonen, and M. Pietikäinen, A novel approach to access control based on face recognition, in *Proceedings of the Workshop on Processing Sensory Information for Proactive Systems (PSIPS 2004)*, 2004, University of Oulu, Finland, pp. 68–74.

[27] A. Hadid, M. Pietikäinen, and T. Ahonen, A discriminative feature space for detecting and recognizing faces, in *IEEE Conference on Computer Vision and Pattern Recognition*, Vol. II, 2004, IEEE Computer Society, pp. 797–804.

[28] P. Sharma and R. Reilly, A colour face image database for benchmarking of automatic face detection algorithms, in *EC-VIP-MC 2003 Fourth EURASIP Conference Focused on Video/Image Processing and Multimedia Communications*, 2003, University of Zagreb, pp. 423–428.

[29] R. Kemp, G. Pike, P. White, and A. Musselman, Perception and recognition of normal and negative faces: The role of shape from shading and pigmentation cues, *Perception*, 25, 37–52, 1996.

[30] L. Torres, J. Reutter, and L. Lorente, The importance of the color information in face recognition, in *IEEE Conference on Image Processing*, IEEE Computer Society, Vol. 3, 1999, pp. 627–631.

[31] C.F. Jones and A.L. Abbott, Optimization of color conversion for face recognition, *EURASIP J. on Applied Signal Process.*, 4, 522–529, 2004.

[32] M. Rajapakse, J. Tan, and J. Rajapakse, Color channel encoding with nmf for face recognition, in *IEEE Conference on Image Processing*, IEEE Computer Society, Vol. 3, 2004, pp. 2007–2010.

[33] C.F. Jones, Color Face Recognition using Quaternionic Gabor Wavelets, Ph.D. thesis, Virginia Polytechnic Institute and State University, Blacksburg, 2005.

[34] E. Marszalec, B. Martinkauppi, M. Soriano, and M. Pietikäinen, A physics-based face database for color research, *J. Electron. Imaging*, 9, 32–38, 2000.

# 13

## Using Colors for Eye Tracking

Dan Witzner Hansen

CONTENTS

## 13.1 Introduction

"The eye is the window to the soul." This familiar proverb is variously attributable to a number of sources: we use our eyes intensively every day for a large variety of purposes: for reading, for watching entertainment, for gathering information to plan actions and movements, and for perceiving and learning new things, for example, on the computer. The eyes play an important role in interpreting and understanding a person's desires, needs, and emotional states. The geometric, photometric, and motion characteristics of the eyes also provide important visual cues for face detection, face recognition, and for facial expression recognition.

As the eye scans the environment or focuses on particular objects in the scene, an eye tracker simultaneously localizes the eye position and tracks its movement over time so as to determine the direction of gaze. Eye tracking is not a new idea. Already in 1878, the first formal eye position recordings were obtained by Delabarre [1], who connected a silk thread between a corneal ring and the recording lever of a smoked-drum recorder. Since then, eye tracking has evolved from being a highly intrusive and time-consuming procedure to nonintrusive and fast, thanks to technological developments. Eye tracking was initially a tool for psychologists to conduct experiments; during the last decade, a tremendous effort has been made on developing robust eye tracking systems and tools for various human–computer interaction applications, such as fatigue and drowsiness detection and eye typing [2], [3], [4], [5], [6]. Current eye tracking methods are not as accurate as the mouse for screen-based applications; however, they have several appealing properties for enhancing computer interaction [7]. The applications of robust eye tracking and gaze estimation methods are therefore growing in importance in many different areas. The tendency is that eye tracking is moving out of laboratories and is aiming toward our homes and vehicles, but contrary to current eye trackers, the mouse is easy to set up, it is cheap, and it can be used almost everywhere we go. Current commercial eye trackers are expensive, and if eye tracking should become another widespread input modality, the price should be lowered [8]. One way to lower the price and increase the availability of eye trackers is through the use of components-off-the-shelf (COTS). Using COTS for eye tracking is appealing, but more care and modeling are needed as knowledge of hardware and geometry of the user, camera, and monitor is *a priori* unknown.

Color perception is essential for humans and, as seen elsewhere in this book, for many vision-based applications. However, eye tracking research and development does not have a tradition of using visible color information. In this chapter, it is shown that color (both in the visible and invisible spectrum) provides valuable information for use in eye trackers. Infrared light (IR) is the most dominant use of "colors" in eye tracking, and its use for eye tracking is described in Section 13.2. The following sections describe the framework for a color-based contour tracker and show that the use of color information promotes higher robustness for eye tracking. One of the limitations of many current systems is their use of thresholds. Thresholds can be difficult to define generically, as the light conditions and head poses may influence the image observations of the eye. The method uses a new likelihood model for the image observations that avoids explicit definition of features and corresponding thresholds. Section 13.3 provides an overview of the method, and Section 13.4 describes the observation model used for color-based eye tracking (without thresholds). Section 13.5 evaluates the method and shows that colors imply better tracking both with and without IR illumination. The chapter concludes in Section 13.6.

## 13.2   Using the IR Colors for Eye Tracking

Eye tracker development has primarily revolved around using the "color" of near-IR light and benefiting from it in practically all stages, starting from the detection, to tracking and gaze estimation [9], [10], [11], [12]. This section presents fundamental properties of the appearance of the pupil when exposed to IR illumination and makes it evident why IR light can be very useful for eye tracking.

Because IR light is not visible to the human eye, the light does not distract the user. The amount of emitted light can therefore be quite high so as to control light conditions. When IR light falls on the eye, part of it is reflected back in a tiny ray pointing directly toward the light source. Actually, several reflections occur on the boundaries of the lens and the cornea (see Figure 13.1), the so-called *Purkinje images* [3], where only one is easily detected (first Purkinje image).

If a light source is located close to the optical axis of the camera (on-axis light), the captured image shows a bright pupil. This effect is similar to the red-eye effect when using flashlight in photography. When a light source is located away from the optical axis of the camera (off-axis), the image shows a dark pupil. An example of dark and bright pupil images is shown in Figure 13.2. Several objects in the background may generate patterns similar to the dark and bright pupil images. The bright and dark pupil effects rarely occur at the

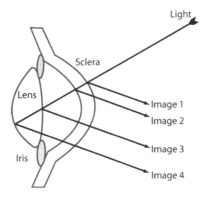

**FIGURE 13.1**
Purkinje images. The four Purkinje images are reflections of the incoming light on the boundaries of the lens and cornea.

same time for other objects than eyes, and therefore, detection and tracking of eyes based on active remote IR illumination is simple and effective. Often, detection and tracking are done through the bright areas in the image resulting from subtracting the dark and bright pupil images. Notice that the changes in intensity as a function of pupil size changes significantly and, furthermore, is correlated with ethnic background [13]. The contour of the iris (limbus) is another prominent feature of the eye which is frequently used in eye tracking. Limbus trackers are generally more influenced by eyelid occlusion than pupil trackers and may thus result in lower accuracy. Temporal filtering and geometric constraints are often incorporated to remove spurious candidates. The use of IR light makes it tempting to use static threshold for feature extraction. However, this approach may be limited if light conditions change.

Reflections (glints) of the IR light source are created at different layers of the eye, but often only the strongest reflection is used. If a user looks directly at the light source, the distance between the glint and the center of the pupil is small, and when the users looks away, the distance is increased. The vector between glint and pupil is therefore directly related to the direction of the gaze. Figure 13.3 shows images with the Purkinje reflections.

Eye tracking for indoor use benefits from using IR light, but sole use of IR also has its limitations. IR is only effective on a limited range of distances and may become unreliable when used outdoors because the atmosphere lets disturbing IR light through. IR light sources should be directed toward the user and may require careful setup.

Obviously, glints are not dependent on IR light — a glint may be generated through visible light. The drawback is that the light may distract the user. By the same token, the use of color imaging does not exclude the simultaneous use of IR light. Besides, systems based on

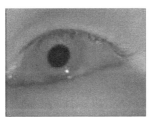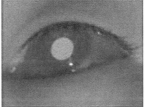

**FIGURE 13.2**
Dark pupil image (left) and corresponding bright image (right). Courtesy of Hitosh Morimoto.

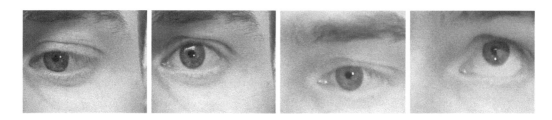

**FIGURE 13.3**
First Purkinje images. Notice the bright spots (glints) close to the pupils.

ambient light typically have a larger working volume than infrared systems. It is, therefore, surprising that the use of visible colors for eye tracking has received little attention, realizing that the region of the eye usually contains different colors than its surroundings.

Using colors for tracking purposes may be employed in various ways. One simple approach compares a color model to regions of the image through a spatially dependent measure of similarity [14], [15]. The advantages of this model are that spatial structures are preserved and the features of the object may be gathered directly from the model. The advantages of these models may be their demise. If the target undergoes drastic spatial changes, an overly committed spatial dependent model will fail. Motivated by the fact that the overall color distribution may be preserved and spatial structures lost, eye tracking can be maintained by removing spatial dependency and working only with color information.

Strict spatial dependencies can be removed by representing the model through color distributions. The obvious limitation of this model is that it is impossible to determine any spatial relations from the model. On the other hand, these models have recently been proven to be robust and versatile at a fairly low computational cost [16], [17], [18]. They are especially appealing for tracking tasks where the spatial structure of the tracked objects exhibits such a dramatic variability that space-dependent appearance trackers would break down very fast. In addition, the methods may be able to handle changes in rotation and scale. Efficiency and robustness toward (partial) occlusion are also some of their advantages. As illustrated in Figure 13.4, such a model is also appealing for eye tracking: if the user rotates the head, the appearance of the eye may change drastically. The spatial information may be lost, but the color distribution only changes slightly. When using an eye tracking system, light may be reflected on the eye, which, in turn, may disrupt some

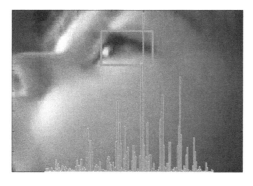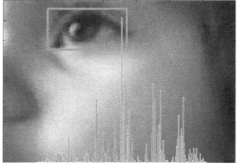

**FIGURE 13.4**
The spatial structure of the eye may change so much under head rotation that the eye becomes difficult to detect when relying on spatial information. The color distribution, on the other hand, is only slightly altered, thus making the representation robust to spatial changes.

of the spatial structures but not severely influence the color distribution. The exact features may, if available, be determined through a spatial dependent model. It is important that the eye tracker maintains track, even though some spatial structures are lost.

## 13.3 Method Overview

In this chapter, we will present an iris tracker based on information from color and gray-level differences. The proposed method is based on recursive estimation of the state variables of the iris. Given a sequence of $T$ frames, at time $t$, only data from the previous $t - 1$ images are available. The states and measurements are represented by $\mathbf{x}_t$ and $\mathbf{y}_t$, respectively, and the previous states and measurements are defined as $\underline{\mathbf{x}}_t = (\mathbf{x}_1, \ldots, \mathbf{x}_t)$ and $\underline{\mathbf{y}}_t = (\mathbf{y}_1, \ldots, \mathbf{y}_t)$. At time $t$, the observation $\mathbf{y}_t$ is assumed to be independent of the previous state $\mathbf{x}_{t-1}$ and previous observation $\mathbf{y}_{t-1}$ given the current state $\mathbf{x}_t$.

Employing these assumptions, the tracking problem can be stated as a Bayesian inference problem in the well-known recursive relation [19]:

$$p(\mathbf{x}_{t+1}|\underline{\mathbf{y}}_{t+1}) \propto p(\mathbf{y}_t|\mathbf{x}_t)\,p(\mathbf{x}_{t+1}|\underline{\mathbf{y}}_t) \tag{13.1}$$

$$p(\mathbf{x}_{t+1}|\underline{\mathbf{y}}_t) = \int p(\mathbf{x}_{t+1}|\mathbf{x}_t)\,p(\mathbf{x}_t|\underline{\mathbf{y}}_t)d\mathbf{x}_t \tag{13.2}$$

The method combines particle filtering with the EM (expectation maximization) algorithm. Particle filtering is used, as it allows for the maintenance of multiple hypotheses that make it robust in clutter and capable of recovering from occlusion. Particle filtering is particularly suitable for iris tracking, because changes in iris position are fast and do not follow a smooth and predictable pattern. Particle filters generally require a large set of particles to accurately determine the pose parameters. By contrast, the method uses a fairly small set of particles to maintain track of the object, while using a variation of the EM contour [20] (MEMC) method for precise pose estimation. In this way, computation time is lowered while maintaining accuracy.

The aim of particle filtering is to approximate the filtering distribution $p(\mathbf{x}_t|\underline{\mathbf{y}}_t)$ by a weighted sample set $\mathbf{S}_t^N = \{(\mathbf{x}_t^{(n)}, \pi_t^{(n)})\}_{n=1}^N$, where $\mathbf{x}_t^{(n)}$ is the $n$th instance of a state at time $t$ with weight $\pi_t^{(n)}$. This sample set will evolve into a new sample set $\mathbf{S}_{t+1}^N$, representing the posterior pdf (probability density function) $p(\mathbf{x}_{t+1}|\underline{\mathbf{y}}_{t+1})$ at time $t + 1$. The object location in the particle filter is usually represented by the sample mean. *Factored sampling* is utilized in the *condensation* approach to particle filtering [19]: the samples are drawn from the prediction prior $p(\mathbf{x}_{t+1}|\underline{\mathbf{y}}_t)$, and sample weights are proportional to the observation likelihood $p(\mathbf{y}_t|\mathbf{x}_t)$. This approach is employed here.

The robustness of particle filters lies in maintaining a set of hypotheses. Generally, the larger the number of hypotheses, the better the chances of getting accurate tracking results, but the slower the tracking speed. Using particle filters in large images may require a large set of particles to sufficiently sample the spatial parameters. Adding samples to the particle set may only improve accuracy slowly due to the sampling strategy employed. This added accuracy may become costly in terms of computation time. To lower the requirements on the number of particles while improving tracking performance, we propose using an image scale space $H_I^M$, with $M$ image scales. Particle filtering is performed at the coarsest scale $H_I^{(0)}$. MEMC is applied to gradually finer image scales $H_I^{(i)}$ ($0 \le i < M$) using the estimate from each scale for initialization at the next finer scale and the sample mean from the particle filter for initialization at the coarsest scale. In this way, the particle filter samples

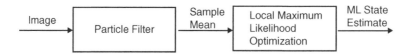

**FIGURE 13.5**
Overall tracking is performed on the coarsest image scale through particle filtering; starting from the weighted mean of the particle states (sample mean); maximum likelihood (ML) estimation of the object state is performed through the EM contour algorithm over gradually finer image scales.

the posterior more effectively, while the MEMC reaches the (local) maximum likelihood estimate of the iris location. Figure 13.5 illustrates the flow diagram of the method, and Figure 13.6 describes the algorithm for a single frame of an image sequence.

### 13.3.1 State Model and Dynamics

The model consists of three components: *a dynamical model* defining the pdf over the eye state at the current image frame given the state in the previous frame, *a geometric model* defining a pdf over contours on the image plane given the iris state at the current frame, and *an observation model* defining a pdf over gray-level differences and colors given the contour. Section 13.4 describes the observation model; the geometric and dynamical models are described below.

The iris appears elliptical on the image plane; therefore, we model it as an ellipse, and the state $\mathbf{x}$ is given by five state variables:

$$\mathbf{x} = (c_x, c_y, \lambda_1 \lambda_2, \theta)$$

where $(c_x, c_y)$ is the center of the iris, $\lambda_1$ and $\lambda_2$ are the major and minor axes, and $\theta$ is the angle of the major axis with respect to the vertical. These are the variables being estimated in the method.

Pupil movements can be very rapid from one image frame to another. The dynamics is therefore modeled as a first-order autoregressive process using a Gaussian noise model:

$$\mathbf{x}_{t+1} = \mathbf{x}_t + \mathbf{v}_t, \qquad \mathbf{v}_t \sim \mathcal{N}(0, \Sigma_t) \tag{13.3}$$

---

*Contour Tracker: operation for a single image frame*

Input: Image scale space $H_I^M$ of $I$, Motion model $\Sigma$ and particle set $S_{t-1}$
Output: Optimized mean state $\bar{\mathbf{x}}$ and new particle set $S_t$

- Obtain the sample set $S_t$ by selecting $N$ samples proportionally to their weight from $S_{t-1}$
- Predict all samples in $S_t$ according to Equation 13.3
- Update weights in $S_t$ according to likelihood model with $H_I^{(0)}$ as reference image.
- Calculate sample mean $\bar{\mathbf{x}}_0 = \dfrac{\sum_{i=1}^{N} \pi_i \mathbf{x}^{(i)}}{\sum_{i=1}^{N} \pi_i}$
- $\widetilde{\mathbf{x}}_0 = \mathcal{O}_0(\bar{\mathbf{x}}_0)$, where $\mathcal{O}_i(\mathbf{x}*)$ represents the EM contour algorithm applied at scale $i$ with initialization given by the argument $\mathbf{x}*$.
- for $i = 1$ to $M$, calculate $\widetilde{\mathbf{x}}_i = \mathcal{O}_i(\widetilde{\mathbf{x}}_{i-1})$
- $\bar{\mathbf{x}} = \widetilde{\mathbf{x}}_M$

---

**FIGURE 13.6**
The Iris Tracker as applied to a single frame of an image sequence.

where $\Sigma_t$ is the time-dependent covariance matrix of the noise $\mathbf{v}_t$. The time dependency is included to compensate for scale changes: when the apparent size of the eye increases, the corresponding eye movements can also be expected to increase. For this reason, the first two diagonal elements of $\Sigma$ (corresponding to the state variables $c_x$ and $c_y$) are assumed to be linearly dependent on the previous sample mean.

## 13.4 Observation Model

This section describes the observation model that defines the pdf $p(\mathbf{y}_t|\mathbf{x}_t)$. The purpose of the likelihood model is to discriminate background from foreground. The likelihood model should use all relevant information while being sufficiently robust to changes but only modeling the class of objects. An example of a model that attempts to do this is the color active appearance models [14]. An active appearance model incorporates both the statistical variation in shape and appearance. Unfortunately, the model is overly committed for the purpose of eye tracking, as it does not handle light coming from the side very well, even though the model has been trained with examples of this kind [21]. One of the problems is that the shape and appearance space becomes very large.

- **Active Contours:** Most active contour methods can be divided into two main classes based on the method for evaluating the image evidence. One class relies on the assumption that object edges generate image features and thus depends on the extraction of features from the image [19], [22]. The pose and shape of contours are estimated by minimizing the squared distances between contours and image features. The assumption behind the feature-based methods is that edges generate image features. From a statistical point of view, this approach throws away information, and from a practical point of view, it is difficult to set appropriate thresholds that apply to large changes in image quality. Apart from the problem of finding correct correspondences, the thresholds necessary for feature detection inevitably make these methods sensitive to noise. Other active contour methods [23], [24], [25] avoid feature detection by maximizing feature values (without thresholding) underlying the contour, rather than minimizing the distance between the locally strongest feature and contour. In this way, there is no information loss. The underlying idea is that a large image gradient is likely to arise from a boundary between object and background. The method introduced here is of the latter class, but smoothing [25] is replaced by marginalization over possible deformations of the object shape.

- **Color Appearance and Shape:** Fixed thresholds may be difficult to define when light condition changes. It is, therefore, important that eye trackers limit the use of thresholds. The proposed model employs shape and shape deformation as well as color appearance. The appearance model is more lenient on the assumptions on spatial dependency than, for example, active appearance models. In particular, the spatial dependencies of the appearance are partially removed, while the overall distribution of the appearance is maintained. In this model, both color and shape are used in the likelihood model. The shape model is used for restricting the possible classes of shapes, while the color model is used for restricting the likelihood in cases where the spatial information is present and where it is not. The color component is described in Section 13.4.6, while the contour model based on gray-level differences is described in Section 13.4.4. Both color and gray-level information avoid the use of thresholds.

### 13.4.1 Assumptions

The model is based on the following assumptions:

- The pdf of the observation depends only on the gray-level differences (GLDs) and color distributions, and these are measured along different lines.
- Gray-level differences between pixels along a line are statistically independent.
- Colors and intensities of nearby pixels are correlated if both belong to the object being tracked or both belong to the background. Thus, *a priori* statistical dependencies between nearby pixels are assumed.
- There is no correlation between pixel values if they are on opposite sides of the object boundary.
- The shape of the contour is subject to random local variability, which means that marginalization over local deformations is required for a Bayesian estimate of the contour parameters.

Similar assumptions can be found separately in the literature (e.g., Reference [26]) for the last assumption. Taking the assumptions together means that no features need to be detected and matched to the model (leading to greater robustness against noise), while at the same time, local shape variations are explicitly taken into account. As shown below, this model leads to a simple closed form expression for the likelihood of the image given the contour parameters [24].

### 13.4.2 Definitions

Define a normal to a given point on the contour as the *measurement line*. Define the coordinate $v$ on the measurement line. Given the position $\mu$ of the contour on the measurement line, the distance from $\mu$ to a point $v$ is $\epsilon = v - \mu$. $\eta(v)$ is a binary indicator variable that is 1 if the boundary of the target is in the interval $[v - \Delta v/2, v + \Delta v/2]$ (with regular interpoint spacing $\Delta v$) on the measurement line; and 0 otherwise. Denote the gray-level difference between two points on the measurement line by $\Delta \mathbf{I}(v) \equiv \mathbf{I}(v + \Delta v/2) - \mathbf{I}(v - \Delta v/2)$, and the *grayscale observation* on a given measurement line by $\mathbf{I} = \{I(i \Delta v) | i \in \mathbb{Z}\}$. These definitions are illustrated in Figure 13.7.

### 13.4.3 Likelihood of the Image

The observations along the measurement line depend on the contour locations in the image. This means that the likelihoods computed for different locations are not comparable, as they are likelihoods of different observations. A better evaluation function is given by the likelihood of the entire image $\mathcal{I}$ given a contour at location $\mu$, as a function $f^*(\mathcal{I}|\mu)$ of the contour location $\mu$ (for simplicity of notation, we do not include the coordinates of the measurement line on which the contour is located).

Denote by $f_a(\mathcal{I})$ the likelihood of the image given no contour and by $f_R(\mathcal{I}|\mu)$ the ratio $f^*(\mathcal{I}|\mu)/f_a(\mathcal{I})$, then the log likelihood of the entire image can be decomposed as follows:

$$\log f^*(\mathcal{I} \mid \mu) = \log f_a(\mathcal{I}) + \log f_R(\mathcal{I} \mid \mu) \tag{13.4}$$

The first term on the right-hand side of Equation 13.4 involves complex statistical dependencies between pixels and is expensive to calculate, as all image pixels must be inspected. Most importantly, the estimation of this term is needless, as it is an additive term that is independent of the presence and location of the contour. Consequently, in order to fit contours

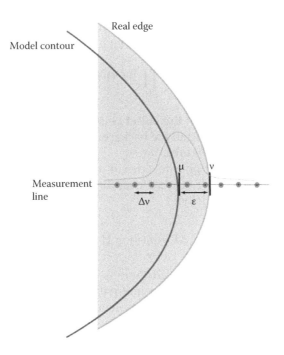

**FIGURE 13.7**
Marginalized contour definitions.

to the image, we consider only the log-likelihood ratio $\log f_R(\mathcal{I}|\mu)$. This derivation is fairly standard in the field of active contours, see for example, References [27], [28].

Note that $f_R(\mathcal{I}|\mu)$ is the ratio between the likelihood of the hypothesis that the target is present, see Equation 13.13; and the null hypothesis that the contour is not present, see Equation 13.7. Hence, the likelihood ratio can also be used for testing the hypothesis of the presence of a contour.

### 13.4.4 Grayscale Model

The pdf of gray-level differences between neighboring pixels is well-approximated by a generalized Laplacian [29]:

$$f_L(\Delta \mathbf{I}) = \frac{1}{Z_L} \exp \left( -\left| \frac{\Delta \mathbf{I}}{\lambda} \right|^\beta \right) \tag{13.5}$$

where $\Delta \mathbf{I}$ is the gray-level difference, $\lambda$ depends on the distance between the two sampled image locations, $\beta$ is a parameter approximately equal to 0.5, and $Z_L$ is a normalization constant. In the following, we assume that $\beta = 0.5$, which implies $Z_L = 4\lambda$.

#### 13.4.4.1 Distributions on Measurement Lines

If there is no known object edge between two points $[v - \Delta v/2, \ v + \Delta v/2]$ on the measurement line, the pdf of the gray levels follows the generalized Laplacian defined in Equation 13.5 as

$$f[\Delta \mathbf{I}(v)|\eta(v) = 0] = f_L[\Delta \mathbf{I}(v)] \tag{13.6}$$

Therefore, assuming statistical independence between gray-level differences,[1] the pdf of the observation in the absence of an edge is given by

$$f_a(\mathbf{I}) \equiv \prod_i f_L[\Delta \mathbf{I}(i \, \Delta v)] \tag{13.7}$$

Note that the absence of an edge of the object being tracked does not imply the absence of any edge: there can be edges within the background as well as within the object due to unmodeled objects and surface features.

Two gray levels observed on opposite sides of an edge are assumed to be statistically independent. The conditional pdf of gray-level differences separated by an edge can be assumed to be uniform for simplicity:

$$f[\Delta \mathbf{I}(v)|\eta(v) = 1] \approx \frac{1}{m} \tag{13.8}$$

where $m$ is the number of gray levels. If there is a known object boundary at location $j \, \Delta v$, then this point on the measurement line will correspond to gray-level differences across the boundary, and the rest will be gray-level differences of either object or background. In this case, the pdf of the observation is given by

$$\begin{aligned} f_c(\mathbf{I}|j \, \Delta v) &= \frac{1}{m} \prod_{i \neq j} f_L[\Delta \mathbf{I}(i \, \Delta v)] \\ &= \frac{1}{m} \frac{f_a(\mathbf{I})}{f_L(\Delta \mathbf{I}(j \, \Delta v))} \end{aligned} \tag{13.9}$$

### 13.4.4.2  Integrating over Deformations

The position of the idealized contour does not exactly correspond to the position of the object boundary, even if the position of the object is known. For simplicity, we assume a Gaussian distribution of geometric deformations of the object at each sample point. In the following, $v$ will denote the location of the object boundary on the measurement line. As mentioned above, $\mu$ is the intersection of the measurement line and the (idealized) contour, and the distance from $\mu$ to $v$ is $\epsilon = v - \mu$. The prior pdf of deformations $f_D(\epsilon)$ is defined by

$$f_D(\epsilon) = \frac{1}{Z_D} \exp\left(\frac{-\epsilon^2}{2\sigma^2}\right) \tag{13.10}$$

where $Z_D = \sqrt{2\pi}\sigma$ is a normalization factor. This assumption is similar to the one proposed in Reference [26], where a contour point generates a feature at a random distance from the contour with a Gaussian pdf.

The likelihood of the observation $\mathbf{I}$ given the contour location $\mu$ and deformation $\epsilon$ is naturally given by

$$f(\mathbf{I}|\mu, \epsilon) = f_c(\mathbf{I}|\mu + \epsilon) \tag{13.11}$$

The joint likelihood of the observation $\mathbf{I}$ and the deformation $\epsilon$ given the contour is

$$f(\mathbf{I}, \epsilon|\mu) = f_c(\mathbf{I}|\mu + \epsilon) f_D(\epsilon) \tag{13.12}$$

---

[1] Dependencies between gray levels are governed by the generalized Laplacian.

Marginalizing over possible deformations, the likelihood is given by

$$f_M(\mathbf{I}|\mu) = \int f_c(\mathbf{I}|\mu + \epsilon) f_D(\epsilon) d\epsilon$$

$$= \frac{1}{m} f_a(\mathbf{I}) \int \frac{f_D(\epsilon)}{f_L(\Delta\mathbf{I}(v))} d\epsilon \qquad (13.13)$$

On the basis of Section 13.4.3, we are interested in the likelihood ratio given by

$$f_R(\mathbf{I}|\mu) = \frac{f_M(\mathbf{I}|\mu)}{f_a(\mathbf{I})} = \frac{1}{m} \int \frac{f_D(\epsilon)}{f_L(\Delta\mathbf{I}(v))} d\epsilon \qquad (13.14)$$

It is convenient to take the logarithm to obtain the log-likelihood ratio:

$$h(\mathbf{I}|\mu) \equiv \log f_R(\mathbf{I}|\mu)$$

$$= -\log(m) + \log \int \frac{f_D(\epsilon)}{f_L(\Delta\mathbf{I}(v))} d\epsilon \qquad (13.15)$$

The integral can be approximated as a finite sum over a discrete set of possible deformations $\epsilon_j = j\Delta v - \mu$:

$$h(\mathbf{I}|\mu) = -\log(m) + \log \sum_j \frac{f_D(\epsilon_j)}{f_L(\Delta\mathbf{I}(j\Delta v))} \Delta v \qquad (13.16)$$

This summation is denoted as the *point-evaluation function*. Note that the integral in Equation 13.15 is defined from minus to plus infinity. However, due to the Gaussian term, the summation in Equation 13.16 only needs to be taken over a finite interval on each side of the contour (e.g., over the interval from $-2\sigma$ to $2\sigma$).

Using the definitions of the generalized Laplacian, $f_L$, and the pdf of the deformation, $f_D$, the point evaluation function above becomes

$$h(\mathbf{I}|\mu) = h_0 + \log \sum_j \exp \left[ \sqrt{\frac{|\Delta\mathbf{I}(j\Delta v)|}{\lambda}} - \frac{\epsilon_j^2}{2\sigma^2} \right] \qquad (13.17)$$

where $h_0 = \log Z_l/m - \log Z_D/\Delta v$.

### 13.4.5 EM Contour Algorithm

Expectation maximization (EM) is an iterative method for maximum likelihood or maximum *a posteriori* estimation. It is useful when the underlying model includes intermediate variables between the observed variables (gray levels) and the state variables to be estimated. The EM contour algorithm is a special case of EM as applied to active contours. A full description is given in Reference [24]. This section gives a short introduction to the algorithm. The way the algorithm is integrated into the iris tracker was described in Section 13.3.

For one sample point, the $k$ iteration of the EM contour algorithm consists of the following steps:

- **E**: Estimate the pdf $p^{(k)}(\epsilon) \equiv f(\epsilon|\mathbf{I}, \mu^{(k-1)})$ of the deformation given the observation and the estimate of the contour in the previous iteration.
- **M**: Maximize the value of the EM functional:

$$\mathcal{F}_p^{(k)}(\mu|\mathbf{I}) \equiv \int_\epsilon p^{(k)}(\epsilon) \log f(\mu^{(k-1)}|\mathbf{I}, \epsilon) d\epsilon \qquad (13.18)$$

Let $p_j$ denote the probability of the deformation taking a value between $(j - \frac{1}{2})\Delta v$ and $(j + \frac{1}{2})\Delta v$ given the observations and the contour:

$$p_j = \frac{f(\epsilon_j|\mathbf{I}, \mu)\Delta v}{\sum_i f(\epsilon_i|\mathbf{I}, \mu)\Delta v} = \frac{f_D(\epsilon_j)f_L^{-1}[\Delta \mathbf{I}(j\Delta v)]}{\sum_i f_D(\epsilon_i)f_L^{-1}[\Delta \mathbf{I}(i\Delta v)]} \tag{13.19}$$

where Equation 13.9 and Equation 13.12 were used in the last step.

As in the case of marginalization by Equation 13.13, the integral in Equation 13.18 will be in the following approximated by a summation. The EM functional can be expanded as follows:

$$\begin{aligned}
\mathcal{F}_p^{(k)}(\mu|\mathbf{I}) &= \sum_j p_j \log f(\mathbf{I}, j\Delta v|\mu) \\
&= \sum_j p_j \log f_c(\mathbf{I}|\mu + \epsilon)f_D(\epsilon) \\
&= h_0 + \sum_j p_j \left[ \sqrt{\frac{|\Delta \mathbf{I}(j\Delta v)|}{\lambda}} - \frac{\epsilon_j^2}{2\sigma^2} \right]
\end{aligned} \tag{13.20}$$

Define the center of mass of the observation: $\hat{v} \equiv \sum p_j j \Delta v$. The definition of the center of mass allows for a simplification of Equation 13.20 to the following expression:

$$\mathcal{F}_p = C - \frac{(\hat{v} - \mu)^2}{2\sigma^2} \tag{13.21}$$

where

$$C \equiv h_0 + \sum_j p_j \left[ \sqrt{\frac{|\Delta \mathbf{I}(j\Delta v)|}{\lambda}} - \frac{(j\Delta v - \hat{v})^2}{2\sigma^2} \right] \tag{13.22}$$

Note that $C$ is constant in the **M** step as the distribution $\{p_j\}$ is determined in the **E** step. The center of mass has the advantage that it integrates over all the image evidence on the measurement line (unlike the strongest feature on the measurement line).

In the case of multiple sample points, the EM iteration is as follows:

- **E**: For all sample points on the contour, estimate the centers of mass.
- **M**: Minimize the sum of squared distances between sample points and corresponding centers of mass.

This algorithm implicitly assumes that the deformations $\epsilon$ at distinct sample points are statistically independent. This assumption depends, of course, on the distance between sample points. However, in general, if prior knowledge is available about statistical dependencies between deformations, then this knowledge should be incorporated into the shape model (i.e., the model should be a deformable template with parameterized deformations). In this case, the independent deformations at each sample point must be considered as additional to the parameterized deformations.

In the EM contour algorithm, the centers of masses are used for minimizing the distance to sample points, and therefore, the algorithm resembles feature-based methods. The main difference lies in the distance measure to be minimized. Partial occlusion of the iris by the eyelids occurs almost constantly, and as a consequence, the set of centers of masses are likely to contain outliers. RANSAC (RAndom Sample Consensus) [30] is used on the centers of masses to remove outliers.

### 13.4.6 Color Model

We represent the color information through the target distribution **q** and a hypothesized distribution **p**($y$) located at position $y$ (the current estimate of the object). The similarity between these distributions is measured through the similarity measure $D(y) = D(\mathbf{p}(y), \mathbf{q})$. As desired, histogramming of spatial data removes the spatial dependency. One way of preserving some spatial locality is by imposing a weighting scheme on the pixels before histogramming. The weighting kernel reflects the importance (or the reliability) of that particular area of the object and is formalized through kernel density estimation [16]. It is generally desirable to choose a kernel that is positive, localized (centered), and differentiable, because the similarity function $D(y)$ inherits the properties of the kernel. In our approach, the kernel is implicitly incorporated through the Gaussian deformation assumption.

Let $x_i^c$ denote the pixel location normalized with respect to the center of the object model. The function

$$\psi : \mathbb{R}^N \rightarrow \{1, \ldots, m\}$$

takes the point of the model and returns the index of the corresponding bin in the histogram. The target model is represented by the spatially weighted distribution of the observations:

$$q_z = C \sum_{i=1}^{n} k\left( \left\| x_i^c \right\|^2 \right) \delta\left( \psi\left( x_i^c \right) - z \right)$$

where $\delta$ is the Kronecker delta function, $k$ is the weighting (kernel) function, and $C$ is a normalizing factor:

$$C = \frac{1}{\sum_{i=1}^{n} k\left( \left\| x_i^c \right\|^2 \right)} \qquad (13.23)$$

Equivalently, the model candidates centered at $y$ with pixel coordinates $\{x_i\}_{i=1}^{n_h}$ is given by

$$p_z(y) = C_h \sum_{i=1}^{n_h} k\left( \left\| \frac{y - x_i}{h} \right\|^2 \right) \delta(\psi(x_i) - z) \qquad (13.24)$$

where $h$ is kernel size, and $C_h$ is

$$C_h = \frac{1}{\sum_{i=1}^{n_h} k\left( \left\| \frac{y - x_i}{h} \right\| \right)^2}$$

The similarity measure $D$ is derived from the Bhattacharyya coefficient, which for $m$ discrete variables is given by Reference [16]:

$$\rho(y) \equiv \rho[p(y), q] = \sum_{z=1}^{m} \sqrt{p_z(y) q_z} \qquad (13.25)$$

The distance between the model and the estimated distributions is defined by

$$D(y) = \sqrt{1 - \rho(y)} \qquad (13.26)$$

The measure Equation 13.26 has several important properties [16] (e.g., that it is a metric and thus symmetric). It is scale invariant, which becomes useful when comparing histograms of regions of different sizes, and even though histograms are not the best representation for nonparametric density estimates, they satisfy the low computational cost imposed by real-time processing. The model given is, in principle, independent of the color space used; however, for simplicity, this approach uses the HSV color space.

## 13.5   Tracking Results

The experiments are conducted using a standard video camera placed on a tripod. The users are sitting at a normal working distance (about 50 cm) from the monitor. They were asked to gaze at a set of predefined regions on the screen while trying to act as if it was a common working situation.

The initial position and the noise model of the dynamics $\Sigma_0$ are set manually as to obtain a sufficient accuracy while still being able to allow some freedom of head movements. The mean of the sample set is optimized until convergence over three image scales with a maximum of five iterations of the MEMC contour algorithm on each image scale, resulting in a total of 12 iterations of the MEMC contour algorithm per frame. The use of the scale space and the RANSAC approach significantly improves accuracy, especially in large images. As evaluating a single iteration in the EM contour method corresponds to an evaluation of a particle, the additional cost required by applying the EM contour method in the image scale space is equivalent to adding 15 particles in the particle filter.

Initialization of the model is done manually, and the method is tested on both Europeans and Asians in live test situations and prerecorded sequences using web and video cameras. In images of sizes $720 \times 576$ (digital video cameras), real-time performance is obtained.

In Figure 13.8 to Figure 13.10, images from testing the method on iris tracking using a standard video and web camera in both indoor and outdoor situations are shown. These images indicate that the method is capable of tracking the iris under scale changes, squinting the eye in various light conditions, under image defocusing, and under moderate head movements. Figure 13.8 shows a sequence in which a video camera is used with built-in IR light emitter that allows a switch between visible light and IR images. Changing between the two modes results in a significant change in image grayscale values. Despite these drastic changes, tracking is maintained without changing the model or any of its parameters.

Due to the changes in image quality, there is a vast difference in the difficulty of tracking eyes in images using web cameras to using video cameras and IR-based images. However, the method is capable of tracking the iris without changing the model for all three types of images. Clearly, tracking accuracy improves with the enhanced image quality.

The number of particles is an important parameter in particle filtering. Too few particles results in insufficient accuracy, while too many particles wastes computation time. Figure 13.11 shows a comparison of accuracy when using contour likelihood and when using the combined color and contour model as a function of the number of particles. The accuracy (Euclidian distance measured in pixels) is measured on the coarsest image level as

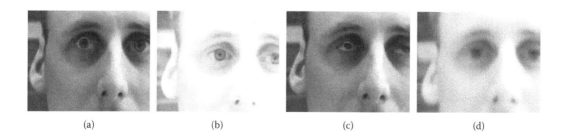

|     (a)     |     (b)     |     (c)     |     (d)     |

**FIGURE 13.8** (See color insert.)
Tracking the iris while staying outdoors and additionally changing the illumination conditions by altering between IR to non-IR lighting. Notice how light conditions change when switching between IR and non-IR light emission (greenish looking images are IR "night vision").

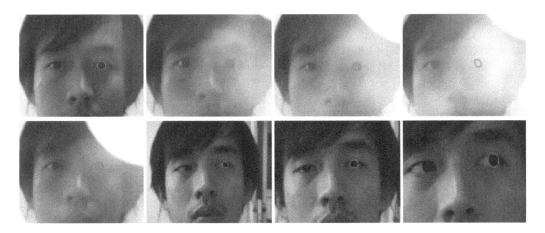

**FIGURE 13.9 (See color insert.)**
Tracking the iris of Asians under scale changes and heavy light disturbances.

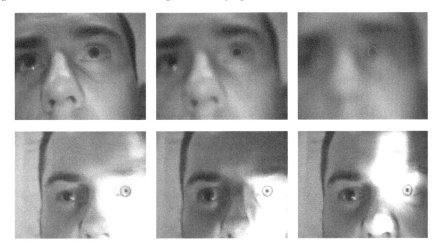

**FIGURE 13.10**
Tracking the iris under various light conditions, head poses, image blurring, and scales.

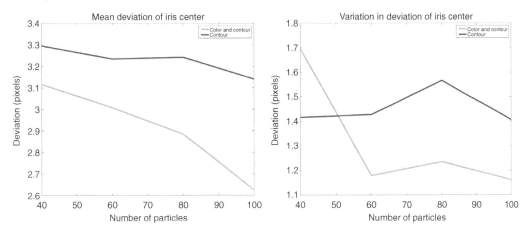

**FIGURE 13.11**
Comparison of contour tracking with and without the use of color information: (left) inaccuracy of the center of the iris, and (right) the corresponding variations in accuracy.

to measure the effects of color without local optimization. The measurement of accuracy is based on a set of 3240 manually annotated images. Not only is the accuracy improved when using color information, but the variance is also reduced. Using a low number of samples results in low accuracy, but accuracy quickly improves with increased sample size. This implies that the number of particles can be reduced while maintaining accuracy when using color information for eye tracking.

## 13.6 Conclusion

Eye tracking is not a new idea, but due to technological developments, it is rapidly moving out of laboratory use and toward a broad range of applications for the general public. IR light is largely dominant in current eye tracker development and commercial systems, but it is also limited by only being reliable indoors. IR light may be potentially uncomfortable (drying the eyes), and to be really efficient, the eye tracker requires novel synchronization schemes to produce dark and bright pupil images. Surprisingly, the use of visible colors have to a large extent been neglected, even though both near-IR light and color information can be used simultaneously in many consumer cameras (i.e., IR glints can be detected in a web camera). We have argued that colors provide valuable information for eye tracking and that IR and color imaging do not exclude each other. In fact, eye trackers may benefit from using both simultaneously as robustness is increased.

In this chapter, we argued that in cases where color information is available, the use of color distributions provides stable information to be used in eye tracking. We have shown that colors provide information to improve tracker robustness and lower the number of particles needed to maintain accuracy. We have also shown that iris tracking can be done without explicit feature detection and thresholds. This is important, because eye trackers should be able to cope with usage in different scenarios, image blurring images, and in both IR and non-IR settings without the user having to define thresholds. This may suggest that eye trackers can be made to work outside constrained laboratory uses and, at the same time, lower the costs by using standard commercially available video and web cameras. Eye tracking using off-the-shelf components holds potential for making eye tracking an input device for the general public. There are still several important issues to be solved due to less *a priori* knowledge of consumer hardware and use scenarios, but the increasing interest in eye tracking as a means for perceptual interfacing in both research and commercial communities [31] may catalyze the process further.

## References

[1] E.B. Delabarre, A method of recording eye-movements, *Am. J. Psychol.*, 9, 572–574, 1898.
[2] P. Majaranta and K.-J. Räihä, Twenty years of eye typing: Systems and design issues, in *Symposium on ETRA 2002: Eye Tracking Research Applications Symposium*, New Orleans, LA, ACM Press, New York 2002, pp. 944–950.
[3] A.T. Duchowski, *Eye Tracking Methodology. Theory and Practice*, Springer, New York, 2003.
[4] A. Hyrskykari, P. Majaranta, A. Aaltonen, and K.-J. Räihä, Design issues of idict: A gaze-assisted translation aid, in *Proceedings of the Symposium on Eye Tracking Research and Applications 2000*, Palm Beach Gardens, FL, ACM Press, New York 2000, pp. 9–14.

[5] D.J. Ward and D.J.C. MacKay, Fast hands-free writing by gaze direction, *Nature*, 418, 838, 2002.

[6] J.P. Hansen, A.S. Johansen, D.W. Hansen, K. Itoh, and S. Mashino, Language technology in a predictive, restricted on-screen keyboard with ambiguous layout for severely disabled people, in *EACL 2003 Workshop on Language Modeling for Text Entry Methods*, 2003.

[7] R. Vertegaal, I. Weevers, and C. Sohn, Gaze-2: An attentive video conferencing system in *CHI'02: Extended Abstracts on Human Factors in Computing Systems*, New York, ACM Press, New York, 2002, pp. 736–737.

[8] J.P. Hansen, D.W. Hansen, A.S. Johansen, and J. Elvsjö, Mainstreaming gaze interaction towards a mass market for the benefit of all, in *Proceedings of the 11th International Conference on Human–Computer Interaction*, CDROM, 2005.

[9] C. Morimoto and M. Mimica, Eye gaze tracking techniques for interactive applications, *Comput. Vis. Image Understand.*, 98, 4–24, April 2005.

[10] Q. Ji and X. Yang, Real time visual cues extraction for monitoring driver vigilance, in *International Workshop of Computer Vision Systems*, London, Springer-Verlag, 2001, pp. 107–124.

[11] Tobii, http://www.tobii.se/, 2005.

[12] Y. Ebisawa, Unconstrained pupil detection technique using two light sources and the image difference method, in *Visualization and Intelligent Design in Engineering and Architecture*, 1995, pp. 79–89.

[13] K. Nguyen, C. Wagner, D. Koons, and M. Flickner, Differences in the infrared bright pupil response of human eyes, in *ETRA'02: Proceedings of the Symposium on Eye Tracking Research and Applications*, New Orleans, LA, ACM Press, New York, 2002, pp. 133–138.

[14] T.F. Cootes, G.J. Edwards, and C.J. Taylor, Active appearance models, in *Proceedings of the European Conference on Computer Vision*, Vol. 2, Springer, New York, 1998, pp. 484–498.

[15] D.W. Hansen, J.P. Hansen, M. Nielsen, A.S. Johansen, and M.B. Stegmann, Eye typing using Markov and active appearance models, in *IEEE Workshop on Applications on Computer Vision*, Orlando, FL, IEEE Computer Society, 2002, pp. 132–136.

[16] D. Comaniciu, V. Ramesh, and P. Meer, Kernel-based object tracking, *IEEE Trans. on Patt. Anal. and Machine Intelligence*, 25, 564–577, 2003.

[17] G. Bradski, Computer vison face tracking as a component of a perceptual user interface, *Workshop on Applications of Computer Vision*, Los Alamitos, CA, IEEE Computer Society, 1998, pp. 214–219.

[18] P. Perez, C. Hue, J. Vermaak, and M. Gangnet, Color-based probabilistic tracking, in *European Conference on Computer Vision*, 2002, pp. 661–675.

[19] M. Isard and A. Blake, Contour tracking by stochastic propagation of conditional density, in *European Conference on Computer Vision*, 1996, pp. 343–356.

[20] D.W. Hansen and A.E. Pece, Eye tracking in the wild, *Comput. Vis. Image Understand.*, 98, 182–210, April 2005.

[21] D.W. Hansen, Comitting Eye Tracking, Ph.D. thesis, IT University of Copenhagen, 2003.

[22] P. Tissainayagam and D. Suter, Tracking multiple object contours with automatic motion model switching, in *International Conference on Pattern Recognition*, 2000, pp. 1146–1149.

[23] M. Kass, A. Witkin, and D. Terzopoulos, Snakes: Active contour models, in *International Conference on Computer Vision*, 1987, pp. 259–268.

[24] A. Pece and A. Worrall, Tracking with the EM contour algorithm, in *European Conference on Computer Vision*, 2002, pp. I: 3–17.

[25] A. Yuille and J. Coughlan, Fundamental limits of Bayesian inference: Order parameters and phase transitions for road tracking, *IEEE Trans. on Patt. Anal. and Machine Intelligence*, 22, 160–173, 2000.

[26] J. MacCormick and A. Blake, A probabilistic contour discriminant for object localisation, in *International Conference on Computer Vision*, 1998, pp. 390–395.

[27] J. Coughlan, A. Yuille, C. English, and D. Snow, Efficient deformable template detection and localization without user initialization, *Comput. Vis. Image Understand.*, 78, 303–319, 2000.

[28] H. Sidenbladh and M.J. Black, Learning the statistics of people in images and video, *Int. J. Comput. Vision*, 54, 183–209, 2003.

[29] J. Huang and D. Mumford, Statistics of natural images and models, in *IEEE Computer Vision and Pattern Recognition (CVPR)*, 1999, pp. I: 541–547.

[30] M.A. Fischler and R.C. Bolles, Random sample consensus: A paradigm for model fitting with applications to image analysis and automated cartography, *Commun. ACM*, 24, 381–395, 1981.

[31] COGAIN, http://www.cogain.org/, 2005.

# 14

## Automated Identification of Diabetic Retinal Exudates in Digital Color Images

Alireza Osareh

### CONTENTS

### 14.1 Introduction

The severe progression of diabetes is one of the greatest immediate challenges to current health care. The number of people afflicted continues to grow at an alarming rate. The World Health Organization expects the number of diabetics to increase from 130 million to 350 million over the next 25 years [1]. However, only one half of the patients are aware of the disease. Diabetes leads to severe late complications including macro- and microvascular changes resulting in heart disease and retinopathy. Diabetic retinopathy (DR) is a common complication of diabetes and the leading cause of blindness in the working populations. It is a silent disease and may only be recognized by the patient when the changes in the retina have progressed to a level at which treatment is complicated and nearly impossible.

Although diabetes cannot be prevented, in many cases, its blinding complications can be moderated if the DR is detected early enough for treatment. Proper screening for retinopathy and then treatment by laser can significantly reduce the incidence of blindness. The aim of laser surgery is to prevent visual loss; thus, the optimal time for treatment is before the patient experiences visual symptoms. It is believed that the screening of diabetics patients for the development of DR potentially reduces the risk of blindness in these patients by 50% [2]. Unfortunately, because visual loss is often a late symptom of advanced DR, many patients remain undiagnosed, even as their disease is causing severe retinal damage.

Nearly all diabetics develop DR within their lifetimes, which represents the importance of annual screening of diabetic patients for this complication. This provides a huge number of retinal images, which need to be reviewed by physicians. The high cost of examination and the shortage of ophthalmologists, especially in rural areas, are prominent factors that hamper patients from obtaining regular examinations [3]. Thus, it would be more cost effective and helpful if the initial task of analyzing the retinal photographs can be automated. In this way, individuals who are diagnosed by the automatic computer system as having early retinal lesions would be referred to an ophthalmologist for further evaluation [4]. This would allow more patients to be screened per year and the ophthalmologists to spend more time on those patients who are actually in need of their expertise.

## 14.2   Background

Background diabetic retinopathy (BDR) is the most common type of DR, accounting for approximately 80% of all patients. It can arise at any point in time after the onset of diabetes. A qualified practitioner, such as a general ophthalmologist, may detect these changes by examining the patient's retina. The physician looks for spots of bleeding, lipid exudation, or areas of retinal swelling caused by the leakage of edema, and will be more concerned if such lesions are found near the central retina (macula), when vision may become affected. Accurate assessment of retinopathy severity requires the ability to detect and record the following clinical features:

- *Microaneurysms*: The earliest clinically recognizable characteristic of DR is microaneurysms. Microaneurysms are focal dilatations of retinal capillaries. They are about 10 to 100 $\mu$ in diameter and appear as small round dark red dots on the retinal surface.

- *Hemorrhages*: As the degree of retinopathy advances, retinal hemorrhages become evident. Retinal hemorrhages appear either as small red dots or blots indistinguishable from microaneurysms or as larger flame-shaped hemorrhages. As the retinal vessels become more damaged and leaky, their numbers increase.

- *Hard exudates*: Intraretinal hard exudates (Figure 14.1a to Figure 14.1c) represent leak from surrounding capillaries and microaneurysms within the retina. They are a visible sign of DR and also a marker for the presence of coexistent retinal edema. If present in the macular area, edema and exudates are a major cause of visual loss in the nonproliferative forms of DR. Retinal edema and exudates in the central area are the clinical signs most closely linked with treatable visual loss. Exudates are associated with patches of vascular damage with leakage and typically manifest as spatially random yellow patches of varying sizes and shapes [5]. The size and distribution of exudates may vary during the progress of the disease.

- *Cotton wool spots*: Cotton wool spots represent a transitional stage between BDR, or *maculopathy*, and proliferative retinopathy. This is sometimes known as preproliferative retinopathy. These abnormalities usually appear as little fluffy round or oval areas in the retina with a whitish color, usually adjacent to an area of hemorrhage (Figure 14.1c).

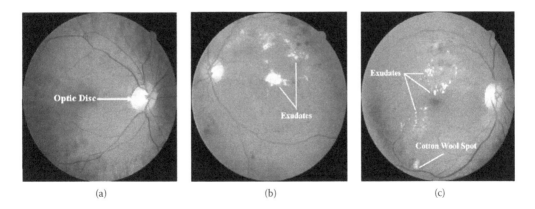

(a)  (b)  (c)

**FIGURE 14.1** (See color insert.)

Normal and abnormal images: (a) a typical normal image with optic disc region, (b) severe retinopathy, with large plaques of exudates, and (c) diabetic retinopathy including retinal exudates and a cotton wool spot.

The application of digital imaging to ophthalmology has now provided the possibility of processing retinal images to assist in clinical diagnosis and treatment. In fact, with the introduction of better and inexpensive ophthalmic imaging cameras, along with the rapid growth of proper software for identifying those at risk of developing DR, as well as the reduction in costs and increase in computational power of computers, an advanced retinal image analysis system can be developed. This will assist ophthalmologists in making the diagnosis more efficiently. Such a system should be able to detect early signs of background retinopathy and provide an objective diagnosis based on criteria defined by the ophthalmologists.

Here, we have concentrated on detecting retinal exudates as the prime marker, because it is likely that accumulating exudates is always associated with retinal edema, and unlike edema, exudates are more visible in color retinal images. Detecting exudates in the retina in a large number of images generated by screening programs, which need to be repeated at least annually, is very expensive in professional time and open to human error. Thus, the main objective of the investigation described here is to contribute novel methods to quantitatively diagnose and classify exudate lesions in color images.

## 14.3  Overview

The overall scheme of the methods used in this work is as follows. The input color retinal image is automatically analyzed, and an assessment of the level of background DR disease is derived after analysis. The proposed method will then choose diabetic patients who need further examination. In the first stage, we put our data through two preprocessing steps, including color normalization and local contrast enhancement. Once the images have been preprocessed, exudate lesions can be identified automatically using the *region-level exudate recognition* approach, which is comprised from two main stages — color retinal image segmentation and region-level classification. Neural network (NN) and support vector machines (SVM) classifiers are employed toward a region-based classification scheme.

Here, we introduce two main criteria for assessing the diagnostic accuracy of our exudate detection technique — lesion based and image based. In lesion-based criteria, each exudate lesion is regarded as an individual connected region, where this region can be comprised of one or more pixels. Each abnormal retinal image can be segmented into a number of exudate regions. By considering a set of retinal images and applying an appropriate segmentation/classification technique, a data set of exudate regions will be created. Then, the lesion-based accuracy is measured in terms of lesion *sensitivity* and *specificity* by comparison of the gained results against the ophthalmologist's outline of the lesions.

The lesion-based accuracy can be assessed either in a pixel resolution basis or alternatively using a bigger collection of pixels, for example, $10 \times 10$ patches (patch resolution). Creating an accurate pixel-based ground-truth by the physician is not an easy task, but a pixel resolution comparison of the results will be more precise than the patch resolution manner. A pixels patch may only be partially covered by exudate pixels. Thus, the effects of misclassification errors for individual patches (exudates/nonexudates) should be taken into consideration when the performance is not measured based on pixel resolution.

In image-based diagnostic-based assessment, each image is examined, and a decision is made to illustrate whether the image has some evidence of DR, purely based on the absence or presence of exudates in the image.

The performance of a medical diagnosis system is best described in terms of sensitivity and specificity. These criteria quantify the system performance according to the false positive ($FP$) and false negative ($FN$) instances. The sensitivity gives the percentage of correctly classified abnormal cases, while the specificity defines the percentage of correctly classified normal cases. Classification of the whole retinal image pixels was required to work on an imbalanced data set of exudate and nonexudate pixels, where the number of true negatives ($TN$) was much higher than the $FP$s. Hence, the specificity measure was mostly near 100% and did not represent an informative measurement. Thus, we used the predictivity measure, which is the probability that a pixel classified as an exudate is really an exudate. This measurement is defined as follows:

$$predictivity = \frac{TP}{TP + FP} \tag{14.1}$$

where $TP$ refers to the true positive criterion.

## 14.4  Previous Works on Exudates Identification

Retinal image analysis is a complicated task, particularly because of the variability of the images in terms of the color, the morphology of the retinal anatomical–pathological structures, and the existence of particular features in different patients. There have been some research investigations to identify retinal main components, such as blood vessels, optic disc, and retinal lesions, including microaneurysms, hemorrhages, and exudates [6], [7], [8], [9], [10], [11]. Here, we review the main works, which have been done in this area with emphasis on exudate detection.

The quantification of DR and detection of exudates on fundus images were investigated by Phillips and Sharp [6]. Global and local thresholding values were used to segment exudate lesions from the red-free images. The lesion-based sensitivity of exudates identification technique was reported between 61% and 100% (mean 87%) [6].

Ege and Hejlesen [7] located the optic disc, fovea, and four red and yellow abnormalities (microaneurysms, hemorrhages, exudates, and cotton-wool-spots) in 38 color fundus images. The abnormalities were detected using a combination of template matching, region growing, and thresholding techniques. During the first stages 87% of exudates were detected in terms of lesion-based criterion. Following preliminary detection of the abnormalities, a Bayesian classifier was engaged to classify the yellow lesions into exudates, cotton wool spots, and noise. The classification performance for this stage was only 62% for exudates and 52% for the cotton wool spots.

Gardner et al. [8] broke down the retinal images into small squares and then presented them to a NN. After median smoothing, the photographed red-free images were fed directly into a large NN with 400 inputs. The NN was trained for 5 days, and the lesion-based sensitivity of the exudate detection method was 93.1%. This performance was the result of classifying all $20 \times 20$ pixel patches rather than pixel resolution.

Sinthanayothin [9] applied a recursive region growing technique using selected threshold values in gray-level images. In this work, it was supposed that the processed retinal images are only including exudates, hemorrhages, and microaneurysms, and other lesions (e.g., cotton wool spots) were not considered. The author reported an accuracy of 88.5% sensitivity and 99.7% specificity for the detection of exudates against a small data set comprising 21 abnormal and 9 normal retinal images. However, these performances were measured based on $10 \times 10$ patches.

In a more recent work, exudates were identified from the green channel of the retinal images, according to their gray-level variation [10]. After initial localization, the exudate contours were subsequently determined by mathematical morphology techniques. This technique achieved a pixel resolution accuracy including 92.8% mean sensitivity and 92.4% mean predictivity against a set of 15 abnormal retinal images. The authors ignored some types of errors on the border of the segmented exudates in their reported performances. A set of 15 normal images was also examined; where in 13 of those, no exudates were found (88.6% specificity in terms of image-based accuracy).

As is apparent from the above reviewed methods, most proposed exudate identification techniques have been assessed only in terms of lesion-based or image-based diagnostic criterion and against an approximately small number of retinal images. The reported lesion-based accuracies are often based on $10 \times 10$ or $20 \times 20$ patches (patch resolution), and no pixel resolution validation has been accomplished except in a couple of works. There are certain errors in reported patch resolution accuracies due to small areas, which some exudates can occupy. In medical decision support systems such as ours, an accurate diagnostic accuracy assessment in terms of both pixel resolution and image-based criteria is important.

One novelty of our proposed method is that we locate exudates at pixel level in color retinal images. We then evaluate the diagnostic accuracy of our techniques in terms of both pixel resolution and image-based criteria against a large set of images. Our technique achieves an image-based diagnostic accuracy of 95.0% sensitivity and 88.9% specificity for the identification of images containing any evidence of retinopathy, where the trade-off between sensitivity and specificity is appropriately balanced for this particular problem. Furthermore, it demonstrates 90.0% mean sensitivity and 89.3% mean predictivity, in terms of pixel resolution exudate identification.

Section 14.5 describes retinal image acquisition and preprocessing methodologies. Section 14.6 briefly introduces region-level exudate recognition based upon fuzzy c-means clustering and region-level classification. The chapter is concluded in Section 14.7.

## 14.5 Data Collection and Preprocessing

Our automated exudate identification system was developed using color retinal images provided by the Bristol Eye Hospital. According to the National Screening Committee standards, all the images are obtained using a Canon CR6-45 nonmydriatic (CR6-45NM)

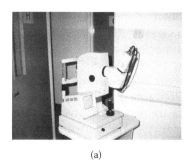
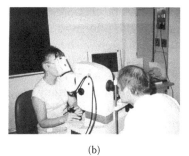

(a)                                                    (b)

**FIGURE 14.2**
Retina screening with a digital camera: (a) Canon CR6-45NM retinal camera, and (b) patient retina screening process.

retinal camera. The acquired image resolution is $760 \times 570$ in 24-bit TIFF format. A total of 142 images were captured by an ophthalmologist of which 90 were abnormal and 52 normal (Figure 14.2). Images were taken with a field of view of $45°$ under the same lighting conditions. All the images were classified by the expert ophthalmologist. Examples of such images were shown in Figure 14.1a to Figure 14.1c.

### 14.5.1   Retinal Color Normalization and Contrast Enhancement

We put our data through two preprocessing steps before commencing the detection of exudates. The retina's color in different patients is variable, being strongly correlated to skin pigmentation and iris color. Thus, the first step is to normalize the color of the retinal images across the data set. We selected a retinal image as a reference and then applied histogram specification [12] to modify the values of each image in the database such that its frequency histogram matched the reference image distribution.

The histogram specification technique was independently applied to each RGB channel to match the shapes of three specific histograms of the reference image. Here, the reference histograms were taken from an image, which represents a frequent retinal pigmentation color among our image data set.

This image was chosen in agreement with the expert ophthalmologist. To demonstrate the color normalization effect, a different color retinal image and its normalized version are shown in Figure 14.3b and Figure 14.3c. As is evident, the normalization process modifies the color distributions of the considered image to match the reference image's distribution.

The color normalization process improves the clustering ability of the different lesion types and removes the variation due to the retinal pigmentation differences between individuals. The retinal images taken at standard examinations are sometimes poorly contrasted due to the intrinsic attributes of lesions, and they can contain artifacts. The retinal image contrast is decreased as the distance of a pixel from the image center increased. Thus, the exudates in such regions are not distinguishable from the background color near the disc. Therefore, preprocessing techniques are necessary to improve the contrast of these images. Here, we apply a local contrast enhancement technique [9]. This enhancement approach is applied only on the intensity channel I of the image after conversion from the RGB (red, green, blue) to the hue-saturation-intensity (HSI) color space [12].

The objective is to apply a transformation of the values inside small windows in the image in a way that all values are distributed around the mean and show all possible intensities. Given each pixel $p$ in the initial image and a small $N \times N$ running window $w$, the image is

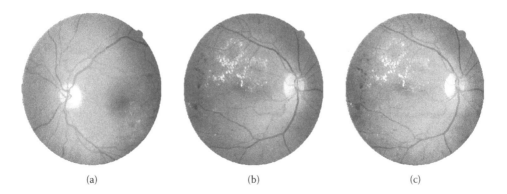

(a)  (b)  (c)

**FIGURE 14.3**
Color normalization: (a) reference image, (b) typical retinal image (including exudates), and (c) color normalized version.

filtered to produce the new image pixel $p_n$:

$$p_n = 255 \left( \frac{[\phi(p) - \phi_w(Min)]}{\phi_w(Max) - \phi_w(Min)]} \right) \tag{14.2}$$

where $\phi$ is defined as

$$\phi_w(p) = \left[ 1 + \exp\left( \frac{\mu_w - p}{\sigma_w} \right) \right]^{-1} \tag{14.3}$$

and *Max* and *Min* are the maximum and minimum intensity values in the whole image, while $\mu_w$ and $\sigma_w$ indicate the local window mean and standard deviation. The exponential function (in Equation 14.3) produces significant enhancement when the contrast is low ($\sigma_w$ is small), while it provides less enhancement if the contrast is already high ($\sigma_w$ is large).

The size of window $N$ should be chosen to be large enough to contain a statistically representative distribution of the local variations of pixels. On the other hand, it must be small enough to not be influenced by the gradual variation of the contrast between the retinal image center and the periphery. We have experimented with different $N$ values.

Figure 14.4a to Figure 14.4c show the result of local contrast enhancement on a retinal image with two different window sizes. As is evident, the image details can be perceived

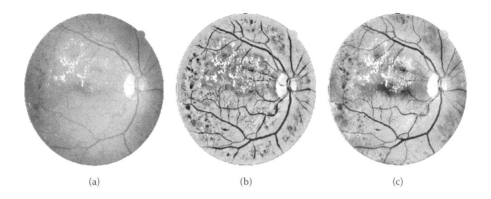

(a)  (b)  (c)

**FIGURE 14.4**
The local contrast enhancement results for different window sizes: (a) a typical retinal image with the color normalized version of the image shown in Figure 14.3b, (b) contrast enhancement with $N = 41$, and (c) contrast enhancement with $N = 69$.

more clearly compared to that of the original image. Here, the window size was empirically set to $69 \times 69$ for our processing, although the other values may also be appropriate. Overall, the preprocessing methods facilitate our subsequent processing by providing better discrimination ability between the exudates and nonexudates.

## 14.6   Region-Level Exudate Recognition

### 14.6.1   Retinal Image Segmentation

While color images contain more information than the gray levels, the additional color information does not necessarily make the segmentation easier. Several color image segmentation methods were developed in the literature [13], [14], [15]. The selection of a segmentation method depends on the type of images and the area that application addresses. Here, investigations are made to identify a robust method to reliably segment the retinal images with some false-positive exudate regions to a moderate extent.

Color image segmentation is frequently based on supervised pixel classification [16], while clustering is the most widely used unsupervised method [17]. In such techniques, clusters are detected in a multidimensional feature space and mapped back to the original image plane, to produce segmentation. Fuzzy c-means (FCM) clustering [18] has received extensive attention in a wide variety of image processing applications, such as medical imaging [19]. The advantages of FCM include a straightforward implementation, fairly robust behavior, applicability to multichannel data, and the ability to model uncertainty within the data.

An efficient color segmentation scheme was proposed in Reference [20]. This utilizes the histogram information of the three color components to estimate the number of valid classes by a statistical evaluation of the histogram compared to the original proposed FCM algorithm by Bezdek et al. Here, we have been inspired by Reference [20] to segment our color retinal images.

### 14.6.2   Color Space Selection

While our color retinal images contain more information about objects and background than the corresponding gray-level images, the additional color information does not necessarily make the process easier, and thus, a careful color modeling is required. There are several different color spaces in the literature [21], and each has its own advantages. To select the most suitable color space for our exudate identification approach, we conducted a quantitative analysis and applied a metric to evaluate the performance of various color spaces. This metric [22] estimated the class separability of our exudate and nonexudate (cotton-wool spots, red lesions, blood vessels, and background) pixel classes in different color spaces and was measured based on within-class and between-class scatter matrices. The within-class scatter matrix ($S_w$) indicates the distribution of sample points around their respective mean vectors and is defined as

$$S_w = \sum_{i=1}^{C} S_i \tag{14.4}$$

$$S_i = \sum_{n \in C_i}(X_n - M_i)(X_n - M_i)^T \quad \text{and} \quad M_i = \frac{1}{N}\sum_{n \in C_i} X_n \tag{14.5}$$

**TABLE 14.1**

Comparative Analysis of Different Color Spaces

| Color Space | YIQ | RGB | HSL | HSI | Lab | Luv |
|---|---|---|---|---|---|---|
| J | 2.20 | 2.25 | 2.64 | 2.81 | 3.32 | 3.67 |

where $C$ is the number of classes, $N_i$ represents the number of examples in class $C_i$, $X_n$ refers to the sample $n$, and $M_i$ is the mean of class $C_i$. The between-class matrix ($S_b$) represents the scatter of samples around the mean vector of the class mixture and is defined as

$$S_b = \sum_{i=1}^{C} N_i (M_i - M)(M_i - M)^T \tag{14.6}$$

$$M = \frac{1}{N} \sum_{n=1}^{N} X_n = \frac{1}{N} \sum_{i=1}^{C} N_i M_i \tag{14.7}$$

while $N = \sum_i N_i$ shows the total number of sample points in the data set. After within-class and between-class matrices are measured, the following metric $J$ can be obtained:

$$J = trace\left(\frac{S_b}{S_w}\right) \tag{14.8}$$

A higher value of $J$ indicates that the classes are more separated, while the members within each class are closer to each other. We experimented with different color spaces using our set of retinal images and found that the color spaces, which separate the luminance and chromaticity of a color, are more successful (Table 14.1).

It is apparent that the *Luv* color space [21] is the most appropriate space for our retinal image analysis. This color space has a good perceptual basis, in the sense that colors, which are equidistant in the Euclidean space, are approximately equidistant in terms of perceived difference. Thus, we choose this color space to carry out our retinal image segmentation task.

### 14.6.3 Retinal Image Coarse Segmentation

The coarse stage attempts to segment the image by using histogram thresholding. The threshold values are determined by the application of scale-space Gaussian filtering to the one-dimensional (1-D) histogram of the three color components. It was identified that the derivatives, the extrema and the interval bounded by the extrema of a histogram, are useful information when carrying out a qualitative analysis of the histograms. A scale-space filter, which is described as a multiscale representation of a signal, is an appealing tool to identify the positions of intervals containing peaks and valleys at different scales. If we can utilize the information, which is embedded in an image histogram, more effectively, we can analyze the correspondent image more accurately. Witkin [23] proposed an approach based on multiscale representation of a measured signal and used the Gaussian function to smooth the curve and detect the peaks and valleys. Suppose we have a signal $f$ and a smoothing kernel $g(x, \sigma)$, the smoothed signal at the scale $\sigma$ is

$$F(x, \sigma) = f(x) * g(x, \sigma) \tag{14.9}$$

where $*$ denotes convolution with respect to $x$. For a Gaussian function as a smoothing kernel, Equation 14.9 is changed to

$$F(x, \sigma) = \int_{-\infty}^{\infty} f(u) \frac{1}{\sigma\sqrt{2\pi}} \exp\left[-\frac{(x - \mu)^2}{2\sigma^2}\right] du \tag{14.10}$$

However, a major problem in Gaussian smoothing is how to determine the scale parameter ($\sigma$) for smoothing a given signal. The Witkin's multiscale representation can extract the features such as peaks and valleys and also determine the scale parameter value. This approach is, however, computationally expensive, because a large number of Gaussian convolutions are required. Here, we determine the optimum scale value ($\sigma$) experimentally and according to our prior knowledge of retinal image characteristics.

Having smoothed the image's histograms, the coarse stage begins to segment the image using the located thresholds. The histogram valley locations can be possible solutions for the thresholds. The valleys and peaks (which represent the number of clusters) are obtained by computing the first and second derivatives of each histogram. The aim of this manipulation is to obtain a set of histogram thresholds that precisely cluster the colors, which emerge in input image. Each of these clusters is separated from its neighbors by a secure-zone parameter as follows:

$$T\_Low(i) = E(i) - secure\_zone$$
$$T\_High(i) = E(i) + secure\_zone \quad (14.11)$$
$$i = 0, 1, \ldots, n$$

where $T\_Low$ and $T\_High$ are the cluster's lower and higher thresholds. The term $E$ represents an extremum (peak), and $n$ is the number of preclusters (classes) that exist in the histogram. The histogram regions, which are not assigned to any cluster, are considered ambiguous regions. These ambiguous regions are then further processed in the fine segmentation stage. The width of the secure-zone is a configurable parameter of the segmentation algorithm (assumed to be between 0 and 1), and it influences the number of pixels, which are passed to the fine segmentation stage.

If we project each color retinal image (which is represented in $Luv$ color space) onto its three color components (i.e., $L$, $u$, and $v$), there will be three 1-D histograms. The histogram analysis of each Gaussian smoothed color component enables reliable detection of meaningful peaks and valleys in the given histogram. At the same time, it determines significant intervals around those peaks. Hence, we can obtain the number of peaks in each color component (i.e., $N_L$, $N_u$, and $N_v$). The maximum number of possible three-dimensional (3-D) peaks is then calculated as the multiplication of the obtained 1-D peak numbers ($N_{max} = N_L.N_u.N_v$).

Thus, we can partition the $Luv$ space into several hexahedra obtained as Cartesian products of peak intervals found for each color component. This can be stated as

$$Cluster(n) = \sum_{L=T\_Low(L_i)}^{T\_High(L_i)} L(x, y) \wedge \sum_{U=T\_Low(u_i)}^{T\_High(u_i)} u(x, y) \wedge \sum_{V=T\_Low(v_i)}^{T\_High(v_i)} v(x, y) \quad (14.12)$$

where $n$ is an index for hexahedral partitioned clustered (i.e., $n = 1, \ldots, N_{max}$); $L, u$, and $v$ are the image's color components; and $\wedge$ is a logical "*and*" operator.

An adjustable threshold (i.e., survival threshold) determines how many and which of these preclusters hexahedra go beyond the fine stage. If a precluster has been assigned fewer pixels than the number required by the survival threshold, then it is eliminated, and its pixels are tagged as ambiguous. Having done this, we can determine the number of valid clusters and their corresponding mean vectors that are then utilized in the fine stage. Those pixels, which are not assigned to any valid clusters, are entered into ambiguous regions, and their fine segmentation is obtained within FCM clustering.

### 14.6.4 Fine Segmentation Using Fuzzy C-Means Clustering

FCM optimizes an objective function based on a weighted similarity measure between the pixels in the image and each of $C$ (e.g., exudates and nonexudates) cluster centers [24].

Local extrema of this objective function are indicative of an optimal clustering of the image. The function is defined as

$$J_{FCM}(U, v; X) = \sum_{k=1}^{n}\sum_{i=1}^{C}(\mu_{ik})^m \|x_k - v_i\|^2, \quad 1 \le m < \infty \qquad (14.13)$$

where $\mu_{ik}$ is the fuzzy membership value of a pixel $k$ to class $i$ and $X = \{x_1, \dots, x_n\}$ is a finite data set in $R^d$, $1 \le k \le n$; is a $d$ dimensional feature vector; and $\|.\|$ is any inner product norm of the form $\|P\| = P^T AP$, $A$ being a positive definite matrix. $v = \{v_1, \dots, v_C\}$ is a set of class centers, where $v_i \in R^d$, $1 \le i \le C$, represents a $d$ dimensional $i$th class center and is regarded as a prototype.

The objective function in Equation 14.13 is minimized when high membership values are assigned to pixels with values close to the centroid for its particular class, and low membership values are assigned when the pixel data are far from the centroid. The parameter $m$ is a weighting exponent that satisfies $m > 1$ and controls the degree of fuzziness in the resulting membership functions. As $m$ approaches unity, the membership functions become crisper (hard clustering) and approach binary functions. As $m$ increases, the membership functions become increasingly fuzzy. In this work, the value of $m$ was assumed to be equal to 2, and the norm operator represented the standard Euclidean distance. For $m > 1$, the local minimum can be defined based on the following equations:

$$\mu_{ik} = \frac{1}{\sum_{j=1}^{C}\left(\frac{\|x_k-v_i\|}{\|x_k-v_j\|}\right)^{2/(m-1)}} \quad \forall i, k \quad v_i = \frac{\sum_{k=1}^{n}(\mu_{ik})^m x_k}{\sum_{k=1}^{n}(\mu_{ik})^m} \qquad (14.14)$$

where the positive definite matrix $U$ is the fuzzy $C$ partition of the input image pixels over the set of $C$ cluster centers treated as vectors, and $v_i$ represents the $i$th class center. An important parameter in an FCM clustering algorithm is the number of classes ($C$) and their corresponding centers that are computed within the coarse segmentation stage, as shown in Section 14.6.3. Hence, there is no need to recompute the class centers $v_i$ for exudate and nonexudate classes by using Equation 14.14 and instead they are considered as sufficiently well approximated within the coarse segmentation stage. At this stage, the pixels stored in the secure-zone (pixels from ambiguous regions and not-valid clusters) are assigned to the remaining clusters.

Thus, for any unclassified pixel $x$ during the coarse stage with the feature vector $x_k$, the fuzzy membership function $\mu_{ik}$ is computed, which evaluates the degree of membership of the given pixel to the given fuzzy class $v_i$, $i = 1, \dots, C$. The resulting fuzzy segmentation is converted to a hard segmentation by assigning each pixel solely to the class that has the highest membership value for that pixel. This is known as the maximum membership rule [25]. Because most pixels are classified in the coarse stage, the significant computation time required for the FCM is saved.

### 14.6.5  Segmentation Results

To investigate the effectiveness of the proposed segmentation technique, 50 abnormal and 25 normal images were considered and then converted from RGB to $Luv$. We use the image shown in Figure 14.4c — which is a typical preprocessed retinal image — as a running example to illustrate each stage of the segmentation process. The segmentation scheme began by Gaussian filtering of $Luv$ histograms of this image to derive the number of clusters and approximate the location of their centers. All the histograms were smoothed using the

**TABLE 14.2**

Coarse Segmentation Results for the Image Shown in Figure 14.4c with $\sigma = 5$

| Initial Nonzero Classes | Number of Pixels | Class Mean Luv Values | | | Assigned Color |
|---|---|---|---|---|---|
| | | $L$ | $u$ | $v$ | |
| 1 | 669 | 2.6 | 4.2 | 20.6 | Green |
| 2 | 214553 | 72.7 | 59.1 | 59.5 | Orange |
| 3 | 4081 | 97.8 | 5.2 | 65.7 | Yellow |

Maximum number of classes = $N_L.N_u.N_v = 3 \times 2 \times 1 = 6$
Number of image pixels = 227,560; unclassified pixels after coarse stage = 8257

same scale parameter equal to 5. The filtered histograms were analyzed separately to find the significant peaks and valleys for each individual smoothed histogram. In this experiment, the secure-zone parameter was set to be equal to 0.3.

We consider a class (cluster) valid if it contained more than 160 (survival threshold) pixels. This threshold was obtained experimentally and in accordance with exudates size facts. Choosing a very small threshold increased the number of valid classes by passing the minor clusters, which were not obviously of interest, to the fine stage. On the other hand, tuning a large threshold could wrongly ignore the main existence clusters, such as exudates, and thus cause a high rate of error. The images' pixels belonging to one of the defined valid clusters were labeled and assigned to the corresponding class, and the remaining pixels fell into the ambiguous regions and were tagged as unclassified in this stage. The invalid identified classes were discarded, and their pixels were tagged as unclassified.

Table 14.2 summarizes the obtained measurements when the coarse stage was finished. In this case, three valid classes were distinguished out of a maximum of six possible classes. These were related to the background, blood vessels/red lesions, and the exudates, respectively. From 227,560 image pixels, the coarse stage assigned 669 pixels to the blood vessels/red lesions class, 214,553 pixels to the background class, and 4081 pixels to the candidate exudates class. Another 8257 pixels were left unclassified at this stage. This table also indicates the mean *Luv* color values of each valid class and the subjective colors that were assigned to the classes.

Table 14.3 represents how the remaining unclassified pixels were assigned to the valid classes based on FCM clustering technique. In fact, within the fine stage, 2865 unclassified pixels were classified as blood vessels/red lesions class, 906 pixels as background, and the remaining 4486 assigned to the exudates class. Figure 14.5c shows the coarse segmentation result for our typical image. There were three final clusters, that is, background (orange), blood vessels/red lesions (green), and exudates (yellow), in addition to the unclassified pixels, which are marked in blue.

The final segmentation result is shown in Figure 14.5d. It is apparent that the actual exudates and some false positives, including optic disc regions, are included in the candidate exudates cluster. To not discard any true exudate pixels, we tuned the segmentation parameters in favor of more false positives than false negatives. The false-positive pixels

**TABLE 14.3**

Fine Segmentation Results ($\sigma = 5$)

| Final Classes | Number of Pixels | Class Mean Luv Values | | |
|---|---|---|---|---|
| | | $L$ | $u$ | $v$ |
| 1 | 669 + 2865 | 18.5 | 27.9 | 30.6 |
| 2 | 214553 + 906 | 72.5 | 59.5 | 59.1 |
| 3 | 4081 + 4486 | 94.5 | 13.9 | 66.9 |

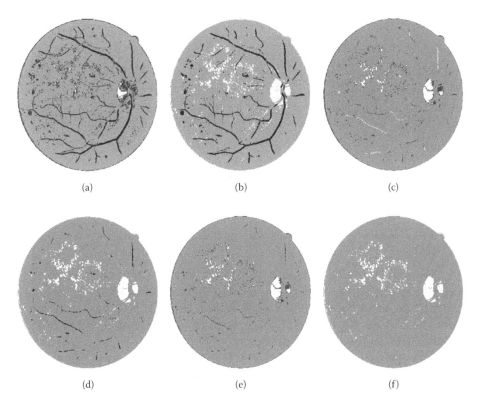

(a)                              (b)                              (c)

(d)                              (e)                              (f)

**FIGURE 14.5**
Color segmentation results for Figure 14.4c: (a) coarse segmentation ($\sigma = 1$), (b) fine segmentation ($\sigma = 1$), (c) coarse segmentation ($\sigma = 5$), (d) fine segmentation ($\sigma = 5$), (e) coarse segmentation ($\sigma = 7$), and (f) fine segmentation ($\sigma = 7$).

are discriminated from true positives using a region-based classification scheme. We return to this issue in Section 14.6.7.

It is expected that the segmentation results degenerate with higher value of $\sigma$, as the smoothing extent is increased and, thus, the histograms' fine structures are more suppressed. To assess this hypothesis, other $\sigma$ values were examined. Figure 14.5a shows the coarse segmentation result for $\sigma = 1$. In this case, the image was segmented into four classes, including background, blood vessels/red lesions, and exudates, which comprised two different clusters. Figure 14.5b illustrates the final segmented image. Here, we would prefer to segment the exudates into one representative cluster; otherwise, the following processing stages can be affected. Thus, it is required to exploit further methods, such as region merging, to cope with the oversegmentation of the exudates.

Figure 14.5e and Figure 14.5f demonstrate the coarse and fine segmentation results for $\sigma = 7$, respectively. In this case, two classes are identified (i.e., background and exudates). Finally, by increasing the $\sigma$ value from 7 to 8, all three $L$, $u$, and $v$ channel histograms became unimodal. Thus, only one valid class was obtained — the background. Therefore, the image fine structures were filtered out too much, and this caused all image pixels to be classified as background. In this case, the exudate pixels were left unclassified after the coarse stage. These exudates were, however, inevitably assigned to the only class (i.e., the background) during the fine stage, and thus, no exudate cluster was identified.

The segmentation algorithm provides a well-founded framework for detecting retinal image structures at multiple scales. According to our segmentation results, choosing an

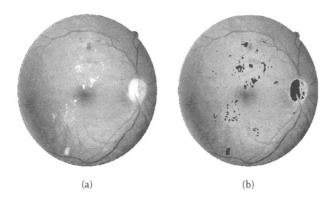

(a)                                    (b)

**FIGURE 14.6**
Color segmentation results with $\sigma = 5$: (a) atypical abnormal image, and (b) exudates cluster superimposed on the original image.

appropriate scale parameter is very important for the success of the algorithm. We apply the segmentation technique to all 75 retinal images using $\sigma = 5$ and secure-zone $= 0.3$ (see Reference [26] for the details of scale and secure-zone parameter selection issues), respectively. This could segment all the images effectively.

Figure 14.6a demonstrates another typical abnormal retinal image from our image data set. The identified exudates cluster, which is superimposed on the original image, can be seen in Figure 14.6b.

### 14.6.6 Feature Selection

Once our color retinal images are segmented, each image is represented by its corresponding segmented regions. The segmented regions, however, need to be identified in terms of exudates and nonexudates. This is attempted, in a bottom-up approach, by extracting a set of features for each region and classifying the regions based on the generated feature vectors.

The performance of the classifiers (i.e., the ability to assign the unknown object to the correct class) is directly dependent on the features chosen to represent the region descriptions. Ideally, the classification process should be based on a small number of significant features that effectively characterize the input data. A review of feature selection techniques is beyond the scope of this section. An overview of feature selection methods can be found in Reference [27].

To select a suitable set of features, it is necessary to take advantage of any prior knowledge of exudates and identify the characteristics that make them distinctive. Here, we used features that correspond to the visual concepts that we, as human beings, typically use to describe exudate lesions. Clinically, ophthalmologists use color to differentiate between various pathological conditions. We also considered region color as one of our main features. Similarly colored objects like exudates and cotton wool spots are differentiated with further features, such as size, edge strength, and shape. We found that features like average color and standard deviation of color are enough to encode appearance in terms of color and texture.

After a comparative study of discriminative attributes of different possible features, 18 were chosen. These include mean $Luv$ color values inside and around (5 pixels distance) the region (6 features); standard deviation of $Luv$ values inside and around (5 pixels distance) the region (6 features); region centroid $Luv$ values (3 features); region size (1 feature); region compactness (1 feature); and region edge strength (1 feature).

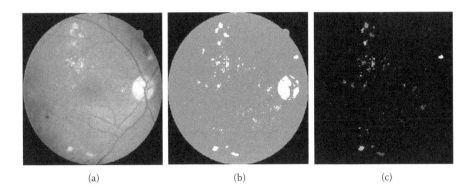

(a)  (b)  (c)

**FIGURE 14.7 (See color insert.)**
Connected component labeling and boundary tracing algorithms results: (a) a typical retinal image, (b) FCM segmented image, and (c) labeled regions using connected component approach.

Having segmented each retinal image into a set of regions, a region identification technique was followed to assign a unique label to each region. We used an eight-neighborhood connected components region identification technique [28]. Figure 14.7a and Figure 14.7b illustrate a retinal image and its segmented version. The connected components are randomly colored and shown in Figure 14.7c. Here, we remove the optic disc regions using an automatic optic disc localization [11].

With the circle being the most compact region in a Euclidean space, a compactness feature gives a measure of about how far an object is from a circular shape. This is given by

$$Compactness = \frac{(region\ border\ length)^2}{area} \tag{14.15}$$

To obtain the region border length, which was necessary for both derivations of compactness feature and region edge strength feature measurement, a boundary-tracing algorithm [28] was employed on the labeled segmented regions. The boundary of each region was traced, and then the information about the position of boundary pixels was collected for the feature evaluation task.

The compactness feature (Equation 14.15) and edge strength features were calculated using localized region's boundary pixels. In order to calculate the region edge strength descriptor, the Prewitt gradient operator was employed. Then, this feature was measured as an average of the region boundary pixels' edge values.

## 14.6.7 Region-Level Classification

The application of the proposed segmentation on our database of 75 retinal images resulted in 3860 segmented regions, including 2366 exudates and 1494 nonexudates that were considered as negative cases. A corresponding 18-D feature vector was measured for each example in the data set. To classify our labeled data set of segmented regions in a region-based framework, we employ two well-known discriminative classifiers — NNs and SVMs.

Discriminative classifiers work on the decision boundary and are more robust against outliers and noise in the training data. These classifiers return the appropriate label for each data point by applying the discrimination functions on that point. Thus, the class posterior probabilities are directly estimated. We briefly review the classifiers theory and assess their performances on our segmented regions data set in the next two sections.

### 14.6.7.1 Neural Network Classifiers

The multilayer perceptrons (MLP) [29] neural networks have been very successful in a variety of applications, producing results that are at least competitive and often exceed other existing computational learning models. One learning algorithm used for MLP is called the backpropagation (BP) rule. This is a gradient descent method based on an error function that represents the difference between the network's calculated output and the desired output.

*The scaled conjugate gradient* (SCG) algorithm is another MLP training rule [30]. Unlike the backpropagation algorithms, which are first-order techniques, SCG methods employ the second derivatives of the cost function. This allows them, sometimes, to find a better way to a minimum than a first-order technique, but at a higher computational cost.

The exudates/nonexudates data set of segmented regions was divided into training, validation, and test sets in a 64:10:26 ratio. The training and validation set contained around 2856 examples; of which 1732 were labeled by an expert ophthalmologist as exudates, and another 1124 examples represented nonexudates. The remaining 1004 (of which 611 are labeled as exudates) were used as an independent test set. The MLP with three layers had an 18-node input layer corresponding to the feature vector. We experimented with hidden layers through a range of 2 to 35 hidden units to find the optimum architecture. A single output node gave the final classification probability. This value was thresholded so that values greater than the defined threshold were assigned to the exudate class, and other values were classified as nonexudates. The MLPs used had sigmoidal activation functions in the hidden and output layers.

All networks were trained using two different learning methods (i.e., BP and SCG). To avoid the local minimum of mean square error function, which can degenerate the performance, several training attempts were conducted, in which the initializations of the weights were varied. A ten-fold cross-validation with early stopping [31] was used to measure the networks' generalization abilities.

The MLPs performances were measured using the previously unseen region examples from the test set in the usual terms of detecting the presence or absence of exudates (i.e., sensitivity and specificity). Another reported measure, the accuracy, is the ratio between the total numbers of correctly classified instances to all the instances that exist in the test set. Table 14.4 summarizes the optimum results obtained on the test set for the various NN configurations. Among several NN containing varying numbers of hidden units that were constructed and trained using the BP learning algorithm, a MLP network, with 15 hidden units, performed best in terms of the overall generalization performance. A cross-validation technique was used to determine the optimum number of hidden units. Similarly, the best generalization accuracy was acquired for a MLP network with 15 hidden units when the SCG learning algorithm was applied.

For each NN classifier in Table 14.4, the threshold giving the best accuracy is shown. By varying this threshold, we can change the misclassification cost associated with exudate or nonexudate class in favor of another class. This leads to a trade-off between sensitivity and specificity criteria. Overall, the BP classifier represented better balance between sensitivity and specificity. On the other hand, SCG achieved a higher level of sensitivity.

**TABLE 14.4**

MLP Neural Networks Accuracy for Region-Based Classification

| Classifier | Threshold | Accuracy | Sensitivity | Specificity |
|---|---|---|---|---|
| BP-NN (15 hidden) | (T = 0.50) | 93.3 | 93.0 | 94.1 |
| SCG-NN (15 hidden) | (T = 0.45) | 92.7 | 97.9 | 85.2 |

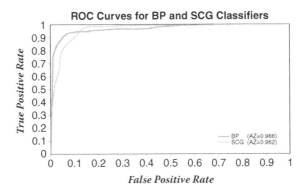

**FIGURE 14.8**
The ROC curves produced for the best BP and SCG neural networks.

The standard tool for controlling the trade-off between the sensitivity and specificity of an algorithm is a receiver operating characteristic (ROC) curve [32]. The ROC curve is a plot of true-positive rate versus false-positive rate. To investigate how changing the output threshold value can affect the performance of our selected NN classifiers, the classifier ROC curves were generated (Figure 14.8). The area under the ROC curve ($A_z$) summarizes the quality of classification over a wide range of misclassification costs [33]. Here, the areas under ROC curves were estimated using the trapezoid rule for the discrete operating points. The bigger the area under the curves, the higher was the probability of making a correct decision.

As apparent from Figure 14.8, the difference between the areas under the curves is not significant (0.966 for the BP algorithm and 0.962 for the SCG algorithm), as the two curves are similar and lie close together. Thus, selection of the best classifier and the optimum threshold value may entirely depend on the sensitivity and specificity requirements as set based on the objective of the task [32], [33]. Overall, the performance of the NN classifiers is very high, with up to 93.3% of segmented regions in the test set correctly classified based on BP, and 92.7% using SCG. We opted for the BP classifier, because it represents a better balance between sensitivity and specificity (an almost equally significant error costs) and also a higher level of generalization ability than the SCG.

### 14.6.7.2 Support Vector Machine Classifiers

Support vector machines [34], [35], [36] have become increasingly popular tools for machine learning tasks involving classification and regression. They have been successfully applied to a wide range of pattern recognition and medical imaging problems. Here, we investigate the application of the SVMs to our medical decision support task of classifying the retinal image segmented regions. The SVMs demonstrate various attractive features, such as good generalization ability, compared to other classifiers. There are relatively few free parameters to adjust, and the architecture does not require them to be found experimentally.

Traditional classifiers such as NNs have suffered from the generalization ability problems and thus can lead to overfitting. This is a consequence of the optimization algorithms used (i.e., empirical risk minimization [ERM]). The main idea behind SVMs is to separate the classes with a surface that maximizes the margin between them [34]. This is an approximate implementation of the structural risk minimization (SRM) principle, which is carried out by achieving a trade-off between the data empirical risk amount and the capacity (complexity) of a set of estimated functions.

For a linearly separable classification task, the idea is to map the training points into a high-dimensional feature space where a separating hyperplane $(w, b)$, with $w$ as the normal and $b$ as the bias to the hyperplane, can be found that maximizes the margin or distance from the closest data points. The optimum separating hyperplane can be represented based on kernel functions:

$$f(x) = sign\left(\sum_{i=1}^{n} \alpha_i y_i K(x, x_i) + b\right) \quad (14.16)$$

where $n$ is the number of training examples, $y_i$ is the label value of example $i$, $K$ represents the kernel, and $\alpha_i$ coefficients must be found in a way to maximize a particular Lagrangian representation. Subject to the constraints $\alpha_i \geq 0$ and $\sum \alpha_i y_i = 0$, there is a Lagrange multiplier $\alpha_i$ for each training point, and only those training examples that lie close to the decision boundary have nonzero $\alpha_i$. These examples are called the support vectors. However, in real-world problems, data are noisy, and in general, there will be no linear separation in the feature space. The hyperplane margins can be made more relaxed by penalizing the training points the system misclassifies. Hence, the optimum hyperplane equation can be defined as

$$y_i(w.x_i + b) \geq 1 - \xi_i, \xi_i \geq 0 \quad (14.17)$$

and the following equation is minimized in order to obtain the optimum hyperplane:

$$\|w\|^2 + C \sum_{i=1}^{n} \xi_i \quad (14.18)$$

where $\xi$ introduces a positive slack variable that measure the amount of violation from the constraints. The penalty $C$ is a regularization parameter that controls the trade-off between maximizing the margin and minimizing the training error. This approach is called *soft margins* [36].

To investigate and compare the SVM classifiers, the same data set of 3860 segmented regions (already used for NNs) was considered for training and testing the SVMs. A ten-fold cross-validation technique was used for estimating the generalization ability of all constructed classifiers. The design of the SVM classifier architecture is simple and mainly requires the choice of the kernel, the kernel-associated parameter, and the regularization parameter $C$ (in a soft margin case). There are currently no techniques available to learn the form of the kernel; thus, we employed a Gaussian RBF kernel function that has been proven successful in a variety of applications (e.g., see Reference [35]). We first constructed a set of SVM classifiers with a range of values for the kernel parameter $\sigma$ and with no restriction on the Lagrange multipliers $\alpha_i$ (i.e., hard margin approach). In this case, the number of RBF centers (number of SVs), the centers or the SVs, $\alpha_i$, and the scalar $b$ were automatically obtained by the SVM training procedure. We found that the best generalization accuracy is achieved when $\sigma = 0.3$, according to the cross-validation results. The performance of the selected SVM classifier was then quantified based on its sensitivity, specificity, and the overall accuracy on the test samples (those samples held out during training). This classifier demonstrates an overall accuracy of 88.6% with 86.2% sensitivity and 90.1% specificity.

Figure 14.9a shows the generalization (i.e., sensitivity, specificity, and overall performance) ability of this classifier versus the kernel parameter $\sigma$. The result indicates good performance over exudate and non-exudate cases. Having chosen the type of kernel function and the optimum $\sigma$ value, we trained another set of SVMs with $\sigma$ fixed at 0.3 and different $C$ values to investigate the effectiveness of the soft-margin-based approaches. A wide range of $C$ values were applied as an upper bound to $\alpha_i$ of both exudate and nonexudate classes (Figure 14.9b). The best overall accuracy, using the soft margin technique (hereafter referred to as SVM*), increased to 90.4% at $C = 1.5$ giving reduced sensitivity of

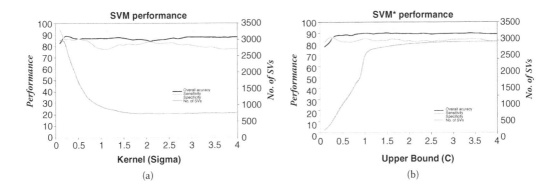

**FIGURE 14.9**
Generalization performance of SVM classifiers: (a) performance against kernel parameter $\sigma$, (b) and the regularization parameter $C$.

83.3% and a higher specificity of 95.5% compared to the result in the case of unrestricted Lagrange multipliers (hard margin). The number of SVs is also shown in Figure 14.9a and Figure 14.9b.

A large number of SVs means that either the training data are complex, or the $C$ constant is too large. As can be seen from Figure 14.9a, by increasing the value of $\sigma$, the number of SVs was significantly dropped due to the smoothness effect of the Gaussian $\sigma$. In contrast, when $C$ was increased, the misclassification error cost became heavier, and thus the separating hyperplane was more complicated. This leads to an increase in the number of SVs that were necessary to construct the decision boundary (Figure 14.9b).

### 14.6.7.3 Comparing SVM and MLP Classifier Results

In the previous two sections, we investigated the application of NN and SVM classifiers toward a region-level classification scheme. Table 14.5 summarizes the best obtained NN and SVM classifiers according to the overall generalization of performance ability.

Although the diagnostic accuracy of the NN classifier is better than the SVM classifier, the performances are close, and there is a good balance between sensitivity and specificity in both cases. To assess and analyze the behavior of these region-level classifiers throughout a whole range of the output threshold values, the ROC curves were produced. The BP classifier shows high performance with an area of 0.966. The SVM* demonstrates slightly lower performance over the entire ROC space with an area of 0.924.

So far, we discussed the region-level classification of a set of segmented regions using NN and SVM classifiers. We can also use our trained classifiers to evaluate the effectiveness of our proposed region-level exudate recognition approach in terms of image-based accuracy. To do that, a population of 67 new retinal images are considered, including 40 abnormal and 27 normal. These new images were all segmented, and the measured feature vectors were separately evaluated using both the BP neural network (BP-NN) and SVM* ($\sigma = 0.3$, $C = 1.5$) classifiers. A final decision was then made as to whether the image had some evidence of retinopathy.

**TABLE 14.5**

Selection of MLP and SVM Classifiers for Region-Level Classification

| Classifier | Threshold | Accuracy | Sensitivity | Specificity |
|---|---|---|---|---|
| BP-NN (15 hidden) | (T = 0.5) | 93.3% | 93.0% | 94.1% |
| SVM* $\sigma = 0.3$, $C = 1.5$ | (T = 0.0) | 90.4% | 83.3% | 95.5% |

**TABLE 14.6**

NN and SVM Classifier Performances for Assessing the Evidence of Diabetic Retinopathy

| Classifier | Image Type | Number of Patients | Detected as Abnormal | Detected as Normal | X = Sensitivity Y = Specificity |
|---|---|---|---|---|---|
| BP-NN | Abnormal | 40 | 38 | 2 | X = 95.0% |
| BP-NN | Normal | 27 | 3 | 24 | Y = 88.9% |
| SVM* | Abnormal | 40 | 35 | 5 | X = 87.5% |
| SVM* | Normal | 27 | 2 | 25 | Y = 92.5% |

As Table 14.6 illustrates, the BP-NN based scheme could identify affected retinal images with 95.0% sensitivity, while it recognized 88.9% of the normal images (i.e., the specificity). On the other hand, the SVM*-based scheme achieved a diagnostic accuracy of 87.5% for abnormal images (sensitivity) and 92.5% specificity for the normal cases.

Figure 14.10a shows a preprocessed abnormal retinal image from our new image data set. This was segmented as shown in Figure 14.10b. The segmented regions are then classified using our trained BP-NN and SVM* classifiers. Figure 14.10c and Figure 14.10d show the final classified exudate regions that are superimposed onto the original image.

To provide an easy way to compare the classifier's behavior on this typical retinal image, we have defined the *TPs*, *FPs*, *TNs*, and *FNs* regions according to the segmented

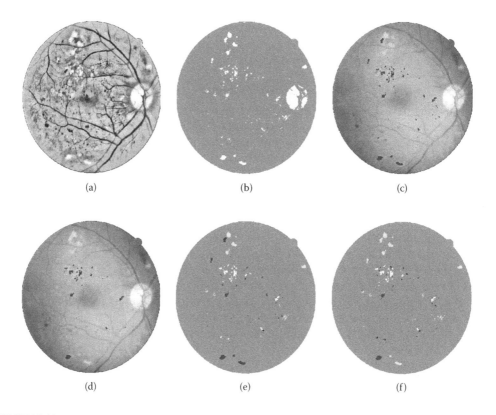

(a)  (b)  (c)

(d)  (e)  (f)

**FIGURE 14.10**

Exudate identification based on *region-level exudate recognition*: (a) a typical preprocessed abnormal retinal image, (b) FCM segmented image, (c) final identified exudate lesions (based on BP-NN) superimposed on the original image, (d) final identified exudate lesions (based on SVM*) superimposed on the original image, (e) classified segmented regions based on BP-NN, and (f) classified segmented regions based on SVM*.

image (Figure 14.10b) and its final classification versions using BP-NN and SVM* classifiers (Figure 14.10c and Figure 14.10d). In Figure 14.10e and Figure 14.10f, which, respectively, indicate the BP-NN and SVM* final results, the yellow, blue, green, and black regions are corresponding to the *TPs*, *FPs*, *TNs*, and *FNs* regions, respectively. As can be seen, the BP-NN classifier provided a higher number of *FP* regions than the SVM* classifier. This can be noticed, for example, from the cotton wool spot regions shown in the bottom part of Figure 14.10a, which have been wrongly classified as exudates in Figure 14.10c. On the other hand, the SVM* classifier demonstrated a higher level of *FNs* compared to the BP-NN classifier.

From Table 14.5 and Table 14.6, it is apparent that the diagnostic accuracies of SVMs and NNs are close in terms of both "region-based" and "image-based" classification tasks. Consequently, both classifiers can be utilized as part of our region-level exudate recognition approach for an automatic identification of retinal exudates. However, assuming that the main objective of our classification task is to achieve maximum overall accuracy (i.e., not taking specifically into account the other issues, such as complexity, training time, etc.), we choose the BP-NN for our region-level classification task.

To evaluate the lesion-based diagnostic accuracy of our region-level exudate recognition approach in a pixel resolution basis, the optimum classifier — BP-NN's output threshold — was changed from 0 to 1. This allows us to achieve different trade-offs between sensitivity and predictivity criteria (defined in Section 14.3) and obtain various points in the ROC space. The procedure was carried out for each image in the data set. Then, we averaged the image's sensitivity and predictivity values to get the final points in the ROC space. Table 14.7 summarizes some typical sensitivity–predictivity values that our region-level exudate recognition approach accomplished.

The highest overall performances based on this approach are including 88.1% sensitivity and 91.2% predictivity, or alternatively, 90.0% sensitivity and 89.3% predictivity. These results also provide a good balance between sensitivity and predictivity measurements. However, according to the requirements of the task, other specifications can be readily utilized. For example, by setting the threshold value equal to 0.6, the sensitivity is increased to 94.5%, with a lower predictivity equal to 82.0%.

The NN and SVM classifiers both achieved a high classification level for distinguishing exudates from the nonexudate segmented regions. Although the selected NN classifier presented slightly better diagnostic accuracy, the SVM classifiers have shown attractive features. For example, the model selection was much easier for SVMs than NNs. Furthermore, SVM classifiers always converged to a unique global optimal, while NNs were prone to overfitting.

**TABLE 14.7**

Sensitivity–Predictivity of our Proposed Region-Level Exudate Recognition Approach for Some Typical Thresholds

| T | Sensitivity | Predictivity |
|------|-------------|--------------|
| 0.1 | 68.4 | 98.5 |
| 0.3 | 83.5 | 93.6 |
| 0.4 | 88.1 | 91.2 |
| 0.45 | 90.0 | 89.3 |
| 0.6 | 94.5 | 82.0 |
| 0.85 | 96.2 | 69.3 |

## 14.7   Summary and Conclusions

In this study, we attempted an automatic exudate identification approach to identify the retinal exudates from color retinal images within an object recognition framework. This was mainly based on color image segmentation, feature selection, and region-level classification techniques. Investigations were made to identify a robust method to segment images with moderate *FP* candidate exudates regions. According to the preprocessed retinal images color distribution, a color image segmentation algorithm, based upon the thresholding and FCM techniques, was found to be very effective.

The obtained regions were required to be identified in terms of exudates and nonexudates. This was attempted, in a bottom-up approach, by extracting a set of features for each region followed by classifying the regions based on the generated feature vectors.

Among several different NN architectures that were constructed and trained, a backpropagation-based NN classifier performed best in terms of the overall generalization performance. This classifier achieved an overall region-based accuracy of 93.3%, including 93.0% sensitivity and 94.1% specificity for the classification of the segmented regions. The use of support vector machines was a particularly attractive approach for our application. According to our best knowledge, this was the first time that SVMs were exploited in the exudate identification context.

A set of SVM classifiers was constructed based on Gaussian kernels with and without any restrictions on the Lagrange multipliers (soft and hard margins). The optimum SVM classifier ($\sigma = 0.3$ and $C = 1.5$) demonstrated an overall region-based accuracy of 90.4%, including 83.3% sensitivity and 95.5% specificity. In order to compare and assess the behavior of NN and SVM classifiers throughout a whole range of the output threshold values, ROC curves were produced. The optimum BP classifier presented a high performance, with the area under the ROC curve of 0.966. Similarly, the optimum SVM demonstrated slightly lower performance over the entire ROC space with an area of 0.924.

Having measured the region-level diagnostic accuracy of our optimum NN and SVM models, we readily utilized the optimum trained classifiers to evaluate the effectiveness of the proposed region-level exudate recognition approach in terms of image-based accuracy. A data set of 67 new retinal images were considered (40 abnormal and 27 normal). A final decision was made as to whether the image had some evidence of retinopathy. The NN-based scheme identified abnormal images with 95.0% sensitivity (correct classification of 38 abnormal images out of 40), while it recognized 88.9% of the images with no abnormality (i.e., the specificity; correct classification of 24 normal images out of 27. On the other hand, the SVM-based scheme illustrated an accuracy including 87.5% sensitivity (correct classification of 35 abnormal images out of 40) and 92.5% specificity (correct classification of 25 normal images out of 27).

To assess the overall performance of our proposed technique in terms of pixel resolution, we constructed a sensitivity–predictivity-based graph against our data set of 67 unseen retinal images. We achieved different trade-offs between the sensitivity and predictivity criteria which, in turn, provided various points in the ROC space. The optimum pixel resolution *sensitivity–predictivity* values were obtained as 90.0% and 89.3%, respectively.

To conclude, the region-level exudate recognition approach provided accurate results toward an automatic approach for the identification of retinal exudates. The study presented here has shown encouraging results and indicates that automated diagnosis of exudative retinopathy based on color retinal image analysis is very successful in detecting exudates. Hence, the system could be used to evaluate digital retinal images obtained in screening programs for diabetic retinopathy and used by nonexperts to indicate which patients require referral to an ophthalmologist for further investigation and treatment. We have shown that we can detect the large majority of exudates, and also most of our normal images can be correctly identified by the proposed system. This provides a huge amount of savings in terms of the number of retinal images that must be manually reviewed by the medical professionals.

# References

[1]  A Newsletter from the World Health Organization, *World Diabetes*, G. Reiber and H. King, Eds., no. 4, pp. 1–78, 1998.

[2]  N. Wareham, Cost-effectiveness of alternative methods for diabetic retinopathy screening, *Diabetic Care*, 844, 1993.

[3]  K. Javitt and A. Sommer, Cost-effectiveness of current approaches to the control of retinopathy in type I diabetics, *Ophthalmology*, 96, 255–264, 1989.

[4]  Early treatment of diabetic retinopathy study group (etdrs). grading diabetic retinopathy from stereoscopic color fundus photographs: An extension of the airlie house classification, *Ophthalmology*, 98, 786–806, 1998.

[5]  I. Ghafour and W. Foulds, Common causes of blindness and visual handicap in the west of Scotland, *Ophthalmology*, 67, 209–213, 1983.

[6]  R. Phillips, J. Forrester, and P. Sharp, Automated detection and quantification of retinal exudates, *Graefe's Arch. for Clinical and Exp. Ophthalmol.*, 231, 90–94, 1993.

[7]  B. Ege, O. Larsen, and O. Hejlesen, Detection of abnormalities in retinal images using digital image analysis, in *Proceedings of the 11th Scandinavian Conference on Image Processing*, B. Ersbell and P. Johansen (Eds.), Kangerlussuaq, Greenland, 1999, pp. 833–840.

[8]  G. Gardner, D. Keating, and A. Elliott, Automatic detection of diabetic retinopathy using an artificial neural network: A screening tool, *Br. J. Ophthalmol.*, 80, 940–944, 1996.

[9]  C. Sinthanayothin, *Image Analysis for Automatic Diagnosis of diabetic Retinopathy*, Ph.D. thesis, King's College, London, 1999.

[10]  T. Walter, J. Klein, and A. Erginary, A contribution of image processing to the diagnosis of diabetic retinopathy, detection of exudates in color fundus images of the human retina, *IEEE Trans. on Medical Imaging*, 21, 1236–1243, 2002.

[11]  A. Osareh, M. Mirmehdi, and R. Markham, Classification and localisation of diabetic related eye disease, in *Proceedings of the 7th European Conference on Computer Vision*, (Springer LNCS 2353), 2002, pp. 502–516.

[12]  J.R. Gonzalez and R. Woods, *Digital Image Processing*, Addison-Wesley, Reading, MA, 1992.

[13]  T. Chen and Y. Lu, Color image segmentation, an innovative approach, *Patt. Recognition*, 35, 395–405, 2002.

[14]  C. Huang and T. Chen, Color images segmentation using scale space filter and Markov random field, *Patt. Recognition*, 25, 1217–1229, 1992.

[15]  Y. Ohta and T. Sakai, Color information for region segmentation, *Comput. Vision, Graphics and Image Processing*, 13, 222–241, 1986.

[16]  A. Osareh and B. Shadgar, Comparative pixel-level exudate recognition in color retinal images, in *Proceedings of the International Conference on Image Analysis and Recognition* M. Kammel and A. Campilho, Eds., Toronto, Canada, (Springer LNCS 3656), Toronto, Canada, 2005, pp. 894–902.

[17]  A.K. Jain and R.C. Dubes, *Algorithms for Clustering Data*, Prentice Hall, New York, 1988.

[18]  J. Bezdek, *Pattern Recognition with Fuzzy Objective Function Algorithms*, Plenum, New York, 1981.

[19]  J. Bezdek and L. Clarke, Review of MR image segmentation techniques using pattern recognition, *Medical Phys.*, 20, 1033–1048, 1993.

[20]  Y. Lim and S. Lee, On the color image segmentation algorithm based on the thresholding and the fuzzy c-means techniques, *Patt. Recognition*, 23, 935–952, 1990.

[21]  S. Sangwine and R. Horne, *The Color Image Processing Handbook*. Chapman & Hall, London; New York, 1998.

[22] K. Fukunaga, *Statistical Pattern Recognition*, Academic Press, New York, 1990.

[23] A. Witkin, Scale space filtering, in *Proceedings of the International Joint Conference on Artificial Intelligence*, Karlsruhe, Germany, 1983, pp. 1019–1022.

[24] R. Krishnapuram and J. Keller, A probabilistic approach to clustering, *IEEE Trans. on Fuzzy Syst.*, 1, 98–110, 1993.

[25] D. Pham and J. Prince, An adaptive fuzzy c-means algorithm for image segmentation in the presence of intensity inhomogeneities, *Patt. Recognition Lett.*, 20, 57–68, 1999.

[26] A. Osareh, *Automated Identification of Diabetic Retinal Exudates and the Optic Disc*, Ph.D. thesis, Bristol, England, 2004.

[27] P. Devijver and J. Kittler, *Pattern Recognition, a Statistical Approach*, Prentice Hall, New York, 1982.

[28] M. Sonka and R. Boyle, *Image Processing, Analysis, and Machine Vision*, PWS Publication, New York, 1999.

[29] D. Rumenhart and R. Williams, Learning internal representations by back-propagating errors, ch., in *Parallel Distributed Processing: Explorations in the Microstructure of Cognition*, MIT Press, Cambridge, MA, 1986, pp. 318–362.

[30] C. Bishop, *Neural Networks for Pattern Recognition*, Oxford University Press, Oxford, 1995.

[31] L. Prechelt, Early stopping but when?, in *Neural Networks: Tricks of the Trade* (Springer LNCS 1524), 1998, pp. 55–69.

[32] C. Metz, Roc methodology in radiological imaging, *Invest. Radiol.*, 21, 720–733, 1986.

[33] J. Hanley and B. McNeil, Method of comparing the areas under receiver operating characteristic curves derived from the same cases, *Radiology*, 148, 839–843, 1983.

[34] V. Vapnik, *The Nature of Statistical Learning Theory*, Springer-Verlag, Heidelberg, 1995.

[35] J. Burges, A tutorial on support vector machines for pattern recognition, *Data Min. and Knowledge Discovery*, 2, 121–167, 1998.

[36] N. Cristianini and J. Shawe-Taylor, *An Introduction to Support Vector Machines and other Kernel-Based Learning Methods*, Cambridge University Press, Cambridge, MA, 2000.

# 15

## Real-Time Color Imaging Systems

**Phillip A. Laplante and Pamela Vercellone-Smith**

## CONTENTS

## 15.1 Introduction

In this chapter, the problem of time as a dimension of color image processing is considered. The purpose here is not to review all color imaging algorithms from a real-time perspective. Instead, the intent is to introduce the reader to the real-time problem so that it may be considered in the discussions in other chapters, as needed.

After describing the nature of real-time and real-time imaging systems, the problems induced are introduced. Then a case study involving experiments using the Java program language and Java3D graphics package are used to illustrate many of the points. Then, a set of recommendations for a real-time color imaging system are given. These recommendations are generic enough to apply in any hardware and software environment and to any type of imaging system.

### 15.1.1 Real-Time Imaging Systems

Real-time systems are those systems in which there is urgency to the processing involved. This urgency is formally represented by a deadline [1]. Because this definition is very broad, the case can be made that every system is real-time. Therefore, the definition is usually specialized.

For example, a "hard," real-time imaging system might involve target tracking for a military weapon, where clearly even one missed deadline can be catastrophic. A "firm" real-time system might involve a video display system, for example, one that superimposes commercial logos, in real-time, on a soccer game broadcast. Here, a few missed deadlines might result in some tolerable flickering, but too many missed deadlines would produce an unacceptable broadcast quality. Finally, a "soft" real-time system might involve the digital processing of photographic images. Here, only quality of performance is at issue.

One of the most common misunderstandings of real-time systems is that their design simply involves improving the performance of the underlying computer hardware or image processing algorithm. While this is probably the case for the aforementioned display or photographic processing systems, this is not necessarily true for the target tracking system. Here, guaranteeing that image processing deadlines are never missed is more important than the average time to process and render one frame.

The reason that one cannot make performance guarantees or even reliably measure performance in most real-time systems is that the accompanying scheduling analysis problems are almost always computationally complex (NP-complete) [1]. Therefore, in order to make performance guarantees, it is imperative that the bounded processing times be known for all functionality. This procedure involves the guarantee of deadline satisfaction through the analysis of various aspects of code execution and operating systems interaction at the time the system is designed, not after the fact when trial-and-error is the only technique available. This process is called a schedulability analysis [2].

The first step in performing any kind of schedulability analysis is to determine, measure, or otherwise estimate the execution of specific code units using logic analyzers, the system clock, instruction counting, simulations, or algorithmic analysis. During software development, careful tracking of central processing unit (CPU) utilization is needed to focus on those code units that are slow or that have response times that are inadequate.

Unfortunately, cache, pipelines, and direct memory access (DMA), which are intended to improve average real-time performance, destroy determinism and thus make prediction of deadlines troublesome, if not impossible. But, schedulability analysis is usually the subject of traditional texts on real-time systems engineering [1]. We confine our discussions in this chapter, therefore, to hardware and software performance optimization, and leave the more fundamental discussions of real-time scheduability analysis for the interested reader to study in other texts.

### 15.1.2 Previous Work

There is very little previous work relating real-time systems concerns to color imaging applications [2]. Typical research in real-time color imaging tends to fall into two categories: algorithmic adaptations of existing color algorithms for fast implementation, and hardware accelerators. Note how these approaches do not directly tackle the problem of predictability of performance — generally speaking, they deal only with accelerating the algorithm. Four relevant papers help to illustrate typical real-time color imaging problems and solutions.

For example, Cheng et al. introduced an image quantization technique involving trellis-coded quantization for both the RGB (red, green, blue) and YUV domains. The performance of their algorithms required no training or look-up tables, which were intended to be suitable for color printing and real-time interactive graphics applications. The speed up that could be obtained for this approach is obvious [3]. Another typical algorithmic approach involves a fast correction method for balancing color appearances in a group of images based on low-degree polynomial functions. The speed enhancement, here, is due to the relatively inexpensive computation of the first- or second-order polynomials [4].

Hardware accelerators are frequently used to improve the performance of high complexity color imaging operations. For example, Andreadis et al. designed an application specific integrated circuit (ASIC) that converts RGB color coordinates to XYZ, YIQ, and YUV, coordinates in real time [5]. This particular device had applications in colorimetry instrumentation for machine vision, measurement, process control, and image compression. Finally, Han introduced a gamut mapping architecture for digital televisions using a hardware-based look-up table, suitable for implementation in either a field-programmable gate array (FPGA) or ASIC [6].

While hardware accelerators and algorithm optimization approaches are very useful in reducing the processing time of real-time color imaging processing, consideration of software issues is also essential. Ultimately, the algorithm must be implemented in some programming language, and the hardware usually has a software interface to the rest of the system. But we know of no work published on software approaches to real-time performance in color imaging systems. This is a research area that warrants investigation.

## 15.2 Hardware and Display Issues

An understanding of the hardware support for color imaging graphics is fundamental to the analysis of real-time performance of the system. Some specialized hardware for real-time imaging applications involves high-performance computers with structural support for complex instruction sets and imaging coprocessors [7]. Inexpensive pixel processors are also available, and scalable structures, such as the *FPGA*, are increasingly being used for real-time imaging applications. But building systems with highly specialized processors is not always easy, particularly because of poor tool support. Therefore, many commonly deployed color imaging systems use consumer-grade personal computers (PCs).

There are many architectural issues relating to real-time performance, such as internal/external memory bus width, natural word size, memory access times, speed of secondary storage devices, display hardware issues, and color representation and storage, to name a few. Collectively, these design issues involve three trade-off problems — schedulability versus functionality, performance versus resolution, and performance versus storage requirements [8]. Real-time design of imaging systems, then, involves making the necessary decisions that trade one quality for another, for example, speed versus resolution.

For example, one of the main performance challenges in designing real-time image processing systems is the high computational cost of image manipulation. A common deadline found in many processing systems involves screen processing and update that must be completed at least 30 times per second for the human eye to perceive continuous motion. Because this processing may involve more than a million pixels, with each color pixel needing one or two words of storage, the computational load can be staggering. For the purposes of meeting this deadline, then, the real-time systems engineer can choose to forgo display resolution, or algorithmic accuracy. Finding improved algorithms or better hardware will also help meet the deadlines without sacrifice — if the algorithms and hardware behavior are bounded, which, as mentioned, is not always the case. In this section, however, we confine our discussion to two important hardware issues.

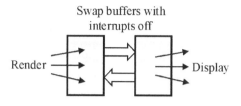

**FIGURE 15.1**
Double buffering configuration. Two identical display memory buffers are rendered or displayed by two different process threads. Switching is accomplished either by a software pointer or hardware discrete.

### 15.2.1   Color Representation and Real-Time Performance

Our interest is in the appropriate representation of color in the physical hardware, because as previously noted, this has real-time performance implications. The color buffer may be implemented using one or more of the following storage formats:

- One byte per pixel (indexed or pseudo-color), which allows $2^8 = 256$ colors
- Two bytes per pixel (high color), which, using 16 bits = 65,536 colors
- Three bytes per pixel (true or RGB color), which yields approximately 16.8 million colors

RGB is often considered the *de facto* standard in many programming languages, and it is used in many important color image data formats, such as JPEG and TIFF. True color uses 24 bits of RGB color, 1 byte per color channel for 24 bits. A 32-bit representation is often used to enhance performance, because various hardware commands are optimized for groups of 4 bytes or more. The extra 8 bits can be used to store the alpha channel giving for an RGBA value [9]. We will refer to RGB True Color format for the remainder of this chapter.

### 15.2.2   Buffering for Speed

A common approach to accelerating image display is to use double buffering or ping-pong buffering. For example, suppose images are rendered directly to the display memory buffer. If the rendering is too slow, then the partial results of the rendering will appear, in sequence, until the frame is completed. If, however, the software renders one screen image to a virtual frame buffer while displaying the other and then flips the virtual and real buffers when the new drawing is complete, the individual rendering commands will not be seen (Figure 15.1). If the screens can be updated at about 30 screens per second, the operator's display will appear fully animated [2].

Triple buffering, in which a third buffer serves to store the second image generation, is also sometimes used, and in theory, $n$-buffering can be implemented where the number of buffers, $n > 3$.

## 15.3   Language Issues

Modern languages for real-time imaging must provide an easy interface to hardware devices and provide a framework for maintainability, portability, and reliability, among many other features. Many programming languages are commonly used to implement color imaging systems, including C, C++, C#, Java, Visual Basic, Fortran, assembly language, and even BASIC.

Poor coding style is frequently the source of performance deterioration in real-time imaging systems. In many cases, the negative effects are due to performance penalties associated with object composition, inheritance, and polymorphism in object-oriented languages. But object-oriented languages are rapidly displacing the lower-level languages like C and assembly language in real-time color imaging systems, and it is probably a good thing because of the accompanying benefits.

Understanding the performance impact of various language features, particularly as they relate to image storage and manipulation, is essential to using the most appropriate construct for a particular situation. For example, in an C++, what is the best way to represent an image? As an object? As a composite object of many pixels? Composed by color plane? There is no clear answer, and experimentation with the language compiler in conjunction with performance measurement tools can be helpful in obtaining the most efficient implementations.

The following list summarizes key issues when implementing real-time imaging systems in a high-level language:

- Use appropriate coding standards to ensure uniformity and clarity.
- Refactor the code continuously (that is, aggressively improve its structure) with an eye to performance improvement.
- Use performance measurement tools continuously to assess the impact of changes to the hardware and software.
- Carefully document the code to enable future developers to make structural and performance enhancements.
- Adopt an appropriate life cycle testing discipline.

Finally, be wary of code that evolved from non-object-oriented languages such as C into object-oriented version in C++ or Java. Frequently, these conversions are made hastily and incorporate the worst of both the object-oriented and non-object-oriented paradigms simultaneously.

In this chapter, however, we focus on Java, because it is highly portable and is widely used in imaging applications. Java is an object-oriented language, with a syntax that is similar to C++ and C#, and to a lesser extent, C. Besides, modern object-oriented languages such as C++ and C# have quite a lot in common with Java.

## 15.3.1 Java

Java is an interpreted language in which the code is translated into machine-independent code that runs in a managed execution environment. This environment is a virtual machine, which executes "object" code instructions as a series of program directives. The advantage of this arrangement is that the Java code can run on any device that implements the virtual machine. This "write once, run anywhere" philosophy has important applications in embedded and portable computing, consumer electronics, image processing, and Web computing. The interpreted nature of Java would ordinarily present significant challenges for real-time rendering. However, a number of enhancements to the standard Java Virtual Machine (JVM) provide for significant performance accelerations. For example, the Java just-in-time (JIT) compiler is a code generator that converts Java byte code into native machine code during program execution. Java programs invoked with a JIT generally run much faster than when the byte code is executed by the interpreter. Other implementations of the JVM involve "hot spot" compilation in which the JVM recognizes that portions of the code are being executed frequently enough that they should be translated directly into the native code. There are also native-code Java compilers, which convert Java directly to assembly code or object code. Finally, there are Java microprocessors that behave precisely as the JVM. These enhancements can help to reduce processing time in Java-based imaging applications.

Another very important Java performance issue involves its garbage collection utility, which can cause serious performance degradation in real-time imaging systems because of the large number of objects to be managed. A discussion of the problem and its solution is outside the scope of this book, but interested readers may refer to Reference [1].

### 15.3.2  Color Image Processing in Java3D

The Java3D applications program interface is a widely used library of software for two (2)- and three (3)-D imaging applications. The following paragraphs provide a basic introduction to color handling in Java3D as a prelude to two real-time color processing experiments. The concepts discussed are similar for other graphics processing packages, such as OpenGL, which can be used with several different programming languages. Much of the foregoing discussion was adapted from Reference [10].

In Java3D, the color of a 3-D object can be specified in three ways: per-vertex, in the shape's material component when a lighting model is applied, or in the shape's coloring attributes when the shape is unlit. Java3D employs the RGB color model. In per-vertex color, the `getColor()` method is used to specify the color per-vertex of a shape object. Color can be applied per-vertex when indexed geometry is specified. Java3D provides classes to support both indexed simple geometry as well as indexed strip geometry. A screenshot of a Java3D application in which a different vertex color was specified for each of the vertices in a triangle is shown in Figure 15.2.

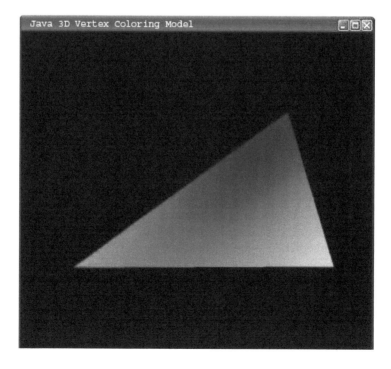

**FIGURE 15.2**
Screenshot of a Gouraud shaded triangle with per-vertex color specified.

The `Material` object is used to define the appearance of an object in the presence of illumination. The `Material` object specifies the ambient, diffuse, specular, and emissive colors, and a shininess value. The ambient, diffuse, and specular colors are used to calculate the corresponding reflection for the lighting model. The shininess value will only be applied for the calculation of a specular color. Emissive colors will simulate a "glow-in-the-dark" effect. The default constructor for a `Material` object sets the following default values:

| | |
|---|---|
| `ambientColor` | $(0.2, 0.2, 0.2)$ |
| `emissiveColor` | $(0, 0, 0)$ |
| `diffuseColor` | $(1, 1, 1)$ |
| `specularColor` | $(1, 1, 1)$ |
| `shininess` | $0.0$ |

Smooth surfaces will behave similarly to a mirror, whereby light will be reflected off the surface without changing the color of the light. As the smoothness of a surface increases, so does the intensity and focus of the specular reflection. The intensity of a specular reflection can be adjusted by changing the specular color. The shininess value is used to control the spread of the specular reflection; the higher the shininess value, the more focused the specular reflection. If a lighting model is applied, the final color will be calculated based on a combination of the material colors specified by the `Material` object.

Finally, the `ColoringAttributes` object defines the intrinsic color and shading model for 3-D shapes. This component object is used only for unlit geometry. The highest priority is given to color that is specified per-vertex for a particular geometry using the `getColor()` method. Color may also be specified in a `Material` object, which will enable lighting (shading) models to be applied. Finally, color may be specified in the `ColorAttributes` object, which should only be used for unlit objects when no material is specified. If textures are applied, they may replace or blend with the object's color.

Although multiple color specifications can be applied to an object, there are several rules that dictate the order of precedence. To enable lighting for an object, only the color of the `Material` object is referenced. Namely,

- Material color, or per-vertex geometry color, will be used in shading.
- To render unlit objects, only the color specified by the `ColoringAttributes` object is used.
- Precedence is always given to per-vertex color specified in the geometry over color specified by either `ColoringAttributes` or material color.

An overview of the specification of color precedence for lit and unlit objects is summarized in Table 15.1 and Table 15.2.

More details can be found at the Java3D API developer's site [10].

**TABLE 15.1**

Lighting Model Enabled `Material` Object is Referenced

| Pre-vertex Geometry Color | `ColoringAttributes` Color | Result |
|:---:|:---:|:---:|
| No | No | Material color |
| Yes | No | Geometry color |
| No | Yes | Material color |
| Yes | Yes | Geometry color |

*Note:* See Bouvier, D., *Getting Started with the Java 3D API*, Sun Microsystems, 1999.

**TABLE 15.2**

Lighting Model Enabled no`Material` Object is Referenced

| Pre-vertex Geometry Color | `ColoringAttributes` Color | Result |
|---|---|---|
| No | No | Flat white |
| Yes | No | Geometry color |
| No | Yes | `Coloring Attributes` color |
| Yes | Yes | Geometry color |

*Note:* See Bouvier, D., Getting Started with the Java 3D API, Sun Microsystems, 1999.

## 15.4 Case Study

The most convenient way to introduce the problems inherent in real-time color imaging systems and discuss their potential resolution, particularly the issue of performance measurement, is through experiments. In this case, we seek to determine the 3-D graphical rendering performance of a color imaging primitive in the Java language on desktop PCs. As previously mentioned, many industrial real-time color imaging systems run on off-the-shelf PCs.

The experiment involved two well-known brand name systems that possessed substantially different graphical rendering pipelines. This comparative evaluation provides an excellent tool for understanding the impact that the rendering pipeline has on real-time performance of a simple color algorithm. Moreover, the experimental approach is the same whether studying a simple color primitive or a much more complex real-time color imaging system. The study is also informative, because it uncovers graphics library, hardware, and software issues in the target systems.

### 15.4.1 Test Configuration

The two systems used in this study were a popular brand desktop computer (Computer A) and the same brand notebook computer (Computer B). An overview of the graphics components for each of the systems is summarized in Table 15.3.

**TABLE 15.3**

Summary of Test System Features

| Feature | Computer A | Computer B |
|---|---|---|
| Processor | 2.8 GHz Pentium 4 | 1.66 GHz Pentium M |
| System RAM | 256 MB | 512 MB |
| Core graphics clock | 200 MHz DDR SDRAM | 400 MHz DDR SDRAM |
| Graphics features | – Intel Extreme Graphics 84G Chipset | – ATI Radeon 9700 |
| | – Integrated Graphics: Dynamic Video Memory Technology — up to 64 MB system memory allocated for graphics | – 128 MB Dedicated VRAM |
| | – 4 × AGP (Accelerated Graphics Processor) Port -200 GB/sec | – 8 × AGP Graphics Port — 200 GB/sec |
| | – Texture engine processes four textures per pixel on a single pass | – Texture engine processes 16 textures per pixels on a single pass |
| | | – Programmable vertex shaders |

Note that Computer A uses integrated graphics components rather than a separate video card. One of the major drawbacks of integrated graphics is that the graphics processing unit (GPU) must share bandwidth with the system memory.

### 15.4.2 Experiment 1

The first experiment involves an investigation of color specification using the Java3D `ColorAttributes` class. To determine whether different shade models affect the rendering performance when color and shading are specified using the `ColorAttributes` class, a simple demonstration program was created in which the frames per second (FPS) was measured for a rotating 3-D sphere and cylinder when Gouraud and flat shading models were applied. For the sphere, the number of divisions was set at 300. For the cylinder, the default number of divisions (50) was used. When using the `ColorAttributes` class, no lighting model is enabled, and no `Material` object is specified. Therefore, the color will represent the intrinsic color set for the shapes. A screenshot is shown in Figure 15.3.

In this simple application, the intrinsic color and shade model were applied to the visual object using a `ColoringAttributes` object. Because the `ColoringAttributes` object can only be used to render unlit objects, a solid color will be rendered (Table 15.4). If lighting is enabled, the intrinsic color set by the `ColoringAttributes` object will be overridden.

It can be seen that there was no difference in the rendering rate between the flat and Gouraud shading models using this color specification method for Computer B. A slight ($\sim 5$ FPS) increase in speed was observed using the Gouraud shading model with

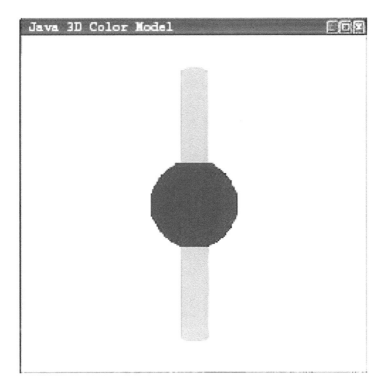

**FIGURE 15.3**
Screenshot of geometric primitives with color specified by the `ColoringAttributes` object used in experiment 1.

**TABLE 15.4**

Rendering Speed with Color Specified by
`ColorAttributes` Object in FPS

| System | Flat Shading | Gouraud Shading |
|---|---|---|
| Computer A | $90.47 \pm 0.02$ | $95.14 \pm 0.09$ |
| Computer B | $404.67 \pm 0.12$ | $404.62 \pm 0.05$ |

Computer A. Computer B rendered this simple scene at an average of 4.25 times faster than Computer A.

### 15.4.3 Experiment 2

The application of lighting, shading, and color models will produce vastly different visual results depending upon the material properties of objects in a Java3D scene. These models will also affect real-time behavior. It is, therefore, important to understand the complexity of the interaction between these models as well as the impact that each will have on performance.

To explore these, another Java experiment, was conducted. In this experiment, the number of FPS rendered was measured for a simple rotating triangle for which the color was specified per-vertex. The screenshots, which are shown in Figure 15.4a and Figure 15.4b, demonstrate the different visual effects of applying the Gouraud and flat shading models using the `ColorAttributes` component to the `Appearance` node. In this program, a rotational behavior was incorporated so that the triangle would rotate about the $y$-axis while the lower right vertex remained fixed.

The shade model for the `ColoringAttributes` component object can also be set as the "FASTEST" available shading method or the "NICEST" shading method, that will produce the highest-quality shading. The Java3D implementor defines which method is the "nicest"

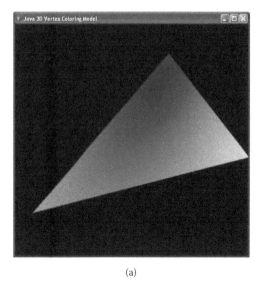
(a)

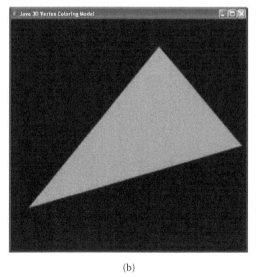
(b)

**FIGURE 15.4**
Screenshot of geometric primitives with color specified by the `ColoringAttributes` object: (a) Gouraud shading, and (b) flat shading.

**TABLE 15.5**

Rendering Speed with Per-Vertex Color
Specified by `ColorAttributes` Object in FPS

| System | Flat Shading | Gouraud Shading |
|---|---|---|
| Computer A | $189.80 \pm 0.30$ | $190.529 \pm 0.29$ |
| Computer B | $1288.22 \pm 0.61$ | $1288.55 \pm 0.99$ |

or "fastest," which, in turn, will be dependent upon the graphics hardware. In this study, setting the shading model to the FASTEST or NICEST resulted in the rendering of Gouraud shading, as shown in Figure 15.4a, for both systems.

The screenshots in Figure 15.4a and Figure 15.4b illustrate the difference in the visual results when the different shading models are applied. Using the Gouraud shading model, the color at each vertex is smoothly interpolated across the primitive (`ColoringAttributes` API). In Java3D, Gouraud shading is the default shading model unless another model is specified. The flat shading model will not interpolate color across a primitive; the color of a single vertex will be used to color all vertices in the primitive. The vertex for which the color is selected for the flat shading model is inherent to the Java3D and cannot be manipulated. In Figure 15.4a and Figure 15.4b, the red vertex color was selected as the color for flat shading.

For Computer B, there was no difference in rendering speed using the two shading models; the Gouraud shaded triangle was rendered at $1288.55 \pm 0.99$ FPS, while the flat shaded triangle was rendered at $1288.22 \pm 0.61$ FPS (Table 15.5).

Clearly, the rendering speed of Computer A was considerably slower, with the Gouraud shaded triangle rendered at $190.52 \pm 0.29$ FPS, and the flat shaded triangle rendered at $189.30 \pm 0.30$ FPS. Although there was no substantial difference in the rendering rate using the two shading models for any individual system, this program illustrates the importance that an optimized graphical pipeline has on rendering speed. For example, Computer B has a significantly enhanced graphical rendering pipeline as compared with Computer A. In addition to having 128 MB dedicated VRAM, and a highly optimized texture rendering engine, the accelerated graphics port ($8 \times$ AGP) can transfer data at a speed of 200 GB/sec, which is twice as fast as Computer A.

Interestingly, the Gouraud and flat shading models produced similar rendering speeds and had no impact on performance in this study. However, Gouraud shading may be faster than flat shading, depending on a variety of factors, such as color model, hardware, and language implementation. This fact alone illustrates the complexity in performance tuning real-time color imaging systems.

## 15.5 Conclusions

In this chapter, the unique problem of real-time processing of images was discussed. Selected issues related to hardware, software, and programming languages were explored, such as hardware and software solutions, and the importance of the programming language.

Two experiments illustrated the impact and linkage between the hardware architecture, color representation, and language features on real-time performance and performance predictability. In doing so, a framework for analyzing other color imaging applications was established.

From a simple design standpoint, the following recommendations will help to ensure that performance is optimal in a real-time color imaging system:

- Understand the color imaging problem. Select the optimal algorithm for the situation.

- Understand the hardware architecture. Select the best hardware for the application, but never more functionality than necessary.

- Understand the programming language. Be sure to use the most efficient language constructs when coding the algorithms.

- Understand operating systems interactions. Know how the system deals with thread synchronization and prioritization.

- Conduct a thorough schedulability analysis to guarantee deadlines.

This sequence is deceptively simplistic, but really is intended to serve as a reminder that there are many issues to be considered in real-time color imaging systems.

One final issue in real-time image processing is that a significant amount of deployed code has been ported from other languages, such as C, Fortran, Visual Basic, and even BASIC, into object-oriented languages such as C++ or Java without thought to redesign to benefit from the object-oriented paradigm. The resultant code often shares the worst characteristics of the object-oriented code (typically, performance degradation) without any of the benefits (e.g., ease of extension and reuse). Therefore, it is highly recommended that when porting legacy code across languages, a complete redesign of the system be considered in order to optimize the real-time performance of the system.

## References

[1] P.A. Laplante, *Real-Time Systems Design and Analysis*, 3rd ed., IEEE Press, Piscataway, NJ, 2005.
[2] P.A. Laplante, A retrospective on real-time imaging, a new taxonomy and a roadmap for the future, *Real-Time Imaging*, 8, 413–425, October 2002.
[3] S.S. Cheng, Z. Xiong, and X. Wu, Fast trellis-coded color quantization of images, *Real-Time Imaging*, 8, 265–275, August 2002.
[4] M. Zhang and N.D. Georganas, Fast color correction using principal regions mapping different color spaces, *Real-Time Imaging*, 10, 23–30, 2004.
[5] I. Andreadis, P. Iliades, and P. Tsalides, A new asic for real-time linear color space transforms, *Real-Time Imaging*, 1, 373–379, November 1995.
[6] D. Han, Real-time color gamut mapping method for digital tc display quality enhancement, *IEEE Trans. on Consumer Electron.*, 50, 691–699, May 2004.
[7] E.R. Dougherty and P.A. Laplante, *Introduction to Real-Time Image Processing*, SPIE Press, Bellingham, WA, 1994.
[8] P.A. Laplante, Real-time imaging, *Potentials*, 23, 8–10, 2005.
[9] T. Moller and E. Haines, *Real-Time Rendering*, A.K. Peters, Natick, MA, 1999.
[10] D. Bouvier, *Getting Started with the Java3D API*, http://java.sun.com/products/java-media/3D/collateral.html, Sun Microsystems, 1999.

# 16

## Single-Sensor Camera Image Processing

**Rastislav Lukac and Konstantinos N. Plataniotis**

## CONTENTS

## 16.1 Introduction

In recent years, a massive research and development effort has been witnessed in color imaging technologies in both industry and ordinary life. Color is commonly used in television, computer displays, cinema motion pictures, print, and photographs. In all these application areas, the perception of color is paramount for the correct understanding and dissemination of the visual information. Recent technological advances have reduced the complexity and the cost of color devices, such as monitors, printers, scanners, and copiers, thus allowing their use in the office and home environment. However, it is the extreme and still increasing popularity of the consumer, single-sensor digital cameras that today boosts the research activities in the field of digital color image acquisition, processing, and storage. Single-sensor camera image processing methods are becoming increasingly important due to the development and proliferation of emerging digital camera-based applications and commercial devices, such as imaging enabled mobile phones and personal digital assistants, sensor networks, surveillance, and automotive apparatus.

This chapter focuses on single-sensor camera image processing techniques with particular emphasis on image interpolation-based solutions. The chapter surveys in a systematic and comprehensive manner demosaicking, demosaicked image postprocessing, and camera image zooming solutions that utilize data-adaptive and spectral modeling principles to produce camera images with an enhanced visual quality. The existence of realistic and efficient design procedures and the variety of processing solutions developed through the presented data-adaptive, spectral model-based processing framework make this family of processing methodologies an indispensable tool for single-sensor imaging.

The chapter begins with Section 16.2, which briefly discusses the digital camera solutions, emphasizing cost-effective hardware architecture for a consumer-grade camera equipped with a color filter array placed on the top of a single image sensor. The most common color filter array layouts are also introduced and commented upon.

The next part of the chapter, Section 16.3, describes the work flow in the single-sensor cameras. Particular emphasis is placed on the essential camera image processing of the sensor data. The second part of this section presents various image processing paradigms that are taxonomized according to their ability to follow the structural and the spectral characteristics of the acquired image. This section also introduces the so-called generalized camera image processing solution and lists the spatial, structural, and spectral constraints imposed on such a solution in practical applications. This part of the chapter also includes Section 16.4, which focuses on an edge-sensing processing mechanism, and Section 16.5, which targets the essential spectral model for single-sensor image processing. The omission of either of these elements during the single-sensor imaging operations results in significant degradation of the visual quality of the full-color camera image.

The main part of the chapter is devoted to single-sensor imaging solutions developed using the concept of image interpolation. The connection between image interpolation operations and the single-sensor imaging solutions that use the edge-sensing mechanism and spectral model is highlighted. Examples and experimental results included in the chapter indicate that the framework is computationally attractive, yields good performance, and produces images of reasonable visual quality. In this part of the chapter, Section 16.6 focuses on the demosaicking process or spectral interpolation, which is used to generate a color image from a single-sensor reading and is an integral processing step in a single-sensor camera pipeline. Because demosaicked images often suffer from reduced sharpness, color shifts, and visual artifacts, demosaicked image postprocessing or full-color image enhancement is often utilized in order to enhance fine details and produce natural colors. This processing step is extensively analyzed and documented in Section 16.7. Finally, image spatial resolution expansion is often implemented in digital cameras with limited optical zooming capabilities. To this end, Section 16.8 focuses on camera image zooming or spatial interpolation, which is to be performed either in the demosaicked image domain or directly on the sensor data. Although based on the same principle, these zooming approaches produce the different visual quality and have the different computational complexity.

The chapter concludes with Section 16.9, which summarizes the main single-sensor camera image processing ideas.

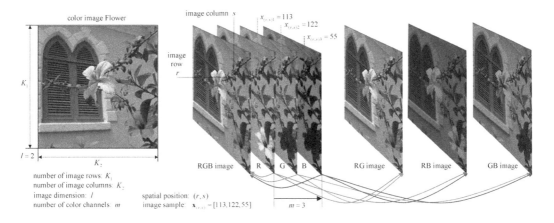

**FIGURE 16.1 (See color insert.)**
Color image representation in the RGB color domain.

## 16.2 Digital Camera Architectures

Digital color cameras [1], [2], [3] capture color images of real-life scenes electronically using an image sensor, usually a charge-coupled device (CCD) [4], [5] or complementary metal oxide semiconductor (CMOS) [6], [7] sensor, instead of the film used in the conventional analog cameras. Therefore, captured photos can be immediately viewed by the user on the digital camera's display, and immediately stored, processed, or transmitted. Without any doubt, this is one of the most attractive features of digital imaging.

The captured photo can be considered a $K_1 \times K_2$ red-green-blue (RGB) digital color image $\mathbf{x} : Z^2 \to Z^3$ representing a two-dimensional matrix of three-component samples (pixels) $\mathbf{x}_{(r,s)} = [x_{(r,s)1}, x_{(r,s)2}, x_{(r,s)3}]^T$, where each individual channel of $\mathbf{x}$ can be considered a $K_1 \times K_2$ monochrome image $x_k : Z^2 \to Z$, for $k = 1, 2, 3$. The pixel $\mathbf{x}_{(r,s)}$ represents the color vector [8] occupying the spatial location $(r, s)$, with $r = 1, 2, \ldots, K_1$ and $s = 1, 2, \ldots, K_2$ denoting the image row and column, respectively. The value of the R ($k = 1$), G ($k = 2$), and B ($k = 3$) component $x_{(r,s)k}$ defined in the integer domain $Z$ is equal to an arbitrary integer value ranging from 0 to 255 in a standard 8-bits per component representation and denotes the contribution of the $k$th primary in the color vector $\mathbf{x}_{(r,s)}$. The process of displaying an image creates a graphical representation of the image matrix where the pixel values represent particular colors in the visible spectrum (Figure 16.1) [8].[1]

Due to the monochromatic nature of the image sensor, digital camera manufacturers implement several solutions to capture the visual scene in color. The following three are the most popular designs currently in use.

- **Three-sensor device** (Figure 16.2) [1], [2], [3]: This architecture acquires color information using a beam splitter to separate incoming light into three optical paths. Each path has its own red, green or blue color filter having different spectral transmittances and sensors for sampling the filtered light. Because the camera color image is obtained by registering the signals from three sensors, precise

---

[1] The figures in this chapter can be seen in color at http://www.dsp.utoronto.ca/~lukacr/CRCcip/CRCchapLukac.pdf.

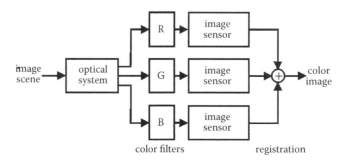

**FIGURE 16.2**
Three-sensor device.

mechanical and optical alignment is necessary to maintain correspondence among the images obtained from the different channels [1]. Besides the difficulties of maintaining image registration, the high cost of the sensor[2] and the use of a beam splitter make the three-sensor architecture available only for some professional digital cameras.

- **X3 technology-based device** (Figure 16.3) [9], [10], [11]: This architecture uses a layered single image sensor that directly captures the complete color information at each spatial location in an image during a single exposure. Color filters are stacked vertically and ordered according to the energy of the photons absorbed by silicon. Taking advantage of the natural light-absorbing characteristics of silicon, each sensor cell records color channels depth-wise in silicon.[3] The drawbacks of the sensor are its noisy behavior (especially for the layers in the base of the chip) and relatively low sensitivity. Furthermore, the sensor usually suffers from intensive optical/eletrical cross talk which, however, can be processed out for natural images by clever signal processing. Specialized X3 technology-based sensors have been used in various medical, scientific, and industrial applications.

- **Single-sensor device** (Figure 16.4) [2], [3]: This architecture reduces cost by placing a color filter array (CFA), which is a mosaic of color filters, on top of the conventional single CCD/CMOS image sensor to capture all three primary (RGB) colors at the same time. Each sensor cell has its own spectrally selective filter, and thus, it stores only a single measurement. Therefore, the CFA image constitutes a mosaic-like grayscale image with only one color element available in each pixel location. The two missing colors must be determined from the adjacent pixels using a digital processing solution called demosaicking [2], [12], [13]. Such an architecture represents the most cost-effective method currently in use for color imaging, and for this reason, it is almost universally utilized in consumer-grade digital cameras.

### 16.2.1 Consumer-Grade Camera Hardware Architecture

Following the block scheme shown in Figure 16.5, the camera acquires the scene by first focusing and transmitting light through the CFA. To reduce the various artifacts present in the demosaicked image due to downsampling the color information performed by the

---

[2] The sensor is the most expensive component of the digital camera and usually takes from 10% to 25% of the total cost [3].
[3] The light directed to the sensor is absorbed first by the blue layer, then by the green layer, and finally by the red layer placed deepest in silicon [9].

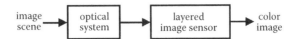

**FIGURE 16.3**
X3 technology-based device.

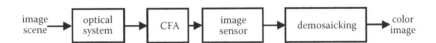

**FIGURE 16.4**
Single-sensor device.

CFA, a blurring filter is placed in the optical path [14]. Because of the presence of blurring filters in a blocking system, both sharpness and resolution of the image captured using a consumer-grade camera is usually lower compared with the architectures depicted in Figure 16.2 and Figure 16.3 [10], [14].

The acquired visual information is sampled using the image sensor and an analog-to-digital (A/D) converter. The DRAM buffer temporally stores the digital data from the A/D converter and then passes them to the application-specific integrated circuit (ASIC) which together with the microprocessor realize the digital data processing operations, such as demosaicking and image resizing. The firmware memory holds the set of instructions for the microprocessor, and along with the ASIC, they are most distinctive elements between the camera manufacturers.

After demosaicking has been completed, the digital image is displayed and stored in memory, often the 16 MB built-in memory or the optional memory supplied by the manufacturers usually in the form of memory stick cards of various types and storage capacities. The end user is often offered the option to reprocess stored images by passing them back to the ASIC unit. The interested reader should refer to References [14], [15], and [16] for additional information on the camera optical and hardware components.

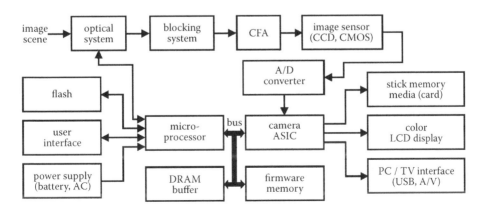

**FIGURE 16.5**
Consumer camera hardware architecture.

### 16.2.2 Color Filter Array (CFA)

Apart from camera firmware, another distinctive element of the consumer-grade digital cameras is the CFA. The type of a color system and the arrangements of the color filters in the CFA significantly vary depending on the manufacturer.

The color systems used in the various CFA designs can be divided into [17] tristimulus (RGB, YMC) systems, systems with mixed primary/complementary colors (e.g., MGCY pattern), and four and more color systems (e.g., those constructed using white and/or colors with shifted spectral sensitivity). Although the last two variants may produce more accurate hue gamut compared to the tristimulus systems, they often limit the useful range of the darker colors [18]. In addition, the utilization of four or more colors in the CFA layout increases computational complexity of the demosaicking operations. For this reason and due to the fact that color images are commonly stored in RGB color format, the tristimulus RGB-based CFAs are widely used by camera manufacturers.

A number of RGB CFAs with the varied arrangement of color filters in the array are used in practice [17], [18], [19], [20], [21]. Key factors that influence this design issue relate to [17] cost-effective image reconstruction, immunity to color artifacts and color moiré, reaction of the array to image sensor imperfections, and immunity to optical/electrical cross talk between neighboring pixels.

The first criterion is essential because of the real-time processing constraints imposed on the digital camera. Among the various CFAs shown in Figure 16.6a to Figure 16.6h, periodic CFAs, such as the Bayer and Yamanaka patterns, enjoy a distinct advantage over pseudo-random (or random) CFAs, because the aperiodic nature of the latter makes the demosaicking process more complex [22]. To reduce the array's sensitivity to color artifacts in the reconstructed image, each pixel of the CFA image should be surrounded in its neighborhood by all three primary colors [18], as it can be seen in the arrays shown in Figure 16.6c to Figure 16.6e. On the other hand, images captured using periodic CFAs (e.g., Bayer and Yamanaka patterns) usually suffer from color moiré effects, which may be reduced by using pseudo-random (or random) CFAs instead [17]. It should also be mentioned that the

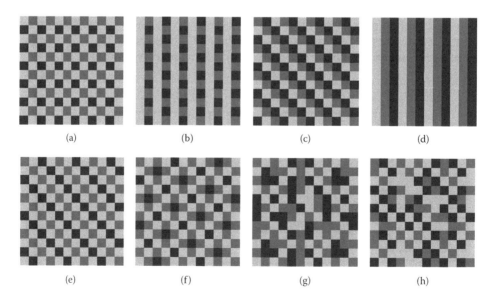

|       |       |       |       |
|:-----:|:-----:|:-----:|:-----:|
| (a)   | (b)   | (c)   | (d)   |
| (e)   | (f)   | (g)   | (h)   |

**FIGURE 16.6** (See color insert.)
Examples of RGB CFAs: (a) Bayer pattern, (b) Yamanaka pattern, (c) diagonal stripe pattern, (d) vertical stripe pattern, (e) diagonal Bayer pattern, (f,g) pseudo-random patterns, and (h) HVS-based pattern.

wavelength of the G color band is close to the peak of the human luminance frequency response, and thus, some CFAs (Figure 16.6a, Figure 16.6b and Figure 16.6e) use the double number of G color filters than that of the R and B filters to reduce the amount of spectral artifacts in the outputted, reconstructed image [23], [24].

CFA designs, such as the diagonal stripe pattern and the diagonal Bayer pattern, are considered to be the best in terms of their robustness against image sensor imperfections, because defects are typically observed along rows or columns of the sensor cells. With respect to immunity to optical/electrical cross talk between neighboring pixels,[4] CFAs with the fixed number of neighbors corresponding to each of the three primary colors significantly outperform pseudo-random CFA layouts.

As can be seen from the above discussion, there is no CFA that satisfies all design constraints. Therefore, camera manufacturers usually select a CFA layout by taking into consideration cost, compatibility with other processing elements, and hardware constraints. Particular attention is devoted to the type and resolution of the image sensor, camera optical system, and image processing capabilities of the device. The intended application (e.g., consumer photography, surveillance, astronomy), in which the single-sensor device will be used, is also an important factor to be considered.

## 16.3   Camera Image Processing

After acquiring the raw sensor data, the image is preprocessed, processed, and postprocessed to produce a faithful digital representation of the captured scene. Figure 16.7 depicts an example flow of the processing steps performed in the consumer-grade camera pipeline. Note that the depicted flow may significantly vary depending on the manufacturer [14], [15].

The preprocessing starts with defective pixel detection and correction of missing pixels by interpolating using the neighboring data. In this way, impairments caused by the failure of certain photo elements in the sensor can be rectified. If the captured data reside in a nonlinear space, often the case due to the electronics involved, then a linearization step is usually implemented. The subsequent dark current compensation reduces the level of dark current noise introduced into the signal through thermally generated electrons in the sensor substrate. This processing step is essential in low exposure images, where both signal and noise levels may be comparable. The last preprocessing step is the so-called white balance that is used to correct the captured image for the scene illuminant by adjusting the image values, thus recovering the true scene coloration. The interested reader can find an overview of the preprocessing steps in References [14], [15], and [16].

After preprocessing, the consumer-grade digital camera performs intensive image processing. Apart from demosaicking, which is a mandatory and integral step in the processing pipeline needed in restoring the color information originally present in the captured image, camera image processing includes some optional steps. For instance, the visual quality of the restored color image can be improved by postprocessing the demosaicked image, whereas the spatial resolution of the captured image can be enhanced by zooming the CFA image or the (postprocessed) demosaicked image. It will be shown in this chapter that these four camera image processing steps are fundamentally different, although they employ similar, if not identical, digital signal processing concepts.

Once the restoration of the full-color information is completed, the captured image enters the postprocessing stage in order to enhance its coloration and transform it to an output

---

[4] Diagonally located neighbors have a lower cross talk contribution than the vertically/horizontally located neighbors [18].

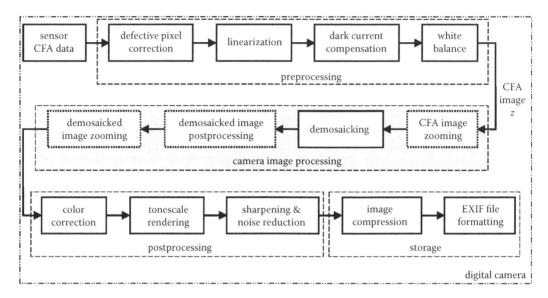

**FIGURE 16.7**
Example image processing flow in a consumer-grade camera.

color encoding, appropriate for displaying and printing purposes [14]. Because the spectral sensitivities of the camera are not identical to the human color matching function [16], the color correction process adjusts the values of color pixels from those corresponding to accurate scene reproduction to those corresponding to visually pleasing scene reproduction. The subsequent tone scale rendering process transforms the color image from the unrendered spaces where a 12 to 16 bit representation was used for calculations to a rendered (mostly sRGB [25]) space with 8-bit representation, as it is required by most output media. The obtained image is then enhanced by sharpening/denoising in order to reduce the low-frequency content in the image and remove insignificant, noise-like details. An overview of the postprocessing steps can be found in References [14], [15], and [16].

The consumer-grade cameras (Figure 16.7) commonly store the rendered/enhanced color image in a compressed format using the Joint Photographic Experts Group (JPEG) standard [14]. However, in recent years, the exchangeable image file (EXIF) format [26] has been popularized due to its convenient implementation and the possibility of storing additional (metadata) information regarding the camera and the environment. High-end single-sensor digital cameras (Figure 16.8) apply image compression onto the preprocessed image, and

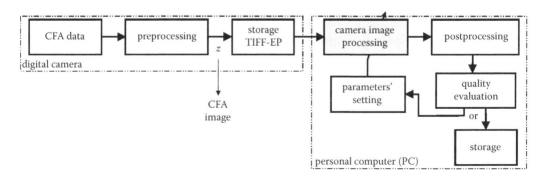

**FIGURE 16.8**
Example image processing flow in a camera interfacing with a companion personal computer.

then the compressed image data are formatted and stored in a tagged image file format for electronic photography (TIFF-EP) [27]. In this format, the image is stored along with additional information, such as the details about camera setting, spectral sensitivities, and illuminant used. Additional information about the methods used for compression and storage of camera images can be found in the literature [28], [29], [30], [31], [32], [33].

As can be seen in Figure 16.7 and Figure 16.8, the camera image processing can be implemented in a conventional digital camera that stores the demosaicked (RGB) output, or in a companion personal computer (PC) that interfaces with the digital camera that stores the images in the CFA-like format. Both above processing pipelines can use the same processing solution. However, the approach depicted in Figure 16.8 allows for the utilization of sophisticated solutions that cannot, due to their complexity, be embedded in the conventional camera image processing pipeline (Figure 16.7), which has to operate under real-time constraints. In addition, due to the utilization of the companion PC in the pipeline, the end user can select different settings of the processing solutions and reprocess the image until certain quality criteria are met. Finally, it should be mentioned that Figure 16.7 and Figure 16.8 depict the basic camera work flow. Both pipelines are flexible enough to accommodate various image, video, and multimedia processing operations, such as video demosaicking [34], CFA video compression [35], and digital rights management (e.g., image indexing by embedding the metadata information into the camera image to allow for securing, and easy organization/retrieval of the captured images in personal or public databases) [36], [37].

## 16.3.1 CFA Data Imaging

For the sake of clarity in the terminology used in the rest of the chapter, it should be emphasized here that the image output by the preprocessing module in Figure 16.7 and Figure 16.8 is called, hereafter, the CFA image, which is a $K_1 \times K_2$ grayscale mosaic-like image $z : Z^2 \to Z$ with the CFA (scalar) data $z_{(r,s)}$. Because information about the arrangements of color filters in the actual CFA is readily available either from the camera manufacturer (Figure 16.7) or obtained from the TIFF-EP format (Figure 16.8), the CFA image $z$ shown in Figure 16.9a can be transformed to a $K_1 \times K_2$ three-channel (color) image $\mathbf{x} : Z^2 \to Z^3$ shown in Figure 16.9b with the RGB pixels $\mathbf{x}_{(r,s)} = [x_{(r,s)1}, x_{(r,s)2}, x_{(r,s)3}]^T$.

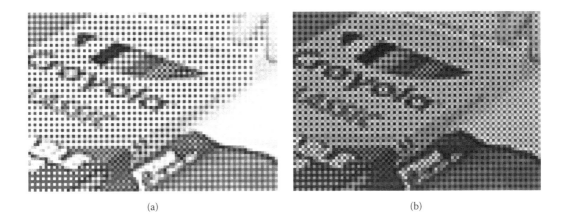

(a)  (b)

**FIGURE 16.9 (See color insert.)**
CFA image obtained using a well-known Bayer CFA with the GRGR phase in the first row: (a) acquired grayscale CFA image and (b) CFA image rearranged as a color image.

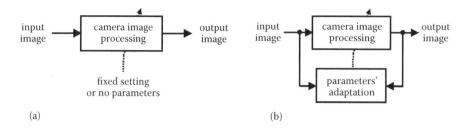

**FIGURE 16.10**
Image processing paradigms divided considering the structural characteristics: (a) nonadaptive processing and (b) data-adaptive processing.

The correspondence between the $z_{(r,s)}$ values and the R ($k = 1$), G ($k = 2$), or B ($k = 3$) color filters at the $(r, s)$ CFA locations can be indicated using spatial location flags [22]. Following the dimensions of the CFA image $z$, a $K_1 \times K_2$ vectorial field $\mathbf{d} : Z^2 \rightarrow Z^3$ of the corresponding location flags $d_{(r,s)k}$ is initialized using the default value $d_{(r,s)k} = 1$ to indicate the presence of a CFA value $z_{(r,s)}$ in the color vector $\mathbf{x}_{(r,s)}$ for the proper value of $k$. For example, if $(r, s)$ corresponds to a G CFA location in the image $z$, then $\mathbf{x}_{(r,s)} = [0, z_{(r,s)}, 0]^T$ and $d_{(r,s)k} = 1$ for $k = 2$ should be used. If $(r, s)$ corresponds to a R (or B) CFA location, then $\mathbf{x}_{(r,s)} = [z_{(r,s)}, 0, 0]^T$ (or $\mathbf{x}_{(r,s)} = [0, 0, z_{(r,s)}]^T$) and $d_{(r,s)k} = 1$ for $k = 1$ (or $k = 3$) should be utilized. In all other cases, the flags are set to $d_{(r,s)k} = 0$, indicating the two missing components in $\mathbf{x}_{(r,s)}$ are set equal to zero to denote their portion to the coloration of the image $\mathbf{x}$ shown in Figure 16.9b. Note that the presented approach is independent from the CFA structure and is thus suitable for an arbitrary CFA shown in Figure 16.6 [22].

### 16.3.2   Structural Information-Based Image Processing

Operating on the CFA image $z$ or its colored variant $\mathbf{x}$, processing solutions included in the camera image processing module in Figure 16.7 and Figure 16.8 can be classified considering the image content (structure) in the two basic paradigms (Figure 16.10): nonadaptive processing, and data-adaptive processing.

The former paradigm (Figure 16.10a) uses no data-adaptive control to follow the structural content of the captured image [38], [39], [40], [41], [42], thus often reducing to a linear processing cycle which is easy to implement. However, it is well known that most image processing tasks cannot be efficiently accomplished by linear techniques. Image signals are nonlinear in nature due to the presence of edges; thus, most of the linear and nonadaptive techniques tend to blur structural elements such as fine image details [43]. It should also be mentioned that images are perceived through the human visual system, which has strong nonlinear characteristics [44].

The latter paradigm (Figure 16.10b) uses the so-called edge-sensing weights to follow structural content of the image [45], [46], [47]. Such a processing solution, often called nonlinear processing, usually results in enhanced performance. Nonlinear, data-adaptive methods are able to preserve important color structural elements and produce sharp looking images.

### 16.3.3   Spectral Information-Based Image Processing

With respect to spectral characteristics, camera image processing can be divided into (Figure 16.11) component-wise processing, spectral model-based processing, and vector processing.

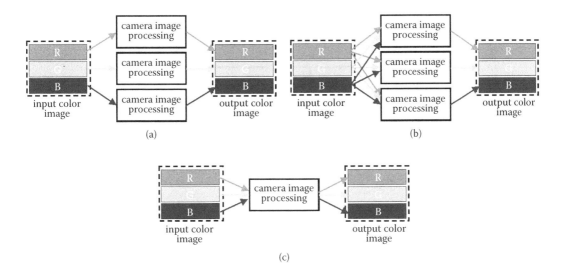

**FIGURE 16.11**

Image processing paradigms divided considering the spectral characteristics: (a) component-wise processing, (b) spectral model-based processing and (c) vector processing.

Component-wise methods (Figure 16.11a), directly adopted from the grayscale imaging, process each channel of the color image separately [38], [39], [48]. By omitting the essential spectral information and thus introducing a certain inaccuracy in the component-wise estimates, the projection of the output color components into the restored RGB image often produces color artifacts (a new color quite different from the neighbors) [8]. On the other hand, component-wise processing methods are usually fast and easy to implement.

Spectral model-based processing methods (Figure 16.11b) use the essential spectral information from the input camera image to reduce, if not eliminate, color shifts and artifacts being produced during processing [2], [49], [50], [51]. This processing paradigm assumes vector (multichannel) samples as the input and generates a single-channel output. Therefore, the procedure has to be repeated for each color channel in order to generate the full-color output. Due to its computational simplicity, the spectral model-based solutions are the most widely used in camera image processing among the paradigms shown in Figure 16.11a to Figure 16.11c.

Similar to the spectral model-based paradigm, vector processing methods (Figure 16.11c) utilize the inherent correlation among the color channels and process the color image pixels as vectors [8], [43]. In this way, color artifacts in the output image are greatly reduced [8]. However, because vector processing methods generate the output color image in a single pass, they are usually computationally expensive compared with the solutions depicted in Figure 16.11a and Figure 16.11b. Therefore, the use of vector processing in camera image processing is rather limited at the moment.

### 16.3.4 Generalized Camera Image Processing Solution

From the discussion in Sections 16.3.2 and 16.3.3, it is evident that an ideal processing solution should be able to follow both the structural content of the image and the spectral characteristics of its color content. To produce visually pleasing output images, it is essential to overcome both the CFA limitations and the spatial, structural, and spectral constraints imposed on the processing solution [52].

Figure 16.12 depicts the block diagram of the so-called generalized processing solution [2], [24], [36]. The characteristics of such a solution are essentially determined by

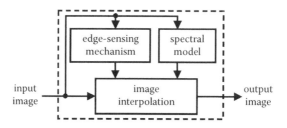

**FIGURE 16.12**
Generalized camera image processing solution suitable for demosaicking, demosaicked image postprocessing, and camera image zooming.

the edge-sensing mechanism (ESM) and the spectral model (SM), which are implemented through the operators $\Lambda$ and $\Psi$, respectively. The ESM operator $\Lambda$ uses both the structural and the spatial characteristics to preserve the sharpness and structural information of the captured image. The SM operator $\Psi$ uses both the spectral and the spatial characteristics of the neighboring color pixels to eliminate spectral artifacts in the output signal. Thus, both the ESM and SM are based on the local neighborhood area determined by parameter $\zeta$.

Spatial constraints imposed on the processing solution relate to the size of an area of support and the form of the shape-mask utilized in processing. By denoting $(r, s)$ as the location under consideration, due to the strong spatial correlation among the neighboring image samples of the natural image, it is commonly expected that the utilization of the closest $3 \times 3$ neighborhood $\{(r \pm u, s \pm v); u, v \in \{-1, 0, 1\}\}$ ensures the faithful reconstruction of the color vector $\mathbf{x}_{(r,s)}$. Because the CFA image has a mosaic-like structure and not all of the neighboring locations correspond to a color channel being reconstructed, operating on the image $\mathbf{x}$ obtained using the well-known Bayer CFA (Figure 16.13a) the local neighborhood described by $\zeta$ is most commonly limited to the shape-masks shown in Figure 16.13b to Figure 16.13e [45], [47], [53].

To quantify the contributions of the adjacent color vectors $\mathbf{x}_{(i,j)} = [x_{(i,j)1}, x_{(i,j)2}, x_{(i,j)3}]^T$ to the vector $\mathbf{x}_{(r,s)}$ under consideration, the so-called data-adaptive concept is used as follows [2], [51], [52]:

$$\mathbf{x}_{(r,s)} = \sum_{(i,j) \in \zeta} \left\{ w'_{(i,j)} \Psi(\mathbf{x}_{(i,j)}, \mathbf{x}_{(r,s)}) \right\} \tag{16.1}$$

where $(i, j) \in \zeta$ denotes the spatial location arrangements on the image lattice, for example $\zeta = \{(r - 1, s), (r, s - 1), (r, s + 1), (r + 1, s)\}$ shown in Figure 16.13b, Figure 16.13d, and Figure 16.13e, and $\zeta = \{(r - 1, s - 1), (r - 1, s + 1), (r + 1, s - 1), (r + 1, s + 1)\}$ shown

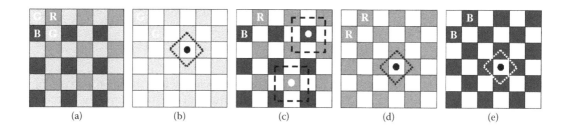

|     |     |     |     |     |
|-----|-----|-----|-----|-----|
| (a) | (b) | (c) | (d) | (e) |

**FIGURE 16.13**
Shape-masks used in restoring the color information in the Bayer CFA image: (a) Bayer CFA with the GRGR phase in the first row, (b) G channel restoration, and (c–e) R and B channel restoration.

in Figure 16.13c. Each of the available color vectors $\mathbf{x}_{(i,j)}$ inside $\zeta$ is associated with the normalized weighting coefficient $w'_{(i,j)}$ defined as

$$w'_{(i,j)} = w_{(i,j)} / \sum_{(i,j) \in \zeta} w_{(i,j)} \tag{16.2}$$

where $w_{(i,j)}$ are the so-called edge-sensing weights. By emphasizing inputs that are not positioned across an edge and directing the processing along the natural edges in the true image, the use of the edge information in the data-adaptive formula in Equation 16.1 preserves the structural image contents, and thus ensures a sharply formed output image.

## 16.4   Edge-Sensing Mechanism (ESM)

Structural constraints of Equation 16.1 relate to the form of the ESM operator $\Lambda$ used to generate the weights in Equation 16.2 as $\{w_{(i,j)}; (i, j) \in \zeta\} = \Lambda(\mathbf{x}, \zeta)$. If the $w_{(i,j)}$ values are not obtained through the function $\Lambda(\cdot)$ of the color components available in the image $\mathbf{x}$, that is, the fixed setting $\{w_{(i,j)} = \xi; (i, j) \in \zeta\}$ to a nonzero constant $\xi$ is used, the data-adaptive solution in Equation 16.1 reduces to nonadaptive schemes, such as those listed in References [38], [40], [42], and [49].

However, such an omission of the structural information in Equation 16.1 leads to the significant degradation of the visual quality [2], [47]. Therefore, most of the available designs employ the data-dependent ESM operator $\Lambda(\mathbf{x}, \zeta)$ which uses some form of inverse gradient of the samples in the image $\mathbf{x}$. Large image gradients usually indicate that the corresponding vectors $\mathbf{x}_{(i,j)}$ are located across edges. Weights $\{w_{(i,j)}; (i, j) \in \zeta\} = \Lambda(\mathbf{x}, \zeta)$ are inversely proportional to gradient values, thus penalizing the corresponding inputs $\mathbf{x}_{(i,j)}$ in Equation 16.1. Because the original CFA components are readably available in the color image $\mathbf{x}$ as explained in Section 16.3.1, in order to increase the accuracy of the adaptive design in Equation 16.1, it is common to restrict $\Lambda(\cdot)$ only on the acquired CFA data $z_{(\cdot,\cdot)}$, that is, edge-sensing weights are obtained as $\{w_{(i,j)}; (i, j) \in \zeta\} = \Lambda(z, \zeta)$.

### 16.4.1   Aggregation Concept-Based ESM

Cost considerations and real-time constraints in digital apparatus necessitate the utilization of a simple and easy to implement ESM $\Lambda(z, \zeta)$, such as the one defined as follows [2], [54]:

$$w_{(i,j)} = 1 / \sum_{(g,h) \in \zeta} |z_{(i,j)} - z_{(g,h)}| \tag{16.3}$$

where $\sum_{(g,h) \in \zeta} |z_{(i,j)} - z_{(g,h)}|$ is the aggregated absolute difference (Figure 16.14a and Figure 16.14b) between the CFA components $z_{(\cdot,\cdot)}$ inside the neighborhood $\zeta$. This approach

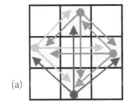
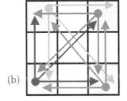

(a)              (b)

**FIGURE 16.14**
Aggregation concept depicted for the shape masks: (a) the shape mask $\zeta = \{(r-1, s), (r, s-1), (r, s+1), (r+1, s)\}$ (see Figure 16.13b, Figure 16.13d, and Figure 16.13e), and (b) $\zeta = \{(r-1, s-1), (r-1, s+1), (r+1, s-1), (r+1, s+1)\}$ (see Figure 16.13c).

significantly reduces memory requirements, because both the ESM operator $\Lambda$ and the data-adaptive estimator (Equation 16.1) use the same inputs occupying the spatial locations $(i, j) \in \zeta$. This also makes the ESM implementation in Equation 16.3 independent from the CFA structure and thus flexible for the use in the imaging pipeline equipped with the CFA other than the Bayer CFA [22]. Thinking in these dimensions, different forms of the ESM $\Lambda(z, \zeta)$ have been proposed in Reference [2].

The framework allows for obtaining the edge-sensing weights in an automated manner (Figure 16.7), with the example of the ESM formulated in Equation 16.3. In addition to this design, the weights can be controlled by the end user, as shown in Figure 16.8 [2]. One of the possible solutions is the utilization of the well-known sigmoidal function. As empirical evidence suggests that the relationship between perception and distances measured in physical units is exponential in nature [55], the weights calculated using

$$w_{(i,j)} = \beta_{(i,j)} \left(1 + \exp\left\{\sum_{(g,h) \in \zeta} |z_{(i,j)} - z_{(g,h)}|\right\}\right)^{-q} \tag{16.4}$$

can lead to some performance improvements in terms of the visual quality [2]. In the definition above, $q$ is a parameter adjusting the weighting effect of the membership function, and $\beta_{(i,j)}$ is a normalizing constant. Within the framework, numerous solutions may be constructed by changing the way the weights are calculated as well as the way the available color components from different color channels are treated. The choice of these parameters determines the characteristics and influences the efficiency of the processing solution.

### 16.4.2　Neighborhood Expansion-Based ESM

On the other hand, the constraint imposed on the size of $\zeta$ in $\Lambda(z, \zeta)$ may reduce the edge-sensing capability of the solution. To overcome the limitation, unfortunately at the expense of an increased implementation complexity and memory requirements, the ESM operator $\Lambda(z, \zeta)$ is modified to $\Lambda(z, \zeta')$ by considering a larger, typically $5 \times 5$ or $7 \times 7$ neighborhood $\zeta' = \{(r \pm u, s \pm v); u, v \in \{-2, -1, \ldots, 2\}\}$ or $\zeta' = \{(r \pm u, s \pm v); u, v \in \{-3, -2, \ldots, 3\}\}$, respectively. In this case, the weights $\{w_{(i,j)}; (i, j) \in \zeta\} = \Lambda(z, \zeta')$, for $\zeta \subset \zeta'$, are calculated using the components $z_{(\cdot,\cdot)}$ in $\zeta'$. The described concept has been employed in various processing solutions, for example, in References [12], [45], [46], [47], [56], and [57]. It should be mentioned that these ESMs may not be directly applicable to non-Bayer CFAs [22], as they implicitly differentiate among the color components corresponding to different color channel is inside $\zeta'$.

To demonstrate the concept, the ESM used in References [52] and [57] is described below. Employing a diamond-shape mask $\zeta = \{(r - 1, s), (r, s - 1), (r, s + 1), (r + 1, s)\}$ in Equation 16.1, the weights $w_{(i,j)}$ for $(i, j) \in \zeta$ are calculated using the original CFA components $z_{(i',j')}$ for $(i', j') \in \zeta'$ as follows (see Figure 16.15a):

$$w_{(r-1,s)} = 1/(1 + |z_{(r-2,s)} - z_{(r,s)}| + |z_{(r-1,s)} - z_{(r+1,s)}|)$$
$$w_{(r,s-1)} = 1/(1 + |z_{(r,s-2)} - z_{(r,s)}| + |z_{(r,s-1)} - z_{(r,s+1)}|)$$
$$w_{(r,s+1)} = 1/(1 + |z_{(r,s+2)} - z_{(r,s)}| + |z_{(r,s+1)} - z_{(r,s-1)}|) \tag{16.5}$$
$$w_{(r+1,s)} = 1/(1 + |z_{(r+2,s)} - z_{(r,s)}| + |z_{(r+1,s)} - z_{(r-1,s)}|)$$

Otherwise, a square-shape mask $\zeta = \{(r - 1, s - 1), (r - 1, s + 1), (r + 1, s - 1), (r + 1, s + 1)\}$ is considered, denoting the weights are obtained as follows (see Figure 16.15b):

$$w_{(r-1,s-1)} = 1/(1 + |z_{(r-2,s-2)} - z_{(r,s)}| + |z_{(r-1,s-1)} - z_{(r+1,s+1)}|)$$
$$w_{(r-1,s+1)} = 1/(1 + |z_{(r-2,s+2)} - z_{(r,s)}| + |z_{(r-1,s+1)} - z_{(r+1,s-1)}|)$$
$$w_{(r+1,s-1)} = 1/(1 + |z_{(r+2,s-2)} - z_{(r,s)}| + |z_{(r+1,s-1)} - z_{(r-1,s+1)}|) \tag{16.6}$$
$$w_{(r+1,s+1)} = 1/(1 + |z_{(r+2,s+2)} - z_{(r,s)}| + |z_{(r+1,s+1)} - z_{(r-1,s-1)}|)$$

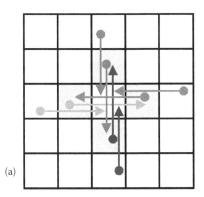 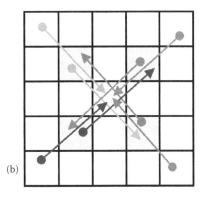

**FIGURE 16.15**
Neighborhood expansion concept depicted for the shape-masks: (a) $\zeta = \{(r-1,s), (r,s-1), (r,s+1), (r+1,s)\}$ (see Figure 16.13b, Figure 16.13d, and Figure 16.13e), and (b) $\zeta = \{(r-1,s-1), (r-1,s+1), (r+1,s-1), (r+1,s+1)\}$ (see Figure 16.13c).

At this point, it should be mentioned that although a significant research effort has been devoted to the development of various ESMs, the latest advances in camera image processing clearly indicate that high-quality camera images are obtained only if the edge-sensing camera image processing solution employs a proper SM [2], [53].

## 16.5 Spectral Model (SM)

In the camera image processing environment, spectral constraints relate to the utilization of the essential spectral characteristics of the captured image during the image interpolation process [52]. Based on the assumption that a typical natural image exhibits significant spectral correlation among its RGB color planes and spatial correlation among the neighboring pixels, a SM is used to support any interpolation operations performed in the single-sensor imaging pipeline.

Following the data-adaptive formula (Equation 16.1), the spectral characteristics of the two neighboring vectors $\mathbf{x}_{(i,j)}$ and $\mathbf{x}_{(r,s)}$ are incorporated into the interpolation process through the SM operator $\Psi(\mathbf{x}_{(i,j)}, \mathbf{x}_{(r,s)})$. If no spectral information is considered during processing, the spectral estimator in Equation 16.1 reduces to component-wise processing:

$$x_{(r,s)k} = \sum_{(i,j)\in\zeta} \{w'_{(i,j)}x_{(i,j)k}\} \tag{16.7}$$

where $x_{(\cdot,\cdot)k}$ denotes the $k$th components of the color vector $\mathbf{x}_{(\cdot,\cdot)}$. By omitting the essential spectral information, the component-wise solutions in References [38], [39], and [48] produce various color shifts and spectral artifacts.

### 16.5.1 Modeling Assumption

The rationale behind the SM construction can be easily explained using the basic characteristics of the color vectors. According to the tristimulus theory of color representation, the three-dimensional RGB vector $\mathbf{x}_{(r,s)} = [x_{(r,s)1}, x_{(r,s)2}, x_{(r,s)3}]^T$ is uniquely defined [8] by its length (magnitude) $M_{\mathbf{x}_{(r,s)}} = \|\mathbf{x}_{(r,s)}\| = \sqrt{x_{(r,s)1}^2 + x_{(r,s)2}^2 + x_{(r,s)3}^2}$ and orientation (direction) $D_{\mathbf{x}_{(r,s)}} = \mathbf{x}_{(r,s)}/\|\mathbf{x}_{(r,s)}\| = \mathbf{x}_{(r,s)}/M_{\mathbf{x}_{(r,s)}}$, where $\|D_{\mathbf{x}_{(r,s)}}\| = 1$ denotes the unit sphere defined in the vector space. Thus, any color image can be considered a vector field where each vector's direction and length are related to the pixel's color characteristics and significantly influence its perception by the human observer [8].

It is well known that natural images consist of small regions that exhibit similar, if not identical, color chromaticity properties [58], [59]. Because color chromaticity relates to the color vectors' directional characteristics determined using $D_{\mathbf{x}_{(\cdot,\cdot)}}$, it is reasonable to assume that two color vectors $\mathbf{x}_{(r,s)}$ and $\mathbf{x}_{(i,j)}$ occupying spatially neighboring locations $(r,s)$ and $(i,j)$ have the same chromaticity characteristics if they are collinear in the RGB color space [52]. Based on the definition of dot product $\mathbf{x}_{(r,s)}.\mathbf{x}_{(i,j)} = \|\mathbf{x}_{(r,s)}\|\|\mathbf{x}_{(i,j)}\|\cos(\langle\mathbf{x}_{(r,s)}, \mathbf{x}_{(i,j)}\rangle)$, where $\|\mathbf{x}_{(\cdot,\cdot)}\|$ denotes the length of $\mathbf{x}_{(\cdot,\cdot)}$ and $\langle\mathbf{x}_{(r,s)}, \mathbf{x}_{(i,j)}\rangle$ denotes the angle between three-component color vectors $\mathbf{x}_{(r,s)}$ and $\mathbf{x}_{(i,j)}$, the enforcement of orientation constraints via the SM operator $\Psi(\mathbf{x}_{(i,j)}, \mathbf{x}_{(r,s)})$ in Equation 16.1 implies that the following condition holds [52]:

$$\langle\mathbf{x}_{(r,s)}, \mathbf{x}_{(i,j)}\rangle = 0 \Leftrightarrow \frac{\sum_{k=1}^{3} x_{(r,s)k} x_{(i,j)k}}{\sqrt{\sum_{k=1}^{3} x_{(r,s)k}^2}\sqrt{\sum_{k=1}^{3} x_{(i,j)k}^2}} = 1 \tag{16.8}$$

Because both the magnitude and directional characteristics of the color vectors are essential for the human perception, the above concept should be extended by incorporating the magnitude information $M_{\mathbf{x}_{(\cdot,\cdot)}}$ into the modeling assumption. Using color vectors $\mathbf{x}_{(i,j)}$ and $\mathbf{x}_{(r,s)}$ as inputs to the so-called generalized vector SM [52], the underlying modeling principle of identical color chromaticity enforces that their linearly shifted variants $[\mathbf{x}_{(r,s)} + \gamma\mathbf{I}]$ and $[\mathbf{x}_{(i,j)} + \gamma\mathbf{I}]$ are collinear vectors:

$$\langle\mathbf{x}_{(r,s)} + \gamma\mathbf{I}, \mathbf{x}_{(i,j)} + \gamma\mathbf{I}\rangle = 0 \Leftrightarrow \frac{\sum_{k=1}^{3} (x_{(r,s)k} + \gamma)(x_{(i,j)k} + \gamma)}{\sqrt{\sum_{k=1}^{3} (x_{(r,s)k} + \gamma)^2}\sqrt{\sum_{k=1}^{3} (x_{(i,j)k} + \gamma)^2}} = 1 \tag{16.9}$$

where $\mathbf{I}$ is a unity vector of proper dimensions, and $x_{(\cdot,\cdot)k} + \gamma$ is the $k$th component of the linearly shifted vector $[\mathbf{x}_{(\cdot,\cdot)} + \gamma\mathbf{I}] = [x_{(\cdot,\cdot)1} + \gamma, x_{(\cdot,\cdot)2} + \gamma, x_{(\cdot,\cdot)3} + \gamma]^T$.

### 16.5.2 Advanced Design and Performance Characteristics

Through the parameter $\gamma$, the model controls the influence of both the directional and the magnitude characteristics of the neighboring vectors in the camera image processing. The scale shift introduced by the parameter $\gamma$ prevents color shifts in flat areas as well as near edge transitions. A number of processing solutions, with different design characteristics and performance, can thus be obtained by modifying the $\gamma$ parameter. The interested reader can find extensive analysis and experimentation, as well as detailed guidelines for the use of the vector SMs in the single-sensor imaging pipeline in Reference [52].

It is also proven in the same work [52] that the vector model defined over the two-dimensional vectors generalizes the previous SMs. Namely, for the parameter $\gamma = 0$, the vector SM reduces to

$$\frac{x_{(r,s)k}}{x_{(i,j)k}} = \frac{x_{(r,s)2}}{x_{(i,j)2}} \tag{16.10}$$

which implements the basic modeling assumption behind the color-ratio model [49]. Using the ratio values in Equation 16.10, the model enforces hue uniformity in localized image areas.

If $\gamma \to \infty$ is considered, the vector SM generalizes the color-difference model that implies uniform image intensity in localized image areas [50]. In this case, the modeling assumption of uniform image intensity is enforced by constraining the component-wise magnitude differences between spatially neighboring color vectors as follows [52]:

$$x_{(r,s)k} - x_{(i,j)k} = x_{(r,s)2} - x_{(i,j)2} \tag{16.11}$$

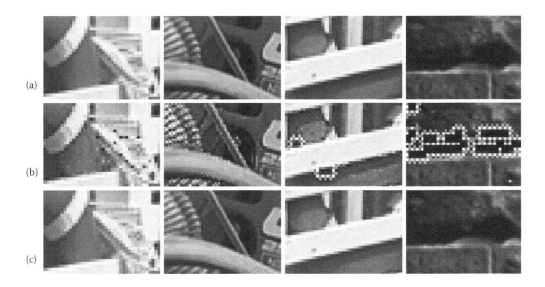

**FIGURE 16.16 (See color insert.)**
Performance improvements obtained by changing the SM: (a) original image, (b) Kimmel algorithm based on the color-ratio model (Kimmel, R., *IEEE Trans. on Image Process.*, 8, 1221, 1999), and (c) Kimmel algorithm based on the normalized color-ratio model (Lukac, R., and Plataniotis, K.N., *IEEE Trans. on Consumer Electron.*, 50, 737, 2004).

Finally, through the simple vectors' dimensionality reduction, the vector generalizes the normalized color-ratio model [51] defined as follows:

$$\frac{x_{(r,s)k} + \gamma}{x_{(i,j)k} + \gamma} = \frac{x_{(r,s)2} + \gamma}{x_{(i,j)2} + \gamma} \tag{16.12}$$

The model above enforces the basic modeling assumption of constant hue both near edge transitions and flat image areas, thus leading to the enhanced performance. For example, Figure 16.16a to Figure 16.16c show that the significant improvements of the visual quality are obtained when the color-ratio model is replaced in the well-known Kimmel demosaicking algorithm with the normalized color-ratio model [51]. Similar conclusions were drawn in Reference [2], where various SMs were tested using the different data-adaptive demosaicking solutions.

## 16.6 Demosaicking

As mentioned in Section 16.3, demosaicking is an integral and probably the most common processing step used in single-sensor digital cameras [2], [12]. The objective of the demosaicking process is to estimate the missing color components of the vectorial pixels $x_{(r,s)}$ obtained using the intermediate step described in Section 16.3.1 and to produce the demosaicked full-color image. Demosaicking performs spectral interpolation $x = f_\varphi(z)$ which transforms a $K_1 \times K_2$ grayscale image $z : Z^2 \rightarrow Z$ shown in Figure 16.9a to a $K_1 \times K_2$ three-channel, full-color image $x : Z^2 \rightarrow Z^3$ depicted in Figure 16.17a [24], [60].

It is well known [8], [43] that natural images are nonstationary due to the edges and fine details, a typical natural image exhibits significant (spectral) correlation among its RGB color planes, and the spatially neighboring pixels are usually highly correlated. Thus, by operating in small localized image areas, each of which can be treated as stationary, a camera

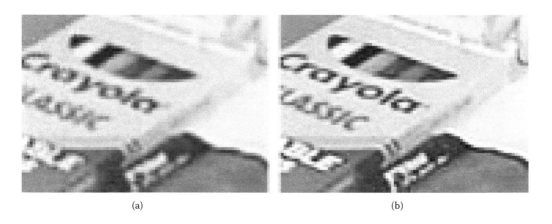

(a)                                                                                (b)

**FIGURE 16.17  (See color insert.)**
Demosaicking process: (a) restoration of the image shown in Figure 16.9a using the demosaicking solution and (b) image shown in Figure 16.17a enhanced using the demosaicked image postprocessor.

image processing solution can minimize local distortion in the output image by utilizing the spatial, structural, and spectral characteristics during processing. Reformulating the spectral interpolation function $f_\varphi(z)$ as $f_\varphi(\Lambda, \Psi, \zeta, z)$ with $z$ denoting the acquired CFA image and $\zeta$ determining the local neighborhood area (Figure 16.13b to Figure 16.13e), the performance of $f_\varphi(\cdot)$ critically depends on the choice of the ESM and SM operators $\Lambda$ and $\Psi$, respectively [2], [52]. As shown in Figure 16.18a to Figure 16.18d, the omission of any of the operators $\Lambda$ and $\Psi$ during demosaicking results in excessive blur, color shifts, and visible aliasing effects [53].

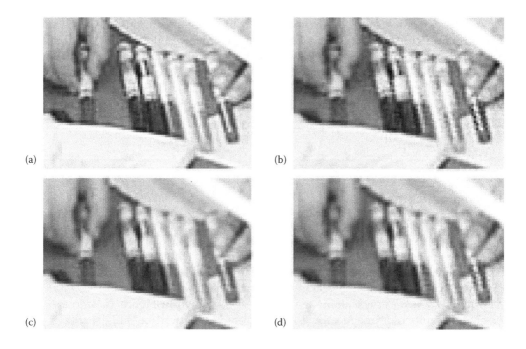

**FIGURE 16.18  (See color insert.)**
Influence of the ESM and SM on the quality of the demosaicked image: (a) used both ESM and SM, (b) omitted ESM, (c) omitted SM, and (d) omitted both ESM and SM.

## 16.6.1   Bayer CFA-Based Demosaicking

Because of the double number of G elements in the Bayer CFA (Figure 16.13a), the conventional practice is to start the demosaicking process by estimating the missing G components in the pixel array [2], [12], [42], [47]. Following the discussion in Section 16.3.1, the $(r, s)$ locations to be demosaicked are readily indicated by the corresponding location flags $d_{(r,s)k} = 0$, with $k = 2$ for the G components. In all such locations, the demosaicking solution updates the color vector $\mathbf{x}_{(r,s)}$ using the component-wise data-adaptive formula (Equation 16.7) with $k = 2$ denoting the G plane and $\zeta = \{(r - 1, s), (r, s - 1), (r, s + 1), (r + 1, s)\}$ indicating the available neighboring locations (Figure 16.13b).[5] At the same time, the solution also updates the location flag for $k = 2$ to $d_{(r,s)k} = 2$, differentiating between the original CFA locations $(d_{(r,s)k} = 1)$, the demosaicked locations $(d_{(r,s)k} = 2)$, and the locations to be demosaicked $(d_{(r,s)k} = 0)$. The procedure is repeated until a fully populated G plane is obtained (i.e., until all the location flags are set to $d_{(\cdot,\cdot)2} \neq 0$).

Because the above processing step makes the G components available at the R and B CFA locations, the missing R and B components can be demosaicked using the spectral model based formula (Equation 16.1). For example, by adopting the color difference model (Equation 16.11), the generalized spectral interpolator in Equation 16.1 is modified to demosaick the R $(k = 1)$ or B $(k = 3)$ component $x_{(r,s)k}$ occupying the location $(r, s)$ with $d_{(r,s)k} = 0$ as follows:

$$x_{(r,s)k} = x_{(r,s)2} + \sum\nolimits_{(i,j)\in\zeta} \left\{ w'_{(i,j)}(x_{(i,j)k} - x_{(i,j)2}) \right\} \tag{16.13}$$

where $\zeta = \{(r - 1, s - 1), (r - 1, s + 1), (r + 1, s - 1), (r + 1, s + 1)\}$ denotes the available locations as shown in Figure 16.13c. The procedure successively updates the flags to $d_{(r,s)k} = 2$ for $k = 1$ and $k = 3$ at each location $(r, s)$ that is being demosaicked via Equation 16.13. In the sequence, Equation 16.13 should be reapplied with $\zeta = \{(r - 1, s), (r, s - 1), (r, s + 1), (r + 1, s)\}$ shown in Figure 16.13d and Figure 16.13e to fully populate both the R and B channels. After demosaicking all available locations and updating all the corresponding flags for $k = 1$ and $k = 3$ to $d_{(\cdot,\cdot)k} \neq 0$, the demosaicking step produces a reconstructed color image, such as the one shown in Figure 16.17a.

If the higher visual quality is required (Figure 16.17b), then both the sharpness and coloration of the demosaicked image can be enhanced by employing a postprocessor in the processing pipeline [60], [61]. Because the postprocessing step can be viewed as a standalone solution, as demonstrated in Figure 16.7, the demosaicked image postprocessing (full-color image enhancement) related issues are discussed in Section 16.7.

## 16.6.2   Universal Demosaicking

By taking advantage of the CFA structure when the demosaicking solution is constructed, the solution becomes too dependent on the particular CFA used, such as the Bayer CFA (Figure 16.6a) in the procedure described above. The dependency mostly relates to the shape masks (Figures 16.13b to Figure 16.13e) and the form of the ESM used during the processing, and it significantly reduces, if not removes altogether, the flexibility of the solution to be employed in the pipeline equipped with a non-Bayer CFA. For instance, the traditional forms of the ESM listed in Reference [12] or the one described in Section 16.4.2, cannot be used in conjunction with the CFAs shown in Figure 16.6b to Figure 16.6h, because each subtraction operation in the gradient calculations requires the presence of the two components from the same color channel. To eliminate these drawbacks, a processing solution must be

---

[5] Some solutions, such as those presented in References [42], [52], [57], use the proper SM in support of this initial processing step to potentially reduce interpolation errors.

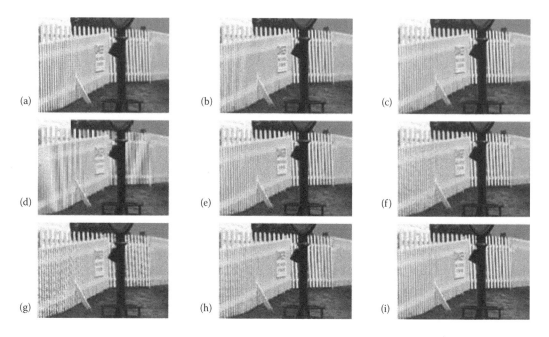

**FIGURE 16.19 (See color insert.)**
Influence of the CFA on the quality of the demosaicked image demonstrated using the same processing solution: (a–h) demosaicked image respectively corresponding to the RGB CFAs shown in Figure 16.6a to Figure 16.6h; and (i) original image.

independent from the arrangement of the color filters in the CFA. This constraint has been addressed in the framework first introduced and analyzed in Reference [22].

The framework employs a $3 \times 3$ sliding window instead of the specialized shape masks (Figure 16.13b to Figure 16.13e) known from the Bayer CFA-based demosaicking procedures. In addition, demosaicking the $k$th channel of the color image $\mathbf{x}$, the framework uses the control mechanism $\sum_{(i,j)\in\zeta} (d_{(i,j)k} = 1) \geq \chi$ over the demosaicking steps in Equation 16.7 and Equation 16.13 to prevent from operating in areas that lack adequate input information [22]. This control is obtained via the design parameter $\chi$ which denotes the minimum number of input values needed to be present when processing the $k$-th color channel in the local neighborhood $\zeta$. Note that the number of color components corresponding to particular color channels and their locations in the processing window vary not only between the CFAs, but often inside the CFA (e.g., for pseudo-random CFAs). Therefore, the framework tracks the structural image characteristics using the aggregation concept-based ESM in Equation 16.3, which obviously constitutes a flexible ESM. The interested reader can find the detailed description of the universal demosaicking framework in Reference [22].

Figure 16.19a to Figure 16.19i demonstrate that the choice of the CFA may be one of the most important factors in designing the single-sensor imaging pipeline [17]. Although the same processing solution has been employed to process the CFA image, results corresponding to the different CFAs differ significantly in terms of aliasing artifacts present in the demosaicked image.

## 16.7 Demosaicked Image Postprocessing

As mentioned in Section 16.6.1 and demonstrated in Figure 16.17a and Figure 16.17b, both the color appearance and the sharpness of the demosaicked image can be further improved by employing a postprocessor in the pipeline to localize and eliminate false colors and other impairments created during demosaicking [60], [61]. Postprocessing the demosaicked image is an optional step, implemented mainly in software and activated by the end user. It performs full color image enhancement $f_\eta(\Lambda, \Psi, \zeta, \mathbf{x})$, because the input of the solution is a fully restored RGB color image $\mathbf{x}$, and the output is an enhanced RGB color image. Unlike demosaicking, postprocessing can be applied iteratively until certain quality criteria are met.

Because there is no method to objectively determine whether or not a color component is inaccurate, the postprocessing framework should utilize the differences between the color components generated by a demosaicking solution and the original CFA components included in the restored color vector $\mathbf{x}_{(r,s)}$ of the demosaicked image $\mathbf{x}$ [60], [61]. If the demosaicked image postprocessing directly follows the demosaicking step in the imaging pipeline, then the location flag values updated during demosaicking to $d_{(r,s)k} = 2$ are restored to $d_{(r,s)k} = 0$, for $r = 1, 2, \ldots, K_1$, $s = 1, 2, \ldots, K_2$, and $k = 1, 2, 3$, to guide the demosaicked image postprocessing step. If the camera stores the demosaicked image, and the demosaicked image postprocessing is to be performed independently from the demosaicking step, then the proper location flags $d_{(r,s)k}$ can be obtained from the metadata information stored in the EXIF format. Finally, it should be mentioned that only the components obtained using the demosaicking process are enhanced by the postprocessing process (i.e., original CFA components are kept unchanged).

Following the Bayer CFA-based demosaicking procedure discussed in Section 16.6.1, postprocessing of the G color plane in all locations $(r, s)$ with the constraints $d_{(r,s)2} = 0$ can be realized using R or B components as follows [60]:

$$x_{(r,s)2} = x_{(r,s)k} + \sum_{(i,j) \in \zeta} \left\{ w'_{(i,j)}(x_{(i,j)2} - x_{(i,j)k}) \right\} \tag{16.14}$$

where $\zeta = \{(r-1, s), (r, s-1), (r, s+1), (r+1, s)\}$ denotes the available G CFA locations (Figure 16.13b). If $(r, s)$ corresponds to the R CFA location $(d_{(r,s)1} = 1)$, then the parameter $k = 1$ should be used in Equation 16.14. Otherwise, Equation 16.14 is used for the B CFA location $(d_{(r,s)3} = 1)$, and the pertinent parameter is $k = 3$. The weights $w'_{(i,j)}$ can be obtained in Equation 16.2 using an arbitrary ESM seen in the demosaicking literature, including ESMs discussed in Section 16.4.

After the G plane is enhanced, the postprocessing step is completed by enhancing the demosaicked R $(k = 1)$ and B $(k = 3)$ components using Equation 16.13, first with $\zeta = \{(r-1, s-1), (r-1, s+1), (r+1, s-1), (r+1, s+1)\}$ shown in Figure 16.13c and then with $\zeta = \{(r-1, s), (r, s-1), (r, s+1), (r+1, s)\}$ shown in Figure 16.13d and Figure 16.13e. This step is performed for R (or B) components only in locations corresponding to G and B (or G and R) CFA values, that is, $d_{(r,s)1} = 0$ (or $d_{(r,s)3} = 0$). The postprocessing process can lead to some significant improvements of the visual quality for most, if not all, demosaicking solutions (Figure 16.20a to Figure 16.20j) [60], [61]. The Bayer CFA-based postprocessing concepts can be easily extended using the control mechanisms described in Section 16.6.2 to complete the demosaicking process for an arbitrary CFA. Such a universal postprocessing solution was introduced in Reference [22].

## 16.8 Camera Image Zooming

Cost-effectiveness considerations in imaging-enabled mobile phones, surveillance, and automotive apparatus often lead to image outputs that do not have sufficient spatial resolution for subsequent image analysis tasks, such as object recognition and scene interpretation [62]. Therefore, digital image zooming is required. In addition, along with the demosaicking,

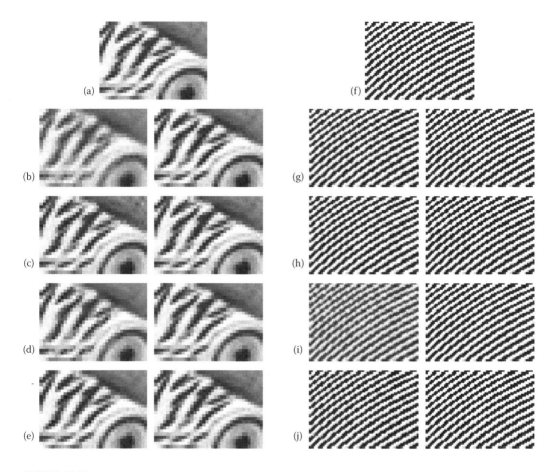

**FIGURE 16.20**
Demosaicked image postprocessing: (a,f) original images; (left) images demosaicked using the solutions presented in (b) Sakamoto, T., Nakanishi, C., and Hase, T., *IEEE Trans. on Consumer Electron.*, 44, 1342, 1998; (c) Kimmel, R., *IEEE Trans. on Image Process.*, 8, 1221, 1999; (d) Kakarala, R., and Baharav, Z., *IEEE Trans. on Consumer Electron.*, 48, 932, 2002; (e) Pei, S.C., and Tam, J.K., *IEEE Trans. on Circuits and Syst. for Video Technol.*, 13, 503, 2003; (g) Kehtarnavaz, N., Oh, H.J., and Yoo, Y., *J. Electron. Imaging*, 12, 621, 2003; (h) Hamilton, J.F., and Adams, J.E., U.S. Patent, 1997; (i) Sakamoto, T., Nakanishi, C., and Hase, T., *IEEE Trans. on Consumer Electron.*, 44, 1342, 1998; (j) Cai, C., Yu, T.H., and Mitra, S.K., *IEE Proceedings — Vision, Image, Signal Processing*, 2001; (right) the corresponding enhanced images obtained by the postprocessing method presented in Lukac, R., and Plataniotis, K.N., *Real-Time Imaging, Spec. Issue on Spectral Imaging II*, 11, 139, 2005.

image zooming is the most commonly performed processing operation in single-sensor digital cameras. Image zooming or spatial interpolation of a digital image is the process of increasing the number of pixels representing the natural scene [8], [63]. Unlike spectral interpolation (demosaicking) $f_\varphi(\cdot)$, spatial interpolation $f_\phi(\cdot)$ preserves the spectral representation of the input. Operating on the spatial domain of a digital image, spatial interpolation [24] transforms a color image $\mathbf{x}$ to an enlarged color image $\mathbf{x}' = f_\phi(\mathbf{x})$, or a grayscale image $z$ to an enlarged grayscale image $z' = f_\phi(z)$.

As shown in Figure 16.7, the spatial resolution of captured camera images can be increased by performing the spatial interpolation $f_\phi(\cdot)$ using the demosaicked image $\mathbf{x}$ (see Figure 16.21a), or the acquired, grayscale CFA image $z$ (see Figure 16.21b). The different order of demosaicking and zooming operations employed in the process significantly influences both the performance (Figure 16.22a to Figure 16.22c) and the cost of the processing pipeline [24], [62], although from the camera user's perspective, both cascades $f_\phi^\tau(f_\varphi(z))$ and

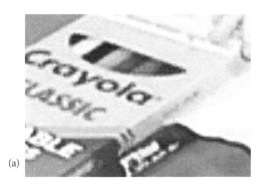 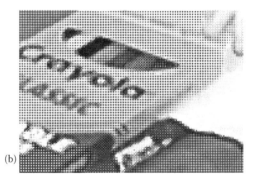

(a) (b)

**FIGURE 16.21**
Spatial interpolation: (a) demosaicked image zooming using the image shown in Figure 16.17b; (b) CFA image zooming using the image shown in Figure 16.9a.

$f_\varphi(f_\phi^\tau(z))$ transform a $K_1 \times K_2$ CFA image $z : Z^2 \to Z$ to an enlarged $\tau K_1 \times \tau K_2$ demosaicked image $\mathbf{x}' : Z^2 \to Z^3$, where $\tau \in Z$ is an integer zooming factor. Other differences result from the capability of a zooming solution to follow the structural content of the captured image and the way the essential spectral information is treated during the processing.

## 16.8.1 Spatial Interpolation of Demosaicked Images

Because the consumer-grade cameras conventionally store the image in the demosaicked full-color format, the spatial resolution of the captured image is most often increased using a color image zooming technique operating on the demosaicked RGB color vectors. For example, assuming the zooming factor $\tau = 2$, the zooming procedure maps the demosaicked

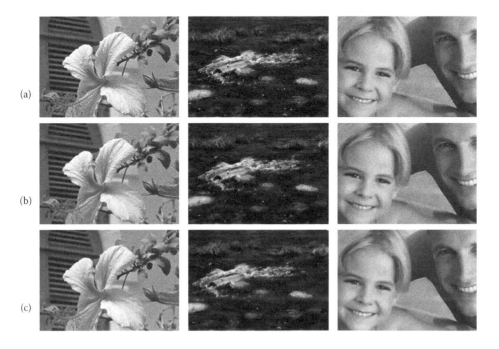

(a)

(b)

(c)

**FIGURE 16.22**
Camera image zooming: (a) original images, (b) demosaicking followed by demosaicked image zooming and (c) CFA image zooming followed by demosaicking.

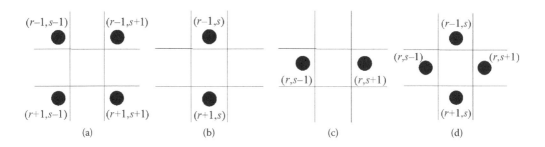

(a)  (b)  (c)  (d)

**FIGURE 16.23**
Demosaicked image zooming with a zooming factor $\tau = 2$. Spatial arrangements obtained by (a–c) mapping the demosaicked image $\mathbf{x}$ into the enlarged image $\mathbf{x}'$, (d) completing the spatial interpolation of $\mathbf{x}'$ using the pattern shown in part (a).

color vectors $\mathbf{x}_{(\cdot,\cdot)}$ into the enlarged image $\mathbf{x}'$ with the pixels $\mathbf{x}'_{(\cdot,\cdot)}$ using $\mathbf{x}'_{(2r-1,2s-1)} = \mathbf{x}_{(r,s)}$, with $r$ and $s$ denoting the spatial coordinates in the demosaicked image [64]. Thus, the pixels $\mathbf{x}'_{(2r,2s)}$ denote the new rows and columns (e.g., of zeros) added to the demosaicked image data $\mathbf{x}_{(r,s)}$, for $r = 1, 2, \ldots, K_1$, and $s = 1, 2, \ldots, K_2$.

The procedure produces the three pixel configurations shown in Figure 16.23a to Figure 16.23c [8], [64], however, configurations depicted in Figure 16.23b and Figure 16.23c lack the available components needed for faithful reconstruction of the enlarged image $\mathbf{x}'$ with the pixels $\mathbf{x}'_{(r,s)}$, for $r = 1, 2, \ldots, 2K_1$ and $s = 1, 2, \ldots, 2K_2$. Therefore, the procedure first interpolates the vector $\mathbf{x}'_{(r,s)}$ located in the center of the four available neighboring vectors $\{\mathbf{x}'_{(i,j)},$ for $(i, j) \in \zeta\}$ with $\zeta = \{(r - 1, s - 1), (r - 1, s + 1), (r + 1, s - 1), (r + 1, s + 1)\}$, as shown in Figure 16.23a. Then, all configurations become similar to the one depicted in Figure 16.23d, and the procedure interpolates the vector $\mathbf{x}'_{(r,s)}$ situated in the center of the four neighboring vectors $\{\mathbf{x}'_{(i,j)},$ for $(i, j) \in \zeta\}$ with $\zeta = \{(r - 1, s), (r, s - 1), (r, s + 1), (r + 1, s)\}$. The process results in the fully populated, enlarged color image $\mathbf{x}'$.

To date, the known color image spatial interpolation methods can be categorized into two classes [24]: component-wise solutions (Figure 16.11a) and vector solutions (Figure 16.11c).

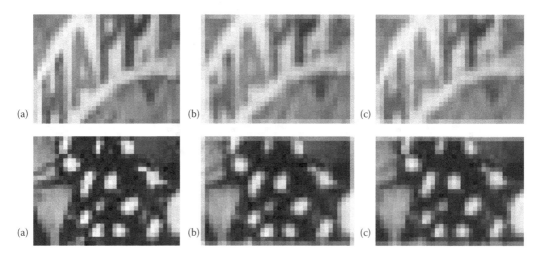

**FIGURE 16.24** (See color insert.)
Median filtering based spatial interpolation (R. Lukac, K.N. Plataniotis, B. Smolka, and A.N. Venetsanopulos, in *Proceedings of the IEEE International Symposium on Industrial Electronics*, III, 1273, 2005). The cropped patterns correspond to: (a) original (small) images, and (b, c) upsampled images obtained using (b) component-wise processing and (c) vector processing.

As shown in Figure 16.24a to Figure 16.24c, the same signal processing concept employed in both the component-wise and vector processing paradigms can lead to different visual quality of the enlarged images, especially in terms of color artifacts and zipper effects.

The component-wise zooming solutions, such as those presented in References [65], [66], and [67], process each color channel of the enlarged image $\mathbf{x}'$ separately, as follows :

$$x'_{(r,s)k} = f\left(\sum_{(i,j)\in\zeta} \{w'_{(i,j)}x'_{(i,j)k}\}\right) \tag{16.15}$$

where $x'_{(\cdot,\cdot)k}$ denotes the $k$th components (i.e., $k = 1$ for R, $k = 2$ for G, and $k = 3$ for B) of the color vector $\mathbf{x}'_{(\cdot,\cdot)}$ and $f(\cdot)$ is a nonlinear function that operates over the weighted average of the input components. The weights $w'_{(i,j)}$ calculated in Equation 16.2 can be obtained using the approaches described in the literature [68], [69], [70], [71]. Due to the component-wise nature of a zooming solution, the enlarged images obtained using Equation 16.15 often suffer from color shifts and artifacts [64]. Moreover, the lack of edge sensing combined with the omission of the spectral information during the processing often results in aliasing, edge burring, jagged lines, or blockiness [63].

Vector techniques process the available color pixels $\mathbf{x}'_{(i,j)}$ as a set of vectors:

$$\mathbf{x}'_{(r,s)} = f\left(\sum_{(i,j)\in\zeta} \{w'_{(i,j)}\mathbf{x}'_{(i,j)}\}\right) \tag{16.16}$$

thus preserving the spectral correlation of the enlarged image's color channels, reducing the presence of most color artifacts, and eliminating shifted color edges [64]. The most popular vector approaches are based on the theory of robust order statistics [8], [63], [64] and data-adaptive concepts [8], [64].

### 16.8.2 Spatial Interpolation of CFA Images

CFA image zooming solutions [24], [62], [72] constitute a novel way of spatial interpolation in single-sensor cameras. By using the zooming solution prior to the demosaicking solution (see Figure 16.7), the zooming approach prevents the amplifying of imperfections and visual impairments introduced in the demosaicking step [24]. Moreover, because the zooming operations are performed on the grayscale CFA image instead of the demosaicked full-color image, the CFA zooming approach is obviously computationally simple and attractive to be embedded in cost-effective devices, such as imaging-enabled mobile phones and pocket-size digital cameras.

The CFA zooming procedure first maps the CFA pixels $z_{(\cdot,\cdot)}$ into the enlarged grayscale image $z'$ with the pixels $z'_{(\cdot,\cdot)}$ and then interpolates the empty positions using the available values. From the first view, the procedure is similar to that used in demosaicked image zooming. However, it is shown in References [24] and [62] that the common mapping step $z'_{(2r-1,2s-1)} = z_{(r,s)}$ used in zooming the demosaicked image with a factor $\tau = 2$ discards the essential mosaic-like structure of the enlarged Bayer CFA image and prohibits the correct use of the demosaicking step. Therefore, zooming the CFA image requires the special, CFA-based approach that maps the CFA values $z_{(r,s)}$, with $r$ and $s$ denoting the spatial coordinates in the CFA image $z$ to $z'_{(2r-1,2s)} = z_{(r,s)}$ for $r$ odd and $s$ even, to $z'_{(2r,2s-1)} = z_{(r,s)}$ for $r$ even and $s$ odd, and $z'_{(2r-1,2s-1)} = z_{(r,s)}$ otherwise [62]. The remaining positions in the enlarged image $z'$ are filled in by zeros.

After the mapping step is completed (Figure 16.25a), the procedure continues by interpolating the pixels corresponding to G CFA locations using $z'_{(r,s)} = \sum_{(i,j)\in\zeta} \{w'_{(i,j)}z'_{(i,j)}\}$ in the two steps due to the lack of spatial information. Thus, $z'_{(r,s)}$ is the center of the four neighboring values $z'_{(i,j)}$ described first by $\zeta = \{(r - 2, s), (r, s - 2), (r, s + 2), (r + 2, s)\}$ depicted in Figure 16.25a, and then by $\zeta = \{(r - 1, s - 1), (r - 1, s + 1), (r + 1, s - 1), (r + 1, s + 1)\}$ in the updated image (Figure 16.25b).

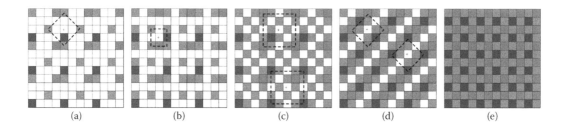

**FIGURE 16.25**
CFA image zooming: (a) mapping step using the CFA image $z$ shown in Figure 16.13a; (b–d) interpolation steps; and (e) enlarged CFA image $z'$.

By populating all G locations in the enlarged image $z'$, the obtained information along with the original CFA values can be used as the basis for the spectral-model-based interpolation operations used to populate R and B locations in the image $z'$. If the color-difference model in Equation 16.11 is employed, then the values corresponding to R locations in the image $z'$ can be obtained as follows:

$$z_{(r,s)} = z_{(r,s-1)} + \sum_{(i,j)\in\zeta} \left\{ w'_{(i,j)}(z'_{(i,j)} - z'_{(i,j-1)}) \right\} \tag{16.17}$$

whereas the values corresponding to B locations are obtained using

$$z_{(r,s)} = z_{(r-1,s)} + \sum_{(i,j)\in\zeta} \left\{ w'_{(i,j)}(z'_{(i,j)} - z'_{(i-1,j)}) \right\} \tag{16.18}$$

In both above equations, the values $z'_{(i,j-1)}$ and $z'_{(i-1,j)}$ represent the spatially shifted neighboring locations used to overcome the lack of spectral information in the locations $(i, j)$. Additional information about these spatial interpolation steps can be found in References [24] and [62]. The weights $w'_{(i,j)}$ in Equation 16.2 can be calculated using the concepts listed in Section 16.4.1. An overview of the other ESM solutions suitable for CFA zooming can be found in Reference [24].

By populating R and B CFA locations using Equation 16.17 and Equation 16.18, respectively, the procedure interpolates the center of the four $z'_{(i,j)}$ values described by $\zeta = \{(r-2, s-2), (r-2, s+2), (r+2, s-2), (r+2, s+2)\}$ shown in Figure 16.25c and then by $\zeta = \{(r-2, s), (r, s-2), (r, s+2), (r+2, s)\}$ in the updated image shown in Figure 16.25d. The process results in the enlarged, mosaic-like image $z'$ (see Figure 16.25e), which is a grayscale image similar to the one shown in Figure 16.21b.

## 16.9   Conclusion

The digital image processing operations that support digital cameras equipped with a color filter array placed on top of a single image sensor were the main focus of this chapter. These consumer-grade cameras capture the natural scene first by producing the grayscale, mosaic-like image, and then use extensive calculations based on the concept of image interpolation to output the full-color, visually pleasing image. Taking into consideration the way the structural content and the spectral characteristics of the captured image are treated during the processing, as well as the nature of the interpolation operations, the chapter provided a taxonomy of single-sensor camera image processing solutions.

Because the edges and fine details (i.e., structural content) are essential for image understanding, and color (i.e., spectral information) plays a significant role in the perception of edges or boundaries between two surfaces, data-adaptive spectral-model-based solutions were the main focus of the chapter. Building on the refined edge-sensing and spectral modeling principles, these solutions constitute a rich and expanding class of tools for demosaicking, demosaicked image postprocessing, and camera image zooming. By utilizing both the structural and spectral characteristics of the samples within the localized image area in cascaded sophisticated processing steps, the presented framework can overcome the spatial, structural, and spectral constraints imposed on the solution; produce sharp-looking, naturally colored camera images; and mimic the human perception of the visual environment.

As shown in this work, image interpolation operators based on the edge-sensing and spectral modeling principles constitute a basis for demosaicking that is the mandatory processing step in single-sensor imaging to obtain the full-color image. The same processing tools can be used to enhance the visual quality of the demosaicked image and to increase the spatial resolution of the captured images. Therefore, it is not difficult to see that single-sensor camera image processing techniques have an extremely valuable position in digital color imaging and will be essential for new-generation imaging-enabled consumer electronics as well as novel multimedia applications.

# References

[1] G. Sharma and H.J. Trussell, Digital color imaging, *IEEE Trans. on Image Process.*, 6(7), 901–932, July 1997.

[2] R. Lukac and K.N. Plataniotis, Data-adaptive filters for demosaicking: A framework, *IEEE Trans. on Consumer Electron.*, 51(2), 560–570, May 2005.

[3] J. Adams, K. Parulski, and K. Spaulding, Color processing in digital cameras, *IEEE Micro*, 18(6), 20–30, November 1998.

[4] P.L.P. Dillon, D.M. Lewis, and F.G. Kaspar, Color imaging system using a single CCD area array, *IEEE J. Solid-State Circuits*, 13(1), 28–33, February 1978.

[5] B.T. Turko and G.J. Yates, Low smear CCD camera for high frame rates, *IEEE Trans. on Nucl. Sci.*, 36(1), 165–169, February 1989.

[6] T. Lule, S. Benthien, H. Keller, F. Mutze, P. Rieve, K. Seibel, M. Sommer, and M. Bohm, Sensitivity of CMOS based imagers and scaling perspectives, *IEEE Trans. on Electron. Devices*, 47(11), 2110–2122, November 2000.

[7] A.J. Blanksby and M.J. Loinaz, Performance analysis of a color CMOS photogate image sensor, *IEEE Trans. on Electron. Devices*, 47(1), 55–64, January 2000.

[8] R. Lukac, B. Smolka, K. Martin, K.N. Plataniotis, and A.N. Venetsanopulos, Vector filtering for color imaging, *IEEE Signal Process. Mag.; Spec. Issue on Color Image Process.*, 22(1), 74–86, January 2005.

[9] R.F. Lyon and P.M. Hubel, Eying the camera: Into the next century, in *Proceedings of the IS&TSID Tenth Color Imaging Conference*, Scottsdale, AZ, November 2002, pp. 349–355.

[10] R.J. Guttosch, Investigation of Color Aliasing of High Spatial Frequencies and Edges for Bayer-Pattern Sensors and Foveon X3 Direct Image Sensor, Technical report, Foveon, San Antonio, TX, 2002.

[11] P.M. Hubel, J. Liu, and R.J. Guttosh, Spatial Frequency Response of Color Image Sensors: Bayer Color Filters and Foveon X3, Technical report ID 6502, Foveon, San Antonio, TX, March 2002.

[12] B.K. Gunturk, J. Glotzbach, Y. Altunbasak, R.W. Schaffer, and R.M. Murserau, Demosaicking: Color filter array interpolation, *IEEE Signal Process. Mag.*, 22(1), 44–54, January 2005.

[13] X. Wu and N. Zhang, Primary-consistant soft-decision color demosaicking for digital cameras, *IEEE Trans. on Image Process.*, 13(9), 1263–1274, September 2004.

[14] K. Parulski and K.E. Spaulding, *Digital Color Imaging Handbook*, ch. Color image processing for digital cameras, G. Sharma Ed., CRC Press, Boca Raton, FL, 2002, pp. 728–757.

[15] J. Holm, I. Tastl, L. Hanlon, and P. Hubel, *Colour Engineering: Achieving Device Independent Colour*, ch. Color processing for digital photography, P. Green and L. MacDonald Eds., Wiley, New York, 2002, pp. 179–220.

[16] R. Ramanath, W.E. Snyder, Y. Yoo, and M.S. Drew, Color image processing pipeline, *IEEE Signal Process. Mag.; Special Issue on Color Image Process.*, 22(1), 34–43, January 2005.

[17] R. Lukac and K.N. Plataniotis, Color filter arrays: Design and performance analysis, *IEEE Trans. on Consumer Electron.*, 51(4), 1260–1267, November 2005.

[18] FillFactory, Technology — Image Sensor: The Color Filter Array Faq, Technical report, Available at: www.fillfactory.com/htm/technology/htm/rgbfaq.htm.

[19] B.E. Bayer, Color imaging array, U.S. Patent 3 971 065, July 1976.

[20] S. Yamanaka, Solid state camera, U.S. Patent 4 054 906, November 1977.

[21] M. Parmar and S.J. Reeves, A perceptually based design methodology for color filter arrays, in *Proceedings of the IEEE International Conference on Acoustics, Speech, and Signal Processing (ICASSP'04)*, Montreal, Canada, Vol. 3, May 2004, pp. 473–476.

[22] R. Lukac and K.N. Plataniotis, Universal demosaicking for imaging pipelines with an RGB color filter array, *Patt. Recognition*, 38(11), 2208–2212, November 2005.

[23] B. Gunturk, Y. Altunbasak, and R. Mersereau, Color plane interpolation using alternating projections, *IEEE Trans. on Image Process.*, 11(9), 997–1013, September 2002.

[24] R. Lukac, K.N. Plataniotis, and D. Hatzinakos, Color image zooming on the Bayer pattern, *IEEE Trans. on Circuit and Syst. for Video Technol.*, 15(11), 1475–1492, November 2005.

[25] M. Stokes, M. Anderson, S. Chandrasekar, and R. Motta, A Standard Default Color Space for the Internet–sRGB, Technical report (www.w3.org/Graphics/Color/sRGB.html), 1996.

[26] T.S.C. on AV & IT Storage Systems and Equipment, Exchangeable Image File Format for Digital Still Cameras: Exif Version 2.2, Technical report JEITA CP-3451, Japan Electronics and Information Technology Industries Association, April 2002.

[27] Technical Committee ISO/TC 42, Photography, "Electronic still picture imaging—Removable memory, Part 2: Image data format—TIFF/EP," ISO 12234-2, January 2001.

[28] Y.T. Tsai, Color image compression for single-chip cameras, *IEEE Trans. on Electron Devices*, 38(5), 1226–1232, May 1991.

[29] T. Toi and M. Ohita, A subband coding technique for image compression in single CCD cameras with Bayer color filter arrays, *IEEE Trans. on Consumer Electron.*, 45(1), 176–180, February 1999.

[30] C.C. Koh, J. Mukherjee, and S.K. Mitra, New efficient methods of image compression in digital cameras with color filter array, *IEEE Trans. on Consumer Electron.*, 49(4), 1448–1456, November 2003.

[31] S. Battiato, A.R. Bruna, A. Buemi, and A. Castorina, Analysis and characterization of JPEG 2000 standard for imaging devices, *IEEE Trans. on Consumer Electron.*, 49(4), 773–779, November 2003.

[32] X. Xie, G.L. Li, X.W. Li, D.M. Li, Z.H. Wang, C. Zhang, and L. Zhang, A new approach for near-lossless and lossless image compression with Bayer color filter arrays, in *Proceedings of the Third International Conference on Image and Graphics (ICIG'04)*, Hong Kong, China, December 2004, pp. 357–360.

[33] A. Bazhyna, A. Gotchev, and K. Egiazarian, Near-lossless compression algorithm for Bayer pattern color filter arrays, in *Proceedings of the SPIE-IS&T Electronic Imaging*, Vol. SPIE 5678, 2005, pp. 198–209.

[34] R. Lukac and K.N. Plataniotis, Fast video demosaicking solution for mobile phone imaging applications, *IEEE Trans. on Consumer Electron.*, 51(2), 675–681, May 2005.

[35] L. Zhang, X. Wu, and P. Bao, Real-time lossless compression of mosaic video sequences, *Real-Time Imaging; Spec. Issue on Multi-Dimensional Image Process.*, 11(5–6), 370–377, October–December 2005.

[36] R. Lukac and K.N. Plataniotis, Digital image indexing using secret sharing schemes: A unified framework for single-sensor consumer electronics, *IEEE Trans. on Consumer Electron.*, 51(3), 908–916, August 2005.

[37] R. Lukac and K.N. Plataniotis, A new approach to CFA image indexing, *Lecture Notes in Comput. Sci.*, 3691, 137–144, September 2005.

[38] T. Sakamoto, C. Nakanishi, and T. Hase, Software pixel interpolation for digital still cameras suitable for a 32-bit MCU, *IEEE Trans. on Consumer Electron.*, 44(4), 1342–1352, November 1998.

[39] P. Longere, X. Zhang, P.B. Delahunt, and D.H. Brainard, Perceptual assessment of demosaicing algorithm performance, *Proceedings of the IEEE*, 90(1), 123–132, January 2002.

[40] D. Alleysson, S. Susstrunk, and J. Herault, Linear demosaicing inspired by the human visual system, *IEEE Trans. on Image Process.*, 14(4), 439–449, April 2005.

[41] W.T. Freeman, Median Filter for Reconstructing Missing Color Samples, U.S. Patent 4 724 395, February 1988.

[42] S.C. Pei and I.K. Tam, Effective color interpolation in CCD color filter arrays using signal correlation, *IEEE Trans. on Circuits and Syst. for Video Technol.*, 13(6), 503–513, June 2003.

[43] K.N. Plataniotis and A.N. Venetsanopoulos, *Color Image Processing and Applications*, Springer-Verlag, Heideberg, 2000.

[44] O. Faugeras, Digital color image processing within the framework of a human visual model, *IEEE Trans. on Acoustics, Speech, and Signal Process.*, 27(4), 380–393, August 1979.

[45] R. Kimmel, Demosaicing: Image reconstruction from color CCD samples, *IEEE Trans. on Image Process.*, 8(9), 1221–1228, September 1999.

[46] R. Lukac, K.N. Plataniotis, D. Hatzinakos, and M. Aleksic, A novel cost effective demosaicing approach, *IEEE Trans. on Consumer Electron.*, 50(1), 256–261, February 2004.

[47] W. Lu and Y.P. Tang, Color filter array demosaicking: New method and performance measures, *IEEE Trans. on Image Process.*, 12(10), 1194–1210, October 2003.

[48] R. Ramanath, W.E. Snyder, G.L. Bilbro, and W.A. Sander III, Demosaicking methods for Bayer color arrays, *J. Electron. Imaging*, 11(3), 306–315, July 2002.

[49] D.R. Cok, Signal processing method and apparatus for producing interpolated chrominance values in a sampled color image signal, U.S. Patent 4 642 678, February 1987.

[50] J. Adams, Design of practical color filter array interpolation algorithms for digital cameras, in *Proceedings of the SPIE*, Vol. 3028, February 1997, pp. 117–125.

[51] R. Lukac and K.N. Plataniotis, Normalized color-ratio modeling for CFA interpolation, *IEEE Trans. on Consumer Electron.*, 50(2), 737–745, May 2004.

[52] R. Lukac and K.N. Plataniotis, A vector spectral model for digital camera image processing, *IEEE Trans. on Circuit and Syst. for Video Technol.*, submitted.

[53] R. Lukac and K.N. Plataniotis, On a generalized demosaicking procedure: A taxonomy of single-sensor imaging solutions, *Lecture Notes in Comput. Sci.*, 3514, 687–694, May 2005.

[54] R. Lukac, K. Martin, and K.N. Plataniotis, Digital camera zooming based on unified CFA image processing steps, *IEEE Trans. on Consumer Electron.*, 50(1), 15–24, February 2004.

[55] K.N. Plataniotis, D. Androutsos, and A.N. Venetsanopoulos, Adaptive fuzzy systems for multichannel signal processing, *Proceedings of the IEEE*, 87(9), 1601–1622, September 1999.

[56] N. Kehtarnavaz, H.J. Oh, and Y. Yoo, Color filter array interpolation using color correlations and directional derivatives, *J. Electron. Imaging*, 12(4), 621–632, October 2003.

[57] L. Chang and Y.P. Tang, Effective use of spatial and spectral correlations for color filter array demosaicking, *IEEE Trans. on Consumer Electron.*, 50(2), 355–365, May 2004.

[58] B. Tang, G. Sapiro, and V. Caselles, Color image enhancement via chromaticity diffusion, *IEEE Trans. on Image Process.*, 10(5), 701–707, May 2001.

[59] P.E. Trahanias, D. Karakos, and A.N. Venetsanopoulos, Directional processing of color images: Theory and experimental results, *IEEE Trans. on Image Process.*, 5(6), 868–881, June 1996.

[60] R. Lukac and K.N. Plataniotis, A robust, cost-effective postprocessor for enhancing demosaicked camera images, *Real-Time Imaging, Spec. Issue on Spectral Imaging II*, 11(2), 139–150, April 2005.

[61] R. Lukac, K. Martin, and K.N. Plataniotis, Demosaicked image postprocessing using local color ratios, *IEEE Trans. on Circuit and Syst. for Video Technol.*, 14(6), 914–920, June 2004.

[62] R. Lukac and K.N. Plataniotis, Digital zooming for color filter array based image sensors, *Real-Time Imaging, Spec. Issue on Spectral Imaging II*, 11(2), 129–138, April 2005.

[63] N. Herodotou and A.N. Venetsanopoulos, Colour image interpolation for high resolution acquisition and display devices, *IEEE Trans. on Consumer Electron.*, 41(4), 1118–1126, November 1995.

[64] R. Lukac, K.N. Plataniotis, B. Smolka, and A.N. Venetsanopulos, Vector operators for color image zooming, in *Proceedings of the IEEE International Symposium on Industrial Electronics (ISIE'05)*, Dubrovnik, Croatia, Vol. III, June 2005, pp. 1273–1277.

[65] R.G. Keys, Cubic convolution interpolation for digital image processing, *IEEE Trans. on Acoustics, Speech and Signal Process.*, 29(6), 1153–1160, December 1981.

[66] R.R. Schultz and R.L. Stevenson, A Bayessian approach to image expansion for improved definition, *IEEE Trans. on Acoustics, Speech and Image Process.*, 3(3), 233–242, May 1994.

[67] S.E. Reichenbach and F. Geng, Two-dimensional cubic convolution, *IEEE Trans. on Image Process.*, 12(8), 857–865, August 2003.

[68] K. Jenseen and D. Anastasiou, Subpixel edge localization and interpolation of still images, *IEEE Trans. on Image Process.*, 4(3), 285–295, March 1995.

[69] S. Thurnhofer and S.K. Mitra, Edge-enhanced image zooming, *Opt. Eng.*, 35(7), 1862–1869, July 1996.

[70] A.M. Darwish, M.S. Bedair, and S.I. Shaheen, Adaptive resampling algorithm for image zooming, *IEE Proceedings — Vision, Image, Signal Processing*, 144(4), 207–212, August 1997.

[71] J.W. Hwang and H.S. Lee, Adaptive image interpolation based on local gradient features, *IEEE Signal Process. Lett.*, 11(3), 359–362, March 2004.

[72] S. Battiato, G. Gallo, and F. Stanco, A locally adaptive zooming algorithm for digital images, *Image and Vision Computing*, 20(11), 805–812, September 2002.

# 17

## Spectral Imaging and Applications

Matthias F. Carlsohn, Bjoern H. Menze, B. Michael Kelm, Fred A. Hamprecht,
Andreas Kercek, Raimund Leitner, and Gerrit Polder

## CONTENTS

## 17.1 Introduction to Spectral Imaging (SI)

Many algorithms are taken from gray-value image processing to deal with color as an additional visual feature for many purposes, however, exceptions have to be regarded. Exploitation of spectral information beyond color needs a generalized view onto the underlying principles extending three color components up to a hundred or more spectral channels in different spectral bands. Although still a large potential for reuse of those methods and algorithms is given, spectral images need particular treatment. This is demonstrated in applications such as waste sorting, medical imaging, and measuring of biochemicals for the entire processing chain from calibration to classification due to the nature of imaging by dedicated sensors in particular spectral ranges.

Spectral imaging is a new and emerging field of applied computer science composed from image processing and spectroscopy. Image processing describes visual information in terms of spatial coordinates and luminance of pixels (intensity), providing additional dimensionality either by depth (three-dimensional [3-D]), time (image sequences), or color (red, green, blue [RGB]) to achieve a representation that is as close to the original scene as necessary with respect to the inspection tasks that have to be performed. The amount of data a system can deal with usually restricts the number of dimensions that can finally be involved. All referred dimensions describe information that can be derived visually by appropriate sensors that optically capture luminance information in the visible range of the electromagnetic spectrum, enabling description of a scene in terms of spatial dimensions like form and shape, surface features as texture and color, movements of objects and their mutual spatial relation in the depth of the 3-D space. Information about the chemical composition of solid objects, the ingredients of chemical compounds or biochemical states of plants cannot be retrieved from previously described imaging of a scene in the visual spectrum. Those indications can only be derived involving information from an extended spectral range in the invisible electromagnetic spectrum (i.e., either from the ultraviolet or the infrared range of the spectrum. The first problem is that typical camera sensors are "blind" with respect to those radiations, because they are insensible (i.e., their sensitivity is very low so that photons emitted in this range neither contribute significantly to the generated image intensity related currents nor do they allow any particular discrimination of specific object properties. The modulation transfer function (MTF) of the sensor determines the weighting of single spectral components to the luminance value of a particular pixel. What we finally see is an integration over spectral components. A discrimination associated with particular properties of the object is no longer possible. In order to achieve a spectral sensitivity of spectral frequency and space, spectral decomposition and additional storage requirements are needed as prerequisites. Spectral decomposition of the light beam can be achieved by involving a dispersive element consisting of a combination of prism, grating, and a second prism. This equipment provides splitting of the light beam into a fan of spectral components, diffraction of these depending on their representing wavelength and recombination of the diffracted light onto a sensor strip for discrete capturing of the particular spectral components.

Current techniques offer two basic approaches to spectral imaging. The first acquires a sequence of two-dimensional images at different wavelengths. This can be implemented by employing a rotating filter wheel or a tunable filter in front of a monochrome camera [1], [2]. The second approach acquires a sequence of line images where for each pixel on the line a complete spectrum is captured. This approach requires an imaging spectrograph [3], [4] coupled to a monochrome matrix camera. One dimension of the camera (spatial axis) records the line pixels and the other dimension (spectral axis) the spectral information for each pixel. To acquire a complete spectral image, either the object, or the spectrograph, needs to be translated in small steps, until the whole object has been scanned.

### 17.1.1 Spectral Imaging as a Generalization of Color Imaging

"Classical" image processing for industrial scene understanding usually exploits luminance information using single shots of gray-scale still images, stereo information from multiple cameras, or spatiotemporal characteristics of image sequences. Color is the supplementary dimension for discrimination of objects by selective features. However, many methods originally developed for gray-value image processing can be applied to multicolor data arrays, although some specific principles have to be regarded with respect to the sensors capturing the data (e.g., single or multichip CCD or CMOS cameras), the illumination (by different color temperature and spectral characteristics), and the color representation system used (RGB, YUV, IHS, or Lab) in which the spectrum is decomposed. Especially in cases where color is used as a major discriminating feature, one has to check if additional information introduced by color is nonredundant and justifies the blow-up of the data amount requiring data reduction and binning of spectral bands afterwards. Alternatively, one should check how spectral bands beyond the visible (VIS) range have the potential to contribute additional information that cannot be gathered otherwise from the VIS range. In principle, SI is an extension of the number of bands subsuming the spectral range from the visible into the invisible bands toward ultraviolet (UV) or infrared (IR) and near-infrared (NIR), and so forth, as visualized in Figure 17.4. Although some researchers working in the field of SI would like to claim this definition exclusively, contributions also dealing with pure color images in the VIS range making use of three spectral channels only (e.g., RGB) can be subsumed as special cases of SI, applying the same methods and principles to few color components only. Initially, multiband spectral data processing was reserved for very few applications, like remote sensing or military surveillance. In the early and mid-1980s, scientists worked on combined spectral–spatial classifiers, in most cases for the analysis of earth observational data. Examples are the ECHO classifier from Kettig and Landgrebe [5], [6], contextual classification from Swain et al. [7] and from Kittler and Föglein [8]. Related defense or space projects usually exceed any industrial or medical budget by orders. Consequently, Figure 17.1 provides a tentative list of technologies and applications focused only on industrial affordable budget levels showing how SI contributes by different imaging principles, spectral ranges, and technologies involved in a wide scope of production fields and sectors for machine vision applications ranging from quality control to chemometry, in order to derive either process decisions or to take quantitative measurements.

The different views on the definition of what SI finally could be is also mirrored in the different contributions of this chapter on spectral imaging. Spectral imaging is progressing well into various application fields, proceeding to mature to allow real-time performance in industrial, agricultural, and environmental applications, where the ratio of price and user benefit defines the commercial margins for successful take-up. This breakthrough has been enabled by the improvements because of developments in novel optical equipment such as Specim's ImSpector[1] [9]. In medical applications, magnetic resonance spectroscopic imaging (MRSI) provides a patient-centric view, and a quite different definition of user benefit lowers the demand for real-time performance compared to typical industrial cycle times for inspection and another calculations based on equipment and connected inspection costs.

### 17.1.1.1 *Time Constraints in SI*

In addition to the major differences in SI applications presented in the subsequent paragraphs and the particular methods used to generate the spectral data, the time requirements that have to be met differ by orders. The harder the real-time constraints given by the application, the faster the standard video speed compliant equipment has to be — give already

---

[1] Imaging spectrograph by Specim, Spectral Imaging Oy Ltd., Oulu, Finland.

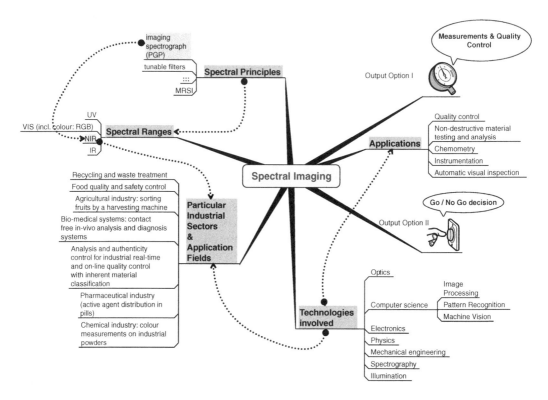

**FIGURE 17.1**
Mind map of spectral imaging.

the preselection for the applied SI principle. The case studies presented here show a significant decrease in real-time demands on one hand, while inspection costs are shown to be inversely proportional (i.e., for waste sorting, quantification of tomato ripeness and brain tumor detection and classification). These differences in real-time performance and cost margins result, on one hand, from the amount of cheap off-the-shelf components that can be used and, on the other hand, from the amount of expensive hardware engineered for boosting processes according to the real-time requirements. This shows a typical dilemma of emergency: medical applications have a patient-centric value scale — processing time and costs can be high, while waste sorting demands for high throughput of the specimen. The food industry is not as quality sensible as the medical sector, but inspection time is as short as in the second case. Answering the question of how ripe is this tomato is not as safety relevant as the decision between benign or malignant brain tissue.

### 17.1.1.2   *The Imaging Principle of SI*

Illuminating one particular SI principle for general consideration in subsequent SI data processing, a combination of geometrical optics and diffractions lead to the ImSpector, a dispersive optical component, which consists of a prism–grating–prism (PGP) arrangement that splits the light of an object-line (1-D row) into its spectral bands, as depicted in Figure 17.2. The second spatial dimension will be generated by moving either the target or the inspection unit perpendicular to the projected object line.

C-mounted between the lens and the CCD camera, this setup generates a spectrophotometer that delivers a new dimension in contact-free inspection techniques beyond simple

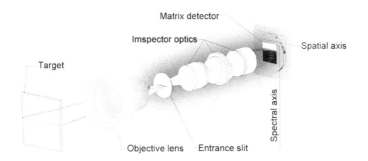

**FIGURE 17.2**

The ImSpector imaging spectrograph showing also the simultaneous spatial (line) and spectral mapping with an area detector. (Courtesy of SPECIM, Spectral Imaging Oy Ltd., Oulu, Finland.)

visual analysis. In addition to spatial features like form, size, position, orientation, or surface properties, such as texture, supplementary spectral data can be exploited for analyzing ingredients and chemical components (i.e., spectral imaging captures both spatial and spectral properties of the specimen). Unfortunately, this leads to an increase in the dimensionality of data that have to be compensated for by data reduction methods or binning of adjacent spectral bands or sophisticated selections techniques in the feature space [10].

### 17.1.1.3 Imaging Techniques in SI

In addition to a couple of alternative imaging techniques for recording full spectral range assigned to each pixel position of an image (forming a data hypercube in the case of SI), two major methods have to be emphasized for industrial applications due to a reasonable recording time and additional constraints given by the cooperating movement behavior of the objects that have to be inspected: either wavelength scanning of so-called "staring imagers" or spatial scanning often referred to as the "push-broom" principle takes place. While the first method records both spatial dimensions simultaneously, subsequent acquisition of spectral bands (e.g., by the use of discrete wavelength filters, particular illumination systems, or by tunable filters), strictly demands a "stop-motion requirement" that inhibits the use of this principle for many applications that inherently have to transport the samples during the inspection process (e.g., by conveyer belts in sorting applications). Although real-time operability is possible, it remains limited by the necessary time consumption that is proportional to the spectral resolution in this case. This limitation can be overcome if one replaces the "staring imager" with a "push-broom recorder." Although the hypercube containing the spectral data intensities should finally be the same as applying the previous recording scheme, the stop-motion requirement can be neglected, exploiting the transport movement of the specimen across the inspection unit via a conveyor belt for recording the second spatial dimension. This imager acquires at any time shot of a picture for all pixels in the first spatial dimension the full spectral range defined by the specified operational range of the dispersive element. Depending on the application in mind, the spectral range has to be carefully selected: UV or VIS (200 to 800 nm) for fluorescence imaging or color imaging with full spectral information compared to simple RGB. The near-infrared (800 to 2500 nm) enables material classification and quantification by its good material specificity and an average sensitivity. Spectrometers operating in the mid-infrared range (2500 to 25,000 nm) improve analysis of structure-specific classification and quantification by excellent material specificity and a good sensitivity. It has to be mentioned that similar to machine vision, the generation of important information by an appropriate illumination can

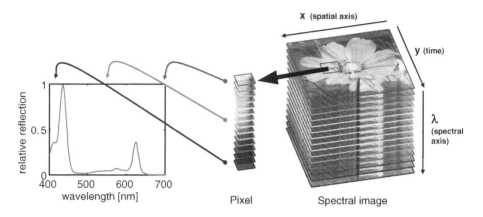

**FIGURE 17.3**
Volume element of the spectral imaging hypercube representing the full spectral range of one single pixel position.

at least simplify and sometimes just enable a reasonable data analysis. Consequently, the SI acquisition mode has to be carefully selected among diffuse reflection, transmission, or different options of transflectance modes using a reflective sample support plus alternative variations in possible illuminations w.r.t. illumination and viewing angles [11].

Recording image data by an aforementioned setup involving a CCD-array camera as a detector, the optical lens projects object reflections as dispersed light via the PGP-device and the slit of the aperture onto the sensor grid. Spatial data parallel to the slit are registered along the $x$-axis of the detector array, while the spectral bands of the dispersed light are recorded along the $y$-axis. Up to this stage of processing, the resulting sensor system could be denoted as a line camera providing full spectral information in each pixel of its line, delivering the spatial and spectral coincidence simultaneously. Moving either the object with respect to the spectral imaging system setup or a spectral imaging system setup with respect to the object perpendicular to the slit allows for the second spatial dimension to be recorded over time into a third dimension of a data array (data cube, see Figure 17.3). Data values represent spectral intensities as the fourth dimension in this hypercube representation, considerably increasing the volume of data compared to conventional gray-value or color-value image processing.

Of course, objects, illumination, and sensors have to be selected and adapted to each other carefully for a particular spectral analysis. Coherent calibration of the setup and normalization of data demand particular adaptation to the task and environmental conditions. Classification of spectral data has to address the extra dimensional semantics of the feature space and has to deal with various problems dedicated to the physical character of the acquired data [10].

This chapter deals with approaches to solve problems ranging from particular recycling of plastic via agricultural applications to medical applications. Classification methods for cellulose-based materials such as pulp, paper, and cardboard could be discussed in the same manner as hardware requirements for industrial use as in the presented plastic sorting application by SI, including adjustment and calibration techniques [12]. Classical color image signal processing can also be embedded in the field of spectral imaging. Unfortunately, in this chapter, we can only spot some aspects of this new and emerging field of spectral imaging applications. This chapter comprises the subject dealing with image spectra in quite different ways that can be clustered due to applications, the spectral bands, and imaging principles used.

**B/W imaging**

One broad spectral band

**RGB color imaging**

Three broad bands
(colors)

**Spectral imaging**

Tnes or hundreds of
narrow spectral bands

**FIGURE 17.4**

Migration from gray value via color imaging to spectral imaging. (Courtesy of SPECIM, Spectral Imaging Oy Ltd.,
Oulu, Finland.)

### 17.1.1.4  SI as Migration from Color Imaging

Emphasizing the focus of the textbook, spectral imaging can be seen either as a generalized processing of color images with a number of channels much larger than three or as
a migration of involving color as a feature for progressing qualification of discrimination
performance. Starting from three-component RGB color space, a migration to SI can be
performed by involving more than three color filters or tunable filters. The principle migration from gray-value image processing to full spectral range as an extension of color
(e.g., RGB) resolution is visualized in Figure 17.4. Plastic sorting is the best example for
the migration, involving principles of all fields (i.e., color processing, spectral imaging, and
pattern recognition).

### 17.1.1.5  Considerations for Practical Setup of SI Systems

All three applications presented here show common features in the processing chain. However, a certain amount of application-specific adaptation, calibration, and normalization
always takes place. This shows the level of engineering that still has to be involved, in
general, influencing the costs considerably.

Raw image data usually has to be preprocessed by well-known image processing methods
as standardization by dark current subtraction and ("white") reference scaling. Normalization and calibration of data are explained in more detail in the following paragraph by an
explicit example, as it is data reduction by "channel and range" selection, global binning
of redundant channels and data, and dimensionality reduction retaining only a few principle components in a PCA while preserving the major signal variance (energy). Gradient
operators can also be applied to spectral images to emphasize structures by generating first-
and second-order derivatives in appropriate intersections of the hypercube. Depending on
the computational performance and the remaining data amount of the spectral hypercube,
evaluation of data either has to be performed off-line or can be applied in real-time [11],
as the quality of data evaluation can range from qualitative classification to semiquantita-
tive analysis (classification). Finally, postprocessing of data for visualization or a simplified
interpretation by men and machines could be necessary. While off-line analysis can make
use of a wide range of possible algorithms, information recovery can be achieved to a
(semi-)optimal level on one hand.

Real-time constraints typically limit the choice of appropriate classifiers, which limits
the information that can be extracted proportionally fast, considering that 10 to 20 ms is
a typical time slot for full processing of one spectral line image (First spatial dimension
only). Adaptation and selection of classification schemes for a particular type of specimen
is of great importance into implementing a real-time classification system. More detailed
insight is given in Reference [11], and concrete examples are provided by the following
case studies: waste sorting, ripeness analysis of tomatoes, and brain inspection by MRSI.
In addition to the examples given in this chapter, it is evident that for other applications,
like, for example, distribution analysis and dissolution studies (in water or gastric juice)

for pharmaceutical products, the implementation could hardly be done online by alternative methods with comparable real-time performance. Similar examples can be given for nondestructive genuine control of semiprecious or material analysis of either surface coatings or in the examination of material behavior of interface reactions of diffusing processes between boundaries of different materials [11].

Next to imaging spectrographs, or tunable filters, other spectral imaging sensors exist (e.g., in magnetic resonance imaging [MRI]. These sensors make use of other physical principles to generate spectral imaging data sets. However, similar pattern recognition methods as the previous ones can be applied, which is described more generally in the following paragraph. Their application to MR-based spectral imaging for the medical sector is presented in Section 17.2.3.

### 17.1.2   Analysis of Spectral Images

All methods for data analysis, including those for spectral imagery, can be broadly classified into three groups, ordered by the amount of prior knowledge that is required:

- Visualization
- Unsupervised learning
- Supervised learning

*Visualization* is an important first step when confronted with a data set of unknown characteristics. In an RGB image, each pixel is associated with three scalar values. Accordingly, and disregarding spatial context for the time being, each pixel can be represented by a point in three-dimensional space. If we plot a point for each pixel in the image, we get a so-called "scatter plot." If the image consists, for instance, of two regions with distinct colors, one expects to observe two distinct clouds of points in the scatter plot. As the complexity of an image increases and as regions slowly change their color over space, the scatter plot becomes more complex and is less easily interpreted. If an image is recorded using four instead of three spectral channels, it becomes less straightforward to produce a scatter plot: we simply cannot plot points in four dimensions. One possible approach is to show only lower-dimensional projections of the point cloud (e.g., plot spectral channels 1 versus 2, 1 versus 3, 1 versus 4, 2 versus 3, etc.). This becomes tedious once the number of spectral channels is very large. Another approach is to resort to dimension reduction, that is, to find a lower-dimensional subspace that "contains" most of the data. The best-known approach, and one of the simplest, is principal components analysis (PCA) — also dubbed the "Karhunen-Loève" or "whitening" transform — which finds the linear subspace with the smallest total squared distance of points to that space. It is well known that finding a basis $\{\alpha_k\}$ of this subspace corresponds to an Eigen-decomposition of the covariance matrix of the spectral signal $x$, thus determining the subspace of maximum variance [13]:

$$\alpha_k = \underset{\substack{||\alpha||=1 \\ \mathrm{Corr}(\alpha^T x, \alpha_j^T x)=0, \ j<k}}{\mathrm{argmax}} \mathrm{Var}(\alpha^T x) \qquad (17.1)$$

The coordinates $s_k = \alpha_k^T x$ of all points within that subspace, also called "scores", can then again be used to produce a scatter plot.

The natural way to visualize an RGB image is just to plot it as one would plot a photo. A spectral image with many spectral channels can be visualized similarly by computing the coordinates of each pixel in an appropriate subspace, and to then plot these "scores" not only in terms of a scatter plot, but also in terms of pictures: either by using a separate (grayscale) image for each component or by combining the three most important components in an RGB or HSV image.

*Unsupervised learning* seeks to uncover the inherent structure in the data. There is overlap with advanced visualization in the sense that the manifold or subspace on which the data mainly lie is an important characteristic of the data. Another important application is the detection of natural groupings or "clusters" in the data. If spatial context is neglected, as in the scatter plots discussed above, this is the subject of cluster analysis [14]. In the spatial domain, the detection of coherent groups of pixels is dubbed "segmentation," and several approaches have been developed that seek to take into account the spectral feature and the spatial context simultaneously [15], [16], [17], [18].

*Supervised learning* aims to predict the class membership — a categorical variable — or a response/dependent variable — which can be ordinal or continuous — from the data. The first task falls in the realm of classification, and a typical example is described in Section 17.2.2. The second task is dubbed "calibration" or "regression" [14], and examples are provided in Section 17.2.1 and Section 17.2.3. In both cases, prior knowledge is required in the form of a training set that comprises, for each object in the data set, both a number of features (independent variables) and the true class membership/response. The goal, then, is to learn a mapping from features to responses that is as reliable as possible, especially for future observations not comprised in the training set. A standard approach in the supervised analysis of spectral data is the use of "regularized" regression methods, in which a bias is traded for variance: a systematic error is knowingly introduced, but the overall procedure becomes more stable and less susceptible to overfitting (e.g., Reference [13]). A common method from chemometrics is partial least squares (PLS) regression, where a linear subspace is determined similar to PCA in Equation 17.2, however, by solving a different optimization problem:

$$\alpha_k = \underset{\substack{||\alpha||=1 \\ \text{Corr}(\alpha^T x, \alpha_j^T x)=0, \ j < k}}{\text{argmax}} \quad \text{Corr}^2(\alpha^T x, y) \, \text{Var}(\alpha^T x) \tag{17.2}$$

Different from the unsupervised and exploratory PCA, PLS also considers the correlation with responses or class labels $y$ when choosing an optimal subspace for the spectral signal $x$. Finally, it is vital to gauge the reliability of the learned model, ideally by means of a separate test set, or, in a data-starved situation, by means of cross-validation [13].

In the context of spectral imagery, both spatial and spectral information should be exploited simultaneously in a supervised learning task; but alas, the field is still in its infancy and no consensus on an optimal processing has been reached as yet.

## 17.2 Applications

### 17.2.1 Calibration of SI Equipment in Measuring of Biochemicals in Food

New consumer demands for food are aimed at taste, ripeness, and health-promoting compounds. These criteria are often related to the presence, absence, and spatial distribution patterns of specific biochemicals, such as chlorophyll, carotenes, plant phenolics, fatty acids, and sugars. All these biochemicals can be measured with analytical chemistry equipment or molecular methods, but such measurements are destructive, expensive, and slow. Color image processing offers an alternative for fast and nondestructive determination of food quality [19], [20], [21], [22]. However, specific biochemicals can often not be visualized in traditional RGB color images.

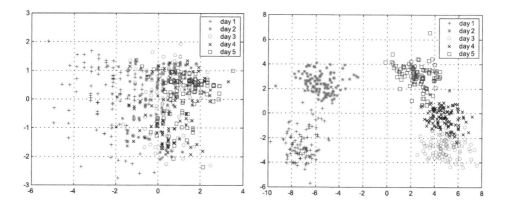

**FIGURE 17.5**
Scatter plot of the first and second canonical variables of the LDA analysis of the RGB (left) and spectral (right) images. Classes 1 to 5 represent the ripeness stages of a tomato during the 5 days after harvest, respectively.

Polder et al. [23] describe an experiment in which tomatoes of close maturity classes are classified using RGB images and spectral images. The resulting classification error is reduced from 51% to 19% when spectral images are used instead of color images. Figure 17.5 shows the resulting scatter plots for individual pixels from RGB and spectral images. From this figure, it is clear that small differences in biochemical concentrations related to ripeness can be measured using spectral images.

Spectral imaging can be seen as an extension of color image processing by employing more wavelength bands. It can also be seen as an extension of spectroscopy by the addition of spatial information. Spectroscopy is the study of light as a function of wavelength that has been transmitted, emitted, reflected, or scattered from an object. Chemical bonds within the food absorb light energy at specific wavelengths. The variety of absorption processes and their wavelength dependency allows us to derive information about the chemistry of the object.

There is a vast literature on spectroscopic methods to measure biochemicals in food and on their relationship to maturity and quality. Among many others, applications are described in peaches [24], [25], apples [26], [27], and tomatoes [28]. Abbott [29] gives a nice overview of quality measurement methods for fruits and vegetables, including optical and spectroscopic techniques.

Conventional spectroscopy gives one spectrum, which is measured on a specific spot, or is a result of an integrated measurement over the whole fruit. Extending this to spectral imaging gives a spectrum at each pixel of the image. This makes it possible to analyze the spatial relationship of the chemistry of the object.

### 17.2.1.1  Equipment Calibration

For the research described in this section, an experimental setup has been built based on an imaging spectrograph. To cover the wavelength range from 400 to 1700 nm, three spectrographs and two cameras are used. Before measurements with this system can be made, it is necessary to calibrate and characterize the system. Equipment calibration is needed in order to know which pixel position matches which wavelength. Characterization is needed to identify the limits of the system. Questions like how sensitive is the system, what is the relation between the signal-to-noise (SNR) ratio to the wavelength, and what is the spectral and spatial resolution need to be answered. These values will be used to choose appropriate binning factors in order to decrease the image size without losing information. A detailed description about characterization and calibration of imaging spectrographs can

**TABLE 17.1**

Mean Concentration and Variation Determined by HPLC, Pixel-Based Classification Error, and Tomato-Based Classification Error

| Calibration Validation Compound | | Pixel Based | | | | Tomato Based | | |
| --- | --- | --- | --- | --- | --- | --- | --- | --- |
| | | Pixel Based | | Tomato Based | | | Tomato Based | |
| | LV | RMSEP/$\mu$ | $Q^2$ | RMSEP/$\mu$ | $Q^2$ | LV | RMSEP/$\mu$ | $Q^2$ |
| Lycopene | 5 | 0.20 | 0.95 | 0.17 | 0.96 | 4 | 0.17 | 0.96 |
| $\beta$-Carotene | 5 | 0.25 | 0.82 | 0.24 | 0.84 | 4 | 0.25 | 0.82 |
| Lutein | 8 | 0.26 | 0.74 | 0.25 | 0.77 | 3 | 0.24 | 0.79 |
| Chlorophyll-a | 6 | 0.30 | 0.73 | 0.27 | 0.79 | 2 | 0.31 | 0.72 |
| Chlorophyll-b | 2 | 0.32 | 0.73 | 0.29 | 0.77 | 2 | 0.29 | 0.77 |

be found in Reference [30]. Due to aberrations in the grating of the spectrograph, the relation between the wavelength and the pixel position shows a slight bending over the spatial axis on the sensor. Therefore, the calibration procedure needs to be carried out at all pixels along the spatial axis. A fully automatic method that simultaneously corrects spectral images for this kind of distortion and yields spectral calibration is described by van der Heijden and Glasbey [31].

### 17.2.1.2 Model Calibration

The next step in measuring the spatial distribution of biochemicals is to build a model in which the spectral data are linked to the concentration of the biochemicals. A regression model relates the spectral information to quantitative information of the measured samples (the concentration of different compounds in the food). In order to build or train such a model, the real concentration of the compounds needs to be measured using analytical chemistry equipment, for instance, HPLC (high-pressure liquid chromatography).

A well-known regression technique is partial least squares (PLS) [32], [33] regression. It is an iterative process where at each iteration, scores, weights, loadings, and inner-coefficients are calculated. Then the **X**- and **Y**-block residuals are calculated, and the entire procedure is repeated for the next factor (commonly called a latent variable [LV] in PLS). The optimal number of LVs used to create the final PLS model is determined by cross-validation. The whole process of calculating the coefficients is known as model calibration.

Ideally, the chemical concentrations should be measured at the same spatial resolution as the spectral images. Obviously this is not possible, and lower resolutions, obtained by extracting small parts from the food, are difficult and expensive. Therefore, the model is often built using the mean compound concentration per object as reference.

We did an experiment in which the concentration of five compounds in a tomato are measured using spectral imaging [34]. Table 17.1 shows the pixel-based and tomato-based PLS regression results for these compounds. For pixel-based calibration, the spectra of individual pixels are used in the **X**-block. For tomato-based calibration, the mean spectrum of all pixels per tomato is used in the **X**-block. In the latter case, the spatial information is lost. The results show that at pixel base, the variation is somewhat larger than at the tomato base. Part of the extra variation at pixel level is due to the variation among pixels not captured in the HPLC analysis.

After the model is built, and the coefficients are known, the concentration of biochemicals of unknown objects can be measured, for instance, in real-time sorting machines. Figure 17.6 shows concentration images of lycopene and chlorophyll in tomatoes of different maturity levels.

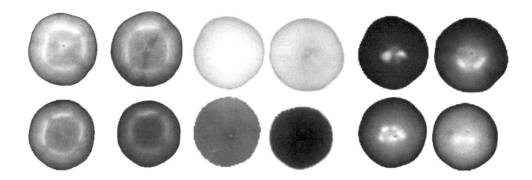

**FIGURE 17.6**
RGB color images (left), lycopene concentration images (middle), and chlorophyll concentration images (right), of tomatoes in four maturity stages.

### 17.2.1.3 Data Reduction

Spectral images with 200 to 300 bands are huge. Capturing and analyzing such data sets currently costs more computing power than available in real-time sorting applications. But as we have seen above, spectral imaging can significantly improve sorting compared to RGB color images. We did a small experiment to study the effect of reducing the number of spectral bands.

The data used in this small experiment are a random selection of 1000 pixels from spectral images of five tomatoes in five ripeness classes (total of 25 images). Each pixel consists of 186 numbers that represent the reflection values between 490 and 730 nm in steps of 1.3 nm. Background and specular parts are removed, and the spectra are made invariant for illumination and object geometry by dividing the spectra through a reference spectrum and normalizing. The ripeness classes are very close, from orange to light red. The Parzen classifier [35] was used for classification. Table 17.2 shows the error rates for all five tomatoes. The original spectra, the smoothed spectra, and the spectra subsampled with a factor ten were analyzed. The processing time is the mean of the elapsed time needed for training the Parzen classifier per tomato.

From this table, we see that the error slightly decreases when the spectra are smoothed, and it decreases even more when the spectra are reduced. From this, we can conclude that the spectra of these tomatoes are so smooth that the number of bands can very well be reduced by a factor of ten. Due to correlation between neighboring bands, reflection values are more or less the same. Hence, taking the means averages out the noise and increases performance. A lower dimensionality also makes the classifier more robust. Because most biological materials have rather smooth reflection spectra in the visible region, we expect

**TABLE 17.2**

Error Rates for Five Tomatoes for a Varying Number of Wavelength Bands (Features), Using Parzen Classification

| Spectra | Error Rate for Tomato | | | | | Processing Time [s] |
|---|---|---|---|---|---|---|
| | 1 | 2 | 3 | 4 | 5 | |
| 186 bands (color constant normalized) | 0.11 | 0.10 | 0.11 | 0.12 | 0.11 | 430 |
| Smoothed (Gauss $\sigma = 2$) | 0.09 | 0.10 | 0.12 | 0.09 | 0.08 | 418 |
| Subsampled to 19 bands | 0.08 | 0.10 | 0.09 | 0.07 | 0.08 | 120 |
| Feature selection (four bands) | 0.12 | 0.13 | 0.15 | 0.11 | 0.13 | |

that spectral sub-sampling or binning can be used in many real-time sorting applications. In case subsampling or binning is done during image recording, both the acquisition and processing speeds can significantly be improved.

When the number of bands is further reduced, to three or four bands, other types of multispectral cameras can be used. The task now is to select those bands that give a maximum separation between classes.

The technique of selecting these bands (features) is known as feature selection and has been studied for several decades [36], [37], [38]. Feature selection consists of a search algorithm for searching the space of feature subsets, and an evaluation function that inputs a feature subset and outputs a numeric evaluation. The goal of the search algorithm is to minimize or maximize the evaluation function.

We did a small experiment in which we tested feature selection methods. The goal was to select four bands of 10 nm bandwidth. Such a setup can easily be implemented in a practical sorting application. In Table 17.2, the resulting error rates are tabulated. We see that the error rate is almost as good as the error rate when using all 186 bands. But a word of caution is needed, because the optimal discriminating wavelength bands are calculated based on these specific tomatoes. The spectrum of the fruit is influenced by the variety and environmental conditions subject to change over the years. For other batches, the selected wavelength bands are presumably less discriminating. When this method is used for selecting filters for implementation in a three- or four-band fixed filter multispectral camera, it is important to do the feature selection on the full range of possible objects that must be sorted in the future. This might not always be possible. More information and additional experiments are described in Reference [39].

### 17.2.2 SI Systems for Industrial Waste Sorting

#### 17.2.2.1 *Sorting of Waste — Why?*

Sorting of waste is one of the major value-adding process steps in recycling, because pure single material fractions serve as high-quality secondary raw materials, whereas mixed fractions are often useless for recycling. Therefore, prices that can be obtained on the market for pure single material fractions are usually much higher than for mixed fractions. Moreover, European Commission (EC) directives force manufacturers to take care of the recycling of their products, especially for "waste electrical and electronic equipment (WEEE)." Recycling is, therefore, a high-potential market. The most prominent examples for recycling, among others, are car recycling, WEEE, paper, polymers, metal, biomass, and so forth. To a large extent, sorting is currently done manually. Automatization of waste-sorting processes makes sense for the following reasons:

- Automatic sorting of waste is cheaper than manual sorting for high volumes of waste.
- The environmental conditions for sorting are very rough (i.e., paper recycling) and extremely unhealthy for persons working in such environments.
- The amount of waste will increase.
- In some countries, funding of recycling will be reduced or abolished (i.e., Germany). As a consequence, recycling companies will have to reduce their costs by enforcing automation.

In the following, we will describe CTR's SpectroSort® as a spectral-imaging-based system for waste sorting.

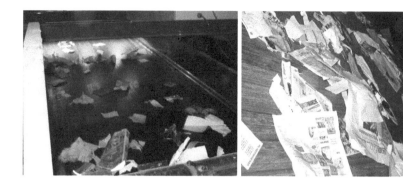

**FIGURE 17.7**
Typical transportation systems applied in sorting facilities.

### 17.2.2.2  Sorting of Paper and Polymers

The main focus of SpectroSort is the sorting of paper and polymers in industrial environments. Paper and polymers waste is produced by both private households and industry and is collected separately from other kinds of waste and recycled in a lot of countries in the world.

Paper waste roughly includes two classes of material that have to be separated, namely, paper that can be freed from ink, so called de-inking paper (i.e., newspapers, catalogs, journals, white office paper, advertisements, etc.) and so-called non-de-inking material, which includes printed or nonprinted cardboard, food packaging (TetraPak®, coated cardboard, etc.), and colored or coated paper. The most desirable fraction is the de-inking paper. Thus, most sorting processes try to get all of the non-de-inking material out of the paper waste in order to produce a pure de-inking fraction.

Among the most common polymers are polyvinyl chloride (PVC), polyethylene (PE), polypropylene (PP), polystyrene (PS), polyethylene terephthalate (PET/PETP), and acrylonitrile butadiene styrene (ABS). Because different polymers have different melting temperatures, different polymers have to be separated in order to feed them into the recycling process. The most common sorting applications are

- Sorting of polymers into single material fractions
- Alternative fuels: removing of polymers that would produce toxic compounds during combustion (i.e., PVC removal because of chlorine content) from a mixed fraction

Apart from the aforementioned purely material-based polymers separation, some niche recycling processes require single color fractions for a given polymer (i.e., natural color PET for the production of noncolored foils, etc.).

### 17.2.2.3  Industrial Requirements for Sorting Systems

Many sorting facilities have to process more than 10 tons of waste per hour. In order to prepare such amounts of waste for optical identification, the waste has to be arranged on conveyor belts in a monolayer. A conveyor belt of 2 m in width can transport 4 to 6 tons of paper waste per hour in a monolayer at a transportation velocity of 3 m/sec. Examples of such transportation systems are shown in Figure 17.7.

Because the objects are usually much smaller than the dimensions of the belt (field of view), a spatially sensitive method must be applied for material localization. Moreover, the data acquisition, data evaluation, and control of a sorting mechanism (in this case, an air-jet array) have to meet real-time requirements.

Additional challenges stem from environmental conditions, such as plenty of dust and dirt. The ambient temperatures vary between $-20°C$ and $+40°C$ depending on the season. Moreover, most of the sorting facilities are neither air-conditioned nor separated from the outside. As a consequence, humidity of the air and the material vary on large scales.

### 17.2.2.4 *Why Spectral Imaging?*

Concerning the sorting of polymers, material properties are not sufficiently correlated to shape and color features, and color image processing is not the appropriate method for polymers recognition. Polymers show absorption bands in the near-infrared (NIR) originating from harmonics (transitions between the ground state of a vibrational mode and its second or higher excited states) and combination vibrations (excitation of two separate vibrational modes by one photon). Thus, NIR spectroscopy can be applied. Mid-infrared (MIR) spectroscopy would be preferred, but the instrumentation is currently too expensive. There are solutions on the market that combine color image processing with NIR spectroscopy. (See, for instance, Reference [40].) Such approaches perform an object recognition via color image processing prior to material classification of the object via NIR-point spectroscopy. A natural spatially resolved extension of point measurement NIR-spectroscopy is NIR spectral imaging. Each pixel of the field of view is spectroscopically assigned to a material property, and afterwards, objects are recognized by gathering pixels of the same material type. With a NIR-SI system, it is possible to identify practically any important polymer [41].

For the sorting of paper, state-of-the-art systems rely on color image processing. This is based on simple assumptions concerning de-inking and non-de-inking fractions. For example, newspapers are preferably printed on grayish paper with black text blocks and contain grayscale or color images. For journals or advertisements, high-quality CMYK printing is applied, whereas color printing of cardboard is done in a three-color system. Uniform gray or brown cardboard or colored paper can sufficiently be identified with a color image processing system.

For the past years, it has been becoming more common to use CMYK printing also for non-de-inking fractions like cardboard and food packaging. Moreover, it is hard to distinguish coated from uncoated material via color image processing. A lot of de-inking base material is coated or wrapped in polymer foils. This can spoil a de-inking fraction.

To overcome those problems, NIR spectroscopy can also be applied here for the followings: coatings are mostly based on polymers, and different sorts of paper and cardboard undergo different production processes, where different chemicals (glues, binders, and whiteners) are used. The corresponding features can be used to distinguish de-inking and non-de-inking materials.

For the sorting of paper, there are also systems on the market that perform object recognition via image processing and, sequentially, NIR spectroscopy for material identification (see, for instance, Reference [40]). The heart of SpectroSort® is a NIR spectral imaging system that is able to distinguish de-inking from non-de-inking material based on those differences. For additional features, the VIS band is also used.

### 17.2.2.5 *SpectroSort® Hardware Setup*

The core module of CTRs waste sorting system SpectroSort is a sensor system containing an SI system that records the spatial information line-wise, while the diffuse reflectance spectrum for each pixel along the sampling line is projected along the second axis of a two-dimensional detector chip. By combining the slices, the second (spatial) axis can be derived, resulting in a full image represented by a spectral hypercube (see Figure 17.8). Such an SI system can be compared to a RGB line-scan system with the difference that a

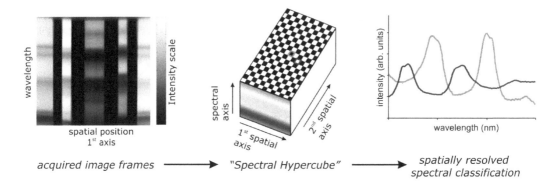

**FIGURE 17.8**
Acquisition of a spectral image following the push-broom scanning principle. The spectral information and one spatial axis are acquired for each frame ($X(x, \lambda)$), and the second spatial axis is derived by combining the frames. The result is a spectral hypercube.

pixel corresponds to a discrete spectrum of up to several hundred reflectance values instead of just the three values of the R, G, and B channels.

The spectral encoding is provided by dispersive optics forming an imaging spectrograph [42]. This imaging spectrograph is based on a direct vision diffraction prism–grating–prism (PGP) component, featuring a transmission volume grating cemented, together with a short-pass and a long-pass filter, between two optically matched prisms. The radiation coming through a line slit is spectrally dispersed by the PGP component and projected onto the camera chip. Attached to the front of the spectrograph or optimized optics, determining the field of view of the first spatial axis and, together with the camera resolution, the spatial resolution. These transfer optics are selected for the specific wavelength ranges. Imaging spectrograph, 2-D detector (camera), and optics form the actual spectral imaging unit as shown in Figure 17.9. An SI system can feature one or several of these units (e.g., to cover

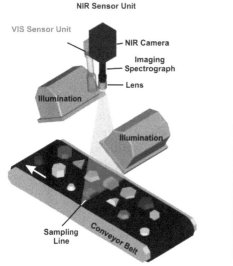

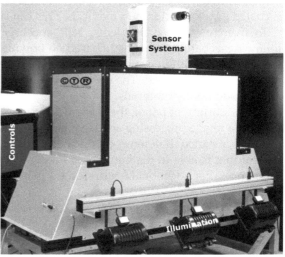

**FIGURE 17.9**
Setup (left) and photograph (right) of an industrial spectral imaging system (CTR SpectroSort®, 1.8 m observation line length).

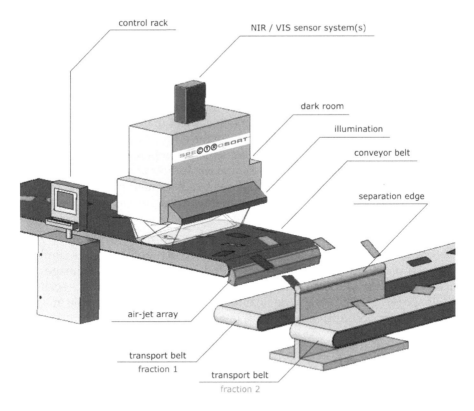

**FIGURE 17.10**
The SpectroSort® hardware setup. (Reproduced from the SpectroSort® product sheet.)

a wider spectral range or to increase the achievable spatial resolution). Imaging spectrographs are commercially available for visible (VIS) and NIR wavelengths (ImSpector from Specim) [9].

The third component is the so-called dark room that avoids stray light from entering the SI system. The fourth building block is the illumination unit. In case of SpectroSort, these are specially modified floodlights. The light sources must provide a spatially sufficiently homogeneous illumination of the sample with sufficient intensity over the required spectral range, as shadows or other inhomogeneities in illumination may lead to erroneous classification results.

The fifth module of SpectroSort is the transport system providing a relative movement of the samples perpendicular to the first spatial axis (sampling line) at a constant speed. By combining the consecutively acquired frames in the computer, the second spatial dimension is obtained, with the resolution in the second spatial axis being determined by the movement velocity and the frame rate of the camera. By varying the two parameters, it can be adapted to meet specific application requirements (material throughput, size of the objects, etc.).

The sixth module is an airjet array that provides the actual separation of material into two material fractions that can be further processed in the recycling chain.

A control rack serves as a seventh module. This module contains the user interface — a standard state-of-the-art industry PC equipped with a suitable frame-grabber card for data acquisition and real-time evaluation. The classification result is transformed into I/O signals that control the air-jet array.

The whole SpectroSort system can be seen in Figure 17.10.

### 17.2.2.6  Data Evaluation — General Remarks

In an industrial system, the data evaluation must be done online and in real-time in contrast to environmental or military remote-sensing applications, where huge amounts of data are stored and processed off-line via highly evolved chemometric algorithms. Hence, application-oriented preprocessing and spectral evaluation with optimized parameters are important factors. For the SpectroSort system, the time for acquisition, processing, data evaluation, and postprocessing of one sample line is less than 15 ms. All operations must be carefully time optimized in order to complete the entire data processing within such a short time using a standard PC. In particular, suitable preprocessing and fast, yet robust and reliable, evaluation algorithms are essential. In addition, the overall system must be easy to use and provide the necessary interfaces to subsequent processing units, like the air-jet array dependent on the sensor data or an integrated process control system.

### 17.2.2.7  Preprocessing

Preprocessing involves three main steps. The first step in preprocessing is similar to what is done in color image processing. This is the standardization of the raw images involving dark current correction (dark-current image $B(x, \lambda)$) and (white) reference scaling (white-standard image ($W(x, \lambda)$) to obtain the final image $R(x, \lambda)$ from the sample image $X(x, \lambda)$, in the case of SpectroSort diffuse reflectance images as follows:

$$R(x, \lambda) = \frac{X(x, \lambda) - B(x, \lambda)}{W(x, \lambda) - B(x, \lambda)} \qquad (17.3)$$

The second step differs from most color image processing systems and is a data reduction (e.g., by spectral range selection or selective binning of redundant data). The algorithms involved herein are optimized to reduce the data that have to be processed to the required minimum without losing relevant information. The proper execution of the data reduction directly influences the real-time capabilities of the system. Data reduction is of particular importance for systems operating in the UV/VIS, as the availability of cameras with millions of pixels allows for the recording of spectral images with much higher spectral and spatial resolution, but at the cost of increasing the data to be processed. Moreover, the spectral resolution of imaging spectrographs is limited.

The final preprocessing step is data preparation for the evaluation. The particular operations are reliant on the chosen evaluation algorithm, but generally, a baseline correction or the calculation of the first- or second-order derivatives of the spectra are involved. In classification applications, a normalization step also can be useful.

### 17.2.2.8  Spectral Data Evaluation

Spatially resolved material identification and the subsequent sorting is currently the prevalent SpectroSort application. We will briefly describe the steps of data evaluation after preprocessing. After preprocessing, each pixel in the spectral image $R(x, \lambda)$ of an object line is associated with a spectrum. An example of different polymer spectra is given in Figure 17.11.

In this figure, reflectance spectra of different polymers are shown in the NIR band between wavelengths of 1000 nm and 1600 nm. All of the spectra show more or less pronounced absorption features around 1200 nm and 1400 nm. These features differ in depth and shape. Such features can be used to distinguish between different polymers with a classification algorithm. In dependence of the particular application, those algorithms have to be carefully selected to produce stable results. As mentioned before, real-time capabilities are vital and pose a hard constraint on classification algorithms and their implementation on certain platforms. Only some types of spectral classifiers can successfully be applied for real-time SI

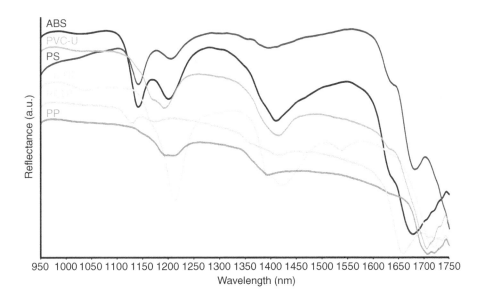

**FIGURE 17.11**
Reflectance spectra of ABS, PVC-U (unplasticized), PS, PE-HD (high-density), PETP and PP in the NIR band.
Strong absorption features can be seen around 1200 nm and 1400 nm.

applications: discriminant classifiers and dissimilarity-based classifiers. In addition, occasionally dedicated algorithms, like fuzzy classifiers, may be useful for special applications (e.g., when there is no *ab-initio* knowledge about number and properties of the classification classes).

Typical discriminant classifiers are the Fisher linear discriminant classifier (FLDC) and the quadratic discriminant classifier (QDC). The FLDC performs a linear mapping to a lower-dimensional subspace optimized for class separability prior to the classification using a linear classifier. During training, the mapping $w$ is optimized for class separability in the subspace by maximizing the criterion:

$$J(\omega) = \frac{\omega^t S_B \omega}{\omega^t S_W \omega} \tag{17.4}$$

with the between-class scatter $S_B$ and the within-class scatter $S_W$. For $c$ classes, the mapping projects the input data on a subspace with $c-1$ dimensions, often called Fisher scores, and subsequently, a conventional linear discriminant classifier is trained on the Fisher scores. The log-likelihood is calculated by

$$ln(p(x)) = -\frac{(x-\mu)^T G^{-1}(x-\mu)}{2} + const \tag{17.5}$$

with the estimated covariance matrix over all classes $G$ and the class mean $\mu$. Each sample is assigned to the class giving the highest log-likelihood.

The QDC calculates the average and the covariance for each class and assigns the spectrum to the class with the highest likelihood. Assignments with likelihoods below a pre-set threshold value are rejected and classified into a common rejection class. By adjusting the rejection threshold, the tolerance of the classification against sample deviations and modifications can be optimized. This algorithm is statistically very powerful, but as usually a PCA of the input data is required to reduce the dimensionality, the algorithm is restricted to applications with lower amounts of data (i.e., slower processes or imaging at comparatively low spatial resolutions).

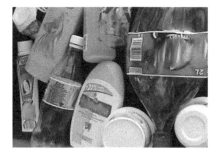 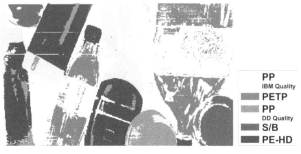

**FIGURE 17.12 (See color insert.)**
Classification of polymer waste: (left) input image, and (right) after classification. The classification image shows the assignment of each pixel to the material PP (injection blow molding [IBM] quality), PETP, PP (deep drawing [DD] quality), S/B (styrenebutadiene copolymer), and PE-HD.

Dissimilarity-based classifiers (DBCs) use a dissimilarity measure $M_D$ to transform the input data into a dissimilarity space, where each trained class represents a separate dimension. Any dissimilarity measure with the following properties can be used:

$$M_D(x, y) = \left\{ \begin{matrix} 0, & x = y \\ > 0, & x \neq y \end{matrix} \right\} \qquad (17.6)$$

By designing the dissimilarity measure, it is possible to use expert knowledge or application-dependent properties to construct an efficient dissimilarity space, where classification is often easier than in the original feature space. For a more detailed discussion of the appropriate classifiers, see References [43], [44], and [45].

Before a classifier is able to classify spectra, it usually has to be trained and parameterized according to expert knowledge and corresponding reference data. The number of classes and the parametrization are strongly application dependent. A certain spectrum can then be assigned to a (material-)class that fits best. In the SpectroSort system, this is done for each pixel of the object.

The result of the classification is a material map of the field of view as indicated in Figure 17.12. Figure 17.12 shows an RGB image of polymer waste and the result of the classification. In the classification image, each pixel is assigned to one of the polymers PP (injection blow molding [IBM] quality), PETP, PP (deep drawing [DD] quality), S/B, PE-HD or "not-recognized" (white), as an example. Before the information can be used to control a sorting mechanism, it can be useful to apply image processing methods to extract the relevant information contained in the material maps. This is valid for any type of waste that can be handled with SpectroSort (i.e., paper waste).

### 17.2.2.9 Integrated Image Processing

From material maps, as shown in Figure 17.12, the objects can be identified and information like position, size, and orientation of an object can be retrieved. Together with the material information, this can serve as control parameters for an automatic sorter, in this case, an air-jet array. For clean, nonoverlapping samples, it is sufficient to determine the center of each object and the approximate size to control the sorting unit. However, frequently, these ideal conditions cannot be guaranteed, as samples overlap or surface adhesions may interfere with the classification. Such artifacts will lead to (partially) false information about size and position of an object and, hence, to incomplete or erroneous sorting [44], [45].

As an example, a PET bottle with a paper label should be detected as one single PET object, not as two separate entities with a piece of paper between, because, based on the classification result, a subsequent sorting or turnout stage has to handle the entire object. This requires a classification system delivering the correct size and shape of the different objects, regardless of the presence of, for example, interfering paper labels that partially occlude the objects' surfaces. To achieve that, an object reconstruction algorithm detects connected components in the material class maps.

Such an image processing stage with careful application-dependent parametrization significantly increases the sorting efficiency and overall process stability [44], [45].

### 17.2.3 Classification of Magnetic Resonance Spectroscopic Images

The diagnosis of an invasive brain tumor is relatively straightforward given conventional T1/T2-weighted magnetic resonance (MR) images. However, a possible recurrence of the tumor after radiation therapy is much more difficult to diagnose reliably; the tissue is obviously perturbed, but differentiating between necrosis, inflammation, or tumor recurrence is difficult. Another related application is the exact localization of the tumor boundaries. Here, infiltrating tumor tissue is only insufficiently mapped by standard imaging modalities.

In both situations, the spectral information from magnetic resonance spectral images (MRSI) can be used to map the disease at a metabolic level. Conventional MR scanners are capable of acquiring sets of spectral images — or even volumes — at $mm^3$ voxel size and up to $32 \times 32 \times 10$ spatial resolution. Technically, they record the excitation states of the hydrogen atomic nucleus — induced by an external magnetic field — as a function of the irradiation wavelength of a second electromagnetic field. Due to differential "shielding" of the nucleus from the external field depending on the local electronic structure, the nuclei absorb energy at different energy levels, or wavelengths. Thus, the resulting spectrum consists of resonance lines in the radio frequency range, which are highly specific to a number of metabolites and freely rotable compounds of the tissue cells (Figure 17.13).

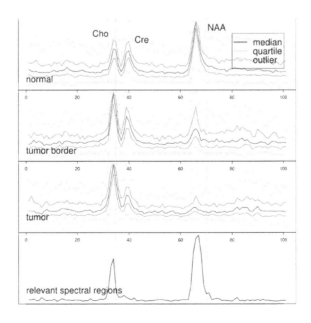

**FIGURE 17.13**
Robust summaries of the spectral patterns that are typical for a tumor, its boundary, and healthy tissue. Also indicated is the relevance of the spectral channels for a prediction of tumor probability, as found by "Random Forest," a nonlinear method for supervised learning.

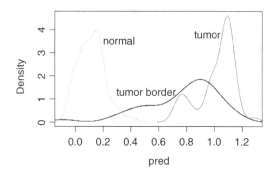

**FIGURE 17.14**
The probability densities indicate the distribution of coordinates of tumor spectra, healthy spectra, and tumor boundary spectra after projection to a one-dimensional subspace.

Their spectral peaks are obscured by a comparatively enormous peak resulting from the hydrogen of the water molecule which is, obviously, much more abundant, and by a very low signal-to-noise ratio.

Under ordinary circumstances, only three metabolites are observable in an MR spectrum of the brain: choline, creatine, and NAA. In the event of a tumor, their ratio is perturbed: choline, as a marker of membrane buildup and degradation, increases in concentration, while the neurotransmitter NAA is depleted. The task, then, is to predict the tumor probability for each region of the brain, given the spectra from the MR spectroscopic image. An automated and reliable prediction is desirable, because a manual analysis of the spectra would be both time-consuming and subjective in the clinical routine, especially in the case of high spatial resolutions.

### 17.2.3.1   *Identification of Noise Spectra*

Due to technical limitations and restrictions on acquisition time, only a fraction of the spectra in an MRSI contain meaningful information, the remainder are deteriorated by high noise levels and a variety of artifacts. As the prediction of tumor probabilities on such spectra will result in random output, a classifier is used to label unreliable regions within the spectral image. The first step in the setup of this classification procedure is the normalization of each spectral vector to unit variance or, due to the positiveness of MR magnitude spectra, to unit area "under" the spectral vector within defined spectral regions. In the next step, either prior knowledge about the spectral data (e.g. positions of known peaks, pattern of common artifacts) or statistical tests (e.g. the univariate $t$-test or multivariate, nonmetric importance measures; see Figure 17.13) can be used to identify relevant spectral regions and to restrict the further data processing on features from these regions. A smoothing and subsampling of the potentially noisy and slightly shifted spectra shows an increase in the performance of the following classifier [46]. Although the continuous degradation of the spectra along a decreasing signal-to-noise ratio can be modeled linearly, the various spectral pattern of the artifacts demands a nonlinear classifier of sufficient flexibility (e.g., decision trees, neural networks, support vector machines). Labeled noise spectra are removed from further processing or at least from the final display within the diagnostic map.

### 17.2.3.2   *Prediction of Tumor Probability*

Ideally, one would like to obtain a crisp classification (i.e., a statement whether a voxel has or has not been invaded by cancer). In practice, however, there is a continuum of spectral

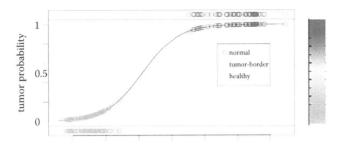

**FIGURE 17.15 (See color insert.)**
Binomial prediction of tumor probability in a one-dimensional subspace resulting from a dimension reduction step (compare densities of Figure 17.14). The predicted tumor probabilities can be mapped out using the color bar shown on the right, see Figure 17.16.

fingerprints ranging from entirely healthy patterns to undoubtedly malignant ones. Among the many reasons [47] is the "partial volume effect" given that the side length of a voxel is several millimeters, the boundary of a tumor will, in most cases, comprise voxels containing both tumorous and healthy tissue. Accordingly, if one wants to do the data and its inherent uncertainty full justice, the only reasonable prediction will be one in terms of a tumor probability (i.e., a scalar prediction for each voxel in the range from zero to one). Because we seek to predict a continuous dependent variable, we are in the realm of regression. Performing an ordinary least-squares regression (Section 17.1.2) using all spectral channels as features is liable to overfitting: the number of parameters (regression coefficients) to be estimated will often be too small compared to the number of observations. Hence, an implicit or explicit dimension reduction is required. In the clinical application described, detailed prior knowledge is available: it is known which metabolites are potential tumor indicators, and what their spectral characteristic is; a spectrum can then be explained as linear combination of these pure spectra, and the linear combination coefficients can used as features for supervised learning. In other situations, such detailed prior knowledge is not available; however, an explicit or implicit dimension reduction can still be performed by methods such as PCA or PLS. It was found that fully automated methods of the type described give excellent results, even when the signal-to-noise ratio is very low [13].

Once the spectra have been projected to a one-dimensional subspace, we have only one scalar value left for each voxel (Figure 17.14). In this one-dimensional subspace, a binomial regression is performed that yields predictions for tumor probability in the range from zero to one (Figure 17.15) and the associated confidence intervals (not shown).[2] The predicted tumor probabilities can then be summarized using a color map or "nosologic image",[3] as shown in Figure 17.16.

The performance of the procedure can be summarized in terms of a receiver–operator characteristic (ROC). It shows the percentage of false positives versus true positives in a dichotomous decision, as a function of the selected threshold on the tumor probability.

A final and important step is to make the automated analysis of a spectral image easily accessible to the practitioner. Figure 17.17 shows the integration of an automated tumor prediction in the prostate [48] in a program for radiation therapy planning [49].

---

[2] It is possible to integrate these two steps and directly perform a binomial partial least squares prediction [48].
[3] Image displaying spatially resolved diagnostic information.

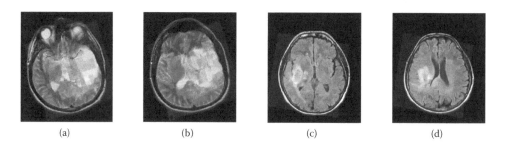

|      |      |      |      |
|:----:|:----:|:----:|:----:|
| (a)  | (b)  | (c)  | (d)  |

**FIGURE 17.16  (See color insert.)**
Color maps indicating the tumor probability computed automatically from MR spectral images (a, c), super-imposed onto morphologic MR images (b, d). The color mapping used is defined on the right-hand side of Figure 17.15.

## 17.3    Conclusion

The analysis of spectral image data still poses numerous open research questions. What is the best way to reduce data dimensionality for storage, transmission, and real-time processing without losing relevant information? How can the hypercube data be visualized

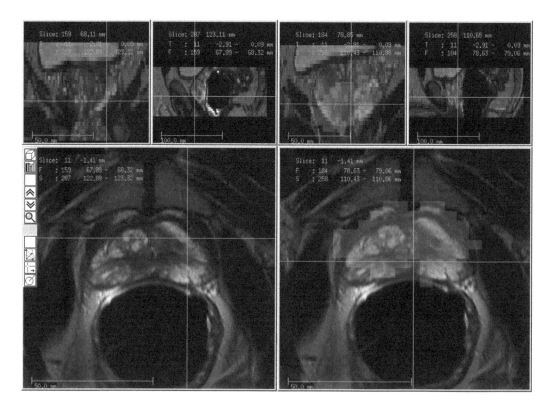

**FIGURE 17.17**
An example of automated tumor detection in the prostate: the entire classification of the spectral image proceeds on the push of a single button; the results are shown on top of a morphologic image in a program for radiation therapy planning.

and analyzed? What is the best way to normalize spectral data in order to compare different recordings (e.g., to preserve high and low influencing PCA components at the same time)? Is it sufficient to describe spectral information by a subset of spectral bands or by choosing a set of basis spectra? Edge pixels are expected in the tails of clusters, but can the tails of clusters, automatically be interpreted as edge pixels? How can edges be detected and characterized in spectral images?

The segmentation of images by a cluster analysis of scores (e.g., from standard PCA), neglects spatial neighborhood relations as well as correlations in adjacent spectral bands. How can both sources of information best be incorporated in a joint analysis? Noise reduction by combining spatial and spectral information for segmentation purposes can reduce the number of clusters and lead to a simplified and more expressive and interpretable visualization of spectral images.

This chapter has illustrated that there is a need to develop special-purpose approaches to spectral image processing. The main goal was to stimulate awareness in the image processing community and make the point that color image processing is still insufficient to capture the potentially rich structure and information contained in spectral images. Although SI enables complete new applications, it also brings a new dimension into the quality of current visual inspection tasks. The added value of spectral information beyond the visual spectrum has been demonstrated in three case studies from areas with completely different requirements (i.e., waste sorting, measurement of biochemicals in food, and tumor detection with MRSI). The experience showed that these solutions cannot be easily transferred to other applications or materials under inspection without investing a reasonable amount of engineering and "trial and error" experimentation.

Spectral imaging should be regarded as a special branch of image processing on its own rather than as an extension to either gray/color-value image processing or spectral analysis. This generalized view on spectral imaging coming from the color image analysis field supports a mutual exchange of mature principles that have already been proven to work under real conditions. The combination of well-studied image processing algorithms with methods from pattern recognition reveals a promising path toward this goal. It is expected to yield even more powerful and innovative SI solutions in the future.

## References

[1] N. Gat, Imaging spectroscopy using tunable filters: A review, in *Wavelet Applications VII*, Vol. 4056 of *Proceedings of the SPIE*, 2000, pp. 50–64.

[2] J. Romier, J. Selves, and J. Gastellu-Etchegorry, Imaging spectrometer based on an acousto-optic tunable filter, *Rev. Sci. Instrum.*, 69, 8, 2859–2867, 1998.

[3] E. Herrala and J. Okkonen, Imaging spectrograph and camera solutions for industrial applications, *Int. J. Patt. Recognition and Artif. Intelligence*, 10, 43–54, 1996.

[4] T. Hyvärinen, E. Herrala, and A. Dall'Ava, Direct sight imaging spectrograph: A unique add-on component brings spectral imaging to industrial applications, in *SPIE Symposium on Electronic Imaging*, Vol. 3302 of *Proceedings of the SPIE*, San Jose, CA, USA, 1998, pp. 165–175.

[5] R. Kettig and D. Landgrebe, Computer classification of remotely sensed multispectral image data by extraction and classification of homogeneous objects, *IEEE Trans. on Geosci. Electron.*, GE-14, 19–26, January 1976.

[6] D. Landgrebe, The development of a spectral-spatial classifier for earth observational data, *Patt. Recognition*, 12, 165–175, 1980.

[7] P. Swain, S. Vardeman, and J. Tilton, Contextual classification of multispectral image data, *Patt. Recognition*, 13, 429–441, 1981.

[8] J. Kittler and J. Föglein, Contextual classification of multispectral pixel data, *Image and Vision Comput.*, 2, 13–29, February 1984.

[9] Imspector Imaging Spectrograph User Manual, Technical report version 2.21, Spectral Imaging Oy Ltd., Oulu, Finland, August 2003.

[10] R. Duin and S.P. Paclik, Oesterreichische Computer Gesellschaft, Vienna, Research challenges in spectral and spatial data analysis, in *Second International Spectral Imaging Workshop — Hyperspectral Data for New Vision Applications*, Villach, Oesterreichische Computer Gesellschaft, Vienna, Austria, 2005.

[11] M. Kraft, Oesterreichische Computer Gesellschaft, Vienna, Spectral imaging in practical applications — an overview, in *Second International Spectral Imaging Workshop — Hyperspectral Data for New Vision Applications*, Villach, Oesterreichische Computer Gesellschaft, Vienna, Austria, 2005.

[12] P. Tatzer, M. Wolf, and T. Panner, *Real Time Imaging — Special Issue on Spectral Imaging II*, vol. 11, ch. Industial application for in-line material sorting using hyperspectral imaging in the NIR range, Elsevier, 2 ed., 2005, pp. 99–107.

[13] T. Hastie, R. Tibshirani, and J. Friedman, *The Elements of Statistical Learning*: Data Minius, Inference, and Prediction, Springer Series in Statistics, Springer, New York, 2001.

[14] R.O. Duda, P.E. Hart, and D.G. Stork, *Pattern Classification*, Wiley, New York, 2000.

[15] C. Noordam and W.H.A.M. van den Broek, Multivariate image segmentation based on geometrically guided fuzzy c-means clustering, *J. Chemometrics*, 16, 1–11, 2002.

[16] T.N. Tran, R. Wehrens, and L.M.C. Buydens, Clustering multispectral images: A tutorial, *Chemom. Intell. Lab. Syst.*, 77, 3–17, 2005.

[17] R.P.M. Paclik, P. Duin, G.M.P. van Kempen, and R. Kohlus, Segmentation of multi-spectral images using the combined classifier approach, *Image and Vision Comput.*, 21, 473–482, 2003.

[18] N. Bonnet, J. Cutrona, and M. Herbin, A "no-threshold" histogram-based image segmentation method, *Patt. Recognition*, 35, 2319–2322, 2002.

[19] K. Choi, G. Lee, Y. Han, and J. Bunn, Tomato maturity evaluation using color image analysis, *Trans. the ASAE*, 38, 171–176, 1995.

[20] K. Liao, J.F. Reid, M.R. Paulsen, and E.E. Shaw, Corn kernel hardness classification by color segmentation, *American Society of Agricultural Engineers*, ps. 14, 913504, 1991.

[21] S. Shearer and F. Payne, Color and defect sorting of bell peppers using machine vision, *Trans. ASAE*, 33, 2045–2050, 1990.

[22] J. Noordam, G. Otten, A. Timmermans, and B. v. Zwol, High-speed potato grading and quality inspection based on a color vision system, in *SPIE, Machine Vision and Its Applications*, K.W. Tobin, Ed., Vol. 3966, San Jose, CA, 2000, pp. 206–220.

[23] G. Polder, G. van der Heijden, and I. Young, Spectral image analysis for measuring ripeness of tomatoes, *Trans. ASAE*, 45, 1155–1161, 2002.

[24] S. Kawano, H. Watanabe, and M. Iwamoto, Determination of sugar content in intact peaches by near-infrared spectroscopy with fiber optics in interactance mode, *J. Jpn. Soc. Hortic. Sci.*, 61, 445–451, 1992.

[25] D. Slaughter, Nondestructive determination of internal quality in peaches and nectarines, *Trans. ASAE*, 38, 617–623, 1995.

[26] J. Lammertyn, A. Peirs, J. De Baerdemaeker, and B. Nicolai, Light penetration properties of NIR radiation in fruit with respect to non-destructive quality assessment, *Postharvest Biol. and Technol.*, 18, 121–132, 2000.

[27] B. Upchurch, J. Throop, and D. Aneshansley, Influence of time, bruise-type, and severity on near-infrared reflectance from apple surfaces for automatic bruise detection, *Trans. ASAE*, 37, 1571–1575, 1994.

[28] D. Slaughter, D. Barrett, and M. Boersig, Nondestructive determination of soluble solids in tomatoes using near infrared spectroscopy, *J. Food Sci.*, 61, 695–697, 1996.

[29] J. Abbott, Quality measurement of fruits and vegatables, *Postharvest Biol. Technol.*, 15, 207–225, 1999.

[30] G. Polder, G. van der Heijden, L. Keizer, and I. Young, Calibration and characterization of imaging spectrographs, *J. Near Infrared Spectrosc.*, 11, 193–210, 2003.

[31] G. van der Heijden and C. Glasbey, Calibrating spectral images using penalized likelihood, *Real-Time Imaging*, 9, 231–236, 2003.

[32] P. Geladi and B. Kowalski, Partial least squares regression: A tutorial, *Analytica Chimica Acta*, 185, 1–17, 1986.

[33] I. Helland, Partial least-squares regression and statistical-models, *Scand. J. Stat.*, 17, 97–114, 1990.

[34] G. Polder, G. van der Heijden, H. van der Voet, and I. Young, Measuring surface distribution of compounds in tomatoes using imaging spectrometry, *Postharvest Biol. and Technol.*, 34, 117–129, 2004.

[35] E. Parzen, On the estimation of a probability density function and the mode, *Ann. Math. Stat.*, 33, 1065–1076, 1962.

[36] T. Cover and J.V. Campenhout, On the possible orderings in the measurement selection problem, *IEEE Trans. on Syst., Man, and Cybernetics*, 7, 657–661, 1977.

[37] K. Fu, *Sequential Methods in Pattern Recognition and Machine Learning*, Academic Press, New York, 1968.

[38] A. Mucciardi and E. Gose, A comparison of seven techniques for choosing subsets of pattern recognition properties, *IEEE Trans. on Comput.*, C-20, 1023–1031, 1971.

[39] G. Polder, *Spectral Imaging for Measuring Biochemicals in Plant Material*, Ph.D. thesis, Delft University of Technology, Delft, The Netherlands, 2004.

[40] O. Løvhaugen, V. Rehrmann, and K. Bakke, Method and Apparatus for Identifying and Sorting Objects, Technical report WO 03/061858, International Patent Publication, 2003.

[41] A. Kulcke, C. Gurschler, G. Spck, R. Leitner, and M. Kraft, On-line classification of synthetic polymers using near infrared spectral imaging, *J. Near Infrared Spectrosc.*, 11, 71–81, February 2003.

[42] M. Aikio, Optical components comprising prisms and a grating, Technical report EP 0635138, European Patent Publication, 1993.

[43] R. Duda, P. Hart, and D. Stork, *Pattern Classification*, 2nd ed., John Wiley & Sons, New York, 2000.

[44] R. Leitner, H. Mairer, and A. Kercek, *Real Time Imaging — Special Issue on Spectral Imaging*, 4th ed., Matthias F. Carlsohn (ed.), Vol. 9, ch. Real-Time Classification of Polymers with NIR Spectral Imaging and Blob Analysis, Elsevier, Amsterdam; New York, 2003, pp. 245–251.

[45] M. Kraft, R. Leitner, and H. Mairer, *Spectrochemical Analyses Using Multichannel Infrared Detectors*, B. Rohit and I. Levin (eds.), ch. Materials analysis systems based on real-time near-IR spectroscopic imaging, Blackwell Scientific Oxford, 2005, pp. 158–174.

[46] B.H. Menze, M. Wormit, P. Bachert, M.P. Lichy, H.-P. Schlemmer, and F.A. Hamprecht, Classification of in vivo magnetic resonance spectra, in C. Weihs, W. Gaul (eds.), *Classification, the Ubiquitous Challenge; Studies in Classification, Data Analysis, and Knowledge Organization;* Springer, Heidelberg; New York, 2005, pp. 362–369.

[47] B.H. Menze, M.P. Lichy, P. Bachert, B.M. Kelm, H.-P. Schlemmer, and F.A. Hamprecht, Optimal classification of in vivo magnetic resonance spectra in the detection of recurrent brain tumors, NMR in Biomedicine, April 2006. [Epub ahead of print]

[48] B. M. Kelm, B.H. Menze, T. Neff, C.M. Zechmann, and F.A. Hamprecht, CLARET: a tool for fully automated evaluation of MRSI with pattern recognition methods, in H. Handels, et al. (eds.); *Proceeding of the BVM 2006*, Hamburg; Springer, Heidelberg; New York, 2006, pp. 51–55.

[49] R. Bendl, J. Pross, A. Hoess, M. Keller, K. Preiser, and W. Schlegel, Virtuos — a program for virtual radiotherapy simulation and verification, in: A.R. Hounsell et al. (eds.), *Proc. 11th Int. Conf. on the Use of Computers in Radiation Therapy*, Manchester, North Western Med. Physics Dept., 1994, pp. 226–227.

# 18

## *Image Enhancement for Plasma Display Panels*

**Choon-Woo Kim, Yu-Hoon Kim, and Hwa-Seok Seong**

## CONTENTS

## 18.1 Introduction

Display technology is changing rapidly to meet market demands. Conventional cathode-ray tube (CRT) technology has been left unchallenged for the last few decades. CRT technology has developed since the 1930s, when the first commercial CRT-based TV was introduced. This technology is regarded as mature. However, the CRT industry has put more effort in improving its technology. Flat-surface CRT technology was introduced in the 1990s and, recently, slim-depth CRT technology was released. Despite the low cost and relatively high picture quality, CRT has considerable disadvantages. Even with the new slim-depth technology, CRT screens are still bulky and heavy. In addition, it is difficult to produce CRT screens larger than 40 in.

Recently, flat display technologies such as plasma display panel (PDP), liquid crystal display (LCD), and organic light emitting device (OLED) are challenging incumbent CRT technology, previously dominating the display markets. LCDs are replacing CRT monitors for computers. LCD and OLED are exclusively utilized in handheld devices, such as cell phones and PDAs. LCD and PDP are competing with each other for flat panel TV market share. PDP is popular for screens larger than 40 in, while LCDs are penetrating TV markets with a display size of around 30 in. When shopping for a large-screen flat TV, consumers examine the price tag, image quality, power consumption, brightness, and so on. PDP and LCD industries have been working hard to improve every aspect of these factors. PDP and LCD will be more popular in large-screen flat high definition (HD) TVs, as the price of large-screen flat TVs is dropping rapidly, and digital TV broadcasting is increasing. In this chapter, color image quality issues that are unique to PDP will be discussed.

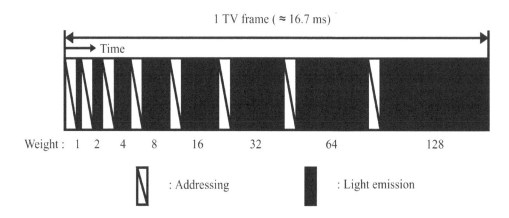

**FIGURE 18.1**
Example of pulse number modulation with eight subfields.

## 18.2    Pulse Number Modulation and Dynamic False Contour

The plasma display panel (PDP) represents gray levels by using the pulse number modulation technique. A TV field, 16.6 ms in case of 60 Hz, is divided into a set of subfields. Figure 18.1 presents an example of a TV field divided into eight subfields. Each subfield consists of addressing and light emission periods. The light emission period is composed of a number of sustaining pulses, proportional to the weights assigned to subfields. Gray-levels are represented by the selected subfields for light emission. Figure 18.2 presents selections of light emitting subfields for gray levels 127 and 128, respectively. Gray-level 127 is represented by turning on subfields [1 2 4 8 16 32 64]. Gray level 128 is represented by selecting subfield 128 only. In the eight subfield case, there is an unique combination of subfields to represent gray levels ranging from 0 to 255. However, when redundancy is permitted, for example, when representing 256 gray levels with more than eight subfields, there are multiple ways of representing the gray levels.

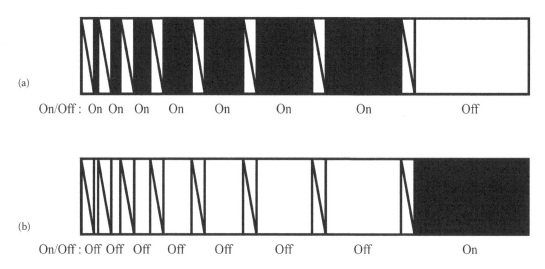

**FIGURE 18.2**
Gray-level representation for gray levels: (a) gray level 127, and (b) gray level 128.

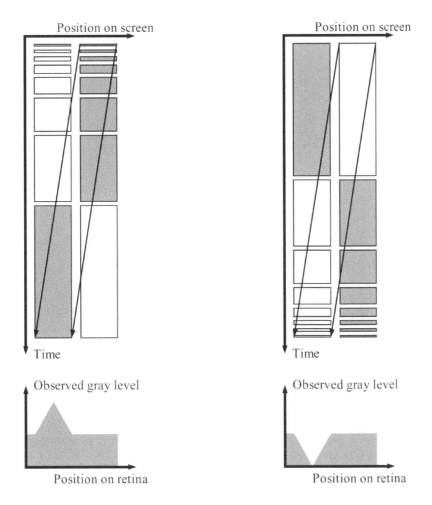

**FIGURE 18.3**
Examples of dynamic false contours for gray levels 127 and 128: (left) subfield [1 2 4 8 16 32 64 128], and (right) subfield [128 64 32 16 8 4 2 1].

Pulse number modulation is suitable for representing gray levels of a still image. However, in case of a moving image, it causes a problem. When an object moves, the human eye follows the motion. The brightness perceived by the human vision system is determined by integrating the light emission over time in the direction of the motion. A false contour would appear when light emission periods for neighboring gray levels are far apart. This is called the dynamic false contour problem of the PDP [1].

Figure 18.3 shows examples of dynamic false contours. Two gray levels 127 and 128 are moving from right to left, one pixel per frame. Slant lines represent lines of human eye integration. For simplicity, only light emission periods are shown. Gray-level 128 is represented by turning on a single subfield with 128 sustained pulses. Gray-level 127 is displayed by turning on seven subfields, excluding the largest one. In the left part of Figure 18.3, subfield [1 2 4 8 16 32 64 128] is applied. Bright false contour appears along the border between gray-levels 127 and 128. In the right of Figure 18.3, subfield of the reversed order [128 64 32 16 8 4 2 1] is employed. In this case, the dark false contour will be visible along the border. Figure 18.4 presents an example of simulated dynamic false contours on the sphere image.

**FIGURE 18.4**
Example of simulated dynamic false contours on a sphere image.

The degree of dynamic false contours depends on the subfield pattern. The number of possible subfield patterns becomes 8!(=40320) (i.e., permutations of [1 2 4 8 16 32 64 128]), when eight subfields are employed for representing 256 gray levels on a PDP. However, when representing 256 gray levels with more than eight subfields, the number of possible subfield patterns reaches an astronomical amount for an exhaustive search. To solve this problem, genetic algorithm-based selection of the optimum subfield pattern was proposed [2]. In Reference [2], a subfield pattern that minimizes quantitative measure of the dynamic false contour is selected as the optimum pattern. The optimization of the subfield pattern is performed by repetitive calculations based on a genetic algorithm. The optimum selection of the subfield pattern reduces the degree of dynamic false contours to some extent, however, it does not eliminate them entirely.

Figure 18.5a represents an original image utilized for the dynamic false contour simulation. Figure 18.5b and Figure 18.5c show the simulated images with subfield patterns [1 2 4 8 16 32 48 48 48 48] and [1 2 4 8 16 32 42 44 52 54], respectively. Subfield [1 2 4 8 16 32 42 44 52 54] is obtained by the genetic optimization method in Reference [2]. When comparing Figure 18.5b and Figure 18.5c, it can be noticed that the optimization of the subfield pattern can reduce the degree of dynamic false contours. However, even with subfield optimization, dynamic false contours are still visible.

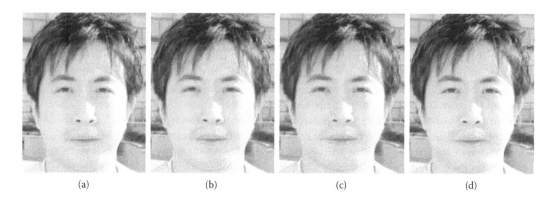

(a)                    (b)                    (c)                    (d)

**FIGURE 18.5 (See color insert.)**
Simulation of dynamic false contours: (a) original image, (b) simulation with [1 2 4 8 16 32 48 48 48 48], (c) simulation with [1 2 4 8 16 32 42 44 52 54], and (d) simulation with error diffusion.

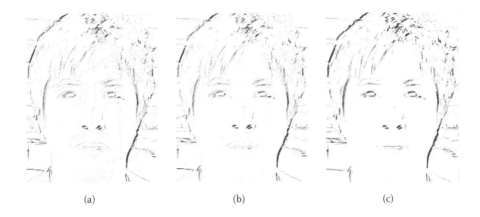

(a)    (b)    (c)

**FIGURE 18.6**
Difference between original (Figure 18.5a) and simulated images shown in (a) Figure 18.5b; (b) Figure 18.5c; and (c) Figure 18.5d.

A number of techniques have been proposed to further reduce dynamic false contours. These include the addition of equalizing pulses [3], the compression of light emission time [4], and error diffusion or dithering [5]. Among these techniques, error diffusion or dithering-based methods have been widely utilized. In these methods, pixels or areas under motion are estimated first. Their gray levels are modified to ensure they would not yield or minimize the dynamic false contour. In order to preserve original tone levels, error diffusion or dithering techniques are applied. Figure 18.5d shows the simulation results with error diffusion. Subfield pattern [1 2 4 8 16 32 42 44 52 54] is utilized in Figure 18.5d. The effect of error diffusion can be easily noticed by comparing Figure 18.5c and Figure 18.5d. Figure 18.6a to Figure 18.6c show the difference between the original image in Figure 18.5a and the simulated images shown in Figure 18.5b to Figure 18.5d. In addition to dynamic false contours, the edge contents are visible in Figure 18.6a to Figure 18.6c. It is due to registration errors during the simulation. By comparing the images shown in Figure 18.6a through Figure 18.6c, the effect of subfield optimization and error diffusion can be verified.

Another popular technique to reduce the dynamic false contour is called stretched-out coding [6]. The number of displayable gray levels is limited to prevent uneven distribution of light emission periods causing dynamic false contours. Table 18.1 presents an example

**TABLE 18.1**

Example of Stretched-Out Coding

| | Subfield Pattern | | | | | | | | | |
|---|---|---|---|---|---|---|---|---|---|---|
| Level | 1 | 2 | 4 | 8 | 16 | 24 | 32 | 40 | 56 | 72 |
| 0 | OFF | OFF | OFF | OFF | OFF | OFF | OFF | OFF | OFF | OFF |
| 1 | ON | OFF | OFF | OFF | OFF | OFF | OFF | OFF | OFF | OFF |
| 3 | ON | ON | OFF | OFF | OFF | OFF | OFF | OFF | OFF | OFF |
| 7 | ON | ON | ON | OFF | OFF | OFF | OFF | OFF | OFF | OFF |
| 15 | ON | ON | ON | ON | OFF | OFF | OFF | OFF | OFF | OFF |
| 31 | ON | ON | ON | ON | ON | OFF | OFF | OFF | OFF | OFF |
| 55 | ON | ON | ON | ON | ON | ON | OFF | OFF | OFF | OFF |
| 87 | ON | ON | ON | ON | ON | ON | ON | OFF | OFF | OFF |
| 127 | ON | ON | ON | ON | ON | ON | ON | ON | OFF | OFF |
| 183 | ON | ON | ON | ON | ON | ON | ON | ON | ON | OFF |
| 255 | ON | ON | ON | ON | ON | ON | ON | ON | ON | ON |

of stretched-out coding with subfield [1 2 4 8 16 24 32 40 56 72]. In stretched-out coding, the number of displayable gray levels equals the number of subfields plus one. The original gray levels ranging from 0 to 255 cannot be fully reproduced, because only the selected gray levels can be displayed. To solve this problem, error diffusion or dithering can be utilized. However, artifacts due to error diffusion or dithering become another impediment to achieving high-quality image representation.

## 18.3 Smooth Gray-Level Reproduction in Dark Areas

CRT technology has a nonlinear light intensity response to input values as demonstrated in Figure 18.7a. However, PDP technology has linear input–output characteristics as presented in Figure 18.7b within a normal operating range [7]. Thus, in order for the PDP to generate images equivalent to those using CRT technology, modification of the input digital values should be made. This process is called inverse gamma correction.

Inverse gamma correction is used to convert the output luminance response of the PDP presented in Figure 18.7b to the shape of the curve presented in Figure 18.7a. In applying inverse gamma correction, the input RGB levels of PDP are modified to the nearest integer values for the desired luminance. In Figure 18.7a, in dark areas (or lower gray-level ranges), the slope of the desired luminance curve is much lower than that of the luminance response of the PDP.

Figure 18.8 presents the result of the inverse gamma correction in dark areas. Horizontal and vertical axes represent input digital values and luminance levels. The smooth curve depicts the desired luminance levels. The staircase-shaped lines represent luminance levels after inverse gamma correction. In Figure 18.8, only six luminance levels can be displayed for input values ranging from 0 to 40. This would result in a loss of details in dark scenes that frequently appear in movies. The reduction in the number of displayable gray levels in dark areas causes false contours. They can appear in both still and moving images. Figure 18.9 presents the result of inverse gamma correction applied to a green ramp image.

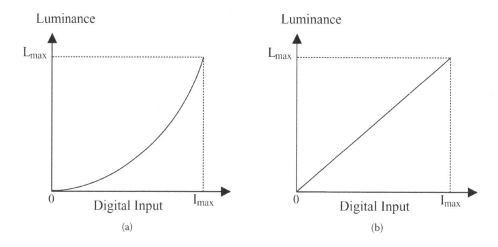

**FIGURE 18.7**
Output luminance response to input digital value: (a) CRT, and (b) PDP.

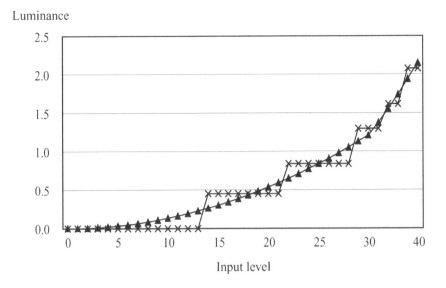

**FIGURE 18.8**
Result of inverse gamma correction for input levels ranging from 0 to 40.

The most popular techniques utilized for smooth representation of the gray levels in dark areas are error diffusion [8] and dithering [9]. The error diffusion-based gray level reproduction technique can be applied as follows: after the inverse gamma correction is applied, the difference between the displayed integer level and ideal gray level yielding the desired luminance level is calculated. The error diffusion technique is applied to the calculated difference. The error, that is, the calculated difference, is propagated to the neighboring pixels after being multiplied by the predetermined weights. The error diffusion method can reproduce gray levels on average. It is important to note that error diffusion could be implemented in terms of luminance levels. In other words, the difference between the desired and displayed luminance levels on a PDP can be utilized for error diffusion instead of the difference in gray levels.

In this section, it is assumed that a constant luminance area is required for display. In addition, assume that the gray level yielding the desired constant luminance level is in the range of [$n, n + 1$], where $n$ is an integer ranging from 0 to 255. The reproduction of the

**FIGURE 18.9**
Result of inverse gamma correction with green ramp image.

desired gray or luminance level is achieved by displaying a portion of area with integer value $n$ and the rest with $(n+1)$. The numbers of pixels displaying levels $n$ and $(n+1)$ are determined such that the average level should be the same or close to the desired gray level. In other words, the decimal fraction of the ideal gray level yielding the desired luminance determines the number of pixels for levels $n$ and $(n+1)$. The pixels of level $(n+1)$ will be called minor pixels, when the decimal fraction is less than 0.5. The pixels of level $n$ become minor pixels, when greater than 0.5.

Instead of error diffusion, dithering has been widely utilized for inverse gamma correction [9]. The principle of utilizing dithering for smooth gray level reproduction is much the same as the error diffusion-based technique. The input gray level is converted according to the desired gamma value. The decimal fraction of the converted level is binarized by comparing it with the contents of a predetermined dithering mask. The thresholded value is added to the integer component. The resulting gray level is displayed on the PDP. By displaying a combination of integer values $n$ and $(n+1)$, the desired level is achieved. However, unlike the error diffusion-based technique, error resulting from the binarization is not compensated.

In the PDP, the smallest difference in luminance levels of two consecutive gray levels is usually much greater than the contrast threshold value of the human visual system. Furthermore, the difference in the luminance levels will be increasing as manufacturers are putting emphasis on making their PDPs brighter. Thus, even though error diffusion or dithering reduces false contours, minor pixels are perceived by human vision as isolated dots. In particular, when minor pixels are not distributed homogeneously, image quality in dark areas deteriorates.

Multiple sustained pulses are usually assigned to represent the digital input level 1. In order to decrease the difference in luminance levels of two consecutive gray levels, utilization of a single-sustained pulse or light emission during the reset and addressing period was proposed for representing digital input level 1 [10]. They would reduce the luminance variation to a certain extent. However, minor pixels would still be noticeable, because the contrast threshold is much smaller than the difference due to a single sustained pulse.

The visibility of minor pixels could be reduced by preventing spatial and temporal overlaps of minor pixels [8]. This idea can be explained by the example shown in Figure 18.10a and Figure 18.10b. Namely, Figure 18.10a demonstrates a method of avoiding temporal

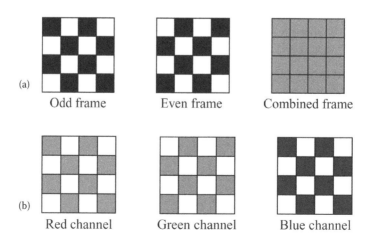

|   | Odd frame | Even frame | Combined frame |
|---|---|---|---|

|   | Red channel | Green channel | Blue channel |
|---|---|---|---|

**FIGURE 18.10**
Concept of minimization of minor pixel overlap: (a) minimization of temporal overlap, and (b) minimization of spatial overlap.

overlaps in minor pixels. For a given color channel, minor pixels (black dots) are turned on at different pixel locations for two consecutive frames. Because the human visual system has low-pass filtering characteristics over time, the combined frame would be perceived as the average of two frames. Figure 18.10b demonstrates an example of spatial distribution of RGB minor pixels. For a given frame, interchannel overlaps are minimized by turning on RGB pixels at different locations. However, it is not possible to place all RGB minor pixels at nonoverlapped locations. The overlaps of green and the other two color channels are minimized first because green is much brighter than red or blue. The overlaps of red and blue channels are allowed only if it is unavoidable. In addition to spatial and temporal overlaps, the spatial distribution of minor pixels is also an important factor in influencing the perceived image quality. Nonhomogeneous distribution of minor pixels would degrade the quality of gray level reproduction. In the subsequent section, error diffusion and dithering-based techniques for solving these problems are described.

### 18.3.1   Error Diffusion-Based Technique

In applying the inverse gamma correction, input RGB gray levels are converted to the nearest integer values for the desired luminance. The difference between the displayed integer level and ideal gray level for the desired luminance is subject to error diffusion. The calculated difference is simply the decimal fraction of the ideal gray level. In this section, it is assumed that the gray level converted by inverse gamma correction would be integer $n$, and the ideal gray level for the desired luminance would be $n.xx$, where $xx$ represents a decimal fraction. The difference between the displayed and ideal gray level becomes $0.xx$.

For the sake of simplicity, it is assumed that the decimal fraction is coded as an 8-bit integer ranging from 0 to 255. The output of error diffusion for the coded decimal fraction will be 0 or 255. The coded decimal fraction is doubled when it is smaller than 128, otherwise, it is doubled, and 255 is subtracted. This process of fraction doubling is demonstrated in Figure 18.11. The effect of doubling can be explained as follows; it is assumed that the coded decimal fraction of a constant image is 20. When doubled, it becomes 40. After error diffusion, the number of minor pixels will be doubled. If the doubled minor pixels were equally divided into two frames, there would be no overlaps over the two frames. Temporal overlaps of minor pixels for a given color channel can be minimized over two consecutive frames. It is assumed that the coded fraction is 204. In this case, it is changed to 153 (= 204*2 − 255) because the value 204 is greater than 128. The coded fraction 204 and 153 corresponds to decimal fractions 0.8 and 0.6, respectively. The number of minor pixels for the coded number 204 should be 20% of the total pixels. When error diffusion is applied, the number of minor pixels becomes 40% of total pixels. The minor pixels per frame will be equal to 20%, when divided into two frames.

It has been known that error diffusion with channel-dependent threshold modulation generates homogeneously distributed minor pixels [11], [12]. This can be described by the following equations:

$$u_i(m, n) = x_i(m, n) + \sum_{(k,l) \in R} w(k, l) e_i(m - k, n - l) \qquad i \in \{r, g, b\} \tag{18.1}$$

$$o_i(m, n) = \begin{cases} 255 & \text{if} \quad u_i(m, n) > T_i(m, n) \\ 0 & \text{else} \end{cases} \tag{18.2}$$

$$e_i(m, n) = u_i(m, n) - b_i(m, n) \tag{18.3}$$

where $x_i(m, n)$ represents the doubled fraction. Subscript $i$ represents one of color channels $r, g, b$. The term $o_i(m, n)$ represents output value, and $u_i(m, n)$ is the updated value, and $e_i(m, n)$ denotes the quantization error defined as the difference between the updated and

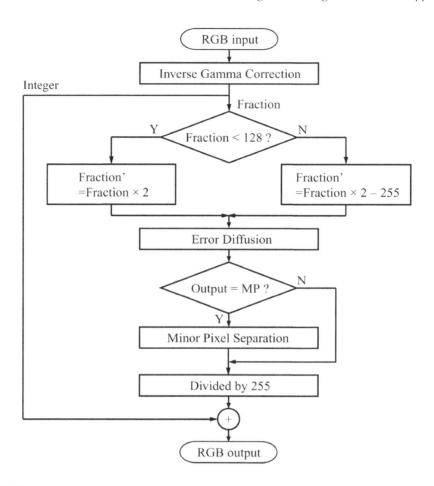

**FIGURE 18.11**
Flow chart of error diffusion-based gray-level reproduction technique.

output value. The term $w(k, l)$ represents the error diffusion kernel, and $R$ denotes the set of neighboring pixels for error propagation. In Equation 18.2, threshold values for green and red channels are respectively determined based on the error values of red and green channels as follows:

$$T_g(m, n) = 128 - \sum_{(k,l) \in R} w(k, l)e_r(m - k, n - l) \tag{18.4}$$

$$T_r(m, n) = 128 - \sum_{(k,l) \in R} w(k, l)e_g(m - k, n - l) \tag{18.5}$$

However, the threshold for B channel remains constant (i.e., $T_b(m, n) = 128$). The details of threshold modulation can be found in Reference [11].

In order to generate homogeneously distributed minor pixels and reduce the spatial inter-channel overlaps (overlaps of color channels within a given frame), error diffusion with decision rules can be applied. It is assumed that R, G, and B denote the doubled fraction. The output values for green and red channels are determined first. The output value of the blue channel is decided next, based on the output values of the green and red channels, because the luminance of the blue channel is the smallest.

The details of the error diffusion process demonstrated in Figure 18.12 can be summarized as follows:

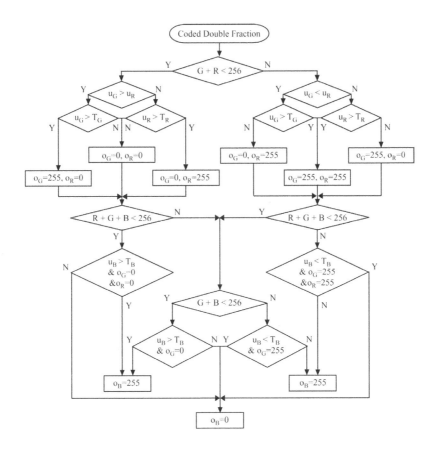

**FIGURE 18.12**
Flow chart of error diffusion process with decision rules.

- When overlaps of minor pixels for green and red channels can be avoided ($G + R < 256$), outputs of green and red channels are decided, such that there will be no overlaps. When overlaps of any two combinations of $RGB$ channels can be avoided ($G + R < 256$ and $R + G + B < 256$), the blue channel is turned on only at the pixel locations where both green and red are in the off state. When overlaps of green and red can be avoided, but overlaps of all $RGB$ values are unavoidable ($G + R < 256$ and $R + G + B \geq 256$), overlaps of red and blue are allowed, but overlaps of green and blue are minimized.
- When there should be some overlaps of green and red ($G+R \geq 256$), their overlaps are minimized. When every pixel is required to be turned on for one or two color channels ($G + R \geq 256$ and $R + G + B < 512$), the output of blue is selected to minimize the overlaps between green and the other two channels. When every pixel is required to be turned on for at least two color channels ($G + R \geq 256$ and $R + G + B > 512$), the number of pixel locations where all three RGB channels are turned on is minimized.

After the error diffusion with decision rules shown in Figure 18.12 is applied, the generated minor pixels should be equally divided into two frames. It is accomplished by utilizing rules listed in Table 18.2, where "R/B" represent the red or blue channel. Note that these rules are applied only to minor pixels. When minor pixels have the value of 255, the top two lines of Table 18.2 can be interpreted as follows: In the odd-numbered row of

**TABLE 18.2**

Rules for Minor Pixel Separation

| Frame | Row | Order of MP | Assigned Output Red/Blue | Green |
|-------|------|-------------|------------|-------|
| Odd | Odd | Odd | On | Off |
| | | Even | Off | On |
| | Even | Odd | Off | On |
| | | Even | On | Off |
| Even | Odd | Odd | Off | On |
| | | Even | On | Off |
| | Even | Odd | On | Off |
| | | Even | Off | On |

an odd-numbered frame, only the even-numbered minor pixels of the green channel are kept. However, in the same row, for the red or blue channel, only the odd-numbered minor pixels are kept. By selecting half of the minor pixels, temporal overlaps are minimized over two consecutive frames.

The decision rules in Table 18.2 are also effective in reducing intechannel overlaps within a given frame. This effect can be explained by the following example: It is assumed that a constant image with the coded fraction $R = G = B = 127$ be chosen for displaying. In this case, the minor pixels for each channel have the value of 255. When doubled, they become $R = G = B = 254$. After error diffusion is applied, all RGB channels will be turned on at almost every pixel location, because this case corresponds to the condition ($G + R \geq 256$ and $R + G + B > 512$), as demonstrated in Figure 18.12. In the odd-numbered row in the odd-numbered frame, only even-numbered minor pixels of the green channel will be kept. However, in the same row, only the odd-numbered minor pixels of R/B will be selected. It is assumed that all pixels in a row have an output value $R = G = B = 255$. Then, green and R/B will be selected alternately by the decision rules in Table 18.2. Thus, it can be said that the rules listed in Table 18.2 are effective in reducing interchannel overlaps, especially in the midtone range. The integer part is incremented by 1 and displayed on the PDP, when the value 255 is selected by the decision rules as presented in Table 18.2; otherwise, the original integer value is displayed on the PDP.

The performance of the described technique is compared with that of conventional error diffusion. In the conventional method, RGB channels are processed independently. Two methods are hardware implemented for a commercial 42-in. sized PDP. The images on the PDP are photographed using a digital camera. The results with a constant gray image whose input gray level $R = G = B = 8$ are presented in Figure 18.13. After inverse gamma correction, the input value is converted into $R = G = B = 0.125$. The 8-bit coded fraction becomes 32. Figure 18.13a and Figure 18.13b show the results of the conventional method. Figure 18.13c and Figure 18.13d shows the results of the described technique. All these images consist of the pixels with value 0 or 1, because the inverse gamma corrected value is 0.125. In Figure 18.13a, all RGB channels are turned on at the same pixel locations. However, in Figure 18.13c, overlaps of minor pixels are minimized. In addition, from Figure 18.13d, it can be noticed that minor pixels are distributed homogeneously. The described techniques can be expanded to reduce temporal overlaps over three or more frames. However, it should be mentioned that as the number of frames considered for reduction of overlaps increases, the degree of flickering may have increased.

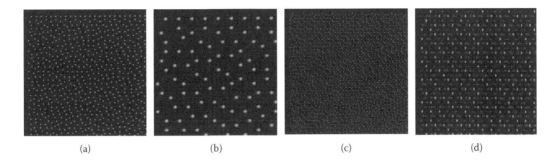

|     |     |     |     |
| :-: | :-: | :-: | :-: |
| (a) | (b) | (c) | (d) |

**FIGURE 18.13 (See color insert.)**
Constant image with 8-bit coded fraction = 32 by error diffusion-based technique: (a, b) result of conventional error diffusion and its enlarged version, and (c, d) result of described technique and its enlarged version.

## 18.3.2 Dithering-Based Technique

Instead of error diffusion, dithering can be utilized for smooth representation of gray levels in dark areas [9]. In the dithering-based approach, the input gray level is converted according to the desired gamma value. The decimal fraction of the converted level is binarized by comparing it with the threshold of a predetermined dithering mask. The quantized value is added to the integer part and subsequently displayed on the PDP. Figure 18.14 shows the flow chart of the dithering-based approach. By displaying a combination of integer value $n$ and $(n + 1)$, the desired level is achieved. The objective of the dithering-based approach would be the same: reduction of minor pixel overlaps and homogeneous distribution of minor pixels.

For simplicity, it is assumed that three frames are considered for a reduction in overlaps, and the decimal fraction is coded as 4-bit integers ranging from 0 to 15. If the coded decimal fraction is less than the threshold value, it is quantized as value 1, otherwise, it will be

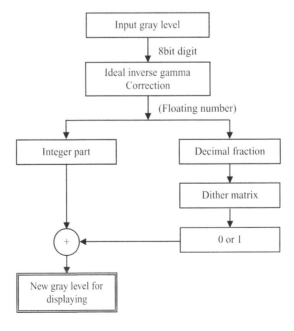

**FIGURE 18.14**
Flow chart of dithering-based technique for gray-level reproduction.

(a)

| 10 | 1 | 11 | 8 | 3 | 15 | 4 | 6 | 3 | 14 |
|---|---|---|---|---|---|---|---|---|---|
| 8 | 3 | 13 | 5 | 10 | 0 | 9 | 2 | 10 | 1 |
| 12 | 15 | 7 | 2 | 14 | 12 | 7 | 15 | 12 | 8 |
| 3 | 0 | 8 | 9 | 3 | 1 | 11 | 4 | 0 | 6 |
| 10 | 4 | 13 | 6 | 11 | 6 | 8 | 3 | 14 | 9 |
| 1 | 11 | 13 | 2 | 15 | 0 | 14 | 10 | 6 | 3 |
| 8 | 5 | 4 | 7 | 12 | 9 | 5 | 2 | 11 | 13 |
| 3 | 14 | 9 | 1 | 5 | 2 | 7 | 15 | 0 | 8 |
| 11 | 0 | 5 | 15 | 11 | 13 | 5 | 10 | 4 | 14 |
| 2 | 12 | 10 | 8 | 4 | 0 | 8 | 14 | 6 | 2 |

(b)

| 3 | 6 | 2 | 14 | 12 | 3 | 13 | 5 | 15 | 2 |
|---|---|---|---|---|---|---|---|---|---|
| 13 | 11 | 9 | 6 | 10 | 6 | 2 | 11 | 0 | 4 |
| 2 | 4 | 0 | 13 | 1 | 8 | 14 | 5 | 7 | 12 |
| 8 | 14 | 11 | 5 | 15 | 4 | 9 | 1 | 13 | 5 |
| 5 | 9 | 7 | 2 | 10 | 13 | 2 | 11 | 9 | 1 |
| 14 | 6 | 0 | 12 | 4 | 6 | 8 | 4 | 15 | 6 |
| 3 | 11 | 15 | 3 | 8 | 14 | 0 | 12 | 3 | 8 |
| 9 | 1 | 12 | 6 | 13 | 9 | 11 | 2 | 7 | 11 |
| 5 | 7 | 10 | 3 | 0 | 7 | 4 | 13 | 12 | 3 |
| 15 | 3 | 14 | 5 | 10 | 15 | 1 | 9 | 5 | 15 |

(c)

| 11 | 14 | 9 | 0 | 7 | 8 | 1 | 13 | 7 | 9 |
|---|---|---|---|---|---|---|---|---|---|
| 0 | 7 | 3 | 15 | 2 | 11 | 14 | 6 | 11 | 14 |
| 6 | 10 | 12 | 4 | 9 | 5 | 0 | 8 | 3 | 1 |
| 13 | 6 | 1 | 11 | 7 | 13 | 4 | 12 | 10 | 15 |
| 10 | 15 | 3 | 14 | 0 | 5 | 15 | 7 | 2 | 7 |
| 2 | 0 | 8 | 6 | 9 | 10 | 1 | 13 | 0 | 12 |
| 12 | 7 | 10 | 14 | 1 | 3 | 11 | 6 | 9 | 4 |
| 15 | 2 | 4 | 11 | 6 | 15 | 4 | 8 | 14 | 2 |
| 10 | 13 | 8 | 2 | 9 | 1 | 13 | 0 | 6 | 10 |
| 8 | 6 | 0 | 14 | 12 | 7 | 10 | 3 | 11 | 7 |

**FIGURE 18.15**
Example of dithering masks to reduce minor pixel overlaps. Portion of dithering mask for: (a) the first frame, (b) the second frame, and (c) the third frame.

assigned as 0. Three different dithering masks can be designed to reduce temporal overlaps. In addition, the order of threshold values can be chosen to yield homogeneous distribution of minor pixels within a frame. Figure 18.15a to Figure 18.15c show a portion of such dithering masks of size $32 \times 32$. Because reduction of temporal overlaps and homogeneous distribution of minor pixels are achieved by the designed dithering masks, only a reduction of interchannel overlaps is left for explanation. The basic principle can be described with a simple $4 \times 4$ mask depicted in Figure 18.16 where the threshold value also represents a pixel location. When the 4-bit coded fraction is $R = G = B = 1$, green, red and blue are turned on at a pixel location with threshold values of 0, 1, and 2, respectively. When $R = G = B = 2$, green is turned on at pixel locations 0 and 1, red is turned on at pixel locations 2 and 3, and blue is turned on at pixel locations 4 and 5.

The flow chart of the described technique is depicted in Figure 18.17, where X_on_pixel_reg is an array representing a 4-bit coded fraction. The values of the array are determined by the following rules:

Coded fraction 0 : X_on_pixel_reg = "0000000000000000"

Coded fraction 1 : X_on_pixel_reg = "1000000000000000"

Coded fraction 2 : X_on_pixel_reg = "1100000000000000"

Coded fraction 3 : X_on_pixel_reg = "1110000000000000"

$$\vdots$$

Coded fraction 15 : X_on_pixel_reg = "1111111111111110"

| 1 | 13 | 3 | 15 |
|---|---|---|---|
| 9 | 5 | 11 | 7 |
| 4 | 0 | 2 | 14 |
| 12 | 8 | 10 | 6 |

**FIGURE 18.16**
Example of $4 \times 4$ mask.

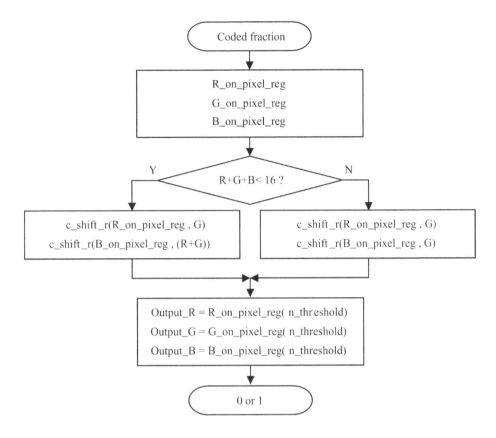

**FIGURE 18.17**
Flow chart of the interchannel overlap reduction technique.

X_on_pixel_reg(n) denotes the value of the *n*th bit of array. For example, X_on_pixel_reg(0) represents the leftmost bit on X_on_pixel_reg. The c_shift_r(m,l) denotes a circular shift right operation for the array *m* by the amount of l bit. The n_threshold is the threshold value at the current pixel location.

If the sum of the 4-bit coded value is less than 16, $R + G + B < 16$, all of three channels can be turned on at different pixel locations. In this case, R_on_pixel_reg is circular shifted to the right by G bits. The B_on_pixel_reg is also circular shifted to the right by $(R + G)$ bits. For example, when $R = G = B = 4$, all of arrays will be "111100000000000". After the shift operation, they are changed to the following values:

$$G\_pixel\_reg = \text{"1111000000000000"}$$

$$R\_pixel\_reg = \text{"0000111100000000"}$$

$$B\_pixel\_reg = \text{"0000000011110000"}$$

If the threshold value under processing is three, n_threhsold = 3, output_G = 1, output_R = 0, output_B = 0. If the sum of the coded value is greater than or equal to 16, overlap of three color channels is unavoidable. Both R_on_pixel_reg and B_on_pixel_reg are circular shifted to the right by G bits. This means that red and blue will be turned on at the same pixel location. In addition, there may be overlaps between green and red/blue channels. It is assumed that the coded values of three channels are of value 10, $R = G = B = 10$.

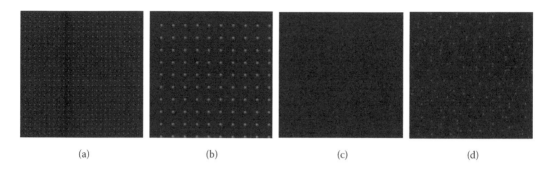

(a)                    (b)                    (c)                    (d)

**FIGURE 18.18** (See color insert.)
Constant image with 4-bit coded fraction = 1 by dithering-based technique: (a, b) result of conventional error diffusion and its enlarged version, and (c, d) result of described technique and its enlarged version.

All the array values would be "1111111111000000". After the shift operation, they are converted into the following values:

$$G\_pixel\_reg = \text{"1111111111000000"}$$

$$R\_pixel\_reg = \text{"1111000000111111"}$$

$$B\_pixel\_reg = \text{"1111000000111111"}$$

The performance of the described technique is compared with that of conventional dithering with the Bayer mask [13]. The two methods are hardware implemented, and images are displayed on a commercial 42-in. PDP. The images on PDP are photographed using a digital camera. The results with a constant gray image with input gray level $R = G = B = 3$ are shown in Figure 18.18a to Figure 18.18d. After inverse gamma correction, the input value is converted into $R = G = B = 0.0625$. The 4-bit coded fraction is 1. Figure 18.18a and Figure 18.8b show results corresponding to the Bayer mask, whereas Figure 18.18c and Figure 18.18d show results of the described dithering technique. As can be seen in Figure 18.18b, the regular structure of the Bayer mask is clearly visible, and all RGB channels are turned on at the same pixel locations. However, in Figure 18.13d, overlaps of minor pixels are reduced, and the regularity of the dithering mask is not clear as in Figure 18.18b. Compared to the results based on the error diffusion-based technique shown in Figure 18.13a to Figure 18.13d, the dithering-based approach lacks the homogeneity of minor pixels.

## 18.4  Color Reproduction on PDP

Faithful color reproduction is another key factor affecting image quality on the PDP. The color coordinates of phosphors utilized for PDP are usually different from those for the CRT or HDTV standard. Figure 18.19 presents chromaticity coordinates of the HDTV standard and those measured from a commercial PDP TV. Table 18.3 lists chromaticity coordinates presented in Figure 18.19.

Figure 18.20 shows the gamut difference in $a^* b^*$ plane of $L^* a^* b^*$ color space between the commercial PDP and CRT monitor. $L^* a^* b^*$ are device-independent color coordinates. $L^*$ represents luminance contents. Chroma can be described by $a^*$ and $b^*$. Gamut of the PDP is larger in the yellow-to-green hue area (left and top area) and smaller in the blue-to-red hue area (right bottom area).

In order to reproduce colors according to HDTV standards, various color matching techniques can be applied. One of these is the vector error diffusion technique [14].

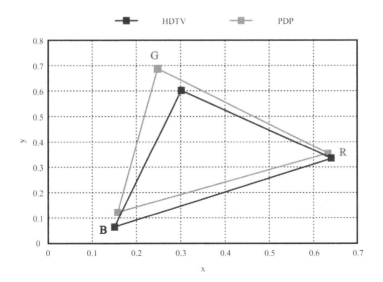

**FIGURE 18.19**
Difference in chromaticity coordinates for PDP and HDTV standard.

Figure 18.21 presents the diagram for the vector error diffusion-based color-matching technique. The vector errors in the XYZ color space are compensated by the error diffusion process. The three color models, reference, forward, and backward color models, are utilized as presented in Figure 18.21. They are determined by the off-line procedure. The reference color model specifies transformation from inverse gamma corrected RGB vector to a desired color vector in the XYZ space. It is determined based on specification of target color, satisfying the HDTV standard and phosphor characteristics of the PDP. The forward and backward color models represent color transformation from XYZ space to RGB space and RGB to XYZ space, respectively. They are calculated based on the colorimetric measurements.

In applying inverse gamma correction, the input RGB vector is changed to a new RGB vector. It is then converted into an ideal color vector in XYZ color space by the reference color model. The following equation specifies transformation from inverse gamma corrected RGB vectors to XYZ vectors when the HDTV standard listed in Table 18.3 is required:

$$\begin{bmatrix} X \\ Y \\ Z \end{bmatrix} = \begin{bmatrix} 41.4815 & 35.2719 & 21.97 \\ 21.3889 & 70.5438 & 8.27 \\ 1.9444 & 11.7573 & 115.7087 \end{bmatrix} \begin{bmatrix} R \\ G \\ B \end{bmatrix} \tag{18.6}$$

**TABLE 18.3**

Chromaticity Coordinates of HDTV Standard and a Typical PDP TV

|  | Chromaticity Coordinates | Red | Green | Blue |
|---|---|---|---|---|
| Measured from PDP | $x$ | 0.63 | 0.24 | 0.15 |
|  | $y$ | 0.35 | 0.68 | 0.11 |
| HDTV standard | $x$ | 0.64 | 0.3 | 0.15 |
|  | $y$ | 0.33 | 0.6 | 0.06 |

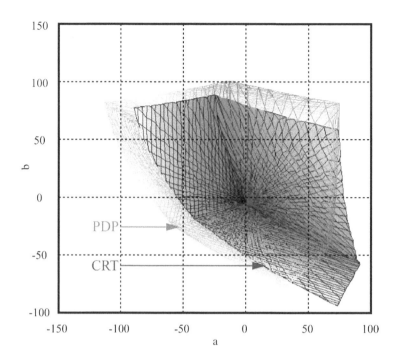

**FIGURE 18.20  (See color insert.)**
Gamut difference between PDP and CRT.

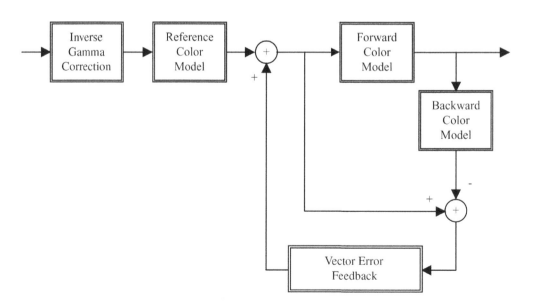

**FIGURE 18.21**
Block diagram of color matching based on vector error diffusion.

The forward color model defines color transformation from the XYZ space to RGB space on the PDP. It can be described by the following linear transformation:

$$
\begin{bmatrix} R \\ G \\ B \end{bmatrix} = \begin{bmatrix} A \end{bmatrix} \begin{bmatrix} f_1(X, Y, Z) \\ f_2(X, Y, Z) \\ \vdots \\ f_n(X, Y, Z) \end{bmatrix}
\tag{18.7}
$$

where $[RGB]^T$ represents input RGB coordinates. $[XYZ]^T$ is measured color coordinates when $[RGB]^T$ is displayed on the PDP. $f_n(X, Y, Z)$ denotes a function of (X,Y,Z). $A$ is the transformation matrix. It is assumed that the input color $[RGB]^T$ and function of the measured output color $[XYZ]^T$ obey linear transformation. The transformation matrix $A$ can be determined by least squares estimation based on a set of measurement data. Table 18.4 lists types of function that can be utilized for color coordinate transformation. The measurement of displayed colors on the PDP is performed based on standardized procedure [15] using a spectroradiometer.

The backward color model specifies color transformation from RGB to XYZ space. It can be formulated as follows:

$$
\begin{bmatrix} X \\ Y \\ Z \end{bmatrix} = \begin{bmatrix} B \end{bmatrix} \begin{bmatrix} f_1(R, G, B) \\ f_2(R, G, B) \\ \vdots \\ f_n(R, G, B) \end{bmatrix}
\tag{18.8}
$$

The transformation matrix $B$ is determined by the same procedure used for the forward color model. When $A$ and $B$ are $3 \times 3$, $A$ will be the inverse of $B$. In order to increase modeling accuracy, piecewise linear transformation can be utilized instead. In this case, the forward and backward models in Equation 18.7 and Equation 18.8 will be specified by multiple transformations.

The online color matching procedure shown in Figure 18.21 can be described as follows: the inverse gamma corrected RGB vectors are converted into the desired XYZ vectors by the reference color model. They are updated based on the weighted vector errors. The updated XYZ color vector is transformed to a RGB vector by the forward color model and displayed on the PDP. Based on the backward color model, the XYZ vector of the displayed color is determined. The difference between updated and displayed color vector in the XYZ space is weighted by the error diffusion kernel and propagated to the neighboring pixels to be processed.

The performance of the described vector error diffusion-based technique can be evaluated by measuring the color difference between the reference and displayed color. Figure 18.22a and Figure 18.22b show 181 samples utilized for evaluation of color reproduction and its distribution in RGB color space. The RGB color coordinates of testing samples are inverse gamma corrected and converted by the reference color model. The resulting XYZ

**TABLE 18.4**

Type of Function for $(X,Y,Z)$ and Size of $A$

| n | $f_n(X, Y, Z)$ | Size of A |
| --- | --- | --- |
| 3 | X,Y,Z | $3 \times 3$ |
| 6 | X, Y, Z, XY, YZ, XZ | $3 \times 6$ |
| 14 | 1, X, Y, Z, XY, YZ, XZ, $X^2$, $Y^2$, $Z^2$, $X^3$, $Y^3$, $Z^3$, XYZ | $3 \times 14$ |

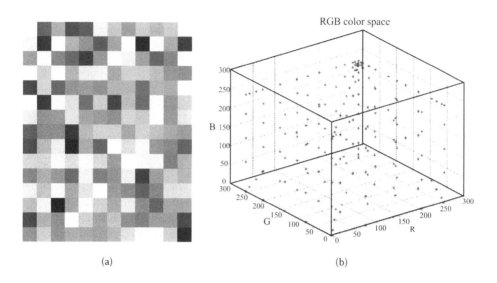

(a)                                            (b)

**FIGURE 18.22**
(a) Testing sample and (b) its distribution in RGB color space.

**TABLE 18.5**

Color Difference Before and After the Described Technique

|  | $\triangle E$ | All Testing Samples (181) | Inside Gamut Samples (106) | Outside Gamut Samples (75) |
|---|---|---|---|---|
| Without color matching | Average | 17.24 | 10.57 | 26.67 |
| With color matching | Average | 8.81 | 2.30 | 18.02 |

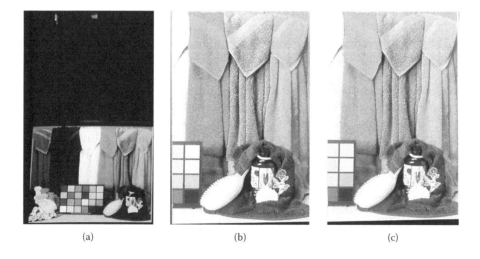

(a)                        (b)                        (c)

**FIGURE 18.23**
(a) Image displayed on CRT, (b) right portion of CRT image displayed on PDP with described color matching technique, and (c) right portion of CRT image displayed on PDP without color matching.

color coordinates are transformed into color coordinates in $L^*a^*b^*$ space. The $L^*a^*b^*$ color coordinates of testing samples displayed on the PDP are measured by spectrora-diometer, after the described technique is applied. Table 18.5 lists average $\triangle E$ before and after applying the described technique. The color difference is dropped by half for all of the 181 testing samples. However, for the inside gamut samples, the color difference is reduced by a factor of 5. Figure 18.23a to Figure 18.23c present the result with a real image. Namely, Figure 18.23a shows the CRT image satisfying the HDTV specification, whereas Figure 18.23b and Figure 18.23c represent the right portion of the CRT image with and without color matching, respectively. The colors of towels after applying the described technique exhibit a closer match with the original colors presented in Figure 18.23a.

## 18.5   Conclusion

The color image quality problems that are unique to the PDP have been discussed. Due to the pulse number modulation and nature of human vision system that follows the motion on the PDP, dynamic false contours appear on the moving image. The degree of dynamic false contour depends on the subfield pattern. Subfield optimization would be the first step for dynamic false contour reduction. In order to further reduce the level of dynamic false contour, gray-level conversion followed by error diffusion or dithering can be applied.

 The smooth reproduction of gray levels in dark areas is an important problem to im-prove image quality on the PDP. The number of displayable gray levels is reduced when inverse gamma correction is applied to generate images equivalent to CRT. Minor pixels ap-pear as isolated noises, when conventional error diffusion or the dithering-based approach is utilized for gray-level reproduction. Minimization of minor pixel overlaps and homo-geneous distribution of minor pixels would yield smoother reproduction of gray levels in dark areas. For error diffusion, threshold modulation provides homogeneous distribu-tion of minor pixels. In doubling the decimal fraction for error diffusion and employing appropriate decision rules, overlaps of minor pixels were reduced. Utilization of different dithering masks generates homogeneous distribution of minor pixels and reduces temporal overlaps, when dithering is chosen for gray-level reproduction. The interchannel overlaps were reduced by arranging image data in the form of an array and employing simple shift operations to the array data.

 Faithful color reproduction is another key factor affecting image quality. The vector error diffusion-based technique was described. Three color models are determined in advance. The difference between the desired and actually displayed color is regarded as error. This is weighted and propagated to neighboring pixels for compensation.

## References

[1] T. Yamaguchi, T. Masuda, A. Kohgami, and S. Mikoshiba, Degradation of moving-image quality in PDPs: Dynamic false contour, *J. SID*, 4/4, pp. 263–270, 1996.

[2] S.H. Park and C.W. Kim, An optimum selection of subfield pattern for plasma displays based on genetic algorithm, in *Spec. Issue on Electron. Displays, IEICE Trans. on Electron.*, E84C, 1659–1666, 2001.

[3] K. Toda, T. Yamaguchi, Y-W Zhu, S. Mikoshiba, T. Ueda, K. Kariya, and T. Shinoda, An equal-izing pulse technique for reducing gray scale disturbances of PDPs below the minimum visual perception level, *Proceedings of Euro Display '96* pp. 39–42, 1996.

[4] T. Yamamoto, Y. Takano, K. Ishii, T. Koura, H. Kokubun, K. Majima, T. Kurita, K. Yamaguchi, K. Kobayashi, and H. Murakami, Improvement of moving-picture quality on a 42-in.-diagonal PDP for HDTV, in *SID'97*, pp. 217–220, 1997.

[5] I. Kawahara and K. Sekimoto, Dynamic gray-scale control to reduce motion picture disturbance for high resolution PDP, in *SID'99 Digest*, pp. 166–169, 1999.

[6] Y. Otobe, M. Yoshida, N. Otaka, M. Tajima, K. Ishida, K. Ogawa, and T. Ueda, Display Driving Method and Apparatus, United States Patent, 6, 144, 364, 2000.

[7] K. Wani, A novel driving scheme and panel design for realization of a picture quality equivalent to CRTs, in *IDW'99*, pp. 775–778, 1999.

[8] J.Y. Cho and C.W. Kim, Error diffusion techniques for reproduction of smooth gray level in dark areas on PDP, in *IDW'03*, pp. 925–928, 2003.

[9] S.H. Park and C.W. Kim, A dithering based technique for reducing false contours in dark areas on plasma displays, in *IMID'01*, pp. 468–471, 2001.

[10] O. Masayuki, Drive system for plasma display, Japanese Patent, 065521, 1999.

[11] H.S. Seo, K.M. Kang, and C.W. Kim, Channel dependent error diffusion algorithm for dot-off-dot printing, in *SPIE'04*, Vol. 5293, pp. 314–321, 2004.

[12] R. Eschbach, Pseudo-vector error diffusion using cross separation threshold imprints, in *Proceedings of the IS&T Symposiun on Electronic Imaging*, pp. 321–323, 1999.

[13] R.A. Ulichney *Digital Halftoning*, MIT Press, Cambridge, MA, USA, 1987.

[14] H. Haneishi, T. Suzuki, N. Shimoyama, and Y. Miyake, Color digital halftoning taking colorimetric color reproduction into account, *J. Electron. Imaging*, 5, pp. 97–106, 1996.

[15] International Electrotechnical Comminssion, Equipment using plasma display panels, in *IEC 61966-5*, 2001.

# 19

# Image Processing for Virtual Artwork Restoration

Alessia De Rosa, Alessandro Piva, and Vito Cappellini

## CONTENTS

## 19.1 Introduction

In the last few years, the development of multimedia technology and the availability of more effective electronic imaging tools attracted the attention of researchers and managers of academy, industry, museums, and government bodies, working in the sector of *cultural heritage*, toward the possibility of applying image processing techniques for the analysis, restoration, archiving, and preserving of artwork. The growing interest for the application of image processing techniques for cultural heritage is due not only to the wider availability of digital computer storage and computational power, but also to the fact that an ever-increasing number of scientists with a background in analytical techniques and interpretation of the produced data have been involved in this field, probably stimulated by several projects founded by national and international governments [1].

Among the recent applications of image processing to the cultural heritage field, it is possible to mention the creation of very high-resolution images of paintings for dissemination or study/research purposes, the evaluation of the quality of digital reproductions of artworks in printed or displayed form, the protection of artwork digital reproductions through data hiding algorithms, the use of three-dimensional (3-D) digital techniques for representation and processing of artworks, automatic tools for better knowledge of conservation materials and processes, art dissemination and fruition, and advanced virtual restoration techniques of artwork [2], [3].

It is the purpose of this chapter to analyze how image processing methods may be used in meaningful applications in the cultural heritage field, with particular focus on the implementation of virtual restoration techniques. It is well known that the present visual appearance of a painting may be altered due to aging or unfortunate events. Because it is questionable whether a real conservation treatment should aim at bringing the artwork back in time at the moment in which the artist completed it, a virtual representation of the artwork can offer a solution to this concern, and at the same time can provide an estimation of the artwork at the time it was created by the artist. On the contrary, with respect to the actual restoration, virtual restoration does not involve the real artwork, so it is possible to perform as many attempts as one wants, resulting in no damage to the artwork and having the possibility of several tests to be compared to point out the best one: it can give useful indications to the restorers who will work on the actual painting or fresco. In particular, image processing tools can be used as a guide to the actual restoration of the artwork, or they can produce a digitally restored version of the work, valuable by itself, although the restoration is only virtual and cannot be reproduced on the real piece of work.

In this chapter, the most important applications of image processing for virtual artwork restoration are reviewed. First, the tools for virtually cleaning dirty paintings will be described in Section 19.2. Several phenomena can degrade the colors of paintings, deteriorating their appearance; cleaning is usually performed by conservation experts with a trial-and-error approach: different chemical cleaning substances are applied in small regions of the painting to select the most appropriate for cleaning the entire painting. A digital color cleaning technique can be used to foresee the final result if the same cleaning methodology is applied to the whole piece of work, so that restorers can use this tool to choose which cleaning procedure is likely to give the best result, thanks to the possibility of analyzing not only the actual cleaned patches, but also the whole virtually cleaned painting.

Next, in Section 19.3, some solutions proposed for the enhancement of the quality of color in images representing paintings, trying to reduce degradations engendered by low-quality acquisition, or by the degradation of the picture with time, will be described.

Section 19.4, reviews the algorithms for removing cracks from paintings and frescos. Cracks are often caused by a rapid loss of water in the painting's varnish: when the painting is located in a dry environment, a nonuniform contraction of the varnish covering can cause the formation of cracks. With image processing tools, it is possible to entirely remove cracks by means of interpolation techniques; in this way, the painting, even if in a virtual version, can again achieve its original appearance as it was in the intent of the artist who created it.

Another technique for virtual artwork restoration is the lacuna filling, reviewed in Section 19.5. Lacunas are a very common damage that can occur to paintings and more often to frescos and wall paintings, when some parts of the fresco collapse and fall down; in this case, the effect is the creation of large areas where the original image is lost. Actual restoration techniques tend to fill in these areas with a uniform color or a set of colors, to give the impression of continuity of image. With image processing tools, it is possible to simulate the same process on the digital version of the artwork.

In addition to the algorithms specifically used for the virtual restoration of artwork digital representations, there are other tasks increasingly pursued for their great benefit in the analysis and preservation of artworks. The first is the mosaicking procedure that can be used to join a certain number of overlapping sub-images, described in Section 19.6. In many cases, the painting to be analyzed is so big that it is not possible to obtain, in a single acquisition, an unique digital image with the desired quality. On the contrary, several images representing subparts of the painting are obtained. In this case, the mosaicking allows for an unique digital image representing the whole scene to be reconstructed. A second task is the registration procedure, reviewed in Section 19.7. Similar to what happens in the medical fields, also in the cultural heritage field it is often needed to observe and integrate several sets of data coming from different sources and stored in various images. Registration is the determination of a geometrical transformation that aligns points in one picture with corresponding points in another picture. It is an useful procedure in all cases in which the analysis of the painting can be performed by gaining the information coming from different images taken at different times (e.g., historical pictures versus current pictures) or from different points of view or by means of different sensors, thus acquiring the images in different spectral bands (e.g., IR-reflectograms, X-radiographies). Another task regards methods for edge extraction, described in Section 19.8. Often, to obtain better knowledge of the artwork, during their work, restorers extract borders or edges of the painting they are dealing with. The revealed features are not only painting's elements (i.e., contours of subjects present in the painting), but also characteristics of the layer, for example, bonds of wood panels, microcracks occurred on the varnish, engravings, and so on. Actually, the restorers usually just draw all the points belonging to borders, manually or with general purpose image processing software, incurring a large waste of time. Image processing tools designed for edge detection can offer assistance in reducing the time to accomplish this task.

## 19.2 Color Cleaning

Varnish oxidation, dirt, smoke, atmospheric pollution, and other phenomena in time can degrade the chemical composition of paintings so that their visual appearance is deteriorated, thus requiring cleaning procedures that try to reverse the aging process. The removal of this dirt layer is usually performed by conservation experts with a trial-and-error approach: different chemical cleaning substances are applied in small regions of the painting to select the most appropriate method for cleaning the whole painting. This operation is very difficult, because it is not reversible, and the amount of cleaning is subjectively decided by the restorer.

A digital color cleaning technique is a tool that, by analyzing the cleaned patches of the painting, can provide an estimate of the final result of the restoration process when the same cleaning methodology is applied to the whole piece of work. Restorers could then use this tool as an aid to choose which cleaning procedure is likely to give the best result.

A digital color cleaning algorithm can work in two different ways. A first class of methods [4], [5], [6] is based on the assumption that there is a digital copy of the painting before the cleaning process, and one of the same painting after some regions have been cleaned chemically; otherwise, let us suppose that there is only the digital image of the painting after the cleaning of the small patches, with the hypothesis that the colors used by the painter, present in the cleaned patches, are also present in other parts of the painting. If $\mathbf{I}$ represents the digital image of the dirty painting, and $\mathbf{I_c}$ the digital image of the same painting after the cleaning process of some patches, it is the aim of the algorithm to find the mathematical color transformation $\mathcal{T}$ that maps the dirty colors into the cleaned ones, such that in the cleaned area $\mathbf{I'} = \mathcal{T}[\mathbf{I}]$ is as close as possible to $\mathbf{I_c}$. Subsequently, the same transformation can be applied to the entire image, obtaining a virtually cleaned image, as represented in Figure 19.1.

The proposed methods in the literature differ with regard to the chosen color coordinates and to the particular model used for the color transformation $\mathcal{T}$.

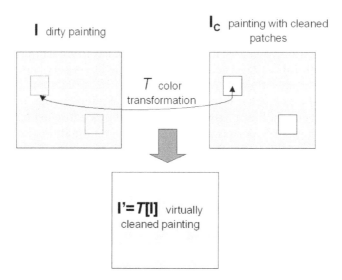

**FIGURE 19.1**
General process of a digital color cleaning technique, based on the comparison between a digital copy of the
painting before the cleaning process, and one of the same painting after some regions have been cleaned chemically.

A second class of methods [7], [8] do not rely on the comparison between cleaned and
dirty regions of the painting, but develop a model trying to estimate the degradation process
occurring in time, and according to this model, they reconstruct the original visual aspect
of uncleaned artwork.

### 19.2.1    Cleaning Based on Two Images

In Barni et al. [4], $\mathcal{T}$ is an operator that acts separately on each image pixel position $p$ of
the image $\mathbf{I}$, that is, on its RGB color coordinates $\mathbf{I}(p) = (P_r, P_g, P_b)$. If $\mathbf{I_c}(p) = (R_r, R_g, R_b)$
are the color coordinates of the corresponding point in $\mathbf{I_c}$, to model the cleaning process,
the algorithm looks for an operator $\mathcal{T}$ such that $\mathcal{T}[(P_r, P_g, P_b)]$ is as close as possible to
$(R_r, R_g, R_b)$. To tune the parameters of $\mathcal{T}$, $N$ pixel positions $\{p_1, p_2, \ldots, p_N\}$ are selected from
the dirty painting $\mathbf{I}$, and the RGB values of the corresponding points in $\mathbf{I_c}$ are considered. By
imposing that $\mathcal{T}[\mathbf{I}(p_i)] = \mathbf{I_c}(p_i)$, for each $i$, the parameters characterizing $\mathcal{T}$ are computed.
In the case that the operator is supposed to be an affine one, we have that

$$\mathcal{T}[(P_r, P_g, P_b)] = \begin{pmatrix} t_{11} & t_{12} & t_{13} \\ t_{21} & t_{22} & t_{23} \\ t_{31} & t_{32} & t_{33} \end{pmatrix} \begin{pmatrix} P_r \\ P_g \\ P_b \end{pmatrix} + \begin{pmatrix} t_{10} \\ t_{20} \\ t_{30} \end{pmatrix} \tag{19.1}$$

In this case, about $N = 20$ pixels are required to estimate all the parameters $t_{ij}$. Otherwise,
the authors propose that color transformation $\mathcal{T}$ be used as a quadratic operator; in this
case, about 60 to 70 reference points are used for the computation of the parameters.

Pitas et al. [5], [6] work in the CIELAB color space coordinates. They assume that the
digital copies of $N$ uniformly colored regions of the painting are available before the cleaning
($\{\mathbf{x_1}, \mathbf{x_2}, \ldots, \mathbf{x_N}\}$) and after the cleaning ($\{\mathbf{s_1}, \mathbf{s_2}, \ldots, \mathbf{s_N}\}$). Let $\mathbf{m_{x_i}}$ and $\mathbf{m_{s_i}}$ (three coordinates
in the CIELAB space) the mean of the $i$th dirty and clean region, and $\Delta\mathbf{m} = \mathbf{m_{s_i}} - \mathbf{m_{x_i}}$ their
difference. The aim is to find the transformation $\mathcal{T}$ from the sample data: $\mathcal{T}[(x_1, x_2, x_3)] =$
$(s_1, s_2, s_3)$, being $(x_1, x_2, x_3)$ and $(s_1, s_2, s_3)$, respectively, the color coordinates of a pixel in
a patch before and after cleaning; then $\mathcal{T}$ is applied on the whole painting. The authors

propose several choices for the operator $T$; the methods showing the best results are the linear approximation method and the white point transformation. In the first case, the transformation is

$$(s_1, s_2, s_3) = T[(x_1, x_2, x_3)] = (\mathbf{A} + \mathbf{B})[(x_1, x_2, x_3)] \tag{19.2}$$

where $\mathbf{B}$ is the $3 \times 3$ identity matrix, and $\mathbf{A}$ a $3 \times 3$ coefficient matrix. The coefficients of $\mathbf{A}$ are computed by polynomial regression.

In the second case, the authors, under the hypothesis that the clean regions and the corresponding dirty ones are viewed under the same lighting conditions, assume that if a clean sample $\mathbf{s}_{LAB}$ is illuminated with a brownish light source, the corresponding dirty sample $\mathbf{x}_{LAB}$ is obtained. Thus, the difference in appearance can be attributed solely to the different white points used for the color transformation. If the light source is characterized by means of its reference white with CIEXYZ tristimulus values, $\mathbf{w}_{XYZ}$, $\mathbf{s}_{LAB}$ denote the CIELAB values of a clean sample, and $\mathbf{x}_{XYZ}$ is the vector of the tristimulus values of the corresponding dirty sample, an estimate of the clean sample will be given by

$$\hat{\mathbf{s}}_{LAB} = T[\mathbf{x}_{XYZ}; \mathbf{w}_{XYZ}] \tag{19.3}$$

where $T[\cdot; \cdot]$ is the nonlinear transformation from CIEXYZ to CIELAB. By minimizing the error between the estimated values and the current values of the clean samples, it is possible to find the white light values. Although this represents a suboptimal solution, it can yield satisfactory results, with little computational overhead.

### 19.2.2   Cleaning Based on One Image

Drago and Chiba [8] propose an algorithm for the automatic removal of the yellowed layers of varnish, the enhancement of chromatic contrast, and the increase of the visibility of some masked details of the painting. The method is based on the retinex theory of human vision [9] that simulates the compensation of the human visual system (HVS) to different conditions of light intensity and chromatic dominance of the illuminant. The authors assume that a dirty painting can be considered as a clean painting displayed in the presence of unknown colored nonuniform illuminants; the cleaning process is then reduced to re-light the painting with a canonical light source, by making use of the retinex algorithm. The method also requires some postprocessing of the reconstructed image, so that it does not appear as a fully automatic algorithm.

Another possible approach for color restoration is described by Li et al. [7]. In this case, a database of all the possible colored pigments that form the Dunhuang frescos has been built; these pigments have been studied in order to understand their physical changes with time and thus to estimate the relationship between the original color and the actual color of each pigment. Thanks to this knowledge, the frescos are segmented into several pigment layers, and into each layer the estimated original color is substituted to the current one, so that the whole image can be seen as it maybe was at its origin.

---

## 19.3   Color Enhancement

Several approaches have been proposed for the enhancement of the color quality of images representing paintings, in order to reduce degradations engendered by low-quality acquisition, or by the degradation of the picture with time. In Reference [10], a color contrast enhancement method based on saturation and desaturation, performed in the $u'v'$ chromaticity diagram of the CIE $Lu'v'$ color coordinate system is presented, in order to change

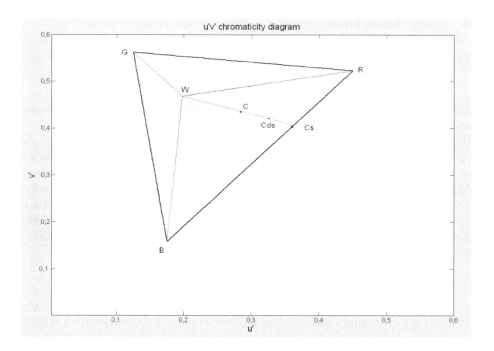

**FIGURE 19.2**
The saturation and desaturation process represented in the $u'v'$ chromaticity domain.

the saturation value and obtain a final image with more appealing colors. The chromaticity values $x'$ and $v'$ can be obtained by means of a linear transformation starting from the XYZ color coordinates; each color can then be represented as a point in the $u'v'$ chromaticity domain, as in Figure 19.2. The method is applied to all the color pixels belonging to the color gamut triangle, except the ones included in the achromatic region, because these pixels are not very colorful, so enhancing these colors should not be useful. Given a color image pixel $C = (u', v', Y)$, the saturation process consists in stretching the line between the white point $W = (u'_w, v'_w, Y_w)$ and $C$ outside the triangle. The intersection between the triangle and this line gives the saturated color $C_s = (u'_s, v'_s, Y)$. Then, after the saturation procedure, all color pixels outside the achromatic triangle are moved to the gamut triangle boundaries. However, this maximally saturated color appears unnatural if displayed in the monitor, so a desaturation step is applied.

Desaturation is applied by using the center of gravity law of color mixing that mixes the chromaticity coordinates of $W$ and $C_s$, resulting in a new color pixel $C_{ds} = (u'_{ds}, v'_{ds}, Y_{ds})$, where

$$u'_{ds} = \frac{u'_s \frac{Y}{v'_s} + u'_w \frac{Y_w}{v'_w}}{\frac{Y}{v'_s} + \frac{Y_w}{v'_w}}, \quad v'_{ds} = \frac{Y + Y_w}{\frac{Y}{v'_s} + \frac{Y_w}{v'_w}} \tag{19.4}$$

Figure 19.2 shows an example of a color pixel that after saturation is moved in the boundaries of the gamut triangle, and next is moved inside the triangle through the desaturation algorithm. Finally, the luminance of the whole image is slightly increased to $Y_{ds} = Y_w + Y$. This proposed color contrast enhancement makes the appearance of the picture more colorful, and consequently, can increase image sharpness.

In Reference [11], a color adjustment process applied to a mosaicking scheme is proposed. As explained in Section 19.6, mosaicking allows a set of partially overlapped color images representing subparts of the same painting to be joined in an automatic way. One of the effects to be considered is the fact that these images are characterized by different

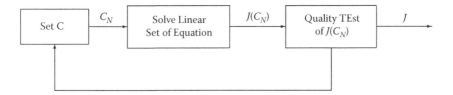

**FIGURE 19.3**
Procedure to estimate the parameters $J$ of the linear affine transformation in the color adjustment process.

acquisition conditions resulting in color distortions. To this aim, a color adjustment algorithm was developed to estimate, through a parametric transformation, the color changes of corresponding pixels belonging to two subimages and then to use this estimation to adjust all colors of the nonreference subimage.

Given a set of corresponding pixels $C$ between two subimages $I_1$ and $I_2$, and a linear affine transformation,

$$\begin{pmatrix} R \\ G \\ B \end{pmatrix} = J \begin{pmatrix} R' \\ G' \\ B' \\ 1 \end{pmatrix} \qquad (19.5)$$

where $J$ is a $3 \times 4$ matrix of real values, the aim of the process is to select those values of $J$ that allow a good color matching to be obtained, so we have to estimate 12 parameters. To achieve this goal, an iterative procedure, described in Figure 19.3, is applied. To solve Equation 19.5, at each iteration of the procedure, a subset of $N$ corresponding pixels $C_N$ is chosen from the elements of $C$.

The goal of the procedure is to find the subset $C_N$ with parameters $J(C_N)$ that obtain the best color matching. In particular, the quality test of $J(C_N)$ is based on the following index:

$$\Delta E^*_{Lab}(P_1, P_2) = \sqrt{(L^*_1 - L^*_2)^2 + (a^*_1 - a^*_2)^2 + (b^*_1 - b^*_2)^2} \qquad (19.6)$$

where $(L^*_1, a^*_1, b^*_1)$ are the color components of $P_1$ (a generic point on a image $I_1$) in the standard, perceptually uniform, color system CIELAB, and $(L^*_2, a^*_2, b^*_2)$ are the corresponding color components of $P_2$, the corresponding pixel in the other subimage $I_2$. $\Delta E^*_{Lab}$ gives a measure of the color difference between $P_1$ and $P_2$ from a perceptual point of view (e.g., a value of $\Delta E^*_{Lab}$ less than three denotes a color difference almost not perceptible by the eye). In order to give a numeric value to compare the quality of $J(C_N)$, the relative $\Delta E^*_{Lab}$ is computed for each correspondence, and all values are summed up:

$$Q_{test} = \sum_{C_N} \Delta E^*_{Lab}(P(I_1), P(I_2, J(C_N))) \qquad (19.7)$$

where $P(I_2, J(C_N))$ represents the color components remapped through $J(C_N)$. We use $Q_{test}$ as a quality measure for $J(C_N)$. As the final estimate of $J$, we take the $J(C_N)$ with the minimum value of $Q_{test}$. Finally, adaptive histogram equalization to adjust the luminance component is adopted. This algorithm is able to give good color adjustment for images with complex, even nonlinear, color distortions (see Figure 19.4).

In the framework of color enhancement, another field is given by the works, see References [12], [13], [14], and [15], that propose different methods for noise suppression in color images representing artwork.

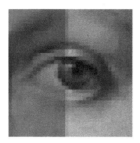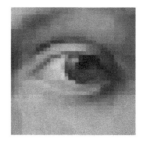

**FIGURE 19.4**
Two joined subimages without (left) and with (right) the color adjustment procedure.

## 19.4   Cracks Removal

Cracks are often caused by a rapid loss of water in the painting's varnish: when the painting is located in a dry environment, a nonuniform contraction of the varnish covering can cause cracks. With image processing tools, it is possible to entirely remove cracks by means of interpolation techniques; in this way, the painting, even if in a virtual version, again achieves its original appearance.

An algorithm for crack removal is usually a two-step procedure: first, the cracks have to be detected; next, the selected cracks are filled in. The crack selection step can be semiautomatic or automatic. In the first case, the aid of the user is requested to let him choose a starting point of the crack; on the contrary, automatic crack selection methods do not require such external help. However, in the latter case, the assistance of the user can be requested later, for distinguishing if some of the automatically selected cracks are really cracks or otherwise different picture elements, like brush strokes.

In the following, the approaches proposed so far for the virtual restoration of cracks will be presented.

### 19.4.1   A Semiautomatic Method

The Image Processing and Communication Lab of the University of Florence, Italy, has developed a technique for virtually removing the cracks from old paintings and frescos [4], [16]. The developed procedure is semi-automatic, that is, the system first asks the user to manually select a point belonging to the crack. It is, in fact, impossible for the system to automatically distinguish between cracks and lines belonging to the drawing. Subsequently, an automatic procedure starts in order to track the crack.

Beginning from the identified starting point, an iterative process is able to identify the whole crack. This is accomplished by assuming the hypothesis that a crack is darker than the background, and it is characterized by a rather elongated structure. After the user has selected a starting point (say $A$), all the pixels (say $B_i$) in a proper neighborhood of $A$ are tested for possible inclusion within the crack. The inquired neighboring pixels belong to the neighborhood of pixel $A$, that is, all the pixels that have a corner or a side in common with $A$. In the following steps, the neighboring pixels refer to the part of the crack already identified by the algorithm. In particular, by referring to Figure 19.5, at the first step, pixels $B_1$ to $B_5$ are analyzed as the neighborhood of pixel $A$ (Figure 19.5a). In the second step (Figure 19.5b), after $B_1$, $B_2$, and $B_3$ have been chosen as belonging to the crack, pixels $C_1$ to $C_6$ are analyzed as in the neighborhood of the present crack. In the third step, pixels $D_1$ to $D_6$ are analyzed as the neighborhood of pixels $A$, $B_1$, $B_2$, $B_3$, $C_5$, and $C_6$, that is, the crack.

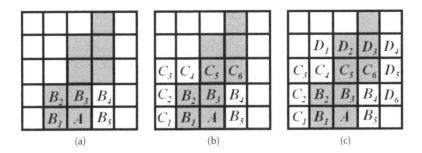

**FIGURE 19.5**
Example of crack tracking: three iterations are presented, in which pixels $B_i$, $C_i$, and $D_i$ are analyzed with respect to the growing crack.

For each step, the pixels are analyzed basing on the following conditions:

$$|f(A) - f(B_i)| \leq T$$
$$f(B_i) \in [T_1, T_2] \tag{19.8}$$

where $f(A)$ and $f(B_i)$ are the gray levels at corresponding pixel positions (e.g., $A = (x_A, y_A)$), while $T$, $T_1$, and $T_2$ are adaptive thresholds computed on the basis of the crack previously classified as such. The first condition means that the crack has to be uniform, while the second means that the gray level of the crack pixels must be included in a given range (i.e., the crack is darker than the background). The advantage of this strategy is that it describes the crack as a sequence of fronts ($\{B_1, B_2, B_3\}$, $\{C_5\}$, and $\{D_2, D_3\}$) which are roughly perpendicular to the crack direction; this helps in passing over gaps [4].

Once the crack is correctly detected, the user can decide to erase it by applying an interpolation algorithm. The proposed method uses the Shepard interpolation technique, in the version of Franke–Little [17]. The interpolation surface $u$ at pixel $(x, y)$, which has to be interpolated, is defined as

$$u(x, y) = \frac{\sum_{j=1}^{N} \left[1 - \frac{r_j(x,y)}{R}\right]^{\mu} \cdot f(x_j, y_j)}{\sum_{j=1}^{N} \left[1 - \frac{r_j(x,y)}{R}\right]^{\mu}} \tag{19.9}$$

where $r_j(x, y)$ is the Euclidean distance from the pixel $(x, y)$ and the interpolation node $(x_j, y_j)$; $R$ is the radius of the circle involving all the interpolation nodes; $f(x_j, y_j)$ is the gray level for pixel $(x_j, y_j)$; $\mu$ is the order of the weighting function (usually equal to 2); and the sum considers all the pixels determined by radius $R$ but not belonging to the crack.

## 19.4.2 Automatic Methods

The first work regarding digital restoration of cracks was proposed in 1998 by the group of Prof. Pitas at the University of Thessaloniki [18]. Such an automatic technique consists of three main steps [6], [18]: the detection of the cracks present in the painting; the elimination of the brush strokes that have been erroneously classified as cracks; the removal, the restoration, of the identified cracks.

Regarding the first phase, the authors consider the fact that cracks are usually darker with respect to the overall painting. By starting from such a consideration, they propose to recover the cracks by searching the minimum values of the luminance of the digital painting, or equivalently, by searching the maximum values after negating the luminance image. In particular, they exploit a morphological filter, called top-hat transform [19], that is a high-pass filter that detects bright details present in the processed image. By considering the image $\mathbf{I}$, after the application of the top-hat filter, it results in

$$\mathbf{I}_{out} = \mathbf{I} - \mathbf{I}_{nB} \qquad (19.10)$$

where $\mathbf{I}_{nB}$ is a low-pass nonlinear filter that erases all peaks of the image, in which the structuring element $nB$, characterizing the morphological opening filter, cannot fit. Hence, in $\mathbf{I}_{out}$, only such peaks will remain, whereas the background has been eliminated. The type and the size of the structuring element can be chosen according to the cracks to be detected; furthermore, the number $n$ of opening $nB$ (i.e., erosion and dilation) can also be chosen. After the application of the top-hat filter, a thresholding operation (globally or locally computed) is applied to $\mathbf{I}_{out}$, in order to select only those pixels with higher values (i.e., pixels belonging, or probably belonging, to a crack), thus producing a binary image indicating crack position.

Before filling the cracks, it is necessary to locate those brush strokes that have been classified as cracks due to their luminance values and thickness. Pitas et al. propose three different approaches for discriminating cracks and dark brush strokes. In the first example, the values of hue ($H$) and saturation ($S$) are used for discerning cracks and dark brush strokes, because the authors observed that different ranges for $H$ and $S$ characterized cracks and brush strokes; in particular, for cracks $\mathbf{H} \in [0\text{--}60]$ and $\mathbf{S} \in [0.3\text{--}0.7]$, while for brush strokes $\mathbf{H} \in [0\text{--}360]$ and $\mathbf{S} \in [0\text{--}0.4]$. By referring to such different values, a classification is then computed by means of a neural network (i.e., the median radial basis function [MRBF]) [18]. Another approach for selecting cracks after the top-hat filter is to start from some sets of pixels (seeds) representing distinct cracks. By referring to each seed (at least one seed for each crack), a simple growth mechanism is applied for selecting the whole crack. The seeds are chosen by the user (in this case, thus, the aid of the user is requested), and because no seeds will be defined for brush strokes, they will not be selected. The last method considers the removal of brush strokes with a specific shape. After defining a structuring element representing the brush strokes (also for this step the aid of the user is requested), a morphological opening operation is applied in order to remove such brush strokes.

The last step in the proposed algorithm is the restoration (i.e., filling) of the identified cracks. First, the image is decomposed in the three RGB channels, and the filling procedure is then applied separately in each channel. Filling is achieved by filtering each channel through proper filters; in particular, the authors propose two different approaches: one based on order statistics (median or trimmed-mean filters) and one based on anisotropic diffusion. In the first case, the idea is to replace values of pixels belonging to a crack with values of pixels in the neighborhood of the crack. With a median filter (or a weighted median filter), the value of the considered pixel is replaced with the median value of a suitable window. By using a trimmed-mean filter, the value of the considered pixel is replaced by the average of the pixel values within the window, but with some of the end-point ranked values properly excluded. On the contrary, by exploiting anisotropic diffusion, luminance values are diffused from neighboring pixels to crack pixels. In particular, by taking into account crack orientation, only those neighboring pixels in the perpendicular orientation are considered, to exclude values of pixels belonging to the crack.

Abas and Martinez, from the University of Southampton (U.K.), studied the problem of crack analysis and classification [20], [21]; such a study was driven by the request, coming from important museums, to classify (automatically or semiautomatically) cracks in paintings as an useful step in art-work preservation. The first step for crack classification, is in regard to their detection. In particular, they propose to recover cracks by working on the

X-radiographs (instead of on the visible images) of the paintings: in fact, in the radiographs, cracks are more evident, because some details in the paint layer are suppressed.

The authors follow two different approaches for detecting cracks: one based on Gabor filters [20] and one based on top-hat transformation [21] that is basically similar to the one presented by Pitas et al. [18] (previously described). Gabor filters are band-pass filters with useful properties of selectivity in frequency and orientation, and good joint resolution in both spatial and frequency domains. By referring to Reference [22], the to be analyzed image $\mathbf{I}$ is convolved by a set of eight Gabor filters with different orientation $\theta$ (i.e., $\theta = [0, 22.5, 45, 67.5, 90, 112.5135, 157.5]$). The other parameters of the filters must be fixed according to the image at hand. The eight output images $\mathbf{I}_{out,i}$, $i = 1 \cdots 8$, are then processed for extracting their maxima that are combined together in one binary image. As a last step a morphological thinning algorithm is applied for producing a thinned version of the detected cracks.

Another approach for crack restoration was proposed by the Pattern Recognition and Image Processing Group, at the University of Technology in Vienna [23], [24]. The aim of the authors is to analyze the underdrawing present in a painting that can be revealed through the infrared reflectograms. For such an analysis, it is fundamental that the cracks affecting the IR images be removed without damaging the boundaries of the drawing. In this case, no color information can be used (the crack restoration technique works on grayscale images), whereas crack characteristics such as thickness and favored orientation are considered as starting points for the *viscous morphological reconstruction* method that authors apply for removing cracks.

The idea is to reconstruct a restored version of the original image $\mathbf{I}$ by starting from a marker image $\mathbf{M}$, which should represent the brush strokes but not the cracks (see Figure 19.6a to Figure 19.6c). The marker image is obtained by eroding the original image with a structuring element $S_e$ suitable with respect to dimensions and orientation of the cracks, in order to eliminate cracks as much as possible:

$$\mathbf{M} = \varepsilon_{S_e}(\mathbf{I}) \tag{19.11}$$

where $\varepsilon_{S_e}$ is the erosion operation using a structuring element $S_e$ applied to $\mathbf{I}$. The reconstruction is achieved by means of dilation (with a structuring element $S_d$) applied to the marker image $\mathbf{M}$ with respect to the mask image (i.e., the original image $\mathbf{I}$), until stability is reached:

$$R_{S_d}(\mathbf{I}, \mathbf{M}) = \delta^i_{S_d}(\mathbf{I}, \mathbf{M}) \tag{19.12}$$

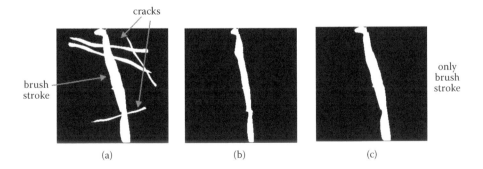

(a)     (b)     (c)

**FIGURE 19.6**

Example of viscous reconstruction: (a) the original image containing both brush strokes and cracks, (b) the marker image obtained by erosion, and (c) the image after viscous reconstruction applied to the marker image with respect to the mask image.

where $\delta^i_{S_d}(\mathbf{I}, \mathbf{M})$ is the dilation operation at the *ith* step, using a structuring element $S_d$, and $i$ is chosen for stability, such that $\delta^i_{S_d}(\mathbf{I}, \mathbf{M}) = \delta^{i+1}_{S_d}(\mathbf{I}, \mathbf{M})$. By starting from such a morphological reconstruction, an opening operation (with a structuring element $S_o$) is applied on the marker image after each dilation reconstruction step. The viscous reconstruction is thus defined as

$$R^v_{S_d, S_o}(\mathbf{I}, \mathbf{M}) = \Delta^i_{S_d, S_o}(\mathbf{I}, \mathbf{M}) \tag{19.13}$$

where $\Delta^i_{S_d, S_o}(\mathbf{I}, \mathbf{M})$ is the dilation operation in Equation 19.12 followed by an opening, with structuring element $S_o$, at $i$th step, and $i$ is chosen for stability, such that $\Delta^i_{S_d, S_o}(\mathbf{I}, \mathbf{M}) = \Delta^{i+1}_{S_d, S_o}(\mathbf{I}, \mathbf{M})$. The additional opening helps to remove from the marker image the remaining cracks, because, step by step, cracks become sufficiently thin to be removed by the opening operation.

The structuring element $S_e$ for the initial erosion producing $\mathbf{M}$ is chosen according to *a priori* information about cracks (also, in this case, help from the user is requested for this choice). For example, in the case that most cracks are horizontal, the erosion of the original image is computed by using a vertical line as structuring element. Then, $S_d$ and $S_o$ are, consequently, fixed. Actually, all the morphological operations are applied after inverting the original image, so that objects to be removed (cracks) became lighter than the background.

## 19.5 Lacuna Filling

Lacunas are a very common damage that can occur to paintings and more often to frescos and wall paintings, when some parts of the fresco collapse and fall down; in this case, the effect is the creation of even large areas where the original image is lost. Actual restoration techniques tend to fill these areas with a uniform color or a set of colors, to give the impression of continuity of the image.

By means of image processing tools, it is possible to accomplish the same task to the digital version of the artwork. In particular, two virtual filling procedures have been proposed so far: the former simulates filling techniques actually performed in the restoration laboratories, in order to simulate and compare real restoration methods; the latter is based on a texture synthesization procedure to fill lacuna regions with the appropriate textures, in order to obtain a restored image where the boundary between original and synthesized paintings is seamless.

### 19.5.1 A Method Based on Restoration Schools

An approach for the virtual restoration of lacunas in artwork digital representations was proposed by De Rosa et al. in 2001 [25]. In particular, the method (that is semiautomatic) consists of two steps: the segmentation of the lacuna and its restoration (i.e., filling). During the first step, the user is asked to choose a pixel belonging to the lacuna, which has to be restored; then, an automatic procedure recovers all the lacuna using an adhoc segmentation algorithm developed for this particular application. During the second step, it is possible for the user to experiment with several implemented filling techniques that simulate restoration techniques actually performed in the restoration laboratories; in fact, the main idea of the proposed algorithm is to provide the user with the possibility of virtually comparing different restoration solutions, in order to select the most suitable one for the specific artwork. In particular, the restoration methods have been implemented by basically referring to two different restoration schools: the "*Scuola Romana*" of Cesare Brandi and the "*Scuola Fiorentina*" of Umberto Baldini [25].

The lacuna segmentation procedure is an adhoc region growing method that starts from the single pixel selected by the user; the neighboring pixels are examined one at a time and added to the growing region if a given homogeneity criterion is satisfied. In particular, an objective function is defined and compared with a threshold. Such a criterion takes into account color features by using the $HVS$ system (hue, value, saturation). The objective function $\gamma$ results in the following:

$$\gamma = \frac{A_1}{\sigma_H^2} + \frac{A_2}{\sigma_V^2} + \frac{A_3}{\sigma_S^2} + A_4 \cdot G_m \tag{19.14}$$

It is based both on the variance values of hue, value, and saturation ($\sigma_H^2, \sigma_V^2, \sigma_S^2$) computed on the present region plus the analyzed pixel $P$ and on the boundary information by means of the mean value of the magnitude of the gradient ($G_m$), computed by the Sobel operator on the same region. The terms $A_1$, $A_2$, $A_3$, and $A_4$ are heuristic constants.

The gradient $G_m$ takes low values everywhere but on region boundaries: hence, at the beginning, the value of $\gamma$ increases, because the considered pixels belong to the lacuna with homogeneous characteristics (low values for variances); then, when pixels belonging to region boundaries are considered, $\gamma$ increases for the term $G_m$; finally, $\gamma$ decreases beyond the region boundaries, and the region growing stops. In particular, the objective function is compared, step by step, with a threshold, which depends on the previous values of $\gamma$. At the $n$-th step, the threshold $T_n$ is

$$T_n = \left(\frac{a}{a+1}\right)^{n-1} \gamma_0 + \frac{1}{a}\left[\sum_{i=1}^{n-1}\left(\frac{a}{a+1}\right)^{n-i}\gamma_i\right] \tag{19.15}$$

where $\gamma_0$ and $\gamma_i$ are the values of the function $\gamma$ at the first and $i$th step, respectively, and $a$ is a constant value. Hence, the $n$th pixel will be added to the segmented region if the value $\gamma_n$ exceeds the threshold $T_n$.

### 19.5.2 A Method Based on Texture Synthesis

In 2004, Pei et al. [10] proposed a new texture synthesis procedure to eliminate, from ancient paintings, undesirable patterns and fill such lacuna regions with the appropriate textures, so that boundaries between original and synthesized painting are seamless.

After the selection of the to-be-restored region, the texture synthesization procedure includes four phases: neighborhood assignment, possible neighborhood collection, auxiliary, and synthesization.

During the neighborhood assignment, a square-window $WS(p)$ of width $L$ is considered for patching the damaged area. The window is centered from time to time on each pixel ($p = (x, y)$) belonging to the lacuna region ($S$), and it consists of two different types of field: the normal field ($WS_n(p)$) and the synthesized field ($WS_s(p)$), so that $WS_n(p) \cup WS_s(p) = WS(p)$ and $WS_n(p) \cap WS_s(p) = 0$. All the $L^2 - 1$ pixels belonging to $WS(p)$ (except the central pixel $p$) are then used for neighborhood searching (see Figure 19.7).

In the second phase, the possible neighborhood is collected from the sample. In this case, a squarewindow ($WN(q)$) is taken into account, the central pixel of which ($q$) moves in the nonlacuna region, that is, in the normal region ($N$). Also, in this case, the considered window is composed of a normal field ($WN_n(q)$) and a synthesized field ($WN_s(q)$).

The auxiliary step considers the case in which the damage area includes different textures (e.g., in the corrupted region a detail of a face, some clothes and background are present together). The idea of the authors is to manually draw the distinct boundary between each of

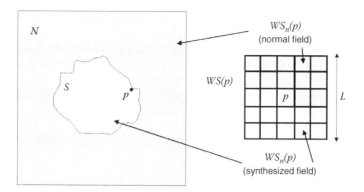

**FIGURE 19.7**
Example of a damaged area with a lacuna region $S$ (left), and the square-window $WS(p)$ of size $L = 5$ centered on $p$ (right).

the different textures: such a step considerably helps the synthesization, because each part of the damaged area can be restored with a different appropriate texture. In the proposed approach, the identification of the corrupt region (i.e., $S$) and decision about using auxiliary is manually computed. Furthermore, pixels belonging to $S$ are analyzed through an annular scanning procedure.

Finally, during the synthesization phase, a neighborhood $WS(p)$ is constructed (where $p$ is a synthesized pixel) and a search is made for the neighborhood $WN(q)$ most similar to $WS(p)$. Then, the value of the central pixel of $WS$ is replaced by the value of the corresponding central pixel of $WN$. A distance measure $d$ between the two neighborhoods is defined for determining their similarity:

$$d(WS(p), WN(q)) = \sum_k w_k [WS(p_k) - WN(q_k)]^2 \qquad (19.16)$$

where the sum is computed on all the corresponding $k$th pixels of the two regions, and $w_k$ is a normalized weight to emphasize the edge connection: in particular, $w_k$ is taken into account if the $k$th pixel in the normal field of $WS$ is or is not a boundary pixel of the synthesized field in the same $WS$ area.

## 19.6 Image Mosaicking

In many cases, the painting to be analyzed is so big that it is not possible to obtain, in a single acquisition, an unique digital image with the desired quality. On the contrary, several images representing subparts of the painting are obtained. In this case, it is possible to reconstruct an unique digital image representing the whole scene by means of mosaicking algorithms that join a certain number of overlapping subimages of the to-be-reproduced scene, in such a way that the target is completely represented with all its details. Generally, mosaicking involves a pair of subimages at a time, which are joined together. This operation is repeated for all the subimages, using the one obtained in the previous step as a reference and joining another one to it: in this way, the whole representation of the painting will be generated in an incremental way using a new subimage a time. The main problem to solve is that the subimages, even if taken in the same acquisition session, can show color variations and small geometric distortions from each other, due to lighting and translation variations.

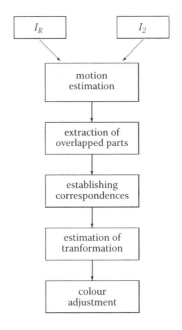

**FIGURE 19.8**
Blocks scheme overview of the mosaicking process in Corsini, M., Bartolini, F., and Cappellini, V., *Proceedings of the Seventh International Conference on Virtual Systems and Multimedia*, 39, 2001.

So, it is easy to understand that joining several subimages together involves a certain number of difficult tasks. A mosaicking procedure starts from the hypothesis that, given two images to be joined (called reference image and nonreference image), the overlapping part of the nonreference image is a transformed version of the same part of the reference image; after having estimated this transformation, it is possible to apply its inverse to the whole subimage, to reduce the geometric distortion between the two images. The possible approaches differ according to the transformations used to model the geometric distortions and to the strategy implemented for estimating it.

In Reference [11], it is assumed to have a set of color images characterized by strong color distortions and small geometric distortions introduced when the operator, taking the pictures, translates the photo camera. The proposed mosaicking method, in the hypothesis that translational motion of the camera is dominant with respect to tilt, slant, and rotation, performs a fully automatic reconstruction of the acquired painting, according to the blocks diagram depicted in Figure 19.8.

First, one of the two images is selected as a reference $I_R$. Then, the nonreference subimage $I_2$ is mapped on the reference (from a geometric viewpoint), and its colors are modified in order to match the colors of the reference subimage. The first step of the mosaicking technique is the estimation of the translational displacement components $(t_x, t_y)$, so that it is possible to extract in the second step the overlapped parts of the two subimages, $I_R^{ov}$ and $I_2^{ov}$. The third step regards the evaluation of a set of pixel correspondences (denoted by $C$) between $I_R^{ov}$ and $I_2^{ov}$. These data are exploited to compute a geometric transformation to map $I_2$ on $I_R$ (fourth step). Because the subimages can be approximated as planar surfaces, homographies (mathematical relationships to model planar perspective transformations) are used for this mapping that not only eliminate the rotational components but also refine the estimation of $(t_x, t_y)$. Finally, color adjustment is performed. All the steps of the local mosaicking process are working on a grayscale version of the two color subimages, but the last one obviously uses the color information.

Mosaicking is also very useful when the need arises to obtain a flattened version of a painting or a fresco applied to a curved surface: the processing allows a view of the artwork as if it was painted on a flat surface and not on a curved one to be obtained. In order to flatten the painting, it is necessary to estimate the parameters of an equation describing the curved surface and the transformation that relates points in the camera coordinate system with the points in the object coordinate system; then, thanks to an iterative process, the acquired image can be backprojected on the surface and subsequently flattened [6], [26], [27].

A problem similar to image mosaicking was proposed in Reference [28]. In this work, a methodology was introduced for the computer-aided reconstruction fragments of wall paintings. According to this methodology, each fragment is photographed, its picture is introduced to the computer, its contour is obtained, and, subsequently, all of the fragments contours are compared to reconstruct the whole wall painting from a set of fragments.

## 19.7 Image Registration

Similar to what happens in the medical fields, for art diagnostics, it is often necessary to observe and integrate several sets of data coming from different sources and stored in various images. The analysis of a painting could be performed, for example, by comparing images taken in different instants (e.g., old pictures versus current pictures) or images acquired from different points of view or by means of different sensors (e.g., IR-reflectograms, X-radiographies, etc.) that thus capture different and often complementary content. In order to successfully integrate these data, pictures corresponding to the same area of the artwork need to be registered. With the term "registration," the determination of a geometrical transformation that aligns points in one picture with corresponding points in another picture is meant. Often, the registration is performed manually by an user iteratively setting the parameters of the geometrical transformation and checking its performance. However, this approach is time consuming and can give subjective results. Thus, it is of interest to design an image registration algorithm, that, in an automatic or a semiautomatic way, is able to determine the parameters of a geometrical transformation mapping points in picture (the so-called *reference* or *target*) with corresponding points in another picture (the so-called *template*) [29]. In general, a registration scheme can be decomposed into the following steps [30]:

- *Feature detection:* by means of this step, it is possible to extract some characteristic features (both manually or automatically) that are then used to find the transformation that occurred between the two images

- *Feature matching:* in this step, the correspondence from the points previously extracted, over both the two images, is established, by means of a given similarity measure

- *Transform model estimation:* with this step, it is possible to estimate the parameters of the geometrical transformation that is able to align the reference and the sensed images

- *Image resampling and transformation:* the sensed image is transformed by means of the transformation parameters estimated in the previous step, to perfectly match the reference image

There are several proposed methods and many ways of classifying them: one is given according to the class of geometrical transformation that we consider in the transform model estimation step: with increasing complexity, we can distinguish between rigid transformations (rotation and translation), nonrigid transformations (scaling, affine, projective, perspective, curved), and rectifications. Another classification can be given according to the registration basis (i.e., the set of features that are involved in the registration task) [29]. According to this, registration methods can be classified in *point-based*, *surface-based*, and *intensity-based methods*. The *point-based methods* identify *a priori* a certain number of points, manually selected or externally superimposed, over both the to-be-registered images; the registration process looks for the displacement between these points. The *surface-based methods* determine corresponding surfaces (instead of points) in the two images and try to find the transformation that best aligns these surfaces. Finally, *intensity-based methods* calculate the transformation using the pixel values alone, with no reference to distinctive points or surfaces, through an iterative optimization of a similarity measure. Within this class, one of the most interesting methods is the one based on the maximization of the mutual information (MMI) [31], which has shown excellent results for the registration of medical images, compared to previously proposed methods that can often fail when dealing with multisource images, for the inherent difference of the image structures and tone dynamics. Moreover, this method is automatic and does not need any preprocessing.

Mutual information (MI), a basic notion of information theory, represents a measure of the amount of information that one source (i.e., an image) contains about another one. The MMI approach states that MI between two images is maximum when the images are correctly registered. Let us suppose that two images $\mathbf{X}$ and $\mathbf{Y}$ are related by the geometric transformation $\mathcal{T}_\alpha$, represented by the geometrical parameters $\alpha = [\alpha_1, \alpha_2, \ldots, \alpha_n]$, such that the pixel $p$ of $\mathbf{X}$ with intensity value $\mathbf{X}(p) = x$ corresponds to the pixel $\mathcal{T}_\alpha(p)$ of $\mathbf{Y}$ with intensity value $\mathbf{Y}(\mathcal{T}_\alpha(p)) = y$. Then, the mutual information between the two images is

$$I(\mathbf{X}, \mathbf{Y}) = \sum_{x,y} p_{\mathbf{XY}}(x, y) log_2 \frac{p_{\mathbf{XY}}(x, y)}{p_{\mathbf{X}}(x) \cdot p_{\mathbf{Y}}(y)} \tag{19.17}$$

where $p_{\mathbf{XY}}(x, y)$ is the joint probability distribution, $p_{\mathbf{X}}(x)$ and $p_{\mathbf{Y}}(y)$ are the marginal ones. The mutual information registration criterion states that the two images are geometrically aligned by the transformation $\mathcal{T}_{\alpha^*}$ such that

$$\alpha^* = \arg \max_{\alpha} I(\mathbf{X}, \mathbf{Y}) \tag{19.18}$$

Estimates for the joint and marginal distributions can be obtained by simple normalization of the joint and marginal histograms of the overlapping parts of both images [32]. The joint histogram $h_\alpha(x, y)$ is obtained by binning the pixel intensity value pairs

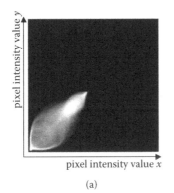
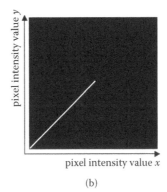

(a)  (b)

**FIGURE 19.9**
Example of the joint histogram $h_\alpha(x, y)$ for two images $\mathbf{X}$ and $\mathbf{Y}$: (a) before, and (b) after images have been registered.

$(\mathbf{X}(p), \mathbf{Y}(\mathcal{T}_\alpha(p)))$ for all the pixels in the overlapping region of $\mathbf{X}$ and $\mathbf{Y}$ (see Figure 19.9a and Figure 19.9b). Because very often the registered pixel position $\mathcal{T}_\alpha(p)$ will not coincide with a grid position, an interpolation of the reference image will be required to obtain the pixel value $\mathbf{Y}(\mathcal{T}_\alpha(p))$. Next, the joint distribution can be estimated as

$$p_{\mathbf{XY},\alpha}(x, y) = \frac{h_\alpha(x, y)}{\sum_{x,y} h_\alpha(x, y)} \tag{19.19}$$

and the marginal ones as $p_{\mathbf{X},\alpha}(x) = \sum_y p_{\mathbf{XY},\alpha}(x, y)$, and $p_{\mathbf{Y},\alpha}(y) = \sum_x p_{\mathbf{XY},\alpha}(x, y)$.

By using the values in Equation 19.17 it is possible to derive the mutual information $I(\mathbf{X}, \mathbf{Y})$, with a maximization that will give the optimal registration parameters $\alpha^*$.

### 19.7.1 Cultural Heritage Applications

In the field of cultural heritage applications, there are few examples of use of image registration methods: they will be briefly described in the following. Martinez et al. [1] describe the activity of color change detection in paintings recorded through the VASARI scanner at different times. In the process of detection, a procedure to cope with possible differences in the geometry of the images due to different imaging equipment and imaging setup is implemented. To correct possible changes in scale, rotation, and perspective, an automatic procedure to compute the coefficients of the transform

$$\begin{aligned}
r' &= r + c_1 + c_2 r + c_3 s + c_4 r s \\
s' &= s + c_5 + c_6 s + c_7 r + c_8 r s
\end{aligned} \tag{19.20}$$

is devised, where $(r', s')$ and $(r, s)$ are the coordinates of the same point in the two corresponding images. The coefficients are computed by minimizing the average difference between the two images.

Zitová et al. [14], [15] present a registration method in the framework of a restoration process of a medieval mosaic. Two pictures of the mosaic are available: an historical black and white photograph taken in 1879, and a current one taken by a digital camera. The availability of these pictures give to the restorers the possibility to compare the conservation of the mosaic at the end of the 19th century and at present. However, to make the comparison, it is required to apply a registration process, because the images were taken from different locations and with a different spatial resolution: in a first step, because the mosaic exhibited distinguishable points like corners and edge endings, a point-based method is used, requiring the manual selection of a set of 20 salient point pairs; the algorithm is exploited to estimate the scale difference between the two pictures, and then to rescale them to the same resolution. Next, a refinement of the selected feature locations is carried out by means of an MMI algorithm; in particular, the method is applied to the windows centered on each selected salient point to find the translation allowing refinement of the position of the salient points in the historical image. The algorithm is successful for 75% of the selected pairs, allowing for the refinement the salient point positions. In the remaining cases, the translation value computed by the MMI algorithm was too far from the initial point, or not found, so that the refinement process was not applied.

Cappellini et al. [33] propose an automatic algorithm, based on the computation of the maximum of the mutual information. In this application, the final aim was to achieve a multispectral calibrated UV fluorescence image of the painting surface and therefore a (undersampled) spectral signature per pixel of the painting. In order to achieve it, data were needed from a set of monochrome images, acquired in different wavebands, both of the UV-induced visible fluorescence images and of the white light radiance.

In particular, 14 multispectral images of the same area of a painting, seven relative to the UV-induced visible fluorescence, and seven relative to the reflectance in the visible range, were acquired with a monochrome CCD camera equipped with a filter wheel, and were slightly misaligned with respect to each other, due to a different optical path and some randomness in the positioning of the filter in front of the camera objective. To combine correctly the different information provided by the multispectral images, a registration algorithm was needed. If only considering the number of images, to be used, an automatic registration was to be preferred. In such a scenario, the transformation the images can undergo is estimated to be a combination of translation, rotation, and scaling, that can be represented as follows [29]:

$$\vec{x}' = \mathbf{S}\mathbf{R}\vec{x} + \vec{t} \tag{19.21}$$

where $\vec{x}$ is the coordinate vector of a single point before transformation and $\vec{x}'$ after it, $\vec{t} = [t_x, t_y]$ is the translational displacement, $\mathbf{R}$ is the 2 by 2 rotation matrix:

$$\mathbf{R} = \begin{bmatrix} cos\theta & sin\theta \\ -sin\theta & cos\theta \end{bmatrix} \tag{19.22}$$

and $\mathbf{S}$ is a diagonal matrix $\mathbf{S} = diag(s_x, s_y)$, whose elements represent the scaling factors along the two axes. In the condition of *isotropic scaling*, assumed by the authors, $s_x = s_y = s$; thus, the previous equation (Equation 19.21) is simplified as follows:

$$\vec{x}' = s\mathbf{R}\vec{x} + \vec{t} \tag{19.23}$$

where $s$ is a scalar value. In the proposed implementation, thus, the geometric parameters were $\alpha = [t_x, t_y, \theta, s]$. The maximization process was an heuristic search procedure, in which the four scalar parameters are iteratively changed by small amounts. In order to make the processing much faster, the procedure was applied only on a small portion of the images, and the estimated transformation $T_{\alpha^*}$ successfully adopted for the whole image. The automatic registration procedure was successful even when the image content was significantly different and when only a small portion of the image was considered.

---

## 19.8   Edge Detection

One of the tasks accomplished by restorers during their work is the extraction of borders or edges of the painting they are dealing with, in order to get a better knowledge of the artwork. The revealed features are not only the painting's elements (i.e., contours of subjects present in the painting), but also characteristics of the layer, for example, bonds of wood panels, microcracks on the varnish, engravings, and so forth. Edge extraction can be useful for monitoring a restoration work, for highlighting some particular features of the painting (e.g., position and size of lacunas), or for studying the geometrical structure of the painting.

The approach of the restorers to this important item is to manually draw all the points belonging to borders; more precisely, very often restorers draw the borders by means of transparent sheets leaned over the painting. It is clear that such an approach is a very time-consuming process, involving restorers working for weeks. Another approach they often follow is to use some general purpose software, like *Autocad*: even if dealing with digital images, the process is similar, involving the restorers pointing out every single border point, by means of a mouse or an optic blackboard instead of a common pen.

Some general purpose image processing software allow the user to find edges in digital images automatically (e.g., *Photoshop, Paint Shop Pro, Corel Photo Paint*); nevertheless, such

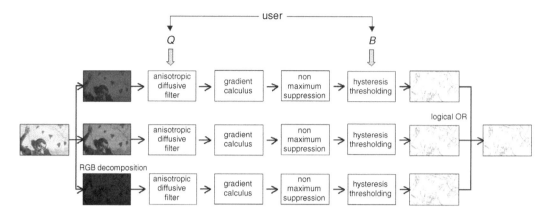

**FIGURE 19.10**
Overall scheme of the proposed edge detection procedure.

tools are too general to provide good results for the cultural heritage applications, because there are no options to calibrate the edge detection algorithms. In the following, an ad hoc technique developed for edge detection in the specific case of artwork will be described.

### 19.8.1   Cultural Heritage Application

The Image Processing and Communication Lab of the University of Florence has developed a procedure for extracting edges in artwork [34]. Starting from a classical edge detection operator (the Canny method [35]), the algorithm asks for the user participation in order to consider peculiarities of the analyzed work: in particular, the user has to tune two parameters, one regarding the level of degradation present in the digital copy of the painting (in other words its "quality" related to the conservation of the good, presenting some cracks, dust, stains, etc.) and one regarding the characteristics of the edges to be revealed (how pronounced are the edges). The first parameter (called $Q$) is used in the setup of the *anisotropic diffusive filter* proposed for noise reduction; the second parameter (called $B$) is used for the computation of the thresholds adopted during the hysteresis thresholding step in the Canny method, as will be described later.

The authors propose separating the image reproducing the painting in the three RGB bands and extracting edges independently in each band; then, the resulting borders are composed through a *logical OR* to obtain a unique overall edge image. In this way, the final edge image will contain all the edges, even if some details are visible only in one of the three bands. The overall scheme of the proposed procedure is shown in Figure 19.10.

To limit the effect of noise, a preprocessing step is applied: an *anisotropic diffusive filter* is used, which smooths the image according to the following iterative rule:

$$[f(n_1, n_2)]_{t+1} = \left[ f(n_1, n_2) + (\Delta T) \sum_{d=1}^{\Gamma} c_d(n_1, n_2) \hat{\nabla} f_d(n_1, n_2) \right]_t \qquad (19.24)$$

where $f(n_1, n_2)$ is the pixel value at position $(n_1, n_2)$ (i.e., the intensity level of the pixel in the considered band); $\hat{\nabla} f_d(n_1, n_2)$ represents the directional derivative of the image $f$, in the direction $d$, which has to be evaluated in $\Gamma$ directions (i.e., $\Gamma = 4$: north, south, east, west are the four directions); $\Delta T = 1/4$ in order to assure stability of the filter; $c_d(n_1, n_2)$ is the diffusion coefficient, which distinguishes this class of filters. It has been fixed to

$$c_d(n_1, n_2) = \frac{1}{1 + \left[\frac{\hat{\nabla} f(n_1, n_2)}{k}\right]^2} \qquad (19.25)$$

where $k$ is a factor that determines the strength of smoothness, depending on the "quality" of the image; the user sets the parameter $Q$, ranging from 1 to 15, choosing higher values for higher quality-images; $k$ is then defined as

$$Q \leq 8 \quad \Rightarrow \quad k = Q \times 3,5$$
$$9 \leq Q \leq 15 \quad \Rightarrow \quad k = Q \times 5,5 \qquad (19.26)$$

Once the diffusive filter has been applied, the three steps of the Canny method are followed [35]: gradient calculus, nonmaximum suppression, and hysteresis thresholding. For each band, the modulus and the phase of the discrete gradient are computed:

$$|\hat{\nabla} f(n_1, n_2)| = \sqrt{D_1(n_1, n_2)^2 + D_2(n_1, n_2)^2}$$
$$\angle \hat{\nabla} f(n_1, n_2) = \arctan\left(\frac{D_1(n_1, n_2)}{D_2(n_1, n_2)}\right) \qquad (19.27)$$

where $D_1$ and $D_2$ represent the two components of the gradient, calculated using standard algorithms (e.g., Sobel, Frei-Chen, or Prewitt methods).

The second step, the *nonmaximum suppression* process, is a preprocessing thinning operation. All the pixels of the gradient modulus matrix $|\hat{\nabla} f|$ are analyzed with respect to the neighboring pixels; if the value of the modulus of the gradient of the considered pixel is lower than the value of the neighboring pixels in the direction of the gradient (specified by the phase), then such a pixel is discarded as a possible border. At the end of such a step, several pixels in the gradient matrix have been set to zero, thus thinning potential edges.

Finally, during the *hysteresis thresholding* procedure, all the nonzero pixels in the gradient matrix are inquired and assigned to be an edge if their modulus satisfies some conditions. In particular, given $T_L$ and $T_H$ (with $T_L < T_H$) two suitable thresholds, then if $|\hat{\nabla} f(n_1, n_2)| > T_H$, the pixel $(n_1, n_2)$ is surely a pixel belonging to a border; if $|\hat{\nabla} f(n_1, n_2)| < T_L$, the pixel $(n_1, n_2)$ is surely not a pixel belonging to a border; if $T_L \leq |\hat{\nabla} f(n_1, n_2)| \leq T_H$, the pixel $(n_1, n_2)$ belongs to a border only if it is connected to a border pixel (belonging to its neighborhood). In this way, connection of the edges is ensured. For the calculus of the thresholds, the authors propose to start from a unique threshold $T$ estimated as

$$T = \mu \cdot \left(1 + \frac{B}{\sigma}\right) \qquad (19.28)$$

hence the thresholds $T_L$ and $T_H$ can be calculated as

$$T_H = T \cdot \text{high}$$
$$T_L = T_H / \text{low} \qquad (19.29)$$

where $\mu$ and $\sigma$ in Equation 19.28 are the mean and the variance of the modulus of the gradient, calculated in a suitable window centered on the processed pixel. $B$ is the parameter chosen by the user, representing how pronounced the borders are, ranging from 50 (slightly pronounced) to 250 (strongly pronounced). According to its value, the coefficients high and low in Equation 19.29 are fixed to

$$
\begin{aligned}
50 \le B < 100 &\Rightarrow \text{high} = 1.1 \quad \text{low} = 3 \\
100 \le B \le 200 &\Rightarrow \text{high} = 1.2 \quad \text{low} = 2.6 \\
200 < B \le 250 &\Rightarrow \text{high} = 1.4 \quad \text{low} = 2.2
\end{aligned}
\tag{19.30}
$$

Subsequently, it is possible to apply a postprocessing procedure, in order to clean the imperfections, such as isolated pixels.

## 19.9 Conclusions

In this chapter, how image processing methods may be used in meaningful applications in the *cultural heritage* field, with particular focus on the implementation of virtual restoration techniques, has been described. Image processing tools can be used as a guide to the actual restoration of the artwork, or they can produce a digitally restored version of the work, valuable by itself, although the restoration is only virtual and cannot be reproduced on the real piece of work.

This research area presents a large number of interesting challenges, of great relevance for the knowledge and dissemination of artwork and of the related culture. Several issues are common to the general research area of digital color imaging. However, the true peculiarity of this field lies in the fact that each work of art is by its nature unique: dimensions, materials, and techniques of artwork may vary enormously, and each object is without equal because of its specific history. Another important issue is the interdisciplinary expertise needed: the research fields involved are optics, image processing, color science, computer science, art history, and painting conservation, so that there is the need to bring together scientists with different backgrounds and belonging to different cultural areas. This aspect is certainly challenging, but in many cases, it also represents the main obstacle to the application of image processing technologies to the art field, due to a sort of cultural clash between researchers with a technical background and researchers belonging to the humanistic area. In spite of the above difficulties, the application of image processing to the processing of visual artwork appears to be one of the most interesting research areas of the future.

## References

[1] K. Martinez, J. Cupitt, D. Saunders, and R. Pillay, Ten years of art imaging research, *Proceedings of the IEEE*, 90, 28–41, January 2002.
[2] V. Cappellini, H. Maitre, I. Pitas, and A. Piva, Guest editorial special issue on image processing for cultural heritage, *IEEE Trans. on Image Process.*, 13, 273–276, March 2004.
[3] M. Barni, A. Pelagotti, and A. Piva, Image processing for the analysis and conservation of paintings: Opportunities and challenges, *IEEE Signal Process. Mag.*, 22, 141–144, September 2005.
[4] M. Barni, F. Bartolini, and V. Cappellini, Image processing for virtual restoration of art-works, *IEEE Multimedia Mag.*, 7, 10–13, April–June 2000.
[5] M. Pappas and I. Pitas, Digital color restoration of old paintings, *IEEE Trans. on Image Process.*, 9, 291–294, February 2000.

[6] N. Nikolaidis and I. Pitas, Digital image processing in painting restoration and archiving, in *Proceedings of IEEE International Conference on Image Processing 2001 (ICIP2001)*, Vol. I, Thessaloniki, Greece, October 7–10, IEEE, 2001, pp. 586–589.

[7] X. Li, D. Lu, and Y. Pan, Color restoration and image retrieval for Dunhuang fresco preservation, *IEEE Multimedia Mag.*, 7, 38–42, April–June 2000.

[8] F. Drago and N. Chiba, Locally adaptive chromatic restoration of digitally acquired paintings, *Int. J. Image and Graphics*, 5, 617–637, July 2005.

[9] E. Land and J. McCann, Lightness and retinex theory, *J. Opt. Soc. Am.*, 61, 1–11, January 1971.

[10] S.-C. Pei, Y.-C. Zeng, and C.-H. Chang, Virtual restoration of ancient Chinese paintings using color contrast enhancement and lacuna texture synthesis, *IEEE Trans. on Image Process., Spec. Issue on Image Process. for Cult. Heritage*, 13, 416–429, March 2004.

[11] M. Corsini, F. Bartolini, and V. Cappellini, Mosaicing for high resolution acquisition of paintings, in *Proceedings of the Seventh International Conference on Virtual Systems and Multimedia (VSMM 2001)*, Berkeley, CA, October 25–27, 2001, IEEE, pp. 39–48.

[12] M. Barni, V. Cappellini, and A. Mecocci, The use of different metrics in vector median filtering: Application to fine arts and paintings, in *Proceedings of the sixth European Signal Processing Conference (EUSIPCO-92)*, Brussels, Belgium, August, 25–28, 1992, Elsevier Science Ltd., pp. 1485–1488.

[13] B. Smolka, M. Szczepanski, K. Plataniotis, and A.Venetsanopoulos, New technique for the restoration of noisy color images, in *Proceedings of 14th International Conference on Digital Signal Processing (DSP 2002)*, Vol. I, Santorini, Greece, July 1–3, 2002, IEEE, pp. 95–98.

[14] B. Zitová, J. Flusser, and F. Lroubek, Application of image processing for the conservation of the medieval mosaic, in *Proceedings of IEEE International Conference on Image Processing 2002 (ICIP2002)*, Rochester, New York, Vol. III, 22-25, September 2002, IEEE, pp. 993–996.

[15] B. Zitová, J. Flusser, and F. Lroubek, An application of image processing in the medieval mosaic conservation, *Patt. Anal. and Appl.*, 7, 18–25, 2004.

[16] V. Cappellini, M. Barni, M. Corsini, A. De Rosa, and A. Piva, Artshop: An art-oriented image processing tool for cultural heritage applications, *J. Visualization and Comput. Animation*, 14, 149–158, July 2003.

[17] R. Franke, Scattered data interpolations: Tests of some methods, *Math. Computation*, 38, 181–200, 1982.

[18] I. Giakoumis and I. Pitas, Digital restoration of painting cracks, in *Proceedings of IEEE International Symposium on Circuits and Systems (ISCAS'98)*, Vol. IV, May 31–June 3, 1998, IEEE, pp. 269–272.

[19] F. Meyer, Iterative image transformations for an automatic screeing of cervical smears, *J. Histochem. and Cytochem.*, 27, 128–135, 1979.

[20] F.S. Abas and K. Martinez, Craquelure analysis for content-based retrieval, in *Proceedings of 14th International Conference on Digital Signal Processing (DSP 2002)*, Vol. I, Santorini, Greece, July 1–3, 2002, IEEE, pp. 111–114.

[21] F.S. Abas and K. Martinez, Classification of painting cracks for content-based retrieval, in *Machine Vision Applications in Industrial Inspection XI, Proceedings of SPIE, Vol. 5011*, Santa Clara, CA, January 23–24, 2003, pp. 149–160.

[22] A. Jain, S. Prabhakar, and L. Hong, An integrated content and metadata based retrieval system for art, *IEEE Trans. on Patt. Anal. and Machine Intelligence*, 21, 348–359, April 1999.

[23] A. Hanbury, P. Kammerer, and E. Zolda, Painting crack elimination using viscous morphological reconstruction, in *Proceedings of 12th International Conference on Image Analysis and Processing (ICIAP2003)*, Mantova, Italy, September 17–19, 2003, IEEE, pp. 226–231.

[24] P. Kammerer, E. Zolda, and R. Sablatnig, Computer aided analysis of underdrawings in infrared reflectograms, in *Proceedings of fourth International Symposium on Virtual Reality, Archaeology and Intelligent Cultural Heritage*, (Brighton, United Kingdom, November 5–7, 2003, pp. 19–27.

[25] A. De Rosa, A.M. Bonacchi, and V. Cappellini, Image segmentation and region filling for virtual restoration of art-works, in *Proceedings of IEEE International Conference on Image Processing 2001 (ICIP2001)*, Thessaloniki, Greece, Vol. I, October 7–10, 2001, IEEE, pp. 562–565.

[26] A.G. Borsand, W. Puech, I. Pitas, and J.-M. Chassery, Mosaicing of flattened images from straight homogeneous generalized cylinders, in *Lecture Notes in Computer Science, Vol. 1296, Seventh*

*International Conference on Computer Analysis of Images and Patterns*, G. Sommer, K. Daniilidis, J. Pauli, and Eds., Kiel, Germany, September 10–12, 1997, Springer, pp. 122–129.

[27] W. Puech, A.G. Bors, I. Pitas, and J.-M. Chassery, Projection distortion analysis for flattened image mosaicing from straight uniform generalized cylinders, *Patt. Recognition*, 34, 1657–1670, August 2001.

[28] C. Papaodysseus, T. Panagopoulos, M. Exarhos, C. Triantafillou, D. Fragoulis, and C. Doumas, Contour-shape based reconstruction of fragmented, 1600 Bc wall paintings, *IEEE Trans. on Signal Process.*, 50, 1277–1288, June 2002.

[29] J. Fitzpatrick, D. Hill, and C.M. Jr., Image registration, in *Handbook of Medical Imaging — Volume 2, Medical Image Processing and Analysis*, M. Sonka and J.M. Fitzpatrick, Eds., SPIE Press, Bellingham, WA, 2000, pp. 488–496, chap. 8.

[30] B. Zitová and J. Flusser, Image registration methods: A survey, *Image and Vision Comput.*, 21, 977–1000, June 2003.

[31] F. Maes, D. Vandermeulen, and P. Suetens, Medical image registration using mutual information, *Proceedings of the IEEE*, 91, 1699–1722, October 2003.

[32] F. Maes, A. Collignon, D. Vandermeulen, G. Marchal, and P. Suetens, Multimodality image registration by maximization of mutual information, *IEEE Trans. on Medical Imaging*, 16, 187–198, 1997.

[33] V. Cappellini, A. Del Mastio, A. De Rosa, A. Piva, A. Pelagotti, and H.E. Yamani, An automatic registration algorithm for cultural heritage images, in *Proceedings of 12th IEEE International Conference on Image Processing 2005 (ICIP2005)*, Genoa, Italy, Vol. 2, September 11–14, 2005, IEEE, pp. 566–569.

[34] A. Del Mastio, V. Cappellini, M. Corsini, F. De Lucia, A. De Rosa, and A. Piva, Image processing techniques for cultural heritage applications, in *Proceedings of the 11th International Conference on Virtual System and Multimedia (VSMM 2005)*, Ghent, Belgium, October 3–7, 2005, Archeolingua (Budapest) pp. 443–452.

[35] J. Canny, A computational approach to edge detection, *IEEE Trans. on Patt. Anal. and Machine Intelligence*, 8, 679–698, 1986.

# 20

## Image and Video Colorization

Liron Yatziv and Guillermo Sapiro

**CONTENTS**

## 20.1   Introduction

Colorization, the art of coloring a grayscale image or video, involves assigning from the single dimension of intensity or luminance a quantity that varies in three dimensions, such as red, green, and blue channels. Mapping between intensity and color is therefore not unique, and colorization is ambiguous in nature, requiring some amount of human interaction or external information. A computationally simple and effective approach of colorization is first presented in this chapter. The method is fast, so it can be used "on the fly," permitting the user to interactively get the desired results promptly after providing a reduced set of chrominance scribbles. Based on concepts of luminance-weighted chrominance blending and fast intrinsic distance computations, high-quality colorization results for still images and video are obtained at a fraction of the complexity and computational cost of previously reported techniques. Extensions of this algorithm include the capability of changing colors of an image or video as well as changing the underlying luminance. We conclude the chapter with a different approach, this time based on variational principles and geometric partial differential equations, that connects image colorization with image inpainting. This algorithm is based on cloning the edges from the provided gray-level image to the color channels.

Colorization is the art of adding color to a monochrome image or movie. The idea of "coloring" photos and films is not new. Ironically, hand coloring of photographs is as old as photography itself. There exist such examples from 1842 and possibly earlier [1]. It was practiced in motion pictures in the early 1900s by the French Company Pathe, where many films were colored by hand. It was widely practiced also for filmstrips into the 1930s.

A computer-assisted process was first introduced by Wilson Markle in 1970 for adding colors to black and white movies [2].

As described by Sykora et al. [3] (this work includes an outstanding overview of the literature on the subject), various early computer-based colorization techniques include straightforward approaches such as luminance keying [4]. This method uses a user-defined look-up table that transforms grayscale into color. Welsh et al. [5], inspired by work of Reinhard et al. [6] and Hertzmann et al. [7], extended this idea by matching luminance and texture rather than just the grayscale values.

Chen et al. [8] used manual segmentation to divide the grayscale image into a set of layers. Then an alpha channel was estimated using Bayesian image matting. This decomposition allows for colorization to be applied using Welsh's approach. The final image is constructed using alpha blending. Recently, Sykora et al. [3] similarly used a segmentation method optimized for the colorization of black-and-white cartoons.

Other approaches, including our own [9], [10], assume that homogeneity of the grayscale image indicates homogeneity in the color. In other words, as detailed in Reference [9], the geometry of the image is provided by the geometry of the grayscale information (see also References [11], [12], [13]). Often in these methods, in addition to the grayscale data, color hints are provided by the user via scribbles. Horiuchi [14] used a probabilistic relaxation method, while Levin et al. [15] solved an optimization problem that minimizes a quadratic cost function of the difference of color between a pixel and its weighted average neighborhood colors. We [9] also proposed to inpaint the colors constrained by the grayscale gradients and the color scribbles that serve as boundary conditions. The method reduces solving linear or nonlinear Poisson equations. This will be detailed later in this chapter.

The main shortcoming of these previous approaches is their intensive computational cost, needed to obtain good-quality results. Horiuchi and Hirano [16] addressed this issue and presented a faster algorithm that propagates colored seed pixels in all directions, and the coloring is done by choosing from a preselected list of color candidates. However, the method produces visible artifacts of block distortion, because no color blending is performed. While Horiuchi's method colorizes a still image within a few seconds, we first present in this chapter a propagation method that colorizes a still image within a second or less, achieving even higher-quality results. In contrast with works such as those in Reference [15], the techniques here described are easily extended to video without the optical flow computation, further improving on the computational cost, at no sacrifice in the image quality.

The first scheme here discussed follows Reference [10] (patent pending) and is based on the concept of color blending. This blending is derived from a weighted distance function efficiently computed (following Reference [17]) from the luminance channel. The underlying approach can be generalized to produce other effects, such as recolorization. In the first part of this chapter, we describe the algorithm and present a number of examples. We then conclude with a different approach, following Reference [9], which is based on variational problems and partial differential equations. This technique connects image colorization with image inpainting.

## 20.2  Fast Colorization Framework

Similar to other colorization methods (e.g., that in Reference [15]), we use luminance/chrominance color systems. We present our method in the $YCbCr$ color space, although other color spaces such as $YIQ$ or $YUV$ could be used as well. Moreover, work can also be done directly on the $RGB$ space. Let $Y(x, y, \tau) : \Omega \times [0, T] \rightarrow \Re^+$ be the given monochromatic image ($T = 0$) or video ($T > 0$) defined on a region $\Omega$. Our goal is to complete the $Cb$ and $Cr$ channels $Cb(x, y, \tau) : \Omega \times [0, T] \to \Re^+$ and $Cr(x, y, \tau) : \Omega \times [0, T] \to \Re^+$, respectively. For clarity of the exposition, we refer to both channels as the chrominance. The proposed technique also uses as input observed values of the chrominance channels in a region $\Omega_c \in \Omega$ which is significantly smaller than $\Omega$ (see Reference [15]). These values are often provided by the user or borrowed from other data.

Let $s$ and $t$ be two points in $\Omega$ and let $C(p) : [0, 1] \to \Omega$ be a curve in $\Omega$. Let also $C_{s,t}$ represent a curve connecting $s$ and $t$ such that $C(0) = s$ and $C(1) = t$. We define the intrinsic (geodesic) distance between $s$ and $t$ by

$$d(s, t) := \min_{C_{s,t}} \int_0^1 |\nabla Y \cdot \dot{C}(p)| dp \qquad (20.1)$$

This intrinsic distance gives a measurement of how "flat" is the flattest curve between any two points in the luminance channel. The integral in the equation above is basically integrating the luminance ($Y$) gradient in the direction of the curve $C(p)$. When considering the minimum over all paths $C_{s,t}$, we then keep the one with the smallest overall gradient in this direction, thereby the flattest path connecting the two points $s$ and $t$ (the path that goes from $s$ to $t$ with minimal overall gradient). Note that the minimal path need not be unique, but we only care about the intrinsic length $d(s, t)$ of this path, so this does not affect the algorithm. Geodesic distances of this type can be efficiently and accurately computed using recently developed fast numerical techniques [17], [18], [19], [20], [21], [22], [23]. We found that for the application at hand, even simpler techniques such as a *best-first* one (in particular, Dijkstra [24]) are sufficient. See Reference [10] for details on this computation.

Even though a mapping between luminance and chrominance is not unique, a close relationship between the basic geometry of these channels is frequently observed in natural images, see, for example, References [11], [12], and [13] and further comments later in this chapter. Sharp luminance changes are likely to indicate an edge in the chrominance, and a gradual change in luminance often indicates that the chrominance is not likely to have an edge but rather a moderate change. In other words, as has been reported in the above-mentioned works, there is a close relationship between the geometry of the luminance and chrominance channels. Exploiting this assumption, a change in luminance causes a related change in chrominance. This has been used in different fashions in References [9] and [15], as well as in Reference [25] for superresolution. From this, for the proposed colorization approach, we assume that the smaller the intrinsic distance $d(s, t)$ between two points $(s, t)$, the more similar chrominance they would have.[1]

Because the chrominance data are often given in whole regions and not necessarily in single isolated points, we would like to get an idea of the distance from a certain known chrominance ("scribbles" with a given uniform color) to any point $t$ in $\Omega$. We then define the intrinsic distance from a point $t$ (to be colored) to a certain chrominance $c$, as the minimum distance from $t$ to any point of the same chrominance $c$ in $\Omega_c$:

$$d_c(t) := \min_{\forall s \in \Omega_c : chrominance(s) = c} d(s, t) \qquad (20.2)$$

This gives the distance from a point $t$ to be colored to scribbles (from the provided set $\Omega_c$) with the same color $c$.

---

[1] It is important to notice that the goal of colorization is not to restore the original color of the image or scene, which is in general not available, but as in image inpainting, to produce visually pleasant and compelling colored images. See also Section 20.4 for more on this.

Our idea for colorization is to compute the $Cb$ and $Cr$ components (chrominance) of a point $t$ in the region where they are missing ($\Omega \backslash \Omega_c$) by blending the different chrominance in $\Omega_c$ according to their intrinsic distance to $t$:

$$chrominance(t) \leftarrow \frac{\sum_{\forall c \in chrominances(\Omega_c)} W(d_c(t)) \ c}{\sum_{\forall c \in chrominances(\Omega_c)} W(d_c(t))} \quad (20.3)$$

where $chrominances(\Omega_c)$ stands for all the different unique chrominances in the set $\Omega_c$, and $W(\cdot)$ is a function of the intrinsic distance that translates it into a blending weight. In words, the above blending expression assigns to any point $t$ to be colored, a color that is a weighted average of the different colors in the provided set of scribbles $\Omega_c$. For every distinct color $c$ in the set $\Omega_c$, the distance to it from $t$ is computed following Equation 20.2 — which uses Equation 20.1 — and this distance is used to define the weight of the color $c$ at the point $t$ (the blending proportion of this color).

The function $W(\cdot)$ should hold some basic properties detailed in Reference [10]. For the experiments reported below, we used

$$W(r) = r^{-b} \quad (20.4)$$

where $b$ is the blending factor, typically $1 \leq b \leq 6$. This factor defines the smoothness of the chrominance transition.

Note that in theory, following the equations above, a point $t$ to be colored will be influenced by all distinct colors $c$ in $\Omega_c$, because $d_c(t) < \infty$.

The described colorization algorithm has average time and space complexity of $O(|\Omega| \cdot |chrominances(\Omega_c)|)$.[2] The algorithm passes over the image/video for each different chrominance observed in $\Omega_c$ and needs a memory in the order of the number of different chrominances observed in $\Omega_c$ times the input image/video size. If there are a large number of scribbles of different chrominances, the algorithm could be relatively slow and pricey in memory (although still more efficient than those previously reported in the literature). Fortunately, because human perception of blending is limited, high blending accuracy is not fully necessary to obtain satisfactory results. Experimental results show that it is enough just to blend the most significant chrominance (the chrominance with the closest intrinsic distance to their observed source). We found that in natural images, it is enough to blend just the two or three most significant chrominances to get satisfactory results. Such a relaxation reduces both time and space complexity to $O(|\Omega|)$, thereby linear in the amount of data. Therefore, we do not include in the blend chrominances that their weight in the blending equation is small relative to the total weight. Additional quality improvements could be achieved if an adaptive threshold following results such as those from the *MacAdam* ellipses [27] is used. Any color lying just outside an ellipse is at the "just noticeable difference" (*jnd*) level, which is the smallest perceivable color difference under the experiment conditions. A possible use of this is to define an adaptive threshold that would filter out chrominance that if added to the blend would not cause a *jnd*. This proposed algorithm relaxation of limiting the number of contributors to the blending equation gives a tight restriction on how far the chrominance will propagate to be included in the blend. The restriction can be easily implemented [10].

## 20.2.1 Colorization Results

We now present examples of our image and video colorization technique. Additional examples, comparisons, and movies, as well as software for testing our approach, can be found on the Internet (http://mountains.ece.umn.edu/~liron/colorization/).

---

[2] Using a priority queue with $O(1)$ average complexity per operation, as done in References [17], [22], and [26], a heap sort data structure as used in the original Dijkstra algorithm would slightly increase the run-time complexity.

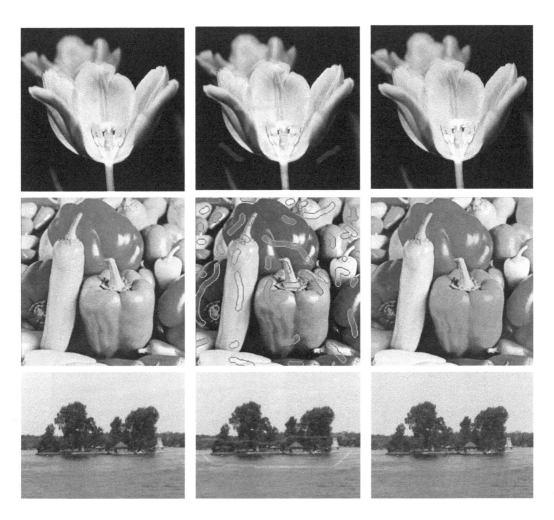

**FIGURE 20.1  (See color insert.)**
Still image colorization examples. Given a grayscale image (left), the user marks chrominance scribbles (center), and our algorithm provides a colorized image (right). The image size/run-times top to bottom are $270 \times 359$/less than 0.83 seconds, $256 \times 256$/less than 0.36 seconds, and $400 \times 300$/less than 0.77 seconds.

The proposed algorithm was implemented in C++ as a stand-alone win32 application so it could be tested for speed and quality. For timing, we used an Intel Pentium III with 512MB RAM running under Windows 2000. Figure 20.1 shows examples of still image colorization using our proposed algorithm. The algorithm run-time for all the examples in Figure 20.1, measured once the images were loaded into memory, is less than 7 $\mu$sec per pixel.

Figure 20.2a to Figure 20.2d and Figure 20.3a to Figure 20.3e compare our method with the one recently proposed by Levin et al. [15] (this work partially inspired our own). The method minimizes the difference between a pixel's color and the weighted average color of its neighboring pixels. The weights are provided by the luminance channel. The minimization is an optimization problem, subject to constraints supplied by the user as chrominance scribbles. Solving this is computationally costly and slower than our proposed technique. First, in Figure 20.2a to Figure 20.2d, we observe that we achieve the same visual quality at a fraction of the computational cost (more comparisons are provided at the above-mentioned Web site, all supporting the same finding). Overall, the method proposed in Reference [15] performs very well on many images, yet Figure 20.3a to Figure 20.3e demonstrate that it can perform poorly when colorizing relatively far from the provided color constraints.

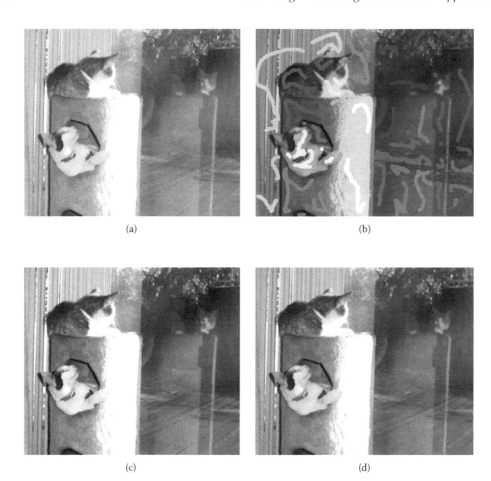

(a)                                                              (b)

(c)                                                              (d)

**FIGURE 20.2**

Comparison of visual quality with the technique proposed in Levin, A., Lischinsk, D., and Weiss, Y., *j-TOG*, 23, 689, 2004. (a) The given grayscale image, (b) the user marks chrominance scribbles (the selected scribbles are obtained from the work in Levin et al. *j-TOG*, 23, 689, 2004), (c) our algorithm results with CPU run-time of 0.54 sec, (d) Levin et al. approach with CPU run-time of 17 sec using their supplied fast implementation based on a multigrid solver. We observe the same quality at a significantly reduced computational cost.

Following the equations in the previous section, see Equation 20.3, even far away pixels will receive color from the scribbles with our approach (in particular from the closest ones, in weighted distance, see section on relaxation above). In order to match visual quality with our technique, the method proposed in Reference [15] needs more user input, meaning additional color scribbles. We also found that the inspiring technique developed in Reference [15] has a sensible scale parameter and often fails at strong edges, because these provide zero or very limited weight/influence in their formulation.

In Figure 20.4, we study the robustness of our proposed approach with respect to the scribbles placement (location of the set $\Omega_c$). Before describing these examples, let us provide some basic comments that will help to understand the observed robustness of this technique. Assume that we know the "ideal" position to place a scribble (see Section 20.4 for more on this). What happens if instead of placing this scribble, we place a different one. If the ideal scribble and the placed one are both inside the same object and the region between them is relatively homogenous, then using our gradient weighted metric, the distance between the two scribbles will be relatively small. From the triangle inequality, we can then bound the distance from the placed scribble to a given pixel to be colored, by simply using the sum

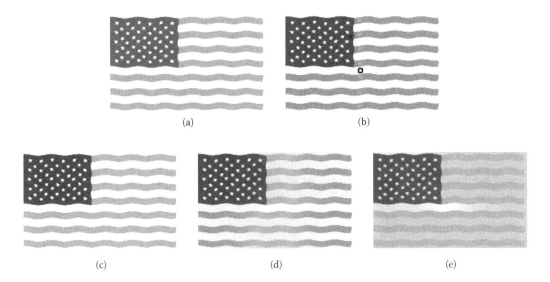

**FIGURE 20.3**
Comparison of visual quality with the technique proposed in Levin, A., Lischinski, D., and Weiss, Y., *j-TOG* 23, 689, 2004. (a) The given grayscale image (200 × 120), (b) the user marks chrominance scribbles, (c) our algorithm results with CPU run-time of 0.3 sec, (d) Levin et al. approach with CPU run-time of 5.7 sec using their supplied fast implementation of multigrid solver, and (e) Levin et al. approach using a slower exact MATLAB least squares solver, also provided by the authors.

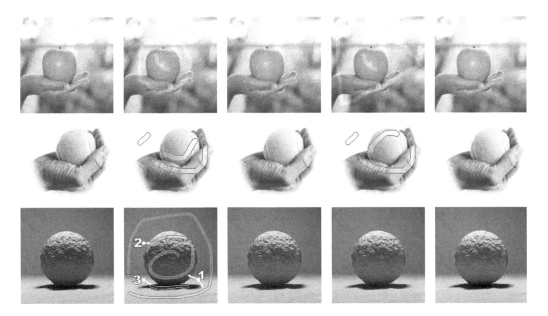

**FIGURE 20.4**
Testing the robustness of the proposed algorithm. The first row shows an example where different sets of scribbles are used, obtaining visually identical results. The original monochromatic image is shown first, followed by the first set of scribbles and the resulting colorized result. This is followed by a second set of scribbles and the corresponding colorized results. Note how the two results are virtually identical. The next row repeats the same experiment for a different image. We next show, third row, how the result is evolving with the addition of new scribbles by the user. The original image is presented first, followed by the set of scribbles labeled by their order of application. The third figure shows the result when only the two scribbles labeled **1** are used. Then scribbled **2** is added to improve the results on the top of the ball, obtaining the fourth figure. Finally, the scribble labeled **3** was added to keep the shadow gray instead of green, and the result is provided in the last figure.

of the distance from the ideal scribble to such pixel and the distance between the scribbles. Because the latter is small, then the distance from the ideal scribble and the one from the placed one to the pixel to be colored are similar, and as such, the result of the colorization algorithm. If the placed scribble is located "on the wrong side of the edge" (or with high gradients between it and the ideal scribble), then of course the distance between the ideal and the placed scribbles will be large, and as such, the algorithm will produce very different results. Of course, this will almost mean an intentional mistake by the user. Moreover, interactive colorization is possible thanks to the fast speed of the proposed technique, thereby permitting the user to correct errors and to add or move scribbles as needed (this can be easily experimented with the public domain software mentioned above). The first row of Figure 20.4 shows an example of an image colored with different sets of scribbles. Notice how the results are visually indistinguishable. This is repeated for a second example in the next row. The last row of the figure shows the evolution of the result as the user adds scribbles, a common working scenario for this type of application, which is allowed by the speed and robustness of our proposed technique (this is also part of the public domain implementation mentioned above).

Figure 20.5a to Figure 20.5d show how our technique can be applied to video, simply by extending the idea into 3-D (space + time) and allowing the colors to propagate in

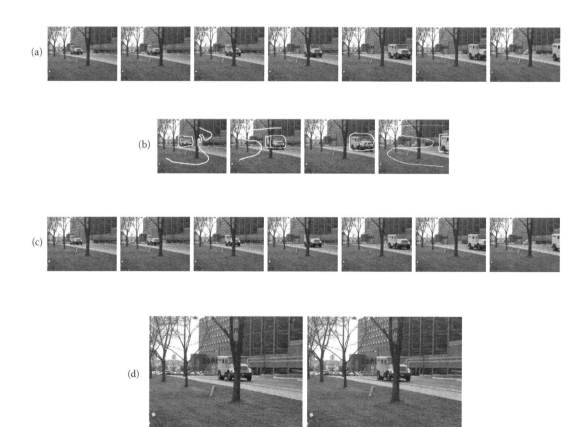

**FIGURE 20.5**
Video colorization example. (a) Given the 75 frame sequence, (b) and four frames with scribbles, (c) our algorithm provides a recolored video of the truck; (d) one of the frames is enlarged to show the recoloring content. The size of each frame is 320 × 240. The movie can be found on the Web site for this project.

the time dimension. Optical flow is optional, and it may improve the quality of the result, especially in videos that have a slow frame rate. Given a grayscale or colored video and some chrominance scribbles anywhere in the video, our algorithm colors the whole video within seconds. This is a significant computational complexity reduction compared to Reference [15] (and Reference [3]), where not only each frame is computed significantly faster, but also there is no need for optical flow (on high frame rate videos). Figure 20.5a to Figure 20.5t demonstrate the colorization of a truck passing an occluder tree. We obtained very good results just by marking a few chrominance scribbles in four frames.

The *blending factor* is the only free parameter of the algorithm as currently implemented. We set it to $b = 4$ for all examples in this paper and the additional ones in the above-mentioned Web page. Better results may have been archived selecting a different value per image and video, although we did not find this necessary to obtain the high-quality results here presented.

## 20.2.2 Recolorization and Extensions

Recolorization is the art of replacing the colors of an image by new colors. Figure 20.6 shows that it is possible to change colors of an existing image or video just by slightly modifying our original colorization algorithm. When colorizing grayscale images, we based the process on the assumption that homogeneity of the grayscale indicates homogeneity in the chrominance. In recolorization, we have more clues about how the chrominance should vary. We assume that homogeneity in the original chrominance indicates homogeneity in the new chrominance. The chrominance propagation can be based on the grayscale assumption or the original color assumption or both, as demonstrated in Figure 20.7. The intrinsic distance can also be measured on the $Cb$ and $Cr$ channels rather than just on the intensity channel as done in Equation 20.1. This is done simply by replacing $Y$ by $Cb$ or $Cr$ in this equation, thereby using the gradients of these (now available) chroma channels to control the blending weight of the new color.

Recolorization is just one possible extension of our method. It is also possible to further generalize it by defining the measurement medium $M(x, y, \tau) : \Omega \times [0, T] \to \Re$ on which the intrinsic distance is measured. $M$ can be any channel of the input image, a mix of the channels, or any other data that will make sense for weighting the intrinsic distance. The blending medium $\mathcal{B}(x, y, \tau) : \Omega \times [0, T] \to \Re$ is then the data that are actually blended.

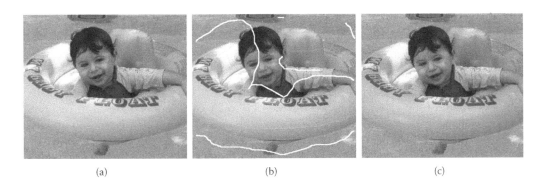

(a)        (b)        (c)

**FIGURE 20.6 (See color insert.)**
Recolorization example. (a) Original color image, (b) shows the scribbles placed by the user, where white is a special scribble used in recolorization that preserves the original colors of the image in selected regions of the image, and (c) is the recolored image. Note that only a few scribbles were used. Applying more scribbles would increase the quality of the result image.

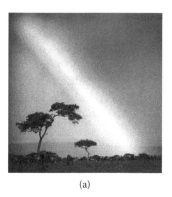 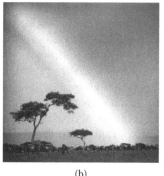 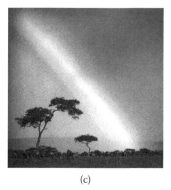

(a)                                   (b)                                   (c)

**FIGURE 20.7** (See color insert.)
Recolorization example using the $Cr$ channel for measurement ($M$) rather than the intensity channel. (a) is the original color image, and (b) is the intensity channel of the image. It can be clearly seen that the intensity image does not contain significant structural information on the red rainbow strip (this is a unique example of this effect). On the other hand, both the $Cb$ and $Cr$ change significantly between the stripes and therefore can be used for recolorization. (c) Recolored image in which the red stripe of the rainbow was replaced by a purple one.

Both in colorization and recolorization, we selected $\mathcal{B}$ to be the chrominance. Yet, $\mathcal{B}$ can be any image processing effect or any data that make sense to blend for a given application. Figure 20.8a to Figure 20.8f follows this idea and gives an example of object brightness change.

Finally, in Figure 20.9a and Figure 20.9b, we show another useful special effect, the removal of color from image regions.

## 20.3   Inpainting the Colors

We will conclude this chapter with a framework for colorization that connects it to *image inpainting*.[3] This is motivated by two main bodies of work, one dealing with the geometry of color images and one dealing with image inpainting, the art of modifying an image in a nondetectable work. Caselles et al. [11] and Chung and Sapiro [12] (see also Reference [28]) have shown that the (scalar) luminance channel faithfully represents the geometry of the whole (vectorial) color image. This geometry is given by the gradient and the level-lines, following the mathematical morphology school. Moreover, Kimmel [13] proposed to align the channel gradients as a way of denoising color images, and showed how this arises naturally from simple assumptions. This body of work brings us to the first component of our proposed technique, to consider the gradient of each color channel to be given (or hinted) by the gradient of the given monochrome data.[4] Similar concepts were used in Reference [25] for increasing the resolution of the spectral channels from a panchromatic image in multispectral satellite data. The second component of our framework comes from inpainting [29]. In addition to having the monochrome (luminance) channel, the user provides a few strokes of color that need to be propagated to the whole color channels, clearly a task of inpainting. Moreover, because from the concepts described above, information on the

---

[3] Similar results are obtained with this framework, but at increased computational cost, when compared with the fast technique just described. The main interest in it is then its connections with image inpainting.
[4] This monochrome image can become the luminance of the reconstructed color data in one possible scenario.

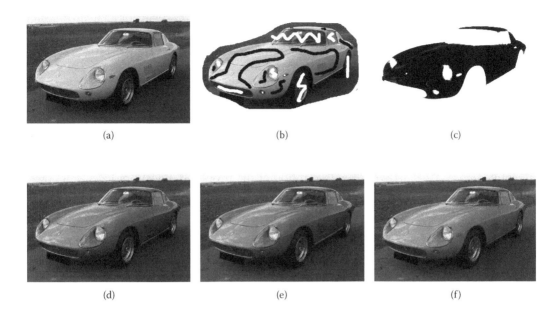

(a)      (b)      (c)

(d)      (e)      (f)

**FIGURE 20.8**

Example of the generalization of our method to other image processing effects. (a) The original color image. Our goal is to change the color of the yellow car into a darker color. (b) We define the blending medium by roughly marking areas we do not wish to change in white and areas we do want to change in black. We do so by placing scribbles or by just marking whole areas. (c) Using our colorization method, we propagate the markings (white and black colors) and get a grayscale matte (we only keep the blending channel). With the matte, it is possible to apply an effect to the original image with a magnitude proportional to the gray-level of the matte. In this case, we chose to change the brightness. (d) Image after applying the darkening. Note that the intensity only changed in the desired parts of the image. The darkening is done simply by subtracting the gray-level matte from the intensity channel, where white means no change and black is the maximum preselected change. It is possible to further process the image using the same matte, (e) and (f) demonstrate this by similarly adding the gray-level matte to the *Cb* and *Cr* channels, respectively.

gradients is also available (from the monochrome channel), this brings us to the inpainting technique described in Reference [25] (see also Reference [30]), where we have interpreted inpainting as recovering an image from its gradients, these obtained via elastica-type interpolation from the available data. Recovering an image from its gradients is, of course a very old subject in image processing and was studied, for example, in Reference [31] for image denoising (see also Reference [32]) and in Reference [33] for a number of very interesting image editing tasks. Combining both concepts, we then obtain that colorizing

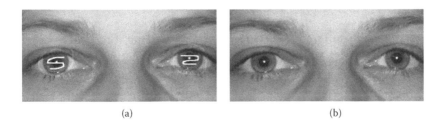

(a)      (b)

**FIGURE 20.9  (See color insert.)**

Using the described technique to remove color from certain image regions: (a) original image, and (b) only the eyes from the original image are preserved.

reduces to finding images (the color channels), provided their gradients (which are derived from the monochrome data) and constrained to color strokes provided by the user. Below we present partial differential equations for doing this, which in its simplest form, is just a Poisson equation with Dirichlet boundary conditions. This puts the problem of colorizing in the popular framework of solving image processing problems via partial differential equations [34], [35], [36].

### 20.3.1   Inpainting Colors from Gradients and Boundary Conditions

We use the same basic notations as for the first algorithm presented above, here repeated for convenience. We start with the description of the proposed algorithm for still images. Let $Y(x, y) : \Omega \to \Re^+$ be the given monochromatic image defined on the region $\Omega$. We will work on the $YCbCr$ color space (other color spaces could be used as well), and the given monochromatic image becomes the luminance $Y$. The goal is to compute $Cb(x, y) :$ $\Omega \to \Re^+$ and $Cr(x, y) : \Omega \to \Re^+$. We assume that colors are given in a region $\Omega_c$ in $\Omega$ such that $|\Omega_c| << |\Omega|$ (otherwise, simple interpolation techniques would be sufficient). This information is provided by the user via color strokes in editing type of applications, or automatically obtained for compression (selected compressed regions) or wireless (nonlost and transmitted blocks) applications. The goal is from the knowledge of $Y$ in $\Omega$ and $Cb, Cr$, in $\Omega_c$ to inpaint the color information $(Cb, Cr)$ into the rest of $\Omega$.[5]

Following the description above, $Cb$ (and similarly $Cr$) is reconstructed from the following minimization problem:

$$\min_{Cb} \int_\Omega \rho(\| \nabla Y - \nabla Cb \|)d\Omega \tag{20.5}$$

with boundary conditions on $\Omega_c$, $\nabla := \left(\frac{\partial}{\partial x}, \frac{\partial}{\partial y}\right)$ is the gradient operator, and $\rho(\cdot) : R \to R$. The basic idea is to force the gradient (and therefore the geometry) of $Cb$ to be as the geometry of the given monochromatic image $Y$ while preserving the given values of $Cb$ at $\Omega_c$. Note that although here we consider these given values as hard constraints, they can be easily included in the above variational formulation in the form of soft constraints. This can be particularly useful for compression and wireless applications, where the given data can be noisy, as well as for editing applications where the user provides only color hints instead of color constraints. For ease of the presentation, we continue with the assumption of hard constraints. In Reference [37], we discussed a number of robust selections for $\rho$ in the case of image denoising, while in Reference [25], we used the $L_1$ norm, $\rho(\cdot) = |\cdot|$, following the work on total variation [38]. Of course, the most popular, though not robust, selection is the $L_2$ norm $\rho(\cdot) = \cdot^2$, which leads via simple calculus of variation to the following necessary condition for the minimizer in Equation 20.5:

$$\Delta Cb = \Delta Y \tag{20.6}$$

with corresponding boundary conditions on $\Omega_c$ and $\Delta$ being the Laplace operator given by $\Delta := (\frac{\partial^2}{\partial x^2} + \frac{\partial^2}{\partial y^2})$. This is the well-known Poisson equation with Dirichlet boundary conditions.

Equation 20.5 and Equation 20.6 can be solved efficiently by a number of well-developed *Poisson solvers* (e.g., see [39]), making our proposed algorithm simple and computationally

---

[5] Note, of course, that exactly the same framework, detailed below, can be used to directly color/inpaint the *RGB* space directly, using the gradients of the given plane $Y$ and the given colors in $\Omega_c$.

efficient. Note that in contrast with the work in Reference [15], our formulation is continuous, and the vast available literature on numerical implementations of these equations accurately handles their efficient solution.

To conclude the presentation, we need to describe how to address the colorization of movies. Although optical flow can be incorporated as in Reference [15], it would be nice to avoid its explicit computation. We could implicitly introduce the concept of motion in the above variational formulation, though we opt for a simpler formulation. Following the color constancy constraint often assumed in optical flow, and if the gradient fields and motion vectors of all the movie channels are the same, then of course we can consider $\frac{\partial Y}{\partial t} = \frac{\partial Cb}{\partial t} = \frac{\partial Cr}{\partial t}$, where $t$ is the time coordinate in the movie. Therefore, Equation 20.5 and Equation 20.6 are still valid constraints for the movie case ($\Omega$ is now a region in $(x, y, t)$ and $\Omega_c$ are 2-D spatial strokes at selected frames), as long as we consider three-dimensional gradients and Laplace operators given by $\nabla := (\frac{\partial}{\partial x}, \frac{\partial}{\partial y}, \frac{\partial}{\partial t})$, $\Delta := (\frac{\partial^2}{\partial x^2} + \frac{\partial^2}{\partial y^2} + \frac{\partial^2}{\partial t^2})$, respectively. Anisotropy between the spatial and temporal derivatives can be easily added to these formulations as well.

### 20.3.2 Comments on Different Variational Formulations

Equation 20.5 and Equation 20.6 represent just one particular realization of our proposed framework. For example (see also comments in the concluding remarks section), we could constrain the color normalized gradients to follow the luminance normalized gradient. In this case, the variational formulation becomes $\min_{Cb} \int_\Omega \rho(\frac{\nabla Y}{\|\nabla Y\|} \cdot \nabla Cb - \| \nabla Cb \|)d\Omega$, with corresponding boundary conditions. From calculus of variations, the corresponding Euler–Lagrange equation is (for an $L_2$ norm) $\text{div}(\frac{\nabla Cb}{\|\nabla Cb\|}) = \text{div}(\frac{\nabla Y}{\|\nabla Y\|})$, which is once again solved using standard efficient numerical implementations [25], [30] (div stands for the divergence). The concepts above transmit to movies as with Equation 20.5 and Equation 20.6.

---

## 20.4 Concluding Remarks

In this chapter, we first described a fast colorization algorithm for still images and video. While keeping the quality at least as good as previously reported algorithms, the introduced technique manages to colorize images and movies within a second, compared to other techniques that may reach several minutes. The proposed approach needs less manual effort than techniques such as those introduced in Reference [15], and can be used interactively due to its high speed. We also showed that simple modifications in the algorithm lead to recolorization and other special effects. We then described a second approach, based on partial differential equations, that connects colorization with image inpainting.

A number of directions can be pursued as a result of the frameworks introduced here. First, as mentioned above, other special effects can be obtained following this distance-based blending of image attributes approach. We are working on including in this framework a crude (fast) computation of optical flow, to use mainly when the motion is too fast for the weighted distance used in the examples presented here. Another interesting problem is to investigate the use of this colorization approach for image compression. As shown in the examples here presented, a few color samples are often enough to produce visually pleasant results. This can be exploited for compression, in the same spirit as done in Reference [40], where the encoder voluntarily drops information that can be efficiently reconstructed by the decoder. In order to do this, we need to understand what is the simplest set of color scribbles that when combined with our algorithm, manages to reconstruct the color without any visual artifacts. In the same spirit, for the colorization of originally monochromatic data, or the recoloring of color data, it is important to understand the best position to place the scribbles so that the user's effort is minimized. For example, an edge map on the luminance data might help to guide the user. Although, as demonstrated with the examples provided in this paper and the additional ones in our Web site, the robustness and speed of the algorithm make it possible to work in an interactive fashion, reducing/minimizing user intervention is always an important goal. Results in these research directions will be reported elsewhere.

## Acknowledgments

The authors would like to thank Gustavo Brown, Alberto Bartesaghi, and Kedar Patwardhan for their inspiring and useful remarks. This work is partially supported by the Office of Naval Research, the National Science Foundation, and the National Geospatial-Intelligence Agency.

## References

[1] P. Marshall, Any Colour You Like, Technical report, http://photography.about.com/library/weekly/aa061002a.htm, June 2002.

[2] G. Burns, Colorization, www.museum.tv/archives/etv/C/htmlC/colorization/colorization.htm.

[3] J.B.D. Sýkora and J. Zára, Unsupervised colorization of black-and-white cartoons, *Proceedings of the Third International Symposium on NPAR'04*, Annecy, France, June 2004, pp. 121–127.

[4] R.C. Gonzalez and R.E. Woods, *Digital Image Processing*, 2nd ed., Addison-Wesley, Reading, MA: 1987.

[5] T. Welsh, M. Ashikhmin, and K. Mueller, Transferring color to greyscale images, *ACM Trans. Graph*, 21, 277–280, 2002.

[6] E. Reinhard, M. Ashikhmin, B. Gooch, and P. Shirley, Color transfer between images, *IEEE Comput. Graphics and Appl.*, 21, 34–41, 2001.

[7] A. Hertzmann, C.E. Jacobs, N. Oliver, B. Curless, and D.H. Salesin, Image analogies, in *SIGGRAPH 2001, Computer Graphics Proceedings*, Annual Conference Series, E. Fiume, Ed., ACM Press/ACM SIGGRAPH, New York, 2001, pp. 327–340.

[8] V.S.T. Chen, Y. Wang, and C. Meinel, Gray-scale image matting and colorization, *Asian Conference on Computer Vision*, 2004, pp. 1164–1169.

[9] G. Sapiro, Inpainting the colors, *IMA Preprint Series*, May 2004 (www.ima.umn.edu), also in *IEEE International Conference Image Processing*, Genoa, Italy, September 2005.

[10] L. Yatziv and G. Sapiro, Fast image and video colorization using chrominance blending, *IEEE Trans. Image Process.*, 15, 5, 1120–1129, May 2006.

[11] V. Caselles, B. Coll, and J.M. Morel, Geometry and color in natural images, *J. Math. Imaging and Vision*, 16, 89–105, March 2002.

[12] D.H. Chung and G. Sapiro, On the level lines and geometry of vector-valued images, *IEEE Signal Process. Lett.*, 7, 241–243, September 2000.

[13]  R. Kimmel, A natural norm for color processing, in *ACCV (1)*, 1998, pp. 88–95.

[14]  T. Horiuchi, Estimation of color for gray-level image by probabilistic relaxation, in *ICPR (3)*, 2002, pp. 867–870.

[15]  A. Levin, D. Lischinski, and Y. Weiss, Colorization using optimization, *j-TOG*, 23, 689–694, August 2004.

[16]  T. Horiuchi and S. Hirano, Colorization algorithm for grayscale image by propagating seed pixels, in *ICIP (1)*, 2003, pp. 457–460.

[17]  L. Yatziv, A. Bartesaghi and G. Sapiro, A Fast O(N) implementation of the fast marching algorithm," *Journal of Computational Physics*, 212, 292–399, 2006.

[18]  P.C.J. Helmsen, E.G. Puckett, and M. Dorr, Two new methods for simulating photolithography development in 3d, in *Proc. SPIE*, 2726, pp. 253–261, 1996.

[19]  S.O. Chiu-Yen Kao and Y.-H. Tsai, Fast sweeping methods for static Hamilton-Jacobi equations, Technical report, Dep. Mathematics, University of California, Los Angeles, 2002.

[20]  J. Sethian, Fast marching level set methods for three-dimensional photolithography development, *Proceedings of the SPIE International Symposium on Microlithography*, Santa Clara, CA, March 1996.

[21]  J.A. Sethian, A fast marching level set method for monotonically advancing fronts, *Proc. Nat. Acad. Sci.* 93, 1591–1595, February 1996.

[22]  J.N. Tsitsiklis, Efficient algorithms for globally optimal trajectories, *IEEE Trans. on Automatic Control*, 40, 1528–1538, 1995.

[23]  H. Zhao, A fast sweeping method for eikonal equations, *j-MATH-COMPUT*, 74, 603–627, April 2005.

[24]  E.W. Dijkstra, A note on two problems in connexion with graphs, *Numerische Mathematik*, 1, 269–271, 1959.

[25]  C. Ballester, M. Bertalmio, V. Caselles, G. Sapiro, and J. Verdera, Filling-in by joint interpolation of vector fields and gray levels, *IEEE Trans. Image Process.*, 10, 1200–1211, August 2001.

[26]  J.B.O.R.K. Ahuja, K. Melhrhorn, and R.E. Tarjan, Faster algorithms for the shortest path problem, *AMC*, 37, 213–223, 1990.

[27]  D. MacAdam, *Sources of Color Science*, MIT Press, Cambridge, MA, 1970.

[28]  G. Sapiro and D.L. Ringach, Anisotropic diffusion of multivalued images with applications to color filtering, *IEEE Trans. Image Process.*, 5, 1582–1586, November 1996.

[29]  V.C.M. Bertalmio, G. Sapiro, and C. Ballester, Image inpainting, *SIGGRAPH Comput. Graphics*, July 2000.

[30]  V.C.C. Ballester and J. Verdera, Disocclusion by joint interpolation of vector fields and gray levels, *SIAM Multiscale Modelling and Simulation*, 2, 80–123, 2003.

[31]  C. Kenney and J. Langan, A new image processing primitive: Reconstructing images from modified flow fields, University of California, Santa Barbara, June 1999, preprint.

[32]  M. Lysaker, S. Osher, and X.C. Tai, Noise removal using smoothed normals and surface fitting, *IEEE Trans. Image Process.*, 13, 1345–1357, October 2004.

[33]  P. Pérez, M. Gangnet, and A. Blake, Poisson image editing, *ACM Transactions on Graphics*, 2(3):313–318, 2003.

[34]  R. Kimmel, *Numerical Geometry of Images: Theory, Algorithms, and Applications*, Springer, 2003.

[35]  S. Osher and N. Paragios, *Geometric Level Set Methods in Imaging, Vision, and Graphics*, Springer-Verlag, Heidelberg, London; New York, July 2003.

[36]  G. Sapiro, *Geometric Partial Differential Equations and Image Processing*, Cambridge University Press, Heidelberg, London; New York, January 2001.

[37]  M.J. Black, G. Sapiro, D.H. Marimont, and D. Heeger, Robust anisotropic diffusion, *IEEE Trans. on Image Process.*, 7, 421–432, March 1998.

[38]  S.O.L.I. Rudin and E. Fatemi, Nonlinear total variation based noise removal algorithms, *Physica D*, 60, 259–268, 1992.

[39]  J. Demmel, *Lecture Notes on Numerical Linear Algebra*, Berkeley Lecture Notes in Mathematics, Mathematics Department, University of California, Berkeley, CA, 1993.

[40]  S.D. Rane, G. Sapiro, and M. Bertalmio, Structure and texture filling-in of missing image blocks in wireless transmission and compression applications, *IEEE Trans. Image Process.*, 12, 296–303, March 2003.

# 21

## Superresolution Color Image Reconstruction

Hu He and Lisimachos P. Kondi

**CONTENTS**

## 21.1 Introduction

In many imaging systems, the resolution of the detector array of the camera is not sufficiently high for a particular application. Furthermore, the capturing process introduces additive noise and the point spread function of the lens and the effects of the finite size of the photo detectors further degrade the acquired video frames. An important limitation of electronic imaging today is that most available still-frame or video cameras can only record images at a resolution lower than desirable. This is related to certain physical limitations of the image sensors, such as finite cell area and finite aperture time. Although high-resolution imaging sensors are being advanced, these may be too expensive or unsuitable for mobile imaging applications.

Superresolution refers to obtaining video at a resolution higher than that of the camera (sensor) used in recording the image. Because most images contain sharp edges [1], they are not strictly band limited. As a result, digital images usually suffer from aliasing due to downsampling, loss of high-frequency detail due to low-resolution sensor point spread function (PSF), and possible optical blurring due to relative motion or out-of-focus, and so forth.

The goal of superresolution (resolution enhancement) is to estimate a high-resolution image from a sequence of low-resolution images while also compensating for the above-mentioned degradations [2], [3]. Superresolution (resolution enhancement) using multiple frames is possible when there exists subpixel motion between the captured frames.

Thus, each of the frames provides a unique look into the scene. An example scenario is the case of a camera that is mounted on an aircraft and is imaging objects in the far field. The vibrations of the aircraft will generally provide the necessary motion between the focal plane array and the scene, thus yielding frames with subpixel motion between them and minimal occlusion effects.

Image/video superresolution relates to some other fields of image processing, and the advance in one field will enrich or promote the study in other fields. For example, the classic image restoration problem [4], [5], [6], [7], [8], [9] is a subset of image/video superresolution. When the input and output lattice are identical, the superresolution problem reduces to an image restoration problem. So, it is not surprising that the superresolution can also be applied to single frame or multiframe image restoration [10], [11]. On the other hand, many techniques in classic image restoration are being extended to image/video superresolution [12], [13], [14], [15], [16], [17], [18]. Such topics range from blind deconvolution [19] to least squares restoration of multichannel images, and so forth. Also, a two-step interpolation/restoration technique is an important branch of superresolution.

The superresolution problem can also be reduced to a noise filtering problem when the input and output lattice are identical and a delta PSF function (no spreading) is assumed. In real applications, noise and outliers usually exist in the acquired low-resolution sequence. A data preprocessing step to remove some types of noise and outliers is very important in superresolution.

Superresolution techniques can benefit other image processing techniques, such as detection, interpretation, recognition, and classification.

Superresolution involves up-conversion of the input sampling lattice as well as reducing or eliminating aliasing and blurring. It can be used to obtain a high-quality output from an interlaced video in high-definition television (HDTV). Other applications include detection of small targets in military or civilian surveillance imaging, detection of small tumors in medical imaging or biological applications [20], and star imaging in astronomy. High-resolution image reconstruction using multiple low-resolution aliased frames is also used in infrared images [21].

## 21.2 Previous Research

The objective of superresolution, or resolution enhancement, is to reconstruct a high-resolution (HR) image from a sequence of low-resolution (LR) images. The LR sequence experiences different degradations from frame to frame, such as point spread function (PSF) blurring, motion, subsampling and additive noise. Each frame of the LR sequence brings only partial information of the original HR image. However, if there exists subpixel motion between these LR frames, each frame will bring unique partial information of the original HR image. Furthermore, if enough of such unique-information-bearing LR frames are available, digital image/video processing can be applied to recover the HR image.

The direct reverse solution from interpolation, motion compensation, and inverse filtering is ill-posed due to the existence of additive noise, even in the cases where perfect motion registration is available and the PSF of the optical lens is known. Under these circumstances, the original HR image cannot be "fully" recovered. Many approaches have been proposed to seek a stable solution with good visual quality to overcome the ill-posedness of the superresolution. The problem of video superresolution is an active research area. We next outline a few of the approaches that have appeared in the literature.

Among the earliest efforts in the field is the work by Tsai and Huang [22]. Their method operates on the noise-free data in the frequency domain and capitalizes on the shifting property of the Fourier transform, the aliasing relationship between the continuous Fourier transform (CFT) and the discrete Fourier transform (DFT), and the fact that the original scene is assumed to be band limited. The above properties are used to construct a system of equations relating the aliased DFT coefficients of the observed images to samples of the CFT of the unknown high-resolution image. The system of equations is solved, yielding an estimate of the DFT coefficients of the original high-resolution image, which can then be obtained using inverse DFT.

This technique was further improved by Tekalp et al. [23] by taking into account a linear shift invariant (LSI) blur point spread function (PSF) and using a least squares approach to solving the system of equations. The big advantage of the frequency domain methods is their low computational complexity. Kim et al. [24] also extended this technique for noisy data and derived a weighted least squares algorithm. However, these methods are applicable only to global motion, and *a priori* information about the high-resolution image cannot be exploited.

Most of the other superresolution (resolution enhancement) techniques that have appeared in the literature operate in the spatial domain. In these techniques, the superresolution reconstruction is processed in two steps: interpolation followed by restoration. These techniques can be further classified to single frame (intraframe) interpolation-restoration methods and multiframe (interframe) interpolation-restoration methods. Superresolution from a single low-resolution, and possibly blurred, image is known to be highly ill-posed (i.e., even a small change in the data may cause a very large change in the result). However, when a sequence of low-resolution frames is available, such as those obtained by a video camera, the problem becomes more manageable. It is evident that the 3-D spatial–temporal sampling grid contains more information than any 2-D still-frame sampling grid. Interframe superresolution methods exploit this additional information, contained in multiple frames, to reconstruct a still high-resolution image.

The most computationally efficient techniques involve interpolation of nonuniformly spaced samples. This requires, that the computation of the optical flow between the acquired low-resolution frames be combined in order to create a high-resolution frame. Interpolation techniques are used to estimate pixels in the high-resolution frame that did not correspond to pixels in one of the acquired frames. Finally, image restoration techniques are used to compensate for the blurring introduced by the imaging device. A method based on this idea is the temporal accumulation of registered image data (TARID) [25], [26], developed by the Naval Research Laboratory (NRL).

Another method that has appeared in the literature is the iterated backprojection method [27]. In this method, the estimate of the high-resolution image is updated by backprojecting the error between motion-compensated, blurred and subsampled versions of the current estimate of the high-resolution image and the observed low-resolution images, using an appropriate backprojection operator.

The method proposed by Stark and Oskoui [28] is the projection onto convex sets (POCS). In this method, the space of high-resolution images is intersected with a set of convex constraint sets representing desirable image characteristics, such as positivity, bounded energy, fidelity to data, smoothness, and so forth. The POCS approach has been extended to time-varying motion blur in References [29] and [30]. Block matching or phase correlation was applied to estimate the registration parameters in Reference [29].

Another proposed method is generalized cross-validation (GCV), which proved to be useful in space-invariant superresolution [31], [32]. To find the matrix trace in a large image system using GCV is not only difficult but also error-prone. The computational cost of GCV is another difficulty for wide application of this method.

Another class of superresolution (resolution enhancement) algorithms is based on stochastic techniques. Methods in this class include maximum likelihood (ML) [33] and maximum a posteriori (MAP) approaches [34], [35], [36], [37], [38], as well as our work in References [39], [40], [41], [42], [43], [44], and [45]. MAP estimation with an edge preserving Huber–Markov random field image prior is studied in References [34], [35], and [36]. MAP-based resolution enhancement with simultaneous estimation of registration parameters (motion between frames) was proposed in References [37] and [41].

In most previous work on image restoration, a special case of resolution enhancement, regularization is widely used to avoid the ill-posed problem of inverse filtering [46], [47], [48], [49]. The regularization parameter [50] of the cost function plays a very important role in the reconstruction of the high-resolution image. The *L*-curve method was used to estimate this parameter in Reference [51], where the desired "*L*-corner," the point with maximum curvature on the *L*-curve, was chosen as the one corresponding to the regularization parameter. However, the computational cost of the *L*-curve method is still huge, even using a spline curve to approximate the *L*-curve for superresolution.

The precise registration of the subpixel motion and knowledge of the PSF are very important to the reconstruction of the HR image. However, precise knowledge of these parameters is not always assured in real applications. Lee and Kang [52] proposed a regularized adaptive HR reconstruction considering inaccurate subpixel registration. Two methods for the estimation of the regularization parameter for each LR frame (channel) were advanced, based on the approximation that the registration error noise is modeled as Gaussian with standard deviation proportional to the degree of the registration error. The convergence of these two methods to the unique global solution was observed experimentally using different initial conditions for the HR image. However, the convergence of these methods was not rigorously proved. Image restoration from partially known blurs was studied in the hierarchical Bayesian framework in References [53], [54], and [55]. The unknown component of the PSF was modeled as stationary zero-mean white noise. Two iterative algorithms were proposed using evidence analysis (EA), which in effect are identical to the regularized constrained total least squares filter and linear minimum mean square-error filter, respectively. However, the random (unknown error) components of the PSF have not been considered in most previous studies on superresolution.

Superresolution/restoration techniques with temporally varying or spatially varying parameters or inaccurate estimates were studied in References [56], [57], [58], [59], and [60]. Robust superresolution techniques have appeared in References [61], [62], and [63] and take into account the existence of outliers (values that do not fit the model very well). In Reference [61], a median filter is used in the iterative procedure to obtain the HR image. The robustness of this method is good when the errors from outliers are symmetrically distributed, which are proved to be, after a biased detection procedure. However, a threshold is needed to decide whether the bias is due to outlier or aliasing information. Also, the mathematical justification of this method is not analyzed. In References [62] and [63], a robust superresolution method was proposed based on the use of the $\mathbf{L}_1$ norm in both the regularization and the measurement terms of the penalty function. Robust regularization based on a bilateral prior was proposed to deal with different data and noise models. Also, the mathematical justification of a "shift and add" was provided and related to $\mathbf{L}_1$ norm minimization when relative motion is purely translational, and the PSF and decimation factor are common and space invariant in all LR images. However, the pure translational assumption of the entire low-resolution image sequence may not be suitable for some real data sequences. Besides the above studies, robust methods for obtaining high-quality stills from interlaced video in the presence of dominant motion are also studied in Reference [64]. Sequential and parallel image reconstruction using neural network implementations was studied in Reference [65].

Efficient methods are also studied in superresolution to reduce the computational cost. Efficient generalized cross-validation was proposed in Reference [31]. It can be used for applications such as parametric image restoration and resolution enhancement. A fast superresolution reconstruction algorithm for pure translational motion and common space-invariant blur was advanced in Reference [66].

The motivation of our method is the successful usage of simultaneous estimation multiple random variables in superresolution fields, for example [37], and the application of regularization in restoration [67].

## 21.3 Generalized Acquisition Model

In the following, we use the same formulation and notation as in Reference [37]. The image degradation process can be modeled by blur due to motion, linear PSF blur, subsampling by pixel averaging, and an additive Gaussian noise process. The blur due to atmospheric turbulence is neglected. We order all vectors lexicographically. We assume that $p$ low-resolution frames are observed, each of size $N_1 \times N_2$. The desired high-resolution image is of size $N = L_1 N_2 L_1 N_2$, where $L_1$ and $L_2$ represent the downsampling factors in the horizontal and vertical directions, respectively. Let the $k$th low-resolution frame be denoted as $\mathbf{y}_k = [y_{k,1}, y_{k,2}, \dots, y_{k,M}]$ for $k = 1, 2, \dots, p$ and where $M = N_1 N_2$. The full set of $p$ observed low-resolution images can be denoted as $\mathbf{y} = [\mathbf{y}_1^T, \mathbf{y}_2^T, \dots, \mathbf{y}_p^T]^T = [y_1, y_2, \dots, y_{pM}]^T$. The observed low-resolution frames are related to the high-resolution image through the following model:

$$y_{k,m} = \sum_{r=1}^{N} w_{k,m,r} z_r + \eta_{k,m} \tag{21.1}$$

for $m = 1, 2, \dots, M$ and $k = 1, 2, \dots, p$. The weight $w_{k,m,r}$ represents the "contribution" of the $r$th high-resolution pixel to the $m$th low-resolution observed pixel of the $k$th frame. The term $\eta_{k,m}$ represents additive noise samples that are assumed to be independent and identically distributed (i.i.d.) Gaussian noise samples with variance $\sigma_\eta^2$.

We can rewrite Equation 21.1 in matrix notation:

$$\mathbf{y} = \mathbf{W}\mathbf{z} + \mathbf{n} \tag{21.2}$$

where matrix

$$\mathbf{W} = \left[ \mathbf{W}_1^T, \mathbf{W}_2^T, \cdots, \mathbf{W}_k^T \right]^T \tag{21.3}$$

contains the values $w_{k,m,r}$ and $\mathbf{n} = [\eta_1, \eta_2, \cdots, \eta_{pM}]^T$.

The $N \times N$ degradation matrix $\mathbf{W}_k$ for channel $k$ can be expressed as the multiplication of subsampling matrix $\mathbf{S}$, blur matrix $\mathbf{B}_k$, and motion matrix $\mathbf{M}_k$, with size $N_1 N_2 \times N$, $N \times N$, $N \times N$, and $N \times N$, respectively:

$$\mathbf{W}_k = \mathbf{S}\mathbf{B}_k\mathbf{M}_k \tag{21.4}$$

This degradation matrix can be further simplified to

$$\mathbf{W}_k = \mathbf{S}\mathbf{B}\mathbf{M}_k \tag{21.5}$$

when the blur is space invariant.

In this work, we assume that no information is lost or added due to motion operation for any specific low-resolution image. Pixel motion within the frame will only exchange pixel locations, for example, but not limited to, translational motion. Matrix $\mathbf{M}_k$ indicates the "new" location of each pixel of frame $k$ on the high-resolution grid after motion operation, with respect to the original high-resolution image. This is a generalized motion model but is suitable for superresolution, because a single high-resolution image is to be reconstructed. The motion here can be per-pixel, global, or block-based translation or in more complex form. In the synthetic tests in this work, without losing any generality, we use pure translation as the registration parameter for easier implementation and understanding, but our method is not limited to pure translation. In this case, the elements of the motion matrix are 0's and 1's, with only one 1 in each column and each row. We can easily verify that $\mathbf{M}_k$ is a unitary matrix (i.e., $\mathbf{M}_k\mathbf{M}_k^T = \mathbf{M}_k^T\mathbf{M}_k = \mathbf{I}$, where $\mathbf{I}$ is the identity matrix).

## 21.4 Joint MAP Registration Algorithm with Gaussian–Markov Random Field as Image Prior

To model the motion, we introduce a vector $\mathbf{s}_k$ for frame $k$. And $\mathbf{s}_k = [s_{k,1}, s_{k,2}, \ldots, s_{k,K}]^T$, where $K$ is the number of registration parameters for frame $k$. Vector $\mathbf{s}_k$ represents translational shift, rotation, affine transformation parameters, or other motion parameters measured in reference to a fixed high-resolution grid.

We rewrite the system model Equation 21.1 to Equation 21.4 with emphasis on the vector $\mathbf{s}$ as follows:

$$y_{k,m} = \sum_{r=1}^{N} w_{k,m,r}(\mathbf{s}_k)z_r + \eta_{k,m} \tag{21.6}$$

$$\mathbf{y} = \mathbf{W}_\mathbf{s}\mathbf{z} + \mathbf{n} \tag{21.7}$$

$$\mathbf{W}_\mathbf{s} = \left[\mathbf{W}_{\mathbf{s},1}^T, \mathbf{W}_{\mathbf{s},2}^T, \ldots, \mathbf{W}_{\mathbf{s},k}^T\right]^T \tag{21.8}$$

$$\mathbf{W}_{\mathbf{s},k} = \mathbf{SB}_k\mathbf{M}_k \tag{21.9}$$

The multivariate p.d.f. of $\mathbf{y}$ given $\mathbf{z}$ and $\mathbf{s}$ is

$$P_r(\mathbf{y}|\mathbf{z}, \mathbf{s}) = \frac{1}{(2\pi)^{pM/2}\sigma_\eta^{pM}} \exp\left\{-\frac{1}{2\sigma_\eta^2}(\mathbf{y} - \mathbf{W}_\mathbf{s}\mathbf{z})^T(\mathbf{y} - \mathbf{W}_\mathbf{s}\mathbf{z})\right\} \tag{21.10}$$

We can form a MAP estimate of the high-resolution image $\mathbf{z}$ and the registration parameters $\mathbf{s}$ simultaneously, given the observed $\mathbf{y}$. The estimates can be computed as

$$\hat{\mathbf{z}}, \hat{\mathbf{s}} = \arg\max P_r(\mathbf{z}, \mathbf{s}|\mathbf{y}) \tag{21.11}$$

Using Bayes' rule, the above equation can be expressed as

$$\hat{\mathbf{z}}, \hat{\mathbf{s}} = \arg\max \frac{P_r(\mathbf{y}|\mathbf{z}, \mathbf{s})P_r(\mathbf{z}, \mathbf{s})}{P_r(\mathbf{y})} \tag{21.12}$$

Clearly, the denominator of the above equation is not a function of $\mathbf{z}$ or $\mathbf{s}$. If we further assume that $\mathbf{z}$ and $\mathbf{s}$ are statistically independent, we have

$$\hat{\mathbf{z}}, \hat{\mathbf{s}} = \arg\max\{P_r(\mathbf{y}|\mathbf{z}, \mathbf{s})P_r(\mathbf{z}, \mathbf{s})\} = \arg\max\{P_r(\mathbf{y}|\mathbf{z}, \mathbf{s})P_r(\mathbf{z})P_r(\mathbf{s})\} \tag{21.13}$$

This can be further simplified to

$$\hat{\mathbf{z}}, \hat{\mathbf{s}} = \arg\max\{P_r(\mathbf{y}|\mathbf{z}, \mathbf{s})P_r(\mathbf{z})\} \tag{21.14}$$

under the assumption that all possible vectors $\mathbf{s}$ are equally probable.

It is very important to choose an appropriate model for the p.d.f of the desired image $\mathbf{z}$. As in Reference [37], we choose Gauss–Markov random field (GMRF) as the image prior, with density of the following form:

$$P_r(\mathbf{z}) = \frac{1}{(2\pi)^{N/2}|\mathbf{C}|^{1/2}} \exp\left\{-\frac{1}{2}\mathbf{z}^T\mathbf{C}^{-1}\mathbf{z}\right\} \tag{21.15}$$

where matrix $\mathbf{C}$ is the $N \times N$ covariance matrix of $\mathbf{z}$. For a specific choice of the covariance matrix $\mathbf{C}$, the above equation can be written as

$$P_r(\mathbf{z}) = \frac{1}{(2\pi)^{N/2}|\mathbf{C}|^{1/2}} \exp\left\{-\frac{1}{2\lambda}\sum_{i=1}^{N}\left(\sum_{j=1}^{N}d_{i,j}z_j\right)^2\right\} \tag{21.16}$$

where $d_i = [d_{i,1}, d_{i,2}, \ldots, d_{i,N}]^T$ is the coefficient vector, and $\lambda$ is called the tuning parameter or temperature parameter of the density. The above equation results if we assume that the elements $C_{i,j}^{-1}$ of the inverse of $\mathbf{C}$ satisfy the following:

$$C_{i,j}^{-1} = \frac{1}{\lambda}\sum_{r=1}^{N}(d_{r,i}d_{r,j}) \tag{21.17}$$

The coefficient $d_{i,j}$ can be chosen as the 2-D Laplacian kernel:

$$d_{i,j} = \begin{cases} 1, & \text{for } i = j \\ -1/4, & \text{for } i, j : z_j \text{ is a cardinal neighbor of } z_i \end{cases} \tag{21.18}$$

Following the same procedure as in Reference [37], we can reach the following regularized cost function to minimize

$$L(\mathbf{z}, \mathbf{s}) = \sum_{m=1}^{pM}(y_m - \sum_{r=1}^{N}w_{m,r}(\mathbf{s})z_r)^2 + \frac{\sigma_\eta^2}{\lambda}\sum_{i=1}^{N}\left(\sum_{j=1}^{N}d_{i,j}z_j\right)^2$$

$$= ||\mathbf{y} - \mathbf{W_s}\mathbf{z}||^2 + \frac{\sigma_\eta^2}{\lambda}||\mathbf{D}\mathbf{z}||^2$$

$$= ||\mathbf{y} - \mathbf{W_s}\mathbf{z}||^2 + \alpha||\mathbf{D}\mathbf{z}||^2 \tag{21.19}$$

where $w_{m,r}$ is the "contribution" of $z_r$ to $y_m$, for $m = 1, 2, \ldots, pM$ and $r = 1, 2, \ldots, N$, and $\alpha$ is the regularization parameter defined as

$$\alpha = \frac{\sigma_\eta^2}{\lambda} \tag{21.20}$$

and $\mathbf{D}$ is the matrix representing the 2-D Laplacian kernel, which is a high-pass filter. We call the term $||\mathbf{y} - \mathbf{W_s}\mathbf{z}||^2$ as the residual norm and the term $||\mathbf{D}\mathbf{z}||^2$ the smoothness norm. We can see that if we set $\alpha = 0$ in Equation 21.19, the smoothness norm disappears. This is equivalent to the maximum likelihood (ML) estimator derived from $\hat{\mathbf{z}}, \hat{\mathbf{s}} = \arg\max\{P_r(\mathbf{y}|\mathbf{z}, \mathbf{s})\}$, dropping the image prior $P_r(\mathbf{z})$ from Equation 21.14. The ML solution may amplify the noise effect due to the ill-posedness of the superresolution problem.

The minimization of Equation 21.19 is

$$\mathbf{z} = \left(\mathbf{W_s}^T\mathbf{W_s} + \alpha\mathbf{D}^T\mathbf{D}\right)^{-1}\mathbf{W_s}^T\mathbf{y} \tag{21.21}$$

But this direct solution is difficult to implement because of large matrix operation, especially the inversion. Instead, the cost function in Equation 21.19 can be minimized using the coordinate-descent method [37]. This iterative method starts with an initial estimate of $\mathbf{z}$ obtained using interpolation from a low-resolution frame.

In order to update the estimate $\mathbf{z}$, we first estimate

$$\hat{\mathbf{s}}_k^n = \arg\min_{\mathbf{s}_k}\left\{\sum_{m=1}^{M}\left(y_{k,m} - \sum_{r=1}^{N}w_{k,m,r}(\mathbf{s}_k)\hat{z}_r^n\right)^2\right\} \tag{21.22}$$

which can be derived via the minimization of the cost function with respect to $\mathbf{s}$ for $\mathbf{z}$ fixed. Thus, the motion of each frame is estimated. The term $n$ is the iteration number starting from 0. Then, for fixed $\mathbf{s}$, a new estimate for $\mathbf{z}$ is obtained as

$$\hat{z}_r^{n+1} = \hat{z}_r^n - \epsilon g_r(\hat{\mathbf{z}}^n\hat{\mathbf{s}}^n) \tag{21.23}$$

for $r = 1, \ldots, N$. This procedure continues until convergence is reached, that is, $\mathbf{z}$ and $\mathbf{s}$ are updated in a cyclic fashion.

The gradient $g_r(\hat{\mathbf{z}}_n, \hat{\mathbf{s}}_n)$ can be obtained from

$$g_r(\mathbf{z}, \mathbf{s}) = \frac{\partial L(\mathbf{z}, \mathbf{s})}{\partial z_r} = 2\left\{\sum_{m=1}^{pM}w_{m,r}(\mathbf{s})\left(\sum_{j=1}^{N}w_{m,j}(\mathbf{s})z_j - y_m\right) + \alpha\sum_{i=1}^{N}d_{i,r}\left(\sum_{j=1}^{N}d_{i,j}z_j\right)\right\} \tag{21.24}$$

Also, the gradient can be obtained by solving

$$\frac{\partial L(\hat{\mathbf{z}}^{n+1}, \hat{\mathbf{s}}^n)}{\partial\epsilon^n} = 0 \tag{21.25}$$

and the solution is

$$\epsilon^n = \frac{\frac{1}{\sigma_\eta^2}\sum_{m=1}^{pM}\gamma_m\left(\sum_{r=1}^{N}w_{m,r}(\hat{\mathbf{s}}^n) - y_m\right) + \frac{1}{\lambda}\sum_{i=1}^{N}\bar{g}_i\left(\sum_{j=1}^{N}d_{i,j}\hat{z}_j^n\right)}{\frac{1}{\sigma_\eta^2}\sum_{m=1}^{pM}\gamma_m^2 + \frac{1}{\lambda}\sum_{i=1}^{N}\bar{g}_i^2} \tag{21.26}$$

where

$$\gamma_m = \sum_{r=1}^{N}w_{m,r}g_r \tag{21.27}$$

is the gradient projected through the degradation operator, and

$$\bar{g}_i = \sum_{j=1}^{N}d_{i,j}g_j \tag{21.28}$$

is a weighted sum of neighboring gradient values.

## 21.5   Regularized Cost Function in Multichannel Form

It can be seen that the cost function in Equation 21.19:

$$L(\mathbf{z}, \mathbf{s}) = ||\mathbf{y} - \mathbf{W_s z}||^2 + \alpha ||\mathbf{Dz}||^2 \qquad (21.29)$$

is a Tikhonov regularization cost function. Thus, for the specific choice of prior model $P_r(\mathbf{z})$ considered here, the MAP formulation is equivalent to a Tikhonov regularization formulation. Equation 21.19 has two terms: a term representing the fidelity of the solution to the received data (residual norm $||\mathbf{y} - \mathbf{W_s z}||^2$) and a term representing *a priori* information about the high-resolution image (smoothness norm $||\mathbf{Dz}||^2$). The latter involves a high-pass filter and thus dictates that the solution be smooth by penalizing discontinuities. The relative weighting of the two terms is determined by a regularization parameter $\alpha$, which is the ratio of the power of noise $\sigma_\eta^2$ over the tuning parameter $\lambda$. In the most general case, we have no prior information for both $\sigma_\eta^2$ and $\lambda$. In this case, the regularization parameter can be explicitly expressed as a function of the original image [67].

We rewrite the regularized cost function as

$$L(\mathbf{z}, \mathbf{s}) = ||\mathbf{y} - \mathbf{W_s z}||^2 + \alpha(\mathbf{z}) ||\mathbf{Dz}||^2 \qquad (21.30)$$

Furthermore, we can rewrite the cost function as the sum of individual smoothing functionals for each of the $p$ low-resolution images as

$$L(\mathbf{z}, \mathbf{s}) = \sum_{k=1}^{p} (||\mathbf{y}_k - \mathbf{W}_{s,k}\mathbf{z}||^2 + \alpha_k(\mathbf{z}) ||\mathbf{Dz}||^2) \qquad (21.31)$$

We drop the subscript $k$ from $\mathbf{D}_k$ in the above equation, because $\mathbf{D}_k = \mathbf{D}$, that is, the same high-pass filter (Laplacian kernel) is used for all low-resolution image $k = 1, 2, \dots, p$. Then, we can define the individual functional for each low-resolution image (channel) as

$$L_k(\alpha_k(\mathbf{z}), \mathbf{z}, \mathbf{s}) = ||\mathbf{y}_k - \mathbf{W}_{s,k}\mathbf{z}||^2 + \alpha_k(\mathbf{z}) ||\mathbf{Dz}||^2 \qquad (21.32)$$

for $k = 1, 2, \dots, p$.

## 21.6   Estimation of the Regularization Parameter

Following the same procedure as in Reference [67], we impose the following requirements for each $\alpha_k(\mathbf{z})$: it should be a function of the regularized noise power of the data, and its choice should yield a convex functional with minimization that would give the high-resolution image. Then, we reach the same iteration expressions as in Equation 21.22, Equation 21.23 and Equation 21.24, except that $\alpha$ is replaced with $\alpha(\mathbf{z}) = \sum_{k=1}^{p} \alpha_k(\mathbf{z})$. The imposed properties on $\alpha(\mathbf{z})$ require a linear function between and each term of the cost function:

$$\alpha_k(\mathbf{z}) = f\{L_k[\alpha_k(\mathbf{z}), \mathbf{z}]\} = \gamma_k\{||\mathbf{y}_k - \mathbf{W}_{s,k}\mathbf{z}||^2 + \alpha_k(\mathbf{z}) ||\mathbf{Dz}||^2\} \qquad (21.33)$$

Thus, the choice of regularization parameter for the multichannel regularization functional is given by

$$\alpha_k(\mathbf{z}) = \frac{||\mathbf{y}_k - \mathbf{W}_{s,k}\mathbf{z}||^2}{\frac{1}{\gamma_k} - ||\mathbf{Dz}||^2} \qquad (21.34)$$

Also, following the same procedure for convergence requirement as in Reference [67], we get

$$\frac{1}{\gamma_k} > \frac{\epsilon p \phi_{max}[\mathbf{D}^T\mathbf{D}]}{2 - \epsilon p \phi_{max}[\mathbf{W}_{\mathbf{s},k}^T\mathbf{W}_{\mathbf{s},k}]} ||\mathbf{y}_k - \mathbf{W}_{\mathbf{s},k}\mathbf{z}||^2 + ||\mathbf{Dz}||^2 \tag{21.35}$$

where $\phi_{max}(\cdot)$ stands for the maximum singular value of a matrix.

From the model of the degradation matrix, with emphasis on the registration parameter **s**, we have

$$\mathbf{W}_{\mathbf{s},k} = \mathbf{SB}_k\mathbf{M}_k \tag{21.36}$$

Therefore, for subsampling by pixel averaging, we can easily verify that

$$\phi_{max}[\mathbf{S}^T\mathbf{S}] = \frac{1}{L_1L_2} \tag{21.37}$$

Because no information is lost or added due to motion operation $\mathbf{M}_k$, the elements of $\mathbf{M}_k$ are "1"s and "0"s, with each column and each row having only a single "1". For such kind of matrix $\mathbf{M}_k$, a special case of the unitary matrix, we can easily verify that

$$\mathbf{M}_k^T\mathbf{M}_k = \mathbf{I} \tag{21.38}$$

where **I** is the identity matrix with size $N \times N$. Thus,

$$\phi_{max}\left[\mathbf{M}_k^T\mathbf{M}_k\right] = 1 \tag{21.39}$$

For a PSF generated from Gaussian blur, we can assume that the impulse response coefficients are normalized to add to 1, which is equivalent to

$$\phi_{max}\left[\mathbf{B}_k^T\mathbf{B}_k\right] = 1 \tag{21.40}$$

By substituting Equation 21.37, Equation 21.39, and Equation 21.40 into Equation 21.36, we have

$$\phi_{max}\left[\mathbf{W}_{\mathbf{s},k}^T\mathbf{W}_{\mathbf{s},k}\right] = \frac{1}{L_1L_2} \tag{21.41}$$

Therefore, the inequality in Equation 21.35 becomes

$$\frac{1}{\gamma_k} > \frac{\epsilon p \phi_{max}[\mathbf{D}^T\mathbf{D}]}{2 - \frac{\epsilon p}{L_1L_2}} ||\mathbf{y}_k - \mathbf{W}_{\mathbf{s},k}\mathbf{z}||^2 + ||\mathbf{Dz}||^2 \tag{21.42}$$

Now, we can select step size $\epsilon$ to make

$$\frac{\epsilon p \phi_{max}[\mathbf{D}^T\mathbf{D}]}{2 - \frac{\epsilon p}{L_1L_2}} = 1 \tag{21.43}$$

That is,

$$\epsilon = \frac{2}{p}\left(\frac{(L_1L_2)}{(L_1L_2)\phi_{max}(\mathbf{D}^T\mathbf{D}) + 1}\right) \tag{21.44}$$

which is consistent with the restoration case $\epsilon = \frac{1}{p}$ in Reference [67], when $\phi_{max}(\mathbf{D}^T\mathbf{D}) = 1$. Then, the inequality (Equation 21.42) becomes

$$\frac{1}{\gamma_k} > ||\mathbf{y}_k - \mathbf{W}_k\mathbf{z}||^2 + ||\mathbf{Dz}||^2 \tag{21.45}$$

Now, $||\mathbf{y}_k||^2 > ||\mathbf{y}_k - \mathbf{W}_k\mathbf{z}||^2$, because the low-resolution image is assumed to have more energy than the additive noise, and $||\mathbf{y}_k||^2 \approx \frac{||\mathbf{z}||^2}{L_1L_2} > ||\mathbf{Dz}||^2$ for small subsampling ratio $L_1 = L_2 = 4$, because **z** is assumed to have much less energy at high frequencies than at low frequencies, and each low-resolution image $\mathbf{y}_k$ has $\frac{1}{L_1 L_2}$ of the energy of $\mathbf{z}$ for noiseless cases. For a subsampling ratio $L_1 = L_2 = 4$, as used in this chapter, we can show that the choice of

$$\frac{1}{\gamma_k} = 2||\mathbf{y}_k||^2 \tag{21.46}$$

satisfies the condition for convergence and also provides a positive $\alpha_k(\mathbf{z})$:

$$\alpha_k(\mathbf{z}) = \frac{||\mathbf{y}_k - \mathbf{W}_{s,k}\mathbf{z}||^2}{2||\mathbf{y}_k||^2 - ||\mathbf{Dz}||^2}. \tag{21.47}$$

We can see from the experimental results that the choice of $\alpha_k(\mathbf{z})$ in Equation 21.46 not only provides a fixed, simple and tight choice for the inequality in Equation 21.45, but also results in good reconstructions. During the iterations, the regularization parameter $\alpha_k(\mathbf{z})$ is adaptively updated according to the current estimate of high-resolution image $\mathbf{z}$.

## 21.7 Extension to the Color Case

Let us now assume that $p_{color}$ color images are observed, each having a red (R), green (G), and a blue (B) component. Thus, our set of LR data consist of $p = 3 \times p_{color}$ images. Furthermore, $\mathbf{z}$ now contains all three color components of the HR image, concatenated in lexicographic ordering:

$$\mathbf{z} = \left[\mathbf{z}_R^T, \mathbf{z}_G^T, \mathbf{z}_B^T\right]^T \tag{21.48}$$

where $\mathbf{z}_R$, $\mathbf{z}_G$, and $\mathbf{z}_B$ are the R, G, and B components of $\mathbf{z}$, which is now of size $3N$. Furthermore, we assume that there is color cross talk in the acquisition process. If $(R_1, G_1, B_1)$ is a color pixel in $\mathbf{z}$ and $(R_2, G_2, B_2)$ is the corresponding pixel after cross talk, then

$$\begin{bmatrix} R_2 \\ G_2 \\ B_2 \end{bmatrix} = \mathbf{A} \cdot \begin{bmatrix} R_1 \\ G_1 \\ B_1 \end{bmatrix} \tag{21.49}$$

where $\mathbf{A}$ is the cross talk matrix with nonnegative elements and the summation of its each row equals 1.0.

The degradation matrix $W_k$ is now of size $3N_1N_2 \times 3N$ and is equal to

$$\mathbf{W}_k = \mathbf{SBM}_k\mathbf{C}_1 \tag{21.50}$$

where $\mathbf{C}_1$ is a $3N \times 3N$ matrix that performs the cross talk operation on the RGB components of $\mathbf{z}$. Now, matrices $\mathbf{S}$, $\mathbf{B}$, and $\mathbf{M}_k$ are of sizes $3N_1N_2 \times 3N$, $3N \times 3N$ and $3N \times 3N$, respectively. Also,

$$\phi_{max}\left[\mathbf{C}_1\mathbf{C}_1^T\right] = 1 \tag{21.51}$$

because of energy conservation of matrix $\mathbf{C}_1$. With this new acquisition model, our superresolution algorithm can be applied to color data.

## 21.8 Experimental Results

A number of experiments were conducted, some of which are presented here. To test the performance of our algorithm, we use the $256 \times 256$ "Lena" and "Flowers" color images for the synthetic test. Four frames were generated with downsampling ratio $L_1 = L_2 = 2$.

We can explicitly express a color image via three correlated channels, that is, RGB (red, green, blue) channels. Therefore, there are 12 channels in total (three color channels multiplied by four frames).

In the test using "Lena", the within-color-channel PSF blur was assumed to have been perfectly estimated, which was a Gaussian blur with support size $15 \times 15$ and standard deviation $\sigma = 1.7$. We assume that the cross talk effect across the RGB channel can be modeled with $\rho$ as

$$\begin{bmatrix} R_2 \\ G_2 \\ B_2 \end{bmatrix} = \begin{bmatrix} 1 - 2\rho & \rho & \rho \\ \rho & 1 - 2\rho & \rho \\ \rho & \rho & 1 - 2\rho \end{bmatrix} \cdot \begin{bmatrix} R_1 \\ G_1 \\ B_1 \end{bmatrix} \tag{21.52}$$

and the cross talk ratio $\rho$ is between 0 and 0.5.

The cross talk ratio between the RGB components was assumed to be $\rho = 0.1$. i.i.d. AWGN noise with same variance $\sigma_\eta^2$ was added to each frame, which corresponds to a signal-to-noise ratio (SNR) of $30 \sim 40$dB. The first R channel is selected as the reference frame, and bilinear interpolation of the first R/G/B channels is chosen as the first estimate of high-resolution image $\mathbf{z}$. The algorithm is carried out for 20 iterations or until convergence is reached when $\frac{\|\hat{\mathbf{z}}^{n+1} - \hat{\mathbf{z}}^n\|}{\|\hat{\mathbf{z}}^n\|} < 10^{-6}$.

In the tests, global shift is implemented as the motion degradation. Therefore, $\mathbf{s}_k = [s_{k,1}, s_{k,2}]^T$, that is, $K = 2$ registration parameters for frame $k$.

The original high-resolution color image, reference frame, reconstructed images from bilinear interpolation (BI) plus de-blurring, the optimal fixed $\alpha$ using exhaustive search in the sense of largest PSNR value, and the proposed "Simultaneous Method" of "Lena" are shown in Figure 21.1a to Figure 21.1e.

To compare, we also run the "Simultaneous Method" and Lee-Kang's method I and II without using the cross-channel information. Reconstructed images from "Simultaneous Method" and Lee-Kang's Methods of "Lena" image are shown in Figure 21.2a to Figure 21.2c. Zoomed versions of the results are shown in Figure 21.3a to Figure 21.3c.

With fine-tuned deblurring, the result using BI can be improved to 25.7220 dB. Also, if post de-cross-talking is processed, the BI+deblur, Lee-Kang's Method I and II can be improved to have PSNR as 27.5250 dB, 26.9808 dB, and 26.4252 dB, respectively.

The PSNR of the reconstructed image for "Lena" using the six methods (bilinear interpolation, simultaneous method with cross-channel information, simultaneous method without cross-channel information, fixed alpha with cross-channel information, Lee-Kang's Method I and II) are listed in Table 21.1.

In the test using "Flowers," the within-color-channel PSF blur was assumed to have been perfectly estimated, which was a Gaussian blur with support size $15 \times 15$ and standard deviation $\sigma = 0.7$. All other settings are the same as those used for "Lena."

The original high-resolution color image, reference frame, reconstructed images from bilinear interpolation (BI) plus deblurring, the optimal fixed $\alpha$ using exhaustive search in the sense of largest PSNR value, and the proposed simultaneous method of "Flowers" are shown in Figure 21.4a to Figure 21.4e.

To compare, we also run the simultaneous method and Lee-Kang's method I and II without using the cross-channel information. Reconstructed images from simultaneous method and Lee-Kang's methods of "Flowers" image are shown in Figure 21.5a to Figure 21.5c.

With fine-tuned deblurring, the result using BI can be improved to 23.5586 dB. Also, if post de-crosstalking is processed, the BI + deblur, Lee-Kang's Method I and II can be improved to have PSNR as 26.3439 dB, 28.7183 dB, and 26.8589 dB, respectively.

The PSNR of the reconstructed image for "Flowers" using the six methods (bilinear interpolation, simultaneous method with cross-channel information, simultaneous method

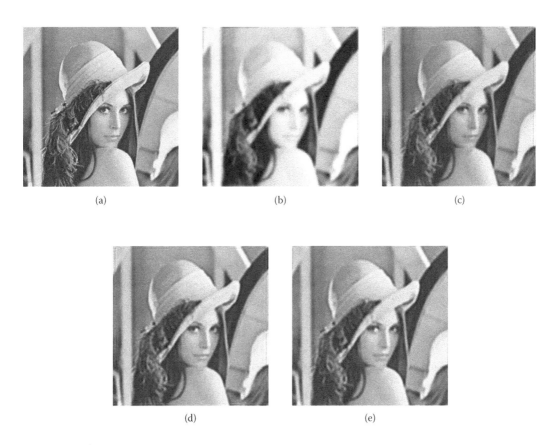

**FIGURE 21.1**
(a) Original high-resolution Lena color image, (b) reference frame of low-resolution Lena color image sequence (first R channel), (c) bilinear interpolation and deblurring of Lena, (d) reconstructed high-resolution Lena image using the optimal fixed $\alpha$, and (e) reconstructed high-resolution Lena image using the simultaneous method.

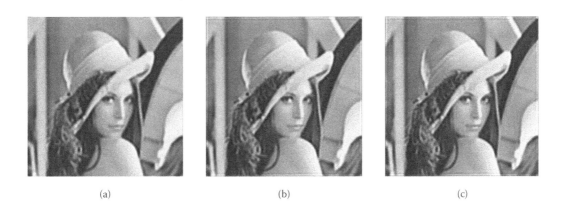

**FIGURE 21.2**
Reconstructed high-resolution Lena image using the (a) simultaneous method without using cross-channel information, (b) using Lee-Kang's Method I, and (c) using Lee-Kang's Method II.

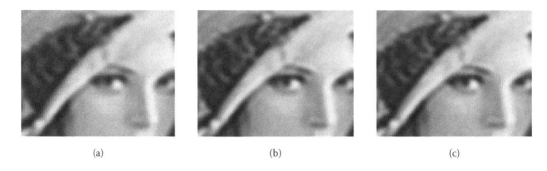

(a)                                           (b)                                           (c)

**FIGURE 21.3**
A zoomed part of the reconstructed high-resolution Lena image using the (a) simultaneous method, (b) Lee-Kang's Method I, and (c) Lee-Kang's Method II.

without cross-channel information, fixed alpha with cross-channel information, Lee-Kang's Method I and II) are listed in Table 21.2.

Next, we used the real image sequence data "sflowg" from the Signal Analysis and Machine Perception Laboratory of the Ohio State University. The reference frame, reconstructed images from bilinear interpolation (BI) plus deblurring, the optimal fixed $\alpha$ using exhaustive search in the sense of largest PSNR value, and the proposed simultaneous method of "sflowg" are shown in Figure 21.6a to Figure 21.6d.

To compare, we also run the simultaneous method and Lee-Kang's method I and II without using the cross-channel information. Reconstructed images from simultaneous method and Lee-Kang's Methods of the "sflowg" image sequences are shown in Figure 21.7a to Figure 21.7c.

From the results, we can see that the proposed simultaneous method using cross-channel information provides the best visual quality among the algorithms. Although some exhaustive search of the regularization space may provide better PSNR for some images (0.2 dB for this test), the reconstructed image is not as good as the simultaneous method, due to noise amplification and color aliasing effects. Also, the adaptive scheme used in the simultaneous method reduces the computational cost to a huge extent, compared to the exhaustive search for a general image used.

Also, the simultaneous method using cross-channel information can greatly recover the color information hidden by the cross talk between the RGB channels, compared to the algorithm without using cross-channel information. The former is more colorful and vivid, while the latter is more close to a "cold" white-and-black image. There is almost a gain of 3.7 dB when cross-channel information is applied.

**TABLE 21.1**

Results of "Lena" Using the Six Methods (values are PSNR in dB)

|  | BI | Method with Optimal Fixed $\alpha$ | SM Method with Cross-Channel Info |
|---|---|---|---|
| Average PSNR (dB) | 23.0653 | 28.4783 | 28.2706 |
|  | SM method without cross-channel info | Lee-Kang I | Lee-Kang II |
| Average PSNR (dB) | 24.5806 | 24.0206 | 23.7412 |

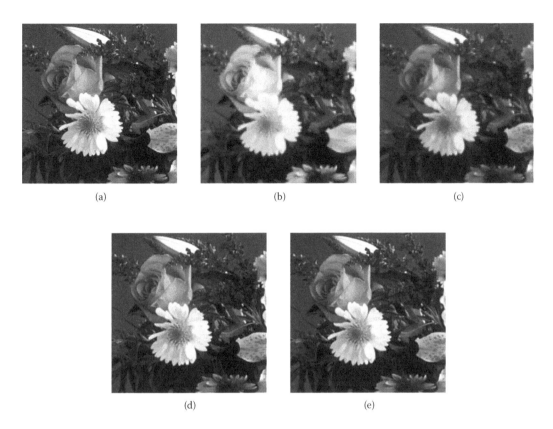

**FIGURE 21.4**

(a) Original high-resolution *Flowers* color image, (b) reference frame of low-resolution *Flowers* color image sequence (first R channel), (c) bilinear interpolation and deblurring of *Flowers*, (d) reconstructed high-resolution *Flowers* image using the optimal fixed $\alpha$, and (e) reconstructed high-resolution *Flowers* image using the simultaneous method.

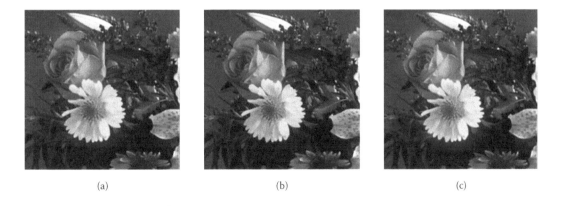

**FIGURE 21.5**

(a) Reconstructed high-resolution *Flowers* image using the simultaneous method, without using cross-channel information. (b) Reconstructed high-resolution *Flowers* image using Lee-Kang's Method I. (c) Reconstructed high-resolution *Flowers* image using Lee-Kang's Method II.

**TABLE 21.2**

Results of "Flowers" Using the Six Methods (values are PSNR in dB)

|                    | BI                                     | Method with Optimal Fixed $\alpha$ | SM Method with Cross-Channel Info |
| ------------------ | -------------------------------------- | ---------------------------------- | --------------------------------- |
| Average PSNR (dB)  | 22.9371                                | 31.2868                            | 33.1362                           |
|                    | SM method without cross-channel info   | Lee-Kang I                         | Lee-Kang II                       |
| Average PSNR (dB)  | 26.1175                                | 24.7419                            | 23.8715                           |

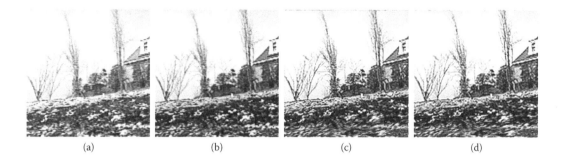

(a)                    (b)                    (c)                    (d)

**FIGURE 21.6**

(a) Reference frame of low-resolution *sflowg* color image sequence (first R channel). (b) Bilinear interpolation and deblurring of *sflowg*. (c) Reconstructed high-resolution *sflowg* image using the optimal fixed $\alpha$. (d) Reconstructed high-resolution *sflowg* image using the simultaneous method.

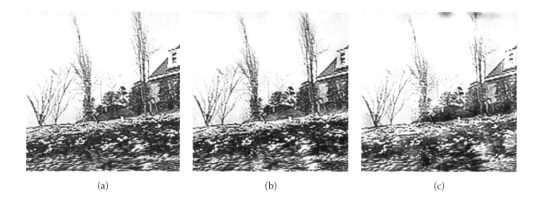

(a)                        (b)                        (c)

**FIGURE 21.7**

Reconstructed high-resolution *sflowg* image using the (a) simultaneous method without using cross-channel information, (b) Lee-Kang's Method I, and (c) Lee-Kang's Method II.

## 21.9 Summary

Superresolution is very useful when the resolution of the camera with which video is captured is not sufficient for a particular application. Using superresolution, it is possible to increase video resolution via the postprocessing of the data. Superresolution capitalizes on the subpixel motion that is usually present between video frames.

In this chapter, we concentrated on superresolution techniques that are based on maximum a posteriori (MAP) estimation. For the Gaussian prior model we utilized, these methods are equivalent to regularization methods. We proposed a technique for the estimation of the regularization parameter for digital image resolution enhancement. Our experimental results demonstrate the performance of the proposed algorithm. Experimental results using synthetic and real image data are presented. The proposed algorithm gives a better reconstruction than results obtained using an optimal fixed-value choice of the regularization parameter, obtained using exhaustive search. The usage of cross-channel information effectively recovers the original color information, providing a pleasant color image, which is a close reproduction of the real object.

We also compared our algorithm with recent methods proposed by Lee and Kang, with or without post de-cross-talking. Our method is better in the sense of PSNR and visual quality and can be successfully applied to color image processing.

## References

[1] J. Immerkaer, Use of blur-space for deblurring and edge-preserving noise smoothing, *IEEE Trans. Image Process.*, 10, 837–840, June 2001.

[2] S. Chaudhuri, *Super-Resolution Imaging*, Kluwer, Dordrecht, 2001.

[3] C.A. Segall, R. Molina, and A.K. Katsaggelos, High resolution images from a sequence of low resolution and compressed observations: A review, *IEEE Signal Process. Maga.*, 20, 37–48, May 2003.

[4] N.P. Galatsanos, A.K. Katsaggelos, R.T. Chin, and A.D. Hillery, Least squares restoration of multichannel images, *IEEE Trans. Acoust. Speech, Signal Process.*, 39, 2222–2236, October 1991.

[5] M.K. Ozkan, A.M. Tekalp, and M.I. Sezan, POCS-based restoration of space-varying blurred images, *IEEE Trans. Image Process.*, 3, 450–454, July 1994.

[6] G.Bonmassar and E.L. Schwartz, Real-time restoration of images degraded by uniform motion blur in foveal active vision systems, *IEEE Trans. Image Process.*, 8, 1838–1842, December 1999.

[7] J.Flusser, T. Suk, and S. Saic, Recognition of blurred images by the method of moments, *IEEE Trans. Image Process.*, 5, 533–538, March 1996.

[8] B.J. Jeffs and M. Gunsay, Restoration of blurred star field images by maximally sparse optimization, *IEEE Trans. Image Process.*, 2, 202–211, April 1993.

[9] W. Chen, M. Chen, and J. Zhou, Adaptively regularized constrained total least-squares image restoration, *IEEE Trans. Image Process.*, 9, 588–596, April 2000.

[10] A.K. Katsaggelos and S.N. Efstratiadis, A class of iterative signal restoration algorithms, *IEEE Trans. Acoust., Speech, Signal Process.*, 38, 778–786, May 1990.

[11] A.K. Katsaggelos, A multiple input image restoration approach, *J. Visual Commun. and Image Representation*, 1, 93–103, September 1990.

[12] M. Elad and A. Feuer, Restoration of a single superresolution image from several blurred, noisy and undersampled measured images, *IEEE Trans. Image Process.*, 6, 1646–1658, December 1997.

[13] V.Z. Mesarovic, N.P. Galatsanos, and A.K. Katsaggelos, Regularized constrained total least squares image restoration, *IEEE Trans. Image Process.*, 4, 1096–1108, August 1995.

[14] A.K. Katsaggelos, J. Biemond, R.W. Schafer, and R.M. Mersereau, A regularized iterative image restoration algorithm, *IEEE Trans. Signal Process.*, 39, 914–929, April 1991.

[15] A.K. Katsaggelos, Iterative image restoration algorithms, *Opt. Eng., Spec. Issue on Visual Commun. and Image Process.*, 28, 735–748, July 1989.

[16] T. Berger, J.O. Stromberg, and T. Eltoft, Adaptive regularized constrained least squares image restoration, *IEEE Trans. Image Process.*, 8, 1191–1203, September 1999.

[17] W. Chen, M. Chen, and J. Zhou, Adaptively regularized constrained total least-squares image restoration, *IEEE Trans. Image Process.*, 9, 588–596, April 2000.

[18] R. Molina, A.K. Katsaggelos, J. Mateos, A. Hermoso, and C.A. Segall, Restoration of severely blurred high range images using stochastic and deterministic relaxation algorithms in compound Gauss-Markov random fields, *Patt. Recognition*, 33, 555–571, April 2000.

[19] T.-H. Li and K.-S. Lii, A joint estimation approach for two-tone image deblurring by blind deconvolution, *IEEE Trans. Image Process.*, 11, 847–858, August 2002.

[20] J. Lehr, J.B. Sibarita, and J.M. Chassery, Image restoration in x-ray microscopy: Psf determination and biological applications, *IEEE Trans. Image Process.*, 7, 258–263, February 1998.

[21] E. Kaltenbacher and R.C. Hardie, High-resolution infrared image reconstruction using multiple low-resolution aliased frames, in *Proceedings of IEEE National Aerospace Electronics Conference.*, Vol. 2, May 1996, pp. 702–709.

[22] R. Tsai and T. Huang, Multiframe image restoration and registration, *Adv. in Comput. Vision and Image Process.*, 1, 317–339, 1984.

[23] A.M. Tekalp, M.K. Ozkan, and M. Sezan, High-resolution image reconstruction from lower-resolution image sequences and space-varying image restoration, *Proceedings of the International Conference on Acoustics, Speech and Signal Processing*, Vol. 3, March 1992, pp. 169–172.

[24] S.P. Kim, N.K. Bose, and H.M. Valenzuela, Recursive reconstruction of high resolution image from noisy undersampled multiframes, *IEEE Trans. on Acoust., Speech, Signal Process.*, 38, 1013–1027, June 1990.

[25] J.M. Schuler, P.R.W.J.G. Howard, and D.A. Scribner, TARID-based image super-resolution, in *Proceedings of SPIE AeroSense*, Orlando, FL, Vol. 4719, April 2002, pp. 247–254.

[26] J. Schuler, G. Howard, P. Warren, and D. Scribner, Resolution enhancement through tarid processing, in *SPIE*, Vol. 4671, January 2002, pp. 872–876.

[27] M. Irani and S. Peleg, Motion analysis for image enhancement: Resolution, occlusion, and transparency, *J. Visual Commun. and Image Representation*, 4, 324–335, December 1993.

[28] H. Stark and P. Oskoui, High-resolution image recovery from imageplane arrays, using convex projections, *J. Opt. Soc. Am. A*, 6, 1715–1726, November 1989.

[29] A.J. Patti, M. Sezan, and A.M. Tekalp, Super-resolution video reconstruction with arbitrary sampling lattices and nonzero apperature time, *IEEE Trans. Image Process.*, 6, 1064–1076, August 1997.

[30] P.E. Erem, M. Sezan, and A.M. Tekalp, Robust, object-based high-resolution image reconstruction from low-resolution video, *IEEE Trans. Image Process.*, 6, 1446–1451, October 1997.

[31] N. Nguyen, P. Milanfar, and G. Golub, Efficient generalized cross-validation with applications to parametric image restoration and resolution enhancement, *IEEE Trans. Image Process.*, 10, 1299–1308, September 2001.

[32] N. Nguyen and P. Milanfar, A computationally efficient superresolution image reconstruction algorithm, *IEEE Trans. Image Process.*, 10, 573–583, April 2001.

[33] B.C. Tom and A.K. Katsaggelos, Reconstruction of a high-resolution image from multiple degraded mis-registered low-resolution images, *Proceedings of the Conference on Visual Communications and Image Processing*, Vol. 2308, September 1994, SPIE, Chicago, IL, pp. 971–981.

[34] R.R. Schultz and R.L. Stevenson, Extraction of high-resolution frames from video sequences, *IEEE Trans. Image Process.*, 5, 996–1011, June 1996.

[35] R.R. Schultz and R.L. Stevenson, Improved definition video frame enhancement, in *Proceedings of IEEE International Conference an Acoustics, Speech, Signal Processing*, Vol. 4, IEEE Press, pp. 2169–2171, May 1995.

[36] R.R. Schultz and R.L. Stevenson, A Bayesian approach to image expansion for improved definition, *IEEE Trans. Image Process.*, 3, 233–242, May 1994.

[37] R.C. Hardie, K.J. Barnard, and E.E. Armstrong, Joint MAP registration and high-resolution image estimation using a sequence of undersampled images, *IEEE Trans. Image Process.*, 6, 1621–1633, December 1997.

[38] L. Guan and R.K. Ward, Restoration of randomly blurred images via the maximum a posteriori criterion, *IEEE Trans. Image Process.*, 1, 256–262, April 1992.

[39] H. He and L.P. Kondi, Resolution enhancement of video sequences with simultaneous estimation of the regularization parameter, *J. Electron. Imaging*, 13, 586–596, July 2004.

[40] H. He and L.P. Kondi, An image super-resolution algorithm for different error levels per frame, *IEEE Trans. Image Process.*, 15, 592–603, March 2006.

[41] L.P. Kondi, D. Scribner, and J. Schuler, A comparison of digital image resolution enhancement techniques, *Proceedings of SPIE AeroSense Conference*, Vol. 4719, April 2002, pp. 220–229.

[42] H. He and L.P. Kondi, Resolution enhancement of video sequences with simultaneous estimation of the regularization parameter, in *Proceedings of SPIE Electronic Imaging*, Santa Clara, CA, Vol. 5022, SPIE, 2003, pp. 1123–1133.

[43] H. He and L.P. Kondi, MAP-based resolution enhancement of video sequences using a Huber-Markov random field image prior model, in *Proceedings of the IEEE International Conference on Image Processing*, Barcelona, Spain, Vol. II, September 2003, IEEE, pp. 933–936.

[44] H. He and L.P. Kondi, Choice of threshold of the Huber-Markov prior in MAP-based video resolution enhancement, in *Proceedings of the IEEE Canadian Conference on Electrical and Computer Engineering*, Niagara Falls, Canada, Vol. 2, May 2004, IEEE, pp. 801–804.

[45] H. He and L.P. Kondi, Resolution enhancement of video sequences with adaptively weighted low-resolution images and simultaneous estimation of the regularization parameter, in *Proceedings of the IEEE International Conference on Acoustics, Speech and Signal Processing*, Montreal, Canada, Vol. 3, May 2004, IEEE, pp. 213–216.

[46] M.K. Ng, R.J. Plemmons, and S. Qiao, Regularization of RIF blind image deconvolution, *IEEE Trans. Image Process.*, 9, 1130–1134, June 2000.

[47] A.M. Tekalp, *Digital Video Processing*, Prentice-Hall, Englewood Cliffs, NJ, 1995.

[48] N.P. Galatsanos and A.K. Katsaggelos, Methods for choosing the regularization parameter and estimating the noise variance in image restoration and their relation, *IEEE Trans. Image Process.*, 1, 322–336, July 1992.

[49] S.J. Reeves and A.C. Higdon, Perceptual evaluation of the mean-square error choice of regularization parameter, *IEEE Trans. Image Process.*, 4, 107–110, January 1995.

[50] J. Mateos, A.K. Katsaggelos, and R. Molina, A Bayesian approach for the estimation and transmission of regularization parameters for reducing blocking artifacts, *IEEE Trans. Image Process.*, 9, 1200–1215, July 2000.

[51] P.C. Hansen, Rank-deficient and discrete ill-posed problems, Society for Industrial & Applied Mathematics (SIAM), Philadelphia, 1997.

[52] E.S. Lee and M.G. Kang, Regularized adaptive high-resolution image reconstruction considering inaccurate subpixel registration, *IEEE Trans. Image Process.*, 12, 826–837, July 2003.

[53] N.P. Galatsanos, V.Z. Mesarovic, R. Molina, and A.K. Katsaggelos, Hierarchical Bayesian image restoration from partially known blurs, *IEEE Trans. Image Process.*, 9, 1784–1797, October 2000.

[54] N.P. Galatsanos, V.Z. Mesarovic, R. Molina, A.K. Katsaggelos, and J. Mateos, Hyperparameter estimation in image restoration problems with partially-known blurs, *Opt. Eng.*, 41, 1845–1854, August 2000.

[55] R. Molina, A.K. Katsaggelos, and J. Mateos, Bayesian and regularization methods for hyperparameter estimation in image restoration, *IEEE Trans. Image Process.*, 8, 231–246, February 1999.

[56] R.K. Ward, Restoration of differently blurred versions of an image with measurement errors in the PSF's, *IEEE Trans. Image Process.*, 2, 369–381, July 1993.

[57] D. Kundur, D. Hatzinakos, and H. Leung, Robust classification of blurred imagery, *IEEE Trans. Image Process.*, 9, 243–255, February 2000.

[58] S.N. Efstratiadis and A.K. Katsaggelos, An adaptive regularized recursive displacement estimation algorithm, *IEEE Trans. Image Process.*, 2, 341–352, July 1993.

[59] H. Zheng and S.D. Blostein, An error-weighted regularization algorithm for image motion-field estimation, *IEEE Trans. Image Process.*, 2, 246–252, April 1993.

[60] S. Koch, H. Kaufman, and J. Biemond, Restoration of spatially varying blurred images using multiple model-based extended kalman filters, *IEEE Trans. Image Process.*, 4, 520–523, April 1995.

[61] A. Zomet, A. Rav-Acha, and S. Peleg, Robust super-resolution, in *Proceedings. of the International. Conference on Computer Vision and Pattern Recognition*, Vol. 1, December 2001, pp. 645–650.

[62] S. Farsiu, D. Robinson, M. Elad, and P. Milanfar, Robust shift and add approach to super-resolution, *Proceedings of the 2003 SPIE Conference on Applications of Digital Signal and Image Processing*, Vol. 5203, August 2003, pp. 121–130.

[63] S. Farsiu, D. Robinson, M. Elad, and P. Milanfar, Fast and robust multi-frame super-resolution, *IEEE Trans. Image Process.*, 13, 1327–1344, October 2004.

[64] A.J. Patti, M. Sezan, and A.M. Tekalp, Robust methods for high quality stills from interlaced video in the presence of dominant motion, *IEEE Trans. on Circuits and Syst. for Video Technol.*, 7, 328–342, April 1997.

[65] M.A.T. Figueiredo and J.M.N. Leitao, Sequential and parallel image restoration: Neural network implementations, *IEEE Trans. Image Process.*, 3, 789–801, November 1994.

[66] M. Elad and Y. Hel-Or, A fast super-resolution reconstruction algorithm for pure translational motion and common space-invariant blur, *IEEE Trans. Image Process.*, 10, 1187–1193, August 2001.

[67] M.G. Kang and A.K. Katsaggelos, Simultaneous multichannel image restoration and estimation of the regularization parameters, *IEEE Trans. Image Process.*, 6, 774–778, May 1997.

# 22

## Coding of Two-Dimensional and Three-Dimensional Color Image Sequences

**Savvas Argyropoulos, Nikolaos V. Boulgouris, Nikolaos Thomos, Yiannis Kompatsiaris, and Michael G. Strintzis**

## CONTENTS

## 22.1   Introduction

Digital color image sequences are used in various applications, like videotelephony, videoconferencing, digital archiving, digital broadcasting, and so forth. The widespread deployment of video sequences was greatly facilitated by the development of video coding

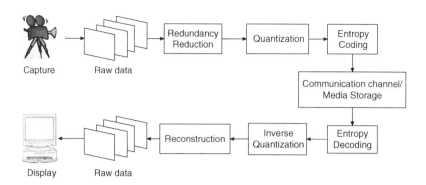

**FIGURE 22.1**
Overview of a video coding system.

schemes, which can provide bandwidth efficiency without sacrificing video quality. Essentially, the ultimate goal of a digital video coding system is to reduce the bit rate needed for the representation of a video sequence, in order to enable the transmission of the stream over a communication channel or its storage in an optical medium.

The main components of a video coding system are depicted in Figure 22.1. Initially, the camera captures a scene at a specific video resolution and frame rate. Subsequently, the frames are processed in order to exploit their inherent spatial and temporal correlation. This processing involves *motion estimation* and *compensation* and the *transformation* of the motion compensated residuals. The next steps include *quantization* and *entropy coding* of the quantized coefficients, which generate the compressed video stream. The resulting compressed bitstream can be stored or transmitted over a communication channel. At the decoder, the inverse processes are applied and, eventually, the image sequence is reconstructed and displayed.

The objective of this chapter is to provide an overview of the techniques for the coding of two- and three-dimensional color image sequences and describe recent developments in this area. First, in Section 22.2, we present a review of the main video coding techniques that have been presented in the literature. Special emphasis is given to the color formats and color spaces used in the existing video coding standards. The motivation for the use of color formats and spaces is explained in detail, because they are of key importance for an efficient video coding system. Section 22.3 outlines the advances and novelties introduced by the latest international video coding standard H.264/MPEG-4 Part 10. A review of three-dimensional (3-D) coding techniques is presented in Section 22.4. In particular, methods for 3-D motion compensation that can be employed for disparity and depth estimation in stereoscopic and multiview sequence processing are described. Furthermore, we illustrate how 3-D model-based coding can be used for segmentation of a 3-D model into rigid objects, which permits model manipulation and more accurate motion estimation.

## 22.2   Overview of Color Video Coding

### 22.2.1   Color Spaces

The understanding of the way the human visual system (HVS) perceives color is necessary in order to develop an efficient color video coding system. The most known color formats used in the international video coding standards are briefly described below, and emphasis is placed on their main attributes.

### 22.2.1.1 RGB Color Format

One of the main color formats is the RGB, which can be defined by using red, green, and blue as primary colors, denoted, respectively, by R, G, and B. Then, a match to an arbitrary color can be obtained by a weighted sum of the three primaries:

$$C = rR + gG + bB \tag{22.1}$$

where $r$, $g$, and $b$ are known as the tristimulus values of $R$, $G$, and $B$ components, and $C$ is the stimulus [1]. The RGB color format is mainly used in computer graphics, because color monitors use red, green, and blue phosphors to generate desired colors.

The main drawback of the RGB format is the equal bandwidths needed to represent the three components. This means that equal pixel depth and display resolution are used for each color component. However, the HVS is actually most sensitive to green and less sensitive to red and blue light.

### 22.2.1.2 YUV Color Format

To alleviate the drawbacks of the RGB color format, most video coding standards use *luminance* and *chrominance* signals. Specifically, luminance refers to the perceived brightness of the light, which is proportional to the total energy in the visible band, while chrominance is characterized by two quantities: *hue* and *saturation*. Hue specifies the color tone, which depends on peak wavelength of the light, whereas saturation denotes the color pureness, which is associated with the bandwidth of the light spectrum. In many applications, it is desirable to describe a color in terms of its luminance and chrominance components separately, to enable more efficient processing and transmission of color signals. To this end, various color coordinates have been proposed, in which the luminance is described by a single component, while hue and saturation are jointly characterized using two components. The most known color coordinate is the YUV, which is used by the NTSC, PAL, and SECAM composite color TV standards. Luminance, which is denoted by Y, and color signals ($U$ and $V$) are combined to create a color representation. YUV signals are derived using the gamma-corrected[1] RGB signal according to the following formula:

$$\begin{bmatrix} Y \\ U \\ V \end{bmatrix} = \begin{bmatrix} 0.299 & 0.587 & 0.114 \\ -0.147 & -0.289 & 0.436 \\ 0.615 & -0.515 & -0.100 \end{bmatrix} \begin{bmatrix} \tilde{R} \\ \tilde{G} \\ \tilde{B} \end{bmatrix} \tag{22.2}$$

where $\tilde{R}$, $\tilde{G}$, and $\tilde{B}$ are the normalized gamma-corrected R, G, and B values [2]. Usually, color-difference signals are subsampled by a factor ranging from two to four, because they are less sensitive to the HVS than the luminance Y. This approach enables reduced bit rate allocation to color information coding in video compression techniques.

### 22.2.1.3 $YC_rC_b$ Color Format

Another color space in which luminance and chrominance are separately represented is the $YC_rC_b$, where $Y$, $C_r$, and $C_b$ components are scaled and shifted versions of the $Y$, $U$, and

---

[1] Usually, display systems, like monitors and televisions, have a nonlinear response to the input voltage signal, which can be approximated by $Y = V^\gamma$, where $Y$ is the displayed value, $V$ is the input voltage signal, and $\gamma$ is a constant ranging from 1.8 to 3.2. This is referred to as gamma correction.

*V* components. The *Y* component takes values from 16 to 235, while $C_b$ and $C_r$ take values from 16 to 240. They are obtained from gamma-corrected R, G, and B values as follows:

$$\begin{bmatrix} Y \\ C_b \\ C_r \end{bmatrix} = \begin{bmatrix} 0.299 & 0.587 & 0.114 \\ -0.169 & -0.331 & 0.500 \\ 0.500 & -0.419 & -0.081 \end{bmatrix} \begin{bmatrix} \tilde{R} \\ \tilde{G} \\ \tilde{B} \end{bmatrix} \tag{22.3}$$

It is worth noting that the first chrominance component, $C_b$, is a scaled version of the difference between the original blue signal, and the luminance signal, and $C_r$ is a red-luminance difference, specifically,

$$C_r = 0.713\,(R - Y) \tag{22.4}$$

$$C_b = 0.564\,(B - Y) \tag{22.5}$$

Thus, the two chrominance components, $C_b$ and $C_r$, represent the extent to which the color deviates from gray toward blue and red, respectively. From the above equations, it is obvious that rounding errors are introduced during both forward and inverse conversion between RGB and $YC_rC_b$ color formats.

#### 22.2.1.4 Color Sampling Formats

Because a viewer is less sensitive to rapid changes in the hue and saturation than to intensity changes, chrominance components are usually subsampled by a factor of two in both the horizontal and the vertical directions, yielding chrominance components consisting of half the number of pixels in each line. This is known as the *4:2:2* format, implying that there are two $C_b$ and two $C_r$ samples for every four *Y* samples. To further reduce the required data rate, the *4:1:1* format was defined, in which chrominance components are subsampled along each line by a factor of four. However, this sampling method yields asymmetric resolutions in the horizontal and the vertical directions. To this end, the *4:2:0* format was developed, in which $C_b$ and $C_r$ are subsampled by a factor of two in both directions.

### 22.2.2 Quantization

As mentioned previously, one of the main tasks of a video coding process is the *quantization*. Quantization represents the sampled data using a finite number of levels according to some metrics, such as minimization of the quantizer distortion. *Scalar quantization* is the most common quantization, in which each sample is quantized independently, according to a codebook. However, all samples in a vector of data can be jointly quantized, rather than individually, and this process is called *vector quantization* [3]. Scalar quantizers are mainly classified as *uniform* and *nonuniform*: a uniform quantizer is fully described by the number of reconstruction levels *L*, the boundary values $b_l, l = 0, 1, \ldots, L$, and the reconstruction values $g_l, l = 1, 2, \ldots, L$, while a nonuniform does not have constant step sizes and has to be specified by the input and output levels. The distance between adjacent boundary values, which is termed *quantization stepsize*, is equal to the distance between adjacent reconstruction values, and the interval around zero is called *dead zone*.[2] A uniform quantizer with an increased dead zone is illustrated in Figure 22.2.

---

[2] Most international video coding standards, such as H.26x and MPEG-x, use a nearly uniform quantizer, with an increased dead zone.

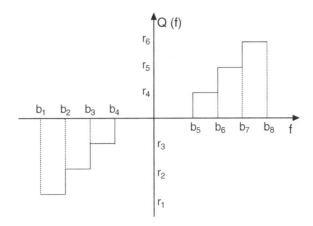

**FIGURE 22.2**
Uniform quantizer with increased dead zone.

### 22.2.3 Motion Compensation

The primary objective of a video coding system is to achieve high compression ratios (or equivalently reduce the size of the compressed stream) while maintaining the desired visual quality. Coding efficiency is achieved by using a number of different redundancy reduction techniques. *Temporal* redundancy is removed by means of *motion estimation* and *compensation*, which exploit the similarities between temporally adjacent video frames. Motion estimation/compensation aims at describing the changes between neighboring frames of a video sequence and forming a prediction of the current frame based on one or more previously coded frames (which are usually termed *reference frames*). It is worth noting that both past and future frames can be used as reference frames, depending on the specific order of the encoding. The prediction frame, which is derived using motion estimation, is subtracted from the current frame, and the residual (difference) frame is encoded along with the motion parameters. Motion estimation techniques are classified as *pixel based* or *block based*. Pixel-based techniques are not used in video coding systems due to their inherent complexity and convergence problems. For this reason, in the sequel, we focus only on block-based methods, which are widely used for motion compensation.

*Block-matching* is the basic process in motion estimation/compensation and is depicted in Figure 22.3. It is based on the fact that if a block is defined as being sufficiently small, then the motion it exhibits can be characterized by a simple parametric model, which describes the motion of all the pixels covered by that block using a single motion vector. Initially, the current frame is split into nonoverlapping rectangular areas of $M \times N$ samples. Each block in the current frame is compared with some or all of the possible blocks (depending on the search window) in the reference frames to determine a block that minimizes a distortion metric, like the sum of absolute differences (SAD), or mean square error (MSE). It must be stressed that most coding schemes examine only the luminance component in the block-matching search and not the chrominance components. Moreover, the search window is usually limited to ±16 pixels. The selected best matching block in the reference frames is subtracted from the current block to produce a residual block. The residual block is encoded and transmitted along with a motion vector.

Because in most cases objects move by a fractional number of pixels between frames, a better prediction may be formed by interpolating the reference frame to subpixel positions before searching these positions for the best match. In the first stage, motion estimation finds the best match on the integer-sample grid. Subsequently, the half-sample positions

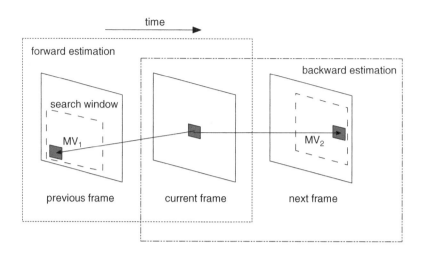

**FIGURE 22.3**
Forward and backward motion estimation.

next to this best match are searched in order to examine whether the integer match can be improved. Similarly, the quarter-samples positions next to the best half-sample position are searched. In general, "finer" interpolation provides better motion estimation performance at the expense of increased complexity. The more accurate the estimation, the less energy is contained in the residual frame, and the more efficiently it can be compressed. However, "finer" estimation requires more bits for the representation of the fractional part of the vector, thus reducing coding efficiency. It is obvious that there is a trade-off in compression efficiency associated with more complex motion compensation schemes, because more accurate motion estimation requires more bits to encode the motion vectors but fewer bits to encode the residual, and *vice versa*.

Block-based motion estimation has several advantages that make it appealing for use in video coding standards. Specifically, it is relatively straightforward, it fits well with rectangular video frames, and it provides a reasonably effective temporal model for many video sequences. Nevertheless, the basic assumption that each block undergoes only a pure translation is not always capable of describing rotation and does not always hold (e.g., in cases of rotation or zooming). For this reason, more sophisticated models have been developed, such as the deformable block-matching algorithm (which maps a block to a nonsquare quadrangle), the mesh-based, and the region-based motion estimation schemes [4].

### 22.2.4 Reconstruction Quality Evaluation

The performance of a video coding system is a trade-off among three parameters: rate, distortion, and computational cost. As explained in the previous sections, distortion is mainly introduced during the quantization step. Both objective and subjective measures have been used in the literature [5], but the former have prevailed, due to comparison issues. Two of the most widely used criteria to measure the distortion of a reconstructed color image sequence are the MSE and the peak signal-to-noise ratio (PSNR) [1]. Usually, only the luminance component is taken into account for the evaluation of the distortion of a video coding system. However, if the color components are also used for the estimation of the distortion, then they have to be weighted due to the difference of perception of color by the HVS.

## 22.3 H.264/MPEG 4 Part 10

The Moving Pictures Experts Group (MPEG) and the Video Coding Experts Group (VCEG) have developed a new standard that aims to outperform previous standards, such as MPEG-4 and H.263/H.263++. The new standard is entitled "Advanced Video Coding" (AVC) and is published jointly as Part 10 of MPEG-4 and ITU-T Recommendation H.264 [6]. In this section, the new features introduced in H.264/AVC are outlined in order to highlight the reasons why it is considered the most attractive candidate for next-generation video services. Moreover, the basic components of an H.264/AVC codec are presented, based on the generic system description of the previous section. It is worth noting that, like previous video coding standards, only the decoder is standardized, by imposing restrictions on bitstream and syntax, and defining the decoding process of the syntax elements. This fact gives the freedom to coding systems designers to optimize their implementations in a manner that is most appropriate for their specific applications.

### 22.3.1 Video Coding Algorithm

The coding structure of the H.264/AVC [7] standard is similar to that of all prior major standards (H.261, MPEG-1, MPEG-2/H.262, H.263/H.263++, and MPEG-4 Part 2). It follows the block-based hybrid video coding approach, in which each coded picture is represented by rectangular blocks of luminance and chrominance samples, called *macroblocks*. The term "hybrid" is due to the deployment of two source coding techniques: *inter-picture prediction*, which exploits temporal statistical dependencies, and *transform coding* of the residual signal, which exploits spatial redundancy.

The block diagram of an H.264/AVC encoder is depicted in Figure 22.4. The color space used by H.264/AVC is the $YC_rC_b$ (although the standard makes provision for other color spaces with the Fidelity Range Extensions, as it will be explained soon). Initially, the picture is partitioned into macroblocks, which consist in a rectangular picture area of $16 \times 16$

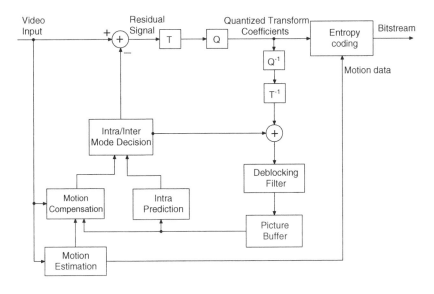

**FIGURE 22.4**
Block diagram of an H.264/AVC encoder.

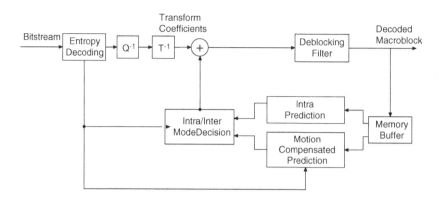

**FIGURE 22.5**
Block diagram of an H.264/AVC decoder.

samples of luminance and $8 \times 8$ samples of each of the two chrominance components.[3] Macroblocks are grouped into slices. A slice is a set of macroblocks processed in raster scan order. A picture may consist of one or more slices, and no prediction is allowed across slice boundaries. This makes slices self-contained, in the sense that their syntax elements can be parsed from the bitstream, and the values of the samples they represent can be correctly decoded without using data from other slices.

After all macroblocks have been associated with slices, all samples of each macroblock are either spatially or temporally predicted, and the resulting prediction error signal (residual) is encoded using transform coding (denoted by $T$ in the block diagram) and quantization (denoted by $Q$). Subsequently, inverse quantization and transform are applied (denoted by $Q^{-1}$ and $T^{-1}$, respectively), the deblocking filter is used to remove blocking artifacts, and the reconstructed macroblock is stored in the memory buffer so that it can be used to predict future macroblocks. Quantized transform coefficients, motion information, and other data that are essential for decoding are entropy coded. The inverse process is followed at the decoder, as depicted in Figure 22.5. In the following, a more thorough analysis of each component of the encoder and the decoder is presented, and the necessary theoretical background is given for a complete understanding.

### 22.3.1.1 Intra Prediction

Intra prediction refers to prediction of macroblock samples by using only the information of already transmitted macroblocks of the same image. Different modes depending on the color component are supported [7]. For the luminance samples, in the first mode, termed INTRA_$4 \times 4$, the macroblock is split into sixteen $4 \times 4$ subblocks, and prediction is applied for each one of them, choosing the best from nine possible directions. This mode is well suited for the coding of parts with significant detail. In the other mode, termed INTRA_$16 \times 16$, prediction is applied for the entire macroblock. Four different prediction modes are supported: vertical, horizontal, DC, and plane prediction. The INTRA_$16 \times 16$ mode is usually employed to code smooth or plane areas, with little detail and limited motion. The intra prediction for the chrominance components of a macroblock is similar to the INTRA_$16 \times 16$ type for the luminance component, because chrominance signals are very smooth in most cases. It is always performed on $8 \times 8$ blocks using vertical, horizontal,

---

[3] This is only true in 4:2:0 sampling; for other sampling formats, the number of chrominance samples in a macroblock is different.

DC, or plane prediction. As mentioned previously, intra prediction across slice boundaries is not allowed in order to keep all slices independent of each other.

#### 22.3.1.2 Inter Prediction

In addition to the intra macroblock coding type, various motion-compensated predictive coding types are specified as $P$ macroblock types, utilizing already transmitted reference images. Each $P$ macroblock type corresponds to a specific partition of the macroblock into the block shapes used for motion-compensated prediction. Partitions with luminance subblock sizes of $16 \times 16$, $16 \times 8$, $8 \times 16$, and $8 \times 8$ samples are supported. In case of a $8 \times 8$ subblock in a $P$-slice, an additional syntax element specifies whether this subblock is further divided into smaller partitions with block sizes of $8 \times 4$, $4 \times 8$, or $4 \times 4$. Unlike previous standards that utilized only $16 \times 16$ and $8 \times 8$ block sizes, the division into smaller partitions is permitted to allow better motion estimation. The accuracy of motion vectors is a quarter of the distance between luminance samples. In case the motion vectors point to an integer position on the sampling grid, the prediction error signal consists of the corresponding samples of the reference pictures; otherwise, the corresponding sample is obtained using interpolation to generate noninteger positions [6].

#### 22.3.1.3 Transform Coding

Two major novelties are introduced in the transform coding component, in order to reduce the spatial correlation of the residual signal. Unlike previous coding standards, which employed a two-dimensional discrete cosine transform (DCT) on $8 \times 8$ blocks as the basic transform, H.264/AVC utilizes three integer transforms [8], depending on the type of the residual data to be coded, on smaller $4 \times 4$ or $2 \times 2$ blocks. The first transform, given by $H_1$ below, is applied to all samples of the prediction error blocks of the luminance and the chrominance component. Its size is $4 \times 4$. If the macroblock is predicted using the INTRA_$16 \times 16$ mode, then a Hadamard transform $H_2$ of size $4 \times 4$ is applied to the first one, to transform all the DC coefficients of the already transformed blocks of the luminance signal. Moreover, the standard specifies a Hadamard transform $H_3$ of $2 \times 2$ size that is applied to the DC coefficients of each chrominance component. Transform coefficients are scanned in zig-zag order, in order to maximize the number of consecutive zero-valued coefficients appearing in the scan:

$$
H_1 = \begin{bmatrix} 1 & 1 & 1 & 1 \\ 2 & 1 & -1 & -2 \\ 1 & -1 & -1 & 1 \\ 1 & -2 & 2 & -1 \end{bmatrix}, \quad H_2 = \begin{bmatrix} 1 & 1 & 1 & 1 \\ 1 & 1 & -1 & -1 \\ 1 & -1 & -1 & 1 \\ 1 & -1 & 1 & -1 \end{bmatrix}, \quad H_3 = \begin{bmatrix} 1 & 1 \\ 1 & -1 \end{bmatrix}
$$

Transforms of smaller size reduce noise around edges, known as *mosquito noise*, and enable the encoder to adapt the residual coding to the boundaries of moving objects and adapt the transform to the local prediction error signal. Furthermore, one of the main advantages of this transform is that it consists of integer numbers ranging from $-2$ to $2$, and therefore, the computation of the forward and the inverse transform is possible in 16-bit arithmetic using only shift, add, and subtract operations.

#### 22.3.1.4 Entropy Coding

Two entropy coding variants are specified in H.264/AVC: a low complexity technique, based on context–adaptively switched sets of variable length coding (CAVLC) [9], and a more demanding algorithm, termed context-based adaptive binary arithmetic coding (CABAC) [10]. Both methods outperform all other techniques of statistical coding used in previous video coding standards, which were based on fixed variable length codes (VLC)

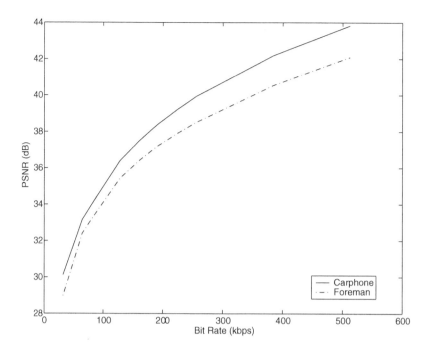

**FIGURE 22.6**
Performance of H.264/AVC encoder for "Foreman" and "Carphone" video sequences.

for each syntax element. In CAVLC, VLC tables for various syntax elements are switched, depending on the already transmitted syntax elements. Because the VLC tables are designed to match the corresponding conditioned statistics, the entropy coding performance is improved in comparison to schemes using a single VLC table. On the other hand, in CABAC, the usage of arithmetic coding allows for the assignment of a noninteger number of bits to each symbol in an alphabet, which is extremely beneficial for symbol probabilities greater than 0.5. In addition to this, adaptive codes permit adaptation to non-stationary symbol statistics. This is of primary importance, because, in general, motion compensation residuals exhibit nonstationary behavior, depending on the video content and the accuracy of the prediction model.

The performance of a Main Profile H.264/AVC encoder is presented for the two QCIF (of size $176 \times 144$) sequences "Foreman" and "Carphone" at a frame rate of 30 frames/sec. Group of Pictures (GOP) of 300 frames and $I\,P\,P\,P\ldots$ structure were encoded at various bit rates, and the results are depicted in Figure 22.6.

### 22.3.1.5  *FREXT (Fidelity Range EXTensions)*

This section discusses fidelity range extensions (FREXT) [11], a recent amendment to the H.264/AVC standard that further improves coding efficiency in some applications and takes care of color-related issues that were underestimated in the initial version. As already discussed, the standard was primarily focused on 8 bits/sample, 4:2:0 sampling, and $YC_rC_b$ color space. However, many applications require more than 8 bits per sample of source video accuracy or higher resolution for color representation, than what is typical in most consumer applications. To address the needs of these demanding applications, the FREXT amendment makes provision for other sampling formats, such as 4:2:2 and 4:4:4, and up to 12 bits of precision per sample.

Another contribution of the FREXT amendment is the support of a new color space, to combat the problems rising from RGB-to-$YC_rC_b$ conversion. As demonstrated in the previous section, both the forward and the inverse transformation from one color space to another introduce rounding errors. Moreover, the trade-off between the complexity of the transformation (which is increased due to the decimal number needed for implementation) and the coding efficiency is suboptimal. To combat these drawbacks, a new color space called $YC_gC_o$ (where $C_g$ stands for green chrominance and $C_o$ for orange chrominance) is supported, which is much simpler and yields equal or better coding efficiency. Its components are derived by the gamma-corrected $\tilde{R}$, $\tilde{G}$, and $\tilde{B}$ values by

$$Y = \frac{1}{2}\left(\tilde{G} + \frac{\tilde{R} + \tilde{B}}{2}\right) \tag{22.6}$$

$$C_g = \frac{1}{2}\left(\tilde{G} - \frac{\tilde{R} + \tilde{B}}{2}\right) \tag{22.7}$$

$$C_o = \frac{\tilde{R} - \tilde{B}}{2} \tag{22.8}$$

It is obvious that rounding errors can be avoided if two additional bits are used for the chrominance components. Instead, a variant of this scheme, which does not introduce any conversion rounding error and does not require adding precision to the luminance samples, is used:

$$C_o = \tilde{R} - \tilde{B}; \quad t = \tilde{B} + (C_o >> 1); \quad C_g = \tilde{G} - t; \quad Y = t + (C_g >> 1) \tag{22.9}$$

where $t$ is an intermediate temporary variable, and $>>$ denotes an arithmetic right shift operation.

## 22.4 Flexible 3-D Motion Estimation for Multiview Image Sequence Coding

This section focuses on motion estimation techniques for multiview image sequences and describes a procedure for model-based coding, using flexible motion estimation of all channels of a three-view image sequence. In a multiview image sequence, each view is recorded with a difference in the observation angle, creating an enhanced 3-D feeling to the observer. The 3-D model is initialized by adapting a 2-D wireframe to the foreground object. Using depth and multiview camera geometry, the 2-D wireframe is reprojected in the 3-D space, forming consistent views. Subsequently, the rigid 3-D motion of each triangle is estimated, taking into account the temporal correlation between adjacent frames. The estimation of rigid 3-D motion vectors for each triangle of the 3-D model is needed before the evaluation of flexible motion estimation is attempted. In order to increase the efficiency and stability of the triangle motion-estimation algorithm, neighborhood triangles are taken into account. This also results in a smoother 3-D motion field, because erroneous large local deformations are suppressed. In the following analysis, the CAHV model, introduced in Reference [12], is used as a camera model, to describe the projection of 3-D points onto a camera target.

### 22.4.1 Rigid 3-D Motion Estimation

In the first frame of each GOP, the rigid motion of each triangle $T_k$, $k = 1, \ldots, K$, where $K$ is the number of triangles in the foreground object, is modeled using a linear 3-D model, with three rotation and three translation parameters [13]:

$$\mathbf{P}_{t+1} = \mathbf{R}^{(k)}\,\mathbf{P}_t + \mathbf{T}^{(k)} \tag{22.10}$$

with $\mathbf{R}^{(k)}$ and $\mathbf{T}^{(k)}$ being of the following form:

$$\mathbf{R}^{(k)} = \begin{bmatrix} 1 & -w_z^{(k)} & w_y^{(k)} \\ w_z^{(k)} & 1 & -w_x^{(k)} \\ -w_y^{(k)} & w_x^{(k)} & 1 \end{bmatrix} \tag{22.11}$$

$$\mathbf{T}^{(k)} = \begin{bmatrix} t_x^{(k)} \\ t_y^{(k)} \\ t_z^{(k)} \end{bmatrix} \tag{22.12}$$

where $\mathbf{P}_t = (x_t, y_t, z_t)$ is a 3-D point on the plane defined by the coordinates of the vertices of triangle $T_k$.

In order to guarantee the production of a homogeneous estimated triangle motion vector field, smoothness neighborhood constraints are imposed for the estimation of the model parameter vector $\mathbf{a}^{(k)} = (w_x^{(k)}, w_y^{(k)}, w_z^{(k)}, t_x^{(k)}, t_y^{(k)}, t_z^{(k)})$. Let $N_k$ be the ensemble of the triangles neighboring the triangle $T_k$, that is, those sharing at least one common node with $T_k$. We define as the neighborhood $TS_k$ of each triangle $T_k$ the set of triangles in

$$TS_k = \{T_j \in N_k\} \cup \{T_k\}$$

For the estimation of the model parameter vector $\mathbf{a}^{(k)}$, the *MLMS* iterative algorithm [14] was used. The *MLMS* algorithm is based on median filtering and is very efficient in suppressing noise with a large amount of outliers (i.e., in situations where conventional least squares techniques usually fail).

At time $t$, each point $\mathbf{P}_t$ in $TS_k$ is projected to points $(X_{c,t}, Y_{c,t})$, $c = l, t, r$ on the planes of the three cameras. Using the equations of the projection of a 3-D point $P$ onto an image plane and Equation 22.10, the projected 2-D motion vector, $\mathbf{d}_c(X_c, Y_c)$ is determined by

$$d_{xc}(X_{c,t}, Y_{c,t}) = X_{c,t+1} - X_{c,t} = \frac{(\mathbf{R}^{(k)} \mathbf{P}_t + \mathbf{T}^{(k)} - \mathbf{C}_c)^T \cdot \mathbf{H}_c}{(\mathbf{R}^{(k)} \mathbf{P}_t + \mathbf{T}^{(k)} - \mathbf{C}_c)^T \cdot \mathbf{A}_c} - \frac{(\mathbf{P}_t - \mathbf{C}_c)^T \cdot \mathbf{H}_c}{(\mathbf{P}_t - \mathbf{C}_c)^T \cdot \mathbf{A}_c} \tag{22.13}$$

$$d_{yc}(X_{c,t}, Y_{c,t}) = Y_{c,t+1} - Y_{c,t} = \frac{(\mathbf{R}^{(k)} \mathbf{P}_t + \mathbf{T}^{(k)} - \mathbf{C}_c)^T \cdot \mathbf{V}_c}{(\mathbf{R}^{(k)} \mathbf{P}_t + \mathbf{T}^{(k)} - \mathbf{C}_c)^T \cdot \mathbf{A}_c} - \frac{(\mathbf{P}_t - \mathbf{C}_c)^T \cdot \mathbf{V}_c}{(\mathbf{P}_t - \mathbf{C}_c)^T \cdot \mathbf{A}_c} \tag{22.14}$$

where $\mathbf{d}_c(X_c, Y_c) = (d_{xc}(X_{c,t}, Y_{c,t}), d_{yc}(X_{c,t}, Y_{c,t}))$.

Using the initial 2-D motion vectors, estimated by applying a block matching algorithm to the images corresponding to the left, top, and right cameras and also using Equations 22.13 and 22.14, a linear system for the global motion parameter vector $\mathbf{a}^{(k)}$ for triangle $T_k$ is formed:

$$\mathbf{b}^{(k)} = \mathbf{D}^{(k)} \mathbf{a}^{(k)} \tag{22.15}$$

Omitting, for notational simplicity, dependence on time $t$, triangle $k$ and camera $c$, $\mathbf{D}$ can be expressed as follows:

$$\mathbf{D} = \begin{bmatrix} d_{x,0}[0] & d_{x,0}[1] & d_{x,0}[2] & d_{x,0}[3] & d_{x,0}[4] & d_{x,0}[5] \\ d_{y,0}[0] & d_{y,0}[1] & d_{y,0}[2] & d_{y,0}[3] & d_{y,0}[4] & d_{y,0}[5] \\ \cdots & \cdots & \cdots & \cdots & \cdots & \cdots \\ d_{x,L}[0] & d_{x,L}[1] & d_{x,L}[2] & d_{x,L}[3] & d_{x,L}[4] & d_{x,L}[5] \\ d_{y,L}[0] & d_{y,L}[1] & d_{y,L}[2] & d_{y,L}[3] & d_{y,L}[4] & d_{y,L}[5] \end{bmatrix} \tag{22.16}$$

where

$$d_{x,l}[0] = -H_y \, z_l + H_z \, y_l + q_{x,l} \, A_y \, z_l - q_{x,l} \, A_z \, y_l$$

$$d_{x,l}[1] = H_x \, z_l - H_z \, x_l - q_{x,l} \, A_x \, z_l + q_{x,l} \, A_z \, x_l$$

$$d_{x,l}[2] = -H_x \, y_l + H_x \, x_l + q_{x,l} \, A_x \, y_l - q_{x,l} \, A_y \, x_l$$

$$d_{x,l}[3] = H_x - q_x \, A_x, \quad d_{x,l}[4] = H_y - q_x \, A_y, \quad d_{x,l}[5] = H_z - q_x \, A_z$$

and

$$q_{x,l} = d_{x,l} + \frac{(\mathbf{P}_l - \mathbf{C})^T \cdot \mathbf{H}}{(\mathbf{P}_l - \mathbf{C})^T \cdot \mathbf{A}}$$

For the $y$ coordinates,

$$d_{y,l}[0] = -V_y \, z_l + V_z \, y_l + q_{y,l} \, A_y \, z_l - q_{y,l} \, A_z \, y_l$$

$$d_{y,l}[1] = V_x \, z_l - V_z \, x_l - q_{y,l} \, A_x \, z_l + q_{y,l} \, A_z \, x_l$$

$$d_{y,l}[2] = -V_x \, y_l + V_x \, x_l + q_{y,l} \, A_x \, y_l - q_{y,l} \, A_y \, x_l$$

$$d_{y,l}[3] = V_x - q_{y,l} \, A_x, \quad d_{y,l}[4] = V_y - q_{y,l} \, A_y, \quad d_{y,l}[5] = V_z - q_{y,l} \, A_z$$

and

$$q_{y,l} = d_{y,l} + \frac{(\mathbf{P}_l - \mathbf{C})^T \cdot \mathbf{V}}{(\mathbf{P}_l - \mathbf{C})^T \cdot \mathbf{A}}$$

Also,

$$\mathbf{b} = \begin{bmatrix} q_{x,0} \cdot (\mathbf{P}_0 - \mathbf{C})^T \cdot \mathbf{A} - (\mathbf{P}_0 - \mathbf{C})^T \cdot \mathbf{H} \\ q_{y,0} \cdot (\mathbf{P}_0 - \mathbf{C})^T \cdot \mathbf{A} - (\mathbf{P}_0 - \mathbf{C})^T \cdot \mathbf{V} \\ \cdots \\ q_{x,L} \cdot (\mathbf{P}_L - \mathbf{C})^T \cdot \mathbf{A} - (\mathbf{P}_L - \mathbf{C})^T \cdot \mathbf{H} \\ q_{y,L} \cdot (\mathbf{P}_L - \mathbf{C})^T \cdot \mathbf{A} - (\mathbf{P}_L - \mathbf{C})^T \cdot \mathbf{V} \end{bmatrix} \tag{22.17}$$

In the above $l = 0, \ldots, L$, where $L$ is the number of 3-D points $\mathbf{P}_l = [x_l, y_l, z_l]^T$ contained in $TS_k$ and $\mathbf{C}$, $\mathbf{A} = [A_x, A_y, A_z]^T$, $\mathbf{H} = [H_x, H_y, H_z]^T$, $\mathbf{V} = [V_x, V_y, V_z]^T$ are the multiview camera parameters. The 2-D motion vectors $[d_{x,l}, d_{y,l}]^T$ correspond to the projected 3-D point $\mathbf{P}_l$.

This is a system of $2 \times 3 \times L$ equations with six unknowns, where $L$ is the number of 3-D points contained in $TS_k$, because for each 3-D point $\mathbf{P}_l$, two equations are formed for the $X$ and $Y$ coordinates for each one of the three cameras. Because $2 \times 3 \times L \geq 6$ for all triangles (in the worst case, $TS_k$ is composed of a single triangle with $L = 3$ and $2 \times 3 \times 3 = 18$), this is overdetermined and can be solved by the robust least median of squares motion-estimation algorithm described in detail in Reference [14]. Erroneous initial 2-D estimates, produced by the block-matching algorithm, will be discarded by the least median of squares motion-estimation algorithm.

## 22.4.2 3-D Motion Tracking Using Kalman Filtering

In order to exploit the temporal correlation between consequent frames, a Kalman filter similar to the one developed in Reference [15] is applied for the calculation of the 3-D rigid motion parameters at every time instant. In this way, the estimation of the motion parameters is honed by additional observations as additional frames arrive. Omitting for the sake of notational simplicity, the explicit dependence of the motion parameters to the triangle $T_k$, thus writing $\mathbf{a}_t$, $\mathbf{b}_t$, $\mathbf{C}_t$ instead of $\mathbf{a}_t^{(k)}$, $\mathbf{b}_t^{(k)}$, $\mathbf{C}_t^{(k)}$, the dynamics of the system are described as follows:

$$\mathbf{a}_{t+1} = \mathbf{a}_t + w \cdot \mathbf{e}_{t+1} \tag{22.18}$$

$$\mathbf{b}_{t+1} = \mathbf{D}_{t+1}\,\mathbf{a}_{t+1} + \mathbf{v}_{t+1} \tag{22.19}$$

where $\mathbf{a}$ is the rigid 3-D motion vector of each triangle, and $\mathbf{e}_t$ is a unit-variance white random sequence. The term $w \cdot \mathbf{e}_{t+1}$ describes the changes from frame to frame, and a high value of $w$ implies small correlation between subsequent frames and can be used to describe fast-changing scenes, whereas a low value of $w$ may be used when the motion is relatively slow and the temporal correlation is high. The noise term $\mathbf{v}_{t+1}$ represents the random error of the formation of the system (Equation 22.15), modeled as white zero mean Gaussian noise, where $E\{\mathbf{v}_n \cdot \mathbf{v}_{n'}\} = \mathcal{R}_v\,\delta(n - n')$, $n$ being the $n$th element of $\mathbf{v}$.

The equations [16], [17] giving the estimated value of $\hat{\mathbf{a}}_{t+1}$ according to $\hat{\mathbf{a}}_t$ are:

$$\hat{\mathbf{a}}_{t+1} = \hat{\mathbf{a}}_t + \mathbf{K}_{t+1} \cdot (\mathbf{b}_{t+1} - \mathbf{D}_{t+1} \cdot \hat{\mathbf{a}}_t) \tag{22.20}$$

$$\mathbf{K}_{t+1} = \left(\mathbf{R}_t + w^2\,\mathbf{I}\right) \cdot \mathbf{D}_{t+1}^T \cdot \mathbf{k}^{-1} \tag{22.21}$$

$$\mathbf{k} = \mathbf{D}_{t+1} \cdot \mathbf{R}_t \cdot \mathbf{D}_{t+1}^T + \mathbf{D}_{t+1} \cdot w^2\,\mathbf{I} \cdot \mathbf{D}_{t+1}^T + \mathcal{R}_v \tag{22.22}$$

$$\mathbf{R}_{t+1} = (\mathbf{I} - \mathbf{K}_{t+1} \cdot \mathbf{D}_{t+1}) \cdot (\mathbf{R}_t + w^2\,\mathbf{I}) \tag{22.23}$$

where $\hat{\mathbf{a}}_{t+1}$ and $\hat{\mathbf{a}}_t$ are the new and old predictions of the unknown motion parameters corresponding to the $t+1$ and $t$th frame, respectively; $\mathbf{K}_{t+1}$ represents the correction matrix; and $\mathbf{R}_t$ and $\mathbf{R}_{t+1}$ describe the old and the new covariance matrix of the estimation error $\mathbf{E}_t$ and $\mathbf{E}_{t+1}$, respectively,

$$\mathbf{E}_t = (\mathbf{a}_t - \hat{\mathbf{a}}_t), \quad \mathbf{R}_t = E\left\{\mathbf{E}_t \cdot \mathbf{E}_t^T\right\}$$

$$\mathbf{E}_{t+1} = (\mathbf{a}_{t+1} - \hat{\mathbf{a}}_{t+1}), \quad \mathbf{R}_{t+1} = E\left\{\mathbf{E}_{t+1} \cdot \mathbf{E}_{t+1}^T\right\}$$

The initial value $\hat{\mathbf{a}}_0$ of the filter (beginning of each GOP) is given by solving Equation 22.15. The correlation matrix $\mathbf{R}_0$ is

$$\mathbf{R}_0 = E\left\{\mathbf{a}_0 \cdot \mathbf{a}_0^T\right\}$$

In the above, $w$ and $\mathbf{v}$ are assumed to be the same for the whole mesh, hence independent of the triangle $T_k$. Notice that Equation 22.15 is solved only once in order to provide the initial values for the Kalman filtering. During the next frames, $\mathbf{D}$ and $\mathbf{b}$ are only formed and used at the Kalman filter procedure. The benefits of using Kalman filtering, rather than simply solving Equation 22.15 for each two consequent frames, are illustrated by the experimental results in Section 22.4.7.

### 22.4.3   Estimation and Tracking of Flexible Surface Deformation Using PCA

The 3-D rigid motion parameters $\mathbf{a}^{(k)}$ estimated from the previously described procedure are input to the 3-D flexible motion estimation procedure. The aim of the 3-D flexible motion estimation is to assign a motion vector to every node of the 3-D model. Then, the 3-D model can be updated at the next frame, and all views can be reconstructed using only the 3-D model, the 3-D flexible motion of each node, and the previous frame information.

### 22.4.4 Estimation of Flexible Surface Deformation

The flexible motion of each node of the wireframe $\mathbf{P}_i$, $\{i = 1, \ldots, P\}$ is affected by the 3-D rigid motion $\mathbf{a}^{(k)}$ of every triangle connected to $\mathbf{P}_i$, with 3-D motion estimated by the procedure described in the preceding sections. We propose the use of PCA in order to determine the best representative motion vector for node $\mathbf{P}_i$.

More specifically, for each node $\mathbf{P}_i$, $\mathbf{a}_i^{(l)}$, $\{l = 1, \ldots, N_i\}$ observations are available, where $N_i$ is the number of triangles containing this node. To form the covariance matrix of $\mathbf{a}_i$, their mean value is found by

$$\bar{\mathbf{a}}_i = \frac{1}{N_i} \sum_{l=1}^{N_i} \mathbf{a}_i^{(l)}$$

The covariance matrix of $\mathbf{a}_i$ is expressed as follows:

$$\mathcal{C}_i = \frac{1}{N_i} \sum_{l=1}^{N_i} \left(\mathbf{a}_i^{(l)} - \bar{\mathbf{a}}_i\right) \left(\mathbf{a}_i^{(l)} - \bar{\mathbf{a}}_i\right)^T$$

Let $\mathbf{u}_{i,k}$ be the eigenvector of the $6 \times 6$ matrix $\mathcal{C}_i$ corresponding to its $k$th highest eigenvalue. The mean value of the projections of all observations to $\mathbf{u}_{i,k}$ is

$$q_{i,k} = \frac{1}{N_i} \sum_{l=1}^{N_i} \mathbf{u}_{i,k}^T \cdot \left(\mathbf{a}_i^{(l)} - \bar{\mathbf{a}}_i\right) \tag{22.24}$$

the best estimated value of the motion parameters for node $i$ based on $M_i$ eigenvectors is:

$$\mathbf{a}_i = \sum_{m=1}^{M_i} q_{i,m} \cdot \mathbf{u}_{i,m} + \bar{\mathbf{a}}_i \tag{22.25}$$

where $M_i \leq 6$. The number $M_i$ used for each node depends on the corresponding number of dominant eigenvalues.

### 22.4.5 Flexible 3-D Motion Tracking Using Kalman Filtering

The previously described flexible motion estimation procedure is applied only at the beginning of each GOP. An iterative Kalman filter is used, for the flexible motion estimation of each node of subsequent frames, taking into account their temporal correlation.

Equation 22.25 with $M = 6$ can be written as

$$\mathbf{Q} = \mathbf{U} \cdot (\Delta \mathbf{a}) \tag{22.26}$$

where $\Delta \mathbf{a} = \mathbf{a} - \bar{\mathbf{a}}$, $\mathbf{Q}$ is the $6 \times 1$ vector with components given by Equation 22.24 for each node $i$, and $\mathbf{U}$ the $6 \times 6$ matrix having as rows the eigenvectors.

Temporal relations can be written as

$$(\Delta \mathbf{a})_{t+1} = (\Delta \mathbf{a})_t + w \cdot \mathbf{e}_{t+1} \tag{22.27}$$

$$\mathbf{Q}_{t+1} = \mathbf{U}_{t+1} \cdot (\Delta \mathbf{a})_{t+1} + \mathbf{v}_{t+1} \tag{22.28}$$

The term $w \cdot \mathbf{e}_{t+1}$ remains the same as in Equation 22.18, because temporal correlation is the same, but the noise term $\mathbf{v}$ now represents the random error of Equation 22.26.

Equations 22.20 to 22.23, with $\mathbf{a}$ replaced by $\Delta \mathbf{a}$, $\mathbf{b}$ replaced by $\mathbf{Q}$ and $\mathbf{D}$ replaced by $\mathbf{U}$ provide the best estimate of the 3-D motion of each node.

### 22.4.6 3-D Flexible Motion Compensation

After the procedure described in the previous section, a 3-D motion vector was assigned to every node of the 3-D model. Using this information, the 3-D model may be updated, and the projected views of the next frame may be found. More specifically, each node of the 3-D model is governed by the following equation:

$$\mathbf{P}_{i,t+1} = \mathbf{R}_i \, \mathbf{P}_{i,t} + \mathbf{T}_i,$$

where $\mathbf{R}_i$ is of the form of Equation 22.11, $\mathbf{T}_i$ is of the form of Equation 22.12, and both are derived from $\mathbf{a}_i$ calculated in the previous section. The 3-D flexible motion vector of each node is given by

$$\mathbf{S}_{i,t} = \mathbf{P}_{i,t+1} - \mathbf{P}_{i,t}$$

In order to assign a 3-D motion vector to every 3-D point, we use the barycentric coordinates of this point. If $\mathbf{P} = (x, y, z)$ is a point on the triangular patch $\widehat{P_1 P_2 P_3} = \{(x_1, y_1, z_1), (x_2, y_2, z_2), (x_3, y_3, z_3)\}$, then the 3-D flexible motion vector of this point is given by

$$\mathbf{S}_t = \mathbf{S}_{1,t} \, g_1(x, y) + \mathbf{S}_{2,t} \, g_2(x, y) + \mathbf{S}_{3,t} \, g_3(x, y) \tag{22.29}$$

The functions $g_i(x, y)$ are the barycentric coordinates of $(x, y, z)$ relative to the triangle, and they are given by $g_i(x, y) = Area(A_i)/Area(\widehat{P_1 P_2 P_3})$, where $Area(A_i)$ is the area of the triangle having as vertices the point $(x, y, z)$ and two of the vertices of $\widehat{P_1 P_2 P_3}$ excluding $P_i$. Each view at the next frame can be reconstructed using

$$I_{c,\, t+1}(p_{c,\, t+1}) = I_{c,\, t}(p_{c,\, t})$$

where $I$ is the intensity of each projected view, and $p_{c,t}$, $p_{c,t+1}$ are the 2-D projected points of $\mathbf{P}_t$, $\mathbf{P}_{t+1}$ using camera $c = left, top, right$ in the camera model equations.

It can be seen from the above discussion that the only parameters with transmission that is necessary for the reconstructing of all but the first frame in each GOP are the 3-D flexible motion vectors of each node of the 3-D wireframe. For the coding of these vectors, a simple DPCM technique is used, coding only the differences between successive nodes. In the beginning of each GOP, the model geometry and the projected views must also be transmitted. For the coding of images at the beginning of each GOP, intraframe techniques are used, as in Reference [18].

### 22.4.7 Experimental Results for Real Multiview Images

The proposed model-based coding was evaluated for the coding of left, top, and right channels of a real multiview image sequence. The interlaced multiview videoconference sequence "Ludo" of size $720 \times 576$ was used.[4] All experiments were performed at the top field of the interlaced sequence, thus using images of size $720 \times 288$.

The 3-D model was formed using the techniques described in Reference [19]. A regular wireframe was first created covering the full size of the top view image, as shown in Figure 22.7a. Only triangles lying on the foreground object (body and desk of "Ludo") were then retained, providing a coarse adaptation to the foreground object Figure 22.7b. The wireframe was then finely adapted to the foreground object Figure 22.7c, and using depth information, the 2-D wireframe was reprojected to the 3-D space, giving the 3-D model (Figure 22.7d).

---

[4] This sequence was prepared by the CCETT for use in the PANORAMA ACTS project.

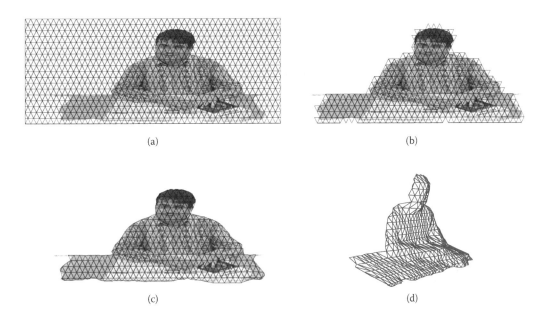

(a)                                          (b)

(c)                                          (d)

**FIGURE 22.7**
(a) Regular wireframe covering the full size of the middle view, (b) coarse adaptation with triangles covering only the foreground object, (c) fine adaption to the foreground object, and (d) the 3-D model produced by reprojecting the 2-D wireframe to the 3-D space.

Because the geometry of the 3-D model is known, the 3-D motion of each triangle can be estimated using the algorithm in Section 22.4.1. The 3-D motion of each triangle was then used as an input to the flexible motion estimation algorithm described in Section 22.4.4. Because a 3-D motion vector is assigned to each node of the wireframe, succeeding frames can be reconstructed using only the 3-D model, the 3-D motion, and the frames of the previous time instant (Section 22.4.6). The flexible motion estimation was performed between frames 0 and 3 (because differences between frames 0 and 1 were negligible). The original top view of frame 0 can be seen in Figure 22.7a to Figure 22.7d and the original left, top and right views of frame 3 are, respectively, shown in Figure 22.8a, Figure 22.8c and Figure 22.8e. The reconstructed left, top, and right views are shown in Figure 22.8b, Figure 22.8d, and Figure 22.8f. The frame differences between the original frames 0 and 3 are given in Figure 22.9a, Figure 22.9c, and Figure 22.9c for all views, while the frame differences between the original frame 3 and reconstructed frame 3 are shown in Figure 22.8b, Figure 22.8d, and Figure 22.8f. As seen, the reconstructed images are very close to original frame 3. The performance of the algorithm was also tested in terms of PSNR, giving an improvement of approximately 4 dB for all views, as compared to the PSNR between frame 0 and 3.

The proposed algorithm was also tested for the coding of a sequence of frames at 10 frames/sec. The model adaptation procedures were applied only at the beginning of each GOP. Each GOP consists of ten frames. The first frame of each GOP was transmitted using intraframe coding techniques. For the rigid 3-D motion estimation of each triangle and for the flexible 3-D motion estimation of each node, between first and second frames in a GOP, the techniques described in Sections 22.4.1 and 22.4.4, respectively, were used. For the rigid 3-D motion estimation of each triangle and for the flexible 3-D motion estimation of each node between subsequent frames, the Kalman filtering approach of Sections 22.4.2

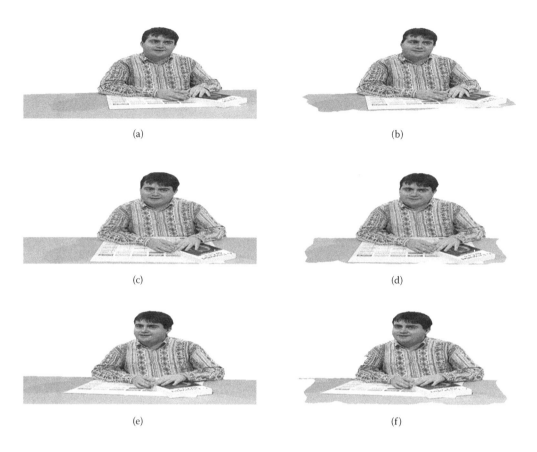

(a)                                                            (b)

(c)                                                            (d)

(e)                                                            (f)

**FIGURE 22.8**
(a,c,e) Original left, top, and right views of frame 3. (b, d, f) Reconstructed left, top, and right views of frame 3.

and 22.4.5 was used. The only parameters that need be transmitted in this case are the 3-D flexible motion vector of each node. The methodology developed in this paper allows left, top, and right images to be reconstructed using the same 3-D flexible motion vectors, thus achieving considerable bitrate savings. The coding algorithm requires a bitrate of 64.4 kbps and produces better image quality compared to a correspondingly simple block matching motion-estimation algorithm. For the block matching scheme, only the first frame of each group of frames was transmitted using intraframe coding. The second frame was reconstructed from the first one using the estimated flexible motion vectors between the first and the second frames, and this procedure was continued for the rest of the group of frames using each previously reconstructed frame for the estimation of the next one. The bitrate required by this scheme with a $16 \times 16$ block size was 68.5 kbps.

In order to demonstrate the benefits of the Kalman filtering approach, we also estimated motion between consequent frames without taking into account the motion information of previous frames. More specifically, for the rigid 3-D motion estimation of each triangle and for the flexible 3-D motion estimation of each node, between all subsequent frames, the techniques described in Sections 22.4.1 and 22.4.4, respectively, were used.

Figure 22.10a to Figure 22.10c show the resulting image quality for every reconstructed frame. The block-based scheme is compared with our approach, with and without use of the Kalman filter, for the left, top, and right views, respectively. As can be seen from the plots,

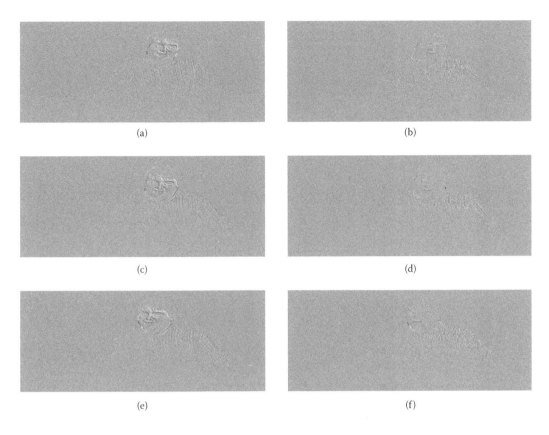

**FIGURE 22.9**
(a, c, e) Difference between original frames 0 and 3 (left, top, and right views, respectively). (b, d, f) Difference between original frame 3 and reconstructed frame 3 (left, top, and right views, respectively).

the proposed approach performs better with the use of Kalman filters. We also note that the additional computational overhead resulting from the use of the Kalman filter, is negligible. The results also demonstrate the robustness of the algorithm for noisy inputs, because the experiments involve real image sequences, where the initial 2-D vector fields are estimated by a simple block-matching algorithm without any special post- or preprocessing, and as a result, they contain many noisy estimates.

## 22.5 Conclusion

In this chapter, we discussed the basic principles for the coding of two- and three-dimensional color image sequences. Initially, we briefly presented the color spaces used for color representation and explained their main attributes. Next, we described the main components of a video coding system. Specifically, we described the scalar quantizers that are employed by most video coding systems. Moreover, we studied the removal of temporal redundancy between successive frames using motion estimation and compensation. Particular emphasis was given to block matching, the most popular block-based technique for motion estimation and compensation.

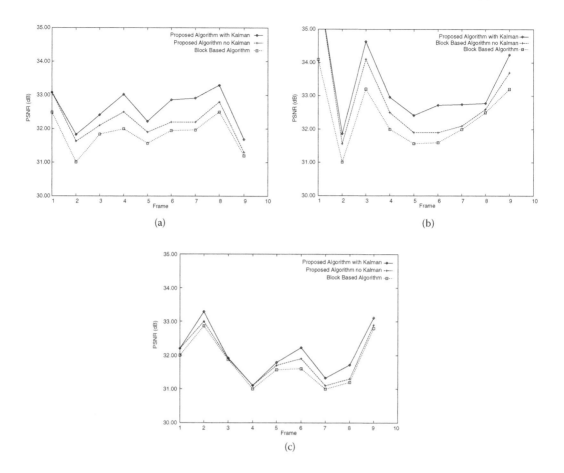

**FIGURE 22.10**
(a) PSNR of each frame of the left channel of the proposed algorithm, compared with flexible motion estimation without Kalman filtering and with the block-matching scheme with a block size of $16 \times 16$ pixels. (b) PSNR of each frame of the top channel. (c) PSNR of each frame of the right channel.

Subsequently, recent advances, such as the latest video coding standard H.264/AVC, were described in detail. The H.264/AVC standard incorporates many novelties, which significantly improve the coding efficiency. In particular, intra- and inter prediction techniques for the generation of low energy residuals were described, along with the integer transform, a variant of the discrete cosine transform, which is used to remove the spatial correlation of the residual signal. In addition, the two entropy coding methods, CAVLC and CABAC, for transmitting the quantized transform coefficients, were analyzed. The section concludes with a brief introduction to FREXT, a recent amendment to H.264/AVC, and a short description of its extensions related to color representation and coding.

Finally, we described in detail a flexible model-based 3-D motion-estimation methodology for multiview image sequence coding. Rigorous parametric models were defined for rigid 3-D motion estimation, which is modeled using a 3-D linear model with three rotation and three translation parameters. A Kalman filter was applied for the 3-D rigid estimation parameters at every time instant. The presented methodology was validated experimentally.

# References

[1] Y. Wang, J. Ostermann, and Y. Zhang, *Video Processing and Communications*, Prentice Hall, Upper Saddle River, NJ, 2002.

[2] K.R. Rao and J. Hwang, *Techniques and Standards for Image, Video, and Audio Coding*, Prentice Hall, Upper Saddle River, NJ, 1996.

[3] R.M. Gray and D.L. Neuhoff, Quantization, *IEEE Trans. on Inf. Theory*, 44, pp. 2325–2383, October 1998.

[4] A. Nostratinia, New kernels for fast mesh-based motion estimation, *IEEE Trans. on Circuits and Syst.*, 11, 40–51, January 2001.

[5] A. Mayache, T. Eude, and H. Cherifi, A comparison of image quality models and metrics based on human visual sensitivity, in *Proceedings of the International Conference on Image Processing (ICIP'98)*, Vol. 3, pp. 409–413, Chicago, IL, October 1998.

[6] ISO/IEC JTC1, *Information Technology — Coding of Audio-Visual Objects — Part 10: Advanced Video Coding. Final Draft International Standard.* ISO/IEC FDIS 14 496–10, 2003.

[7] T. Wiegand, G.J. Sullivan, G. Bjntgaard, and A. Luthra, Overview of the h.264/avc video coding standard, *IEEE Trans. Circuits and Syst. for Video Technol.*, 13, 560–576, July 2003.

[8] H. Malvar, A. Halappuro, M. Karczewicz, and L. Kerofsky, Low-complexity transform and quantization in h.264/avc, *IEEE Trans. Circuits and Syst. for Video Technol.*, 13, 598–603, July 2003.

[9] G. Bjontegaard and K. Lillevold, Context-Adaptive VLC Coding of Coefficients, Technical report ID 6502, JVT Document JVT-C028, Fairfax, VA, May 2002.

[10] D. Marpe, H. Schwarz, and T.Wiegand, Context-adaptive binary arithmetic coding in the h.264/avc video compression standard, *IEEE Trans. on Circuits and Syst. for Video Technol.*, 13, 620–636, July 2003.

[11] G.J. Sullivan, P. Topiwala, and A. Luthra, The h.264/avc advanced video coding standard: Overview and introduction to the fidelity range extensions, in *SPIE Conference on Applications of Digital Image Processing XXVII*, Vol. 5558, August 2004, Denver, CO, pp. 53–74.

[12] Y. Yakimovski and R. Cunningham, A System for Extracting 3D Measurements from a Stereo Pair of TV Cameras, *CGVIP*, 7, 195–210, 1978.

[13] G. Adiv, Determining three-dimensional motion and structure from optical flow generated by several moving objects, *IEEE Trans. on Patt. Anal. and Machine Intelligence*, 7, 384–401, July 1985.

[14] S.S. Sinha and B.G. Schunck, A two-stage algorithm for discontinuity-preserving surface reconstruction, *IEEE Trans. on PAMI*, 14, 36–55, January 1992.

[15] L. Falkenhagen, 3D object-based depth estimation from stereoscopic image sequences, in *Proceedings of International Workshop on Stereoscopic and 3D Imaging '95*, pp. 81–86, Santorini, Greece, September 1995.

[16] A.K. Jain, *Fundamentals of Digital Image Processing*, Prentice Hall, Englewood Cliffs, NJ, 1986.

[17] A.P. Sage and J.L. Melsa, *Estimation Theory with Applications to Communications and Control*, McGraw-Hill, New York, 1971.

[18] MPEG-2, Generic Coding of Moving Pictures and Associated Audio Information, technical report, ISO/IEC 13818, 1996.

[19] I. Kompatsiaris, D. Tzovaras, and M.G. Strintzis, Flexible 3d motion estimation and tracking for multiview image sequence coding, *Signal Process.: Image Commun. J., Spec. Issue on 3D Video Technol.*, 14, 95–110, November 1998.

# 23

## Color-Based Video Shot Boundary Detection

Costas Cotsaces, Zuzana Cernekova, Nikos Nikolaidis, and Ioannis Pitas

## CONTENTS

## 23.1 Introduction

One of the defining characteristics of video is its temporal nature. This is what gives it its semantic richness, as semantic content can vary enormously over the duration of a video sequence. Conversely, exactly because of the variability of video semantic content with respect to time, any attempt to exact semantics from the video necessitates the temporal segmentation of the video. The basic concepts and principles that are involved in the temporal segmentation of digital video are derived from the art of creating motion pictures. There, directors and film editors perceptually segment their motion pictures into a hierarchy of scenes and shots. Scenes (also called story units) are a concept that is much older than motion pictures, ultimately originating in the theater. Traditionally, a scene is a continuous sequence that is temporally and spatially cohesive in the real world, but not necessarily cohesive in the projection of the real world on film. Shots originate with the invention of motion cameras and are defined as the longest continuous sequence that originates from a single camera take, which is what the camera images in an uninterrupted run, as shown in Figure 23.1. A video (or film) is completely and disjointly segmented into a sequence of scenes, which are subsequently segmented into a sequence of shots. Finally, frames are the most basic temporal component of a film or video.

Temporal segmentation of video is often a necessary first step for many video processing tasks. For example, a video index is much smaller if it refers to the video segments rather than single frames. Likewise, the limits of video segments provide convenient jump points for video browsing. Video segmentation into coherent segments (especially shots) also enables the extraction of a larger range of video features, for example, camera and object motion patterns. Other applications are the extraction of condensed representations for video, which is often based on extracting keyframes from shots, and fingerprinting, where shots provide an effectively invariant basis on which to make the comparison between two videos.

At the current moment, the automatic segmentation of a video into scenes is considered to be very difficult or even intractable. One reason for this is the subjectivity of this task, because it depends on human cultural conditioning, professional training, and intuition. Another reason is its focus on real-world actions and temporal and spatial configurations of objects and people, requiring the ability to extract semantic meaning from images, a task well known to be extremely difficult for computers.

In contrast, video segmentation into shots is exactly defined and also characterized by distinctive features of the video stream. This stems from the fact that changes within a shot can arise from two factors: changes in the camera parameters or changes in the physical scene being captured. Changes in the captured physical scene are generally localized only in parts of the frame and are usually due to object motion. In addition, both the camera parameters and the captured physical scene change continuously in time. The above ensure that changes between adjacent video frames within the same shot are temporally continuous or spatially localized, and that quantities like texture, motion, and color distribution are likely to be continuous over time. On the other hand, the camera parameters and the physical scenes of two distinct shots do not exhibit any specific continuity. Thus, adjacent frames that belong to different shots do not exhibit any content continuity over time. Therefore, in principle, the detection of a shot change between two adjacent frames simply requires computation of an appropriate continuity or similarity metric.

Not all shot changes are abrupt. Using motion picture terminology, changes between shots can belong to the following categories:

- *Cut*: This is the classic abrupt change case, where one frame belongs to the disappearing shot and the next one to the appearing shot.

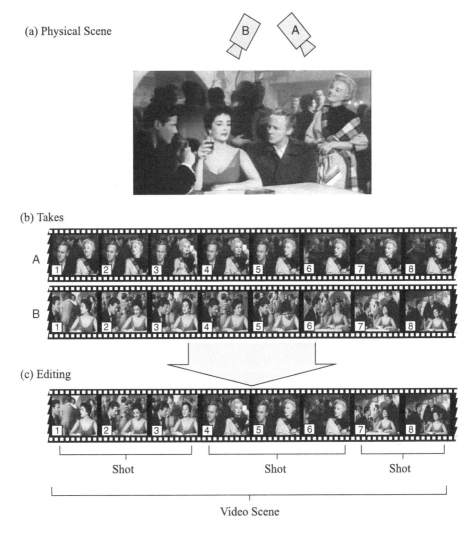

**FIGURE 23.1**
Sketch of scenes and shots as defined by the film industry: (a) imaged objects comprising a *scene*, (b) *takes* imaged by different cameras, and (c) *shots* created from takes.

- *Dissolve* (Figure 23.2a): In this case, the last few frames of the disappearing shot overlap temporally with the first few frames of the appearing shot. During the overlap, the intensity of the disappearing shot gradually decreases from normal to zero (fade out), while that of the appearing shot gradually increases from zero to normal (fade in).
- *Fade* (Figure 23.2b): Here, first the disappearing shot fades out into a blank frame, and then the blank frame fades in into the appearing shot. In other words, a fade is like a dissolve without temporal overlap between the two shots.
- *Wipe* (Figure 23.2c and Figure 23.2d): This is actually a set of shot change techniques, where the appearing and disappearing shots coexist in different spatial regions of the intermediate video frames, and the area occupied by the former shot grows until it entirely replaces the latter. The movement may be vertical, horizontal, diagonal, or from multiple directions. This category includes various

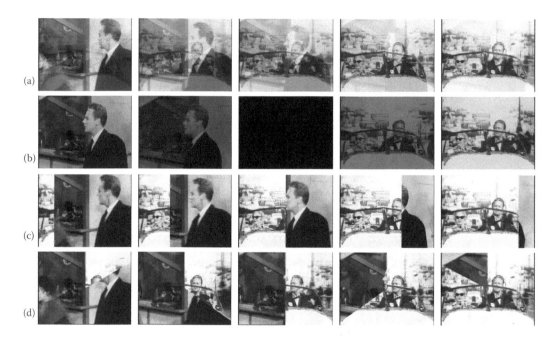

**FIGURE 23.2** (See color insert.)
Examples of gradual transitions: (a) dissolve, (b) fade, (c) a classical wipe, and (d) a wipe of the "curtain" variety.

transition techniques like push, slide, stretch, door, flip, drop, grill, page turn, dither, mosaic, iris, and others.

- *Other transition types*: There is a multitude of inventive special effects techniques used in motion pictures that usually take a feature from one shot and merge or morph it into the next one. These are, in general, very rare and difficult to detect.

Hampapur et al. [1] classify the above categories more rigorously, depending on the spatial and chromatic/luminance constancy of the shots. Let $S(x, y, t)$ be the video, $S_1(x, y, t)$, $t \in [0, T_1]$ the disappearing shot, and $S_2(x, y, t)$, $t \in [0, T_2]$ the appearing shot. Then the resulting classes are the following:

- *Identity class*, where the shots remain both spatially and chromatically unchanged:

$$S(x, y, t) = (1 - u(t - t_{change}))S_1(x, y, t) + u(t - t_{change})S_2(x, y, t)$$

Only cuts belong to this class.

- *Spatial class*, where the position/occlusion of the shots are altered but their color/luminance are not:

$$S(x, y, t) = (1 - u(t - t_{change}(x, y)))S_1(f_{1x}(x, y, t), f_{1y}(x, y, t), t)$$
$$+ u(t - t_{change}(x, y))S_2(f_{2x}(x, y, t), f_{2y}(x, y, t), t)$$

This is essentially the same as the wipe category.

- *Chromatic class*, where color/luminance are altered but their position is not:

$$S(x, y, t) = (1 - u(t - t_{end}))f_1(S_1(x, y, t), t) + u(t - t_{start})f_2(S_2(x, y, t), t)$$

It includes fades and dissolves.

- *Spatio chromatic class*, where no special consistency with the constituent shots is observed. This contains the "other transitions" category.

A number of different surveys on the subject have been published in the last decade, all before 2002. The work by Lienhart [2] analyzes different basic algorithmic strategies for cut and dissolve detection. In his previous work [3], four specific shot boundary detection algorithms are compared in depth. Koprinska and Carrato [4] summarize a great volume of previous work, focusing especially on shot change detection in MPEG compressed video data, while Ford et al. [5] focus on the description and performance comparison of the classic features and metrics commonly used for shot change detection. Finally, Gargi et al. [6] focus exclusively on histogram-based methods, exploring their performance when using different color spaces and histogram difference metrics.

Color information is often used for shot boundary detection. Some of the most commonly used features are the ones based on color, such as the color statistics in a frame, or its color histogram. There are two reasons for the popularity of this approach. First, color is a special characteristic of a physical scene. Second, it varies more smoothly over time than other features, because color content rarely changes as a result of the action that occurs in the physical scene. In this chapter, we will discuss the basic principles of shot boundary detection and provide a review of recent algorithms, with emphasis on color.

This chapter is organized in the following way. First, in Section 23.2, we present a typology of the various types of shot boundary detection algorithms found in the literature. Then, in Sections 23.3 and 23.4, we review several important contributions to the field in recent years. Section 23.4 focuses on the TREC Video Evaluation. We then compare the performance of the above methods in Section 23.5. In Sections 23.6 and 23.7, we review in detail two robust shot boundary detection algorithms that we proposed. These can be optionally combined, as described in Section 23.8. Finally, in Section 23.9, we present some conclusions.

## 23.2 Typology of Shot Boundary Detection Algorithms

Shot boundary detection algorithms work by extracting one or more features from a video frame or a subset of it, called a *region of interest* (ROI). An algorithm can then use different methods to detect a shot change from these features. Because there are many different ways the above components can be combined, we have chosen not to provide a hierarchical decomposition of different classes of algorithms. Instead, we present below the different choices that can be made for each component. These can then be combined to design a shot detection algorithm.

### 23.2.1 Features Used for Shot Boundary Detection

Almost all shot change detection algorithms reduce the large dimensionality of the video domain by extracting a small number of features from one or more regions of interest in each video frame. The simplest of such features is the average grayscale luminance [7], [8] in a ROI, but it has problems in many cases, because its dimensionality is too low to provide adequate discriminance between shots and is also susceptible to illumination changes within a shot. A common alternative is the use of average color values [9], [10], [11], which have a larger range of possible values and are more discriminant. In addition, they make it possible to achieve illumination invariance by using appropriate channels of certain color spaces. For example, it is possible to use the $H$ and $S$ channels of the HSV color space, or the $a*$ and $b*$ components in the L*a*b* color space.

However, because different shots can contain similar averages of color values, color histograms are often selected as a feature in order to give a better representation of the distribution of color in a frame [12], [13]. By varying the number of bins, it is possible to fine-tune the dimensionality of the histogram. In color-based shot boundary detection, it is common to use either a set of one-dimensional histograms, for example, $H_R(i)$, $H_G(i)$, $H_B(i)$ for the RGB color space, or a single two- or three-dimensional histogram, for example, $H_{HS}(i, j)$ for the HSV color space.

Other features that can be used are image edges [14], [15], [16] and frequency transform coefficients (e.g., from DFT, DCT, or wavelets) [17]. Of course, it is also possible to combine different features, as in References [18], [19], [20], [21], and [22].

The size of the region from which individual features are extracted plays an important role in the overall performance of shot change detection. A small region tends to reduce detection invariance with respect to motion, while a large region might lead to missed transitions between similar shots. The various possible choices of the region used for the extraction of a single feature are a single pixel (e.g., luminance of a single pixel [23] or edge strength at a single pixel [14]); a rectangular block [7], [9], [10], [11], [17], [18]; an arbitrarily shaped region [24]; and the entire frame [13], [21]. Obviously, not all types of ROIs make sense for all types of features (e.g., a histogram is meaningless for a single pixel).

### 23.2.2 Feature Similarity Metrics

In order to evaluate discontinuity between frames based on the selected features, an appropriate similarity/dissimilarity metric needs to be chosen. Assuming that a frame $i$ is characterized by $K$ scalar features $F_i(k)$, $k = 1, \ldots, K$, the most traditional choice for finding its distance from frame $j$ is to use the $L_n$ norm:

$$D_{L_n}(i, j) = \left( \sum_{k=1}^{K} |F_i(k) - F_j(k)|^n \right)^{1/n} \tag{23.1}$$

An example of the above is squared image difference, where $F(k)$ are the pixels of the (usually subsampled) image, and $n = 2$. Another choice is to use a weighted metric:

$$D_{weighted}(i, j) = \left( \sum_{m=1}^{K} \sum_{k=1}^{K} W(k, m) |F_i(k) - F_j(m)|^n \right)^{1/n} \tag{23.2}$$

In the case of histograms, a number of specialized similarity measures are used, for example, the $L_1$ metric, as described above, where we substitute the histogram bins $H_i(k)$ of frame $i$ for the feature vector $F_i(k)$. Sometimes a locally weighted version is used, similar to Equation 23.2 but with $W(k, m) = 0$ when $|k - m| > d$, where $d$ is a small number [4]. Another commonly used measure is the chi-square ($\chi^2$) metric:

$$D_{\chi^2}(i, j) = \sum_{k=1}^{K} \frac{(H_i(k) - H_j(k))^2}{H_i(k)}$$

A rather different measure is *histogram intersection* [25]:

$$D_{int}(i, j) = 1 - \frac{\sum_{k=1}^{K} \min(H_i(k) - H_j(k))}{\sum_{k=1}^{K} \max(H_i(k) - H_j(k))}$$

Additionally, the computation of all the above similarity measures can be preceded by the equalization of the histograms used, in order to reduce the disproportionate effect that

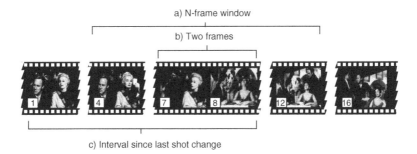

**FIGURE 23.3**
Possible choices of temporal window for shot detection between frames 7 and 8.

less prevalent colors in the image have on the value of the metric, due to the large number of bins that are allotted to them.

Another important aspect of shot boundary detection algorithms is the temporal window that is used to perform shot change detection, as illustrated in Figure 23.3. In general, the objective is to select a temporal window that contains a representative amount of video activity. Thus, a transition can be detected using the features in two frames [20], [26], [27], [28]; within an $N$-frame window [9], [13], [21], [22]; or in the interval that has been processed since the last detected transition [11], [14], [18], [29]. In addition, it is possible to take the characteristics of the entire video (or at least the part of the video that has been processed) into consideration when detecting a shot change, as in Reference [21]. The problem in this case is that the video can have great variability between shots, making the use of global statistics precarious.

Having defined a feature (or a set of features) computed on one or more ROIs for each frame, a shot change detection algorithm needs to detect where these exhibit discontinuity. This can be done by using a static threshold [14], [29] or an adaptive threshold [8], [17], [18] over the discontinuity metric. Alternatively, it is possible to model the pattern of shot transitions and, presupposing specific probability distributions for the feature difference metrics in each shot, to perform optimal *a posteriori* shot change estimation [9], [11]. Finally, the problem can be formulated as a classification task, where frames are classified into two classes, namely, "shot change" and "no shot change," and then train a classifier to distinguish between the two classes [21].

## 23.3 Survey of Shot Boundary Detection Algorithms

In the following, some of the more interesting recent publications on the subject of shot boundary detection are reviewed. The focus is placed on methods that utilize color information. However, we should note that many of the presented methods use other types of features in addition to color. The publications reviewed below were chosen either because they introduce novel components or because they present the most advanced variant of an established method.

### 23.3.1 Classifier Trained by Dissolve Synthesizer

This approach, developed by Lienhart [21], focuses on detecting dissolves. This is achieved by a neural network (or any type of learning classifier), which is used to detect possible dissolves at multiple temporal scales. The features used by the classifier are either color histograms or edge-based image contrast. The results of the classifier are then merged using a winner-take-all strategy. A significant novelty of this method is that the classifier is trained using a *dissolve synthesizer* that creates artificial dissolves from any available set of video sequences. Performance is shown to be superior to the simple edge-based methods commonly used for dissolve detection (e.g., Reference [30]), although the videos used for experimental verification are nonstandard.

### 23.3.2   Temporal Splitting and Merging

The approach presented by Janvier et al. [31] performs shot boundary detection in three independent steps. First, the existence of a cut is detected by estimating the probability that a shot boundary exists between two frames. The various probability functions are derived experimentally, and their parameters are computed from training data. Then the derived "shots" are further segmented into pieces that exhibit greater continuity using a linear model of homogeneous segments and applying dynamic programming with a minimum message length criterion to fit this model. In order to get acceptable results in the task of shot boundary detection, these segments are then merged using two-class $K$-means clustering. This operates on color histograms and mutual information of frames [32] within a window around the segment change and classifies them into "shot change" and "no shot change" categories. The main strength of the work is the statistically robust method for temporal segmentation, which, however, results in segments that are smaller than a shot. Its main problem is that the criterion for segment merging is heuristic and also inappropriate for long transitions. The authors have run their experiments on the AIM video corpus [33].

### 23.3.3   Dual Classifier

Qi et al. [19] use two binary classifiers trained with manually labeled data: one for separating cuts from noncuts and one for separating abrupt from gradual cuts. These are either $K$-nearest-neighbor classifiers, Bayesian networks, or support vector machines. The gradual/abrupt classifier input is preprocessed by wavelet smoothing. The input of the classifiers is a vector composed of whole-frame and block YUV color histogram differences from 30 neighboring frames, camera motion estimations derived from MPEG2 features, and frame blackness. The value of this work lies in the comparison of the different types of classifiers for the task and the fact that the experimental results are on the standard TRECVID 2001 data. The optimal cumulative recall precision is obtained using $K$-nearest-neighbor classifiers.

### 23.3.4   Coupled Markov Chains

The method proposed by Sánchez and Binefa [18] models each shot as a coupled Markov chain (CMC), encoding the probabilities of temporal change of a set of features. Here, hue and motion from $16 \times 16$ image blocks are used. For each frame, two CMCs are computed, one from the shot start up to and including that frame and one from that frame and the next one. Then the Kullback–Leibler divergence between the two distributions is compared with a threshold, which is adaptively (but heuristically) computed from the mean and standard deviation of the changes encoded in the first CMC. The fact that the dynamics of the disappearing shot are inherently taken into consideration for detecting shot changes gives strength and elegance to this method. However, the assumption made by the author — that these dynamics are consistently different between shots — and the anticipated performance remain to be proven, especially because the data volume used for verification was very small (less than 20 transitions), and the data were not particularly representative.

### 23.3.5 Gaussian Random Distribution Modeling

The statistical approach presented by Lelescu and Schonfeld [11] is designed to operate on MPEG-compressed videos. The luminance and chrominance for each block in every $I$ and $P$ frame is extracted, and then PCA is performed on the resulting feature vectors. The eigenvectors are computed based only on the $M$ first frames of each shot. A Gaussian random distribution is used to model resulting vectors, and its mean and covariance matrix are estimated, also from the $M$ first frames of each shot. What is interesting about this method is that a change statistic is estimated for each new frame by a maximum likelihood methodology, the generalized likelihood ratio algorithm. If this statistic exceeds an experimentally determined threshold, a new shot is started. A number of videos originating from news, music clips, sports, and other video types, where gradual transitions are common, have been used by the authors to test the algorithm. The greatest problem of this algorithm is that the extraction of the shot characteristics (eigenspace, mean, and covariance) happens at its very beginning (first $M$ frames). This means that in the case of long and nonhomogeneous shots, like the ones common in motion pictures, the values calculated at the start of the shot would be irrelevant at its end. This is also demonstrated by the fact that the test videos used have a short average shot duration. Finally, it must be noted that the subject of the work is not *scene* but *shot* change detection, despite the authors' claims.

### 23.3.6 Color Anglogram and Latent Semantic Indexing

Zhao and Grosky [28] first split each frame into blocks and computed the average hue and saturation for each. Then they computed, for every pair of hue and saturation values, the angles of the Delaunay triangulation of the blocks that have these values. The histogram of the angles of the triangulation was then used as a feature vector, with a dimensionality (for each frame) of 720 (10 hue values × 36 angle bins + 10 saturation values × 36 angle bins = 720). The option of applying latent semantic indexing (LSI) is also explored. This is essentially a SVD dimensionality reduction of the frame vectors, which is followed by normalization and frequency-based weighting. Two thresholds are used for shot change detection. The first is used to detect a shot change, which happens if the magnitude of the feature vector difference (histogram, anglogram, or LSI of either) exceeds this threshold. If the difference is between the two thresholds, then the shot change is verified semiautomatically. Experiments were run on a set of eight videos containing 255 cuts and 60 gradual transitions. The application of the color anglogram and of LSI to the shot boundary detection problem have not been tried before, and it is clear that they present an improvement over the classic histogram method. It is not shown that the color anglogram at least would function well in cases where color information alone is insufficient to detect a shot transition. However, the biggest drawback of this work is the necessity of user interaction for the detection of gradual transitions.

### 23.3.7 Gradual Shot Change Boundary Refinement

The work of Heng and Ngan [34] addresses the novel task of the accurate detection of the exact gradual transition limits, when its approximate location is given. They derive a change indicator from each specific frame which is either the mean of color difference, the difference of color means, the difference of color histograms, or the difference of luminance histograms. This indicator function is approximately constant during each shot but becomes a ramp during a transition. They heuristically estimate the slope of the ramp and the mean deviation of the indicator in the parts of the shots adjacent to a transition. These are then used to probabilistically find the transition boundaries. With the optimal configuration, their method gives an average transition boundary location error as 10% of the length of the transition.

### 23.3.8 Joint Probability Image and Related Statistics

Li et al. [26] define the joint probability image (JPI) of two frames as a matrix with a $(i, j)$ element that contains the probability that a pixel with color $i$ in the first image has color $j$ in the second image. The joint probability projection vector (JPPV) and the joint probability projection centroid (JPPC) are then defined as vector and scalar statistics of the JPI. It is observed that specific JPI patterns are associated with specific types of transition (dissolve, fade, dither). To detect shot changes, possible locations are first detected by using the JPPC, and then they are refined and validated by matching the JPPV with specific transition patterns. Results are given for a relatively small number of abrupt and gradual transitions. This method has obvious problems with large object or camera motion, a fact which is admitted by the authors.

### 23.3.9 Projection into Principal Component Eigenspace

A method that can function with any feature is presented by Liu and Chen [29], but it is tested by default on color histograms. A modified PCA algorithm is used on the part of each shot that has been processed, in order to extract its principal eigenspace. Two novel algorithms are presented to facilitate the incremental computation of the eigenspace and also to place greater weight on the most recent frames. A set of heuristics is used to compute these weights. A cut is detected when the difference between a frame and its projection into the eigenspace is above a static threshold. Experimental results, however, show only a small qualitative improvement over classical algorithms, except for a dramatic improvement in precision for very high recall rates.

### 23.3.10 Probabilistic Modeling of Discontinuities

A probabilistic algorithm for shot boundary detection is described by Hanjalic [9]. It is also accompanied by a thorough analysis of the shot boundary detection problem. The algorithm works by segmenting each video frame into blocks, and by extracting the average YUV color components from each block. Block similarity is used to match blocks between each pair of adjacent frames. The discontinuity value is then defined as the average difference between the color components in matching blocks. Abrupt transitions are detected by comparing adjacent frames, while gradual ones are detected by comparing frames that are apart by the minimum shot length. Manually labeled data are used for deriving the *a priori* likelihood functions of the discontinuity metric, but the choice of these functions is largely heuristic. Modeling the *a priori* probability of shot boundary detection conditional on the time from last shot boundary detection as a Poisson distribution was observed to produce good results. Then the shot boundary detection probability is refined with a heuristic derived from either the discontinuity value pattern (for cuts and fades) or from in-frame variances (for dissolves), in both cases, extracted from a temporal window around the current frame. Thus, in effect, a different detector is implemented for each transition type. In conclusion, although the proposed method claims to offer a rigorous solution to the shot boundary detection problem, it is still quite heuristic. Yet, the probabilistic analysis of the problem is valid and thorough. Additionally, experimental results are very satisfactory, being perfect for cuts and having good recall and precision for dissolves.

---

## 23.4   TREC Shot Boundary Detection Task

Because of the richness and variety of digital video content, the effective quantitative (and even qualitative) comparison of the results of different video-related algorithms is meaningless if they are derived from different video corpora. To alleviate this problem, the TREC Video Retrieval Evaluation[1] (*TRECVID*) was organized with the sponsorship of the National Institute of Standards and Technology of the United States and other organizations. Before the year 2003, it was a part ("track") of TREC (Text Retrieval Conference), but in 2003, it was first organized as a separate event (although still affiliated with TREC). The goal of TRECVID is not only to provide a common corpus of video data as a testbed for different algorithms but also to standardize and oversee their evaluation and to provide a forum for the comparison of the results. As for shot boundary detection, or "shot boundary determination," it is one of the four tasks that comprise TRECVID, the other three being story segmentation, high-level feature extraction, and shot search.

### 23.4.1   Description of the Evaluation Procedure

The test collection for the TRECVID 2005 shot boundary detection task was 12 videos lasting approximately 6 h and containing 744,604 frames and 4535 transitions, of which 2759 (60.8%) were cuts, 1382 (30.5%) were dissolves, 81 (1.8%) were fades, and 313 (6.9%) were other transition types. The transitions were determined manually and then used as a reference for the evaluation of the results of the participants' algorithms. Participants in the evaluation were allowed to submit up to ten versions of their algorithms for evaluation, in order to compensate for the effect of parameter choice on algorithm performance. Success of detection (recall and precision) was measured separately for cuts and for gradual transitions (which includes all transition types other than cuts). In addition, the localization accuracy of gradual transitions was evaluated, as was the computational performance of the algorithms.

### 23.4.2   Algorithms Participating in TRECVID

Below, we review the most important color-based contributions to the TRECVID shot boundary detection task. It should be noted that, in general, the contributors to TRECVID place greater importance on the quality and stability of their results than on the originality and the theoretical foundation of their methods.

#### 23.4.2.1   *Graph Partitioning and Support Vector Machines*

Some of the best results in the shot detection task were produced by Yuan et al. at Tsinghua University [35]. The color feature they use for all the stages of their algorithm are RGB histograms with 16 bins per channel. Their first step is to detect fades by finding dark frames, which are those that have their pixels gathered in the dimmest 1/4 of the color bins. The limits of detected fades are then found, overlapping fades are merged, and the fades are removed from the video. Cuts are detected by creating a graph with nodes that are

---

[1] URL: http://www-nlpir.nist.gov/projects/trecvid/.

frames and with links that are the histogram differences between frames and finding the partition cost at each frame. At the local minima of the partitioning cost, a feature vector is created from the partition costs of nearby frames and is fed to a support vector machine (SVM) classifier that decides if there is a cut. Gradual transitions are detected in exactly the same way as cuts, except that previously detected cuts are removed from consideration, the detection process is repeated for different temporal scales, and of course, the SVMs used for the decision are trained on gradual transitions instead of cuts.

### 23.4.2.2 Finite State Machine

The basic features used in the work by Amir et al. at IBM Research [22] are RGB color histograms, motion magnitude in 64 image blocks, gray-level thumbnails, and a number of global detectors (whether a frame is blank, etc.). Differences with a number of previous frames and an adaptive threshold based on average values in a 61-frame window are computed. These features are then fused by a completely heuristic finite-state machine. The system has only received minor modifications in the last 3 years, such as ignoring the color content of the bottom 20% of the frame in order not to be confused by subtitles.

### 23.4.2.3 Moving Query Windows

The work of Volkmer et al. at RMIT University [13] begins by defining the dissimilarity between frames as the distance of their three-dimensional HSV color histograms. Then, for each frame, it ranks adjacent frames by similarity and checks what proportion of the top half frames are before and after the current frame in this ranking (called preframes and postframes). A cut is detected when a frame with a large proportion of preframes is followed by a frame with a large proportion of postframes. To eliminate false cuts, the average distance between the frame and the top-ranked and bottom-ranked half-windows is also used. For gradual transitions, the ratio of the average distance of the frame and the postframes to the average distance between the frame and the preframes (called pre–post ratio) is used. The frames that are too close to the frame are excluded from the computation. The average distance between the frame and all frames in the window is also used. A transition start is detected when the pre–post ratio exceeds an adaptive lower threshold, and the transition end is detected when it falls below a (higher) upper threshold. The thresholds are adjusted according to a noise factor computed from the entire video. Additionally, if the sum of the area between the pre–post ratio curve and the upper threshold and the area between the average frame distance curve and its own adaptive upper threshold is too small, the transition is rejected. Detected gradual transitions are also verified by comparing the frames immediately before and after them.

### 23.4.2.4 Similarity Matrices and k-Nearest Neighbor Classifiers

The entry by Adcock et al. from the FX Palo Alto Laboratory [36] is a variant of the work of Qi et al. [19], which is reviewed in the previous section. Like in Reference [19], global and block-based YUV histograms are extracted from each frame, and the $\chi^2$ metrics between nearby frames is computed. But here the metrics are used to create two frame similarity matrices, which are then processed by correlating with a checkerboard kernel in order to detect structures similar to transitions. These are then fed into a k-nearest neighbor (kNN) classifier in order to detect transitions.

### 23.4.2.5 Motion-Compensated Frame Difference and Temporal Derivatives

Similar to previous CLIPS TREC systems, the system described by Quenot et al. [37] detects cuts by employing a subsampled image difference after motion compensation using optical flow. A heuristic flash detector is also incorporated. Additionally, a dissolve is detected if the metric of the first temporal derivative of the image is large while that of the second derivative is small over an appropriate number of frames.

## 23.5 Performance Review

The basic measures in detection and retrieval problems in general are recall, precision, and sometimes *temporal accuracy*. Recall, also known as the true positive function or sensitivity, corresponds to the ratio of correct experimental detections over the number of all true detections. Precision corresponds to the accuracy of the method considering false detections, and it is defined as the number of correct experimental detections over the number of all experimental detections. Therefore, if we denote by $D$ the shot transitions correctly detected by the algorithm, by $D_M$ the number of missed detections, that is, the transitions that should have been detected but were not, and by $D_F$ the number of false detections, that is, the transitions that should not have been detected but were, we have

$$\text{Recall} = \frac{D}{D + D_M} \tag{23.3}$$

$$\text{Precision} = \frac{D}{D + D_F} \tag{23.4}$$

Temporal accuracy reflects the temporal correctness of the detected results, that is, if a correctly identified transition location is correct. In Table 23.1, we summarize the results given by the authors of the algorithms we reviewed in Section 23.3. It should be noted that the results were not verified experimentally by us, that they depend on the authors' choice of video data and other factors, and that they are thus not directly comparable and are only included to give a rough estimation of performance. On the other hand, the results given in Table 23.2, referring to the methods reviewed in Section 23.4, are taken directly from TRECVID 2005 and are thus completely reliable. Because, as we noted above, each participant in TRECVID submitted up to ten different runs of their algorithm, we selected for the sake of brevity only the overall best run of their algorithm, chosen as the one that has the highest recall–precision score.

**TABLE 23.1**

Reported Results of Shot Boundary
Detection Algorithms

| Algorithm | Precision | Recall |
|---|---|---|
| Lienhart | 0.72 | 0.62 |
| Janvier | 0.76 | 0.97 |
| Qi et al. | 0.94 | 0.82 |
| Sánchez and Binefa | 1.00 | 0.81 |
| Lelescu and Schonfeld | 0.92 | 0.72 |
| Li et al. | 0.90 | 0.93 |
| Zhao and Grosky (cuts) | 0.91 | 0.83 |
| (gradual) | 0.88 | 0.73 |
| Liu and Chen | 1.00 | 0.75 |
| Hanjalic (cuts) | 0.79 | 0.83 |
| (dissolves) | 0.79 | 0.83 |

**TABLE 23.2**

Results of the TRECVID 2005 Shot Boundary
Detection Task

| | Cut | | Gradual | |
|---|---|---|---|---|
| Algorithm | Precision | Recall | Precision | Recall |
| Adcock et al. | 0.87 | 0.87 | 0.76 | 0.76 |
| Amir et al. | 0.89 | 0.93 | 0.72 | 0.84 |
| Quenot et al. | 0.91 | 0.91 | 0.79 | 0.73 |
| Volkmer et al. | 0.93 | 0.91 | 0.65 | 0.74 |
| Yuan et al. | 0.94 | 0.93 | 0.79 | 0.79 |

Having given a broad introduction to the problem of shot boundary detection and a short overview of work in the area, in the following three sections, we will provide a more detailed look at three algorithms that were developed by the authors.

## 23.6 Information Theory-Based Shot Cut/Fade Detection

The first presented approach to shot transition detection is based on the mutual information and the joint entropy between two consecutive video frames. Mutual information is a measure of the information transported from one frame to the next. It is used within the context of this method for detecting abrupt cuts, where the image intensity or color changes abruptly, leading to a low mutual information value. Joint entropy is used for detecting fades. The entropy measure produces good results, because it exploits the interframe information flow in a more compact way than a frame subtraction. A more detailed description of this work is presented in Reference [32].

### 23.6.1 Background and Definitions

Let $X$ be a discrete random variable with a set of possible outcomes $A_X = \{a_1, a_2, ..., a_N\}$, having probabilities $\{p_1, p_2, ..., p_N\}$, with $p_X(x = a_i) = p_i$, $p_i \geq 0$ and $\sum_{x \in A_X} p_X(x) = 1$. Entropy measures the information content or "uncertainty" of $X$, and it is given by the following [38], [39]:

$$H(X) = - \sum_{x \in A_X} p_X(x) \log p_X(x) \tag{23.5}$$

The *joint entropy* (JE) of discrete random variables $X$ and $Y$ is expressed as

$$H(X, Y) = - \sum_{x,y \in A_X, A_Y} p_{XY}(x, y) \log p_{XY}(x, y) \tag{23.6}$$

where $p_{XY}(x, y)$ is the joint probability density function. For two random variables $X$ and $Y$, the *conditional entropy* of $Y$ given $X$ is written $H(Y|X)$ and is defined as

$$H(Y|X) = \sum_{x \in A_X} p_X(x) H(Y|X = x) = - \sum_{x,y \in A_X, A_Y} p_{XY}(x, y) \log p_{XY}(x|y) \tag{23.7}$$

where $p_{XY}(x|y)$ denotes conditional probability. The conditional entropy $H(Y|X)$ is the uncertainty in $Y$ given knowledge of $X$. It specifies the amount of information that is gained by measuring a variable when already knowing another one, and it is very useful if we want to know if there is a functional relationship between two data sets.

The *mutual information* (MI) between the random variables $X$ and $Y$ is given by

$$I(X, Y) = - \sum_{x, y \in A_X, A_Y} p_{XY}(x, y) \log \frac{p_{XY}(x, y)}{p_X(x) p_Y(y)} \qquad (23.8)$$

and measures the amount of information conveyed by $X$ about $Y$. The relation between the mutual information and the joint entropy of random variables $X$ and $Y$ is the following:

$$I(X, Y) = H(X) + H(Y) - H(X, Y) \qquad (23.9)$$

where $H(X)$ and $H(Y)$ are the marginal entropies of $X$ and $Y$. Mutual information is a measure of the additional information that we obtain about one random variable when given another one:

$$I(X, Y) = H(X) - H(X|Y) \qquad (23.10)$$

According to Equation 23.9, mutual information not only provides us with a measure of correspondence between $X$ and $Y$ but also takes into account the information carried at their overlap. This way, mutual information decreases when the amount of shared information between $H(X)$ and $H(Y)$ is small. We can also see from Equation 23.10 that mutual information will decrease if $X$ carries no information about $Y$.

## 23.6.2 Shot Detection Using Entropy Measures

In this approach, the mutual information and the joint entropy between two successive frames is calculated separately for each of the RGB components. Let the pixel values in each color component vary from 0 to $N - 1$. At frame $\mathbf{f}_t$, three $N \times N$ matrices $\mathbf{C}^R_{t,t+1}$, $\mathbf{C}^G_{t,t+1}$ and $\mathbf{C}^B_{t,t+1}$ carrying information about the color value transitions between frames $\mathbf{f}_t$ and $\mathbf{f}_{t+1}$ are created. In the case of the $R$ component, the element $\mathbf{C}^R_{t,t+1}(i, j)$, with $0 \leq i \leq N - 1$ and $0 \leq j \leq N - 1$, corresponds to the probability that a pixel with value $i$ in frame $\mathbf{f}_t$ has value $j$ in frame $\mathbf{f}_{t+1}$. In other words, $\mathbf{C}^R_{t,t+1}(i, j)$ is the number of pixels that change from value $i$ in frame $\mathbf{f}_t$ to value $j$ in frame $\mathbf{f}_{t+1}$, divided by the number of pixels in the video frame. Following Equation 23.8, the mutual information $I^R_{t,t+1}$ of the transition from frame $\mathbf{f}_t$ to frame $\mathbf{f}_{t+1}$ for the $R$ component is expressed by

$$I^R_{t,t+1} = - \sum_{i=0}^{N-1} \sum_{j=0}^{N-1} \mathbf{C}^R_{t,t+1}(i, j) \log \frac{\mathbf{C}^R_{t,t+1}(i, j)}{\mathbf{C}^R_t(i) \mathbf{C}^R_{t+1}(j)} \qquad (23.11)$$

The total mutual information is defined as $I_{t,t+1} \triangleq I^R_{t,t+1} + I^G_{t,t+1} + I^B_{t,t+1}$. By using the same considerations, the joint entropy $H^R_{t,t+1}$ of the transition from frame $\mathbf{f}_t$ to frame $\mathbf{f}_{t+1}$, for the $R$ component, is given by

$$H^R_{t,t+1} = - \sum_{i=0}^{N-1} \sum_{j=0}^{N-1} \mathbf{C}^R_{t,t+1}(i, j) \log \mathbf{C}^R_{t,t+1}(i, j) \qquad (23.12)$$

The total joint entropy is defined as

$$H_{t,t+1} \triangleq H^R_{t,t+1} + H^G_{t,t+1} + H^B_{t,t+1} \qquad (23.13)$$

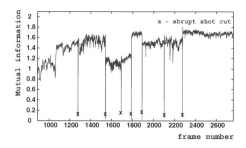

**FIGURE 23.4**
Time series of the mutual information from "ABC News" video sequence showing abrupt cuts (marked with "X").

### 23.6.2.1 Abrupt Shot Cut Detection

The existence of a shot cut between frames $f_t$ and $f_{t+1}$ is indicated by a small value of the mutual information $I_{t,t+1}$. An adaptive thresholding approach is employed to detect possible shot cuts. For every temporal window $W$ of size $N_W$ centered at $t_c$, a mutual information mean value $\bar{I}_{t_c}$ is calculated, without taking into account the value $I_{t_c,t_c+1}$ corresponding to time instant $t_c$ [40]:

$$\bar{I}_{t_c} = \frac{1}{N_W} \sum_{\substack{t \in W \\ t \neq t_c}} I_{t,t+1} \qquad (23.14)$$

In order to detect shot cuts, the time series of $\bar{I}_{t_c}$ is used. When the value $\bar{I}_{t_c} / I_{t_c,t_c+1}$ exceeds an experimentally chosen threshold $\epsilon_c$, a cut is detected. An example of abrupt cut detection using mutual information is illustrated in Figure 23.4.

### 23.6.2.2 Fade Detection

Mutual information decreases when little information is transmitted from one frame to another, a phenomenon that characterizes both cuts and fades. Thus, in order to efficiently distinguish fades from cuts, joint entropy Equation 23.13 is employed. Joint entropy measures the amount of information carried by the union of these frames. Thus, its value decreases only during fades, where a weak amount of interframe information is present. Therefore, only the values of $H_{t,t+1}$ that are below a threshold $\epsilon_f$ are examined. These values correspond to black frames. A pattern showing a fade out and a fade in is presented in Figure 23.5. The point where the joint entropy reaches a local minimum corresponds to the end point $t_e$ of the fade-out. At this point, the frame has become black and does not

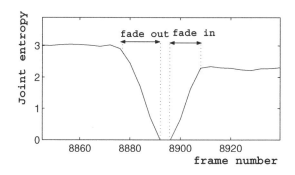

**FIGURE 23.5**
The joint entropy signal from "CNN News" video sequence showing a fade-out and fade-in to the next shot.

**TABLE 23.3**

The TREC2003 Video Sequences Used in Our Experiments

| Video | Frames | Cuts | Fade-ins | Fade-outs | Other Transitions |
|-------|--------|------|----------|-----------|-------------------|
| 6 debate videos | 125,977 | 230 | 0 | 0 | 0 |
| 4 CNN News | 209,978 | 1,287 | 57 | 57 | 464 |
| 4 ABC News | 206,144 | 1,269 | 64 | 69 | 553 |

provide any information. The next step consists of searching for the fade-out start point $t_s$ in the previous frames, using the following criterion:

$$\frac{H_{t_s,t_s+1} - H_{t_s-1,t_s}}{H_{t_s-1,t_s} - H_{t_s-2,t_s-1}} \geq T \tag{23.15}$$

where $T$ is a predefined threshold that guarantees that the joint entropy starts decreasing at the start point, $t_s$. The same procedure also applies for fade-in detection (with $t_s$ being detected at first). Finally, because the fade is spread across a number of frames, the segment is considered to be a fade only if $t_e - t_s \geq 2$, otherwise, it is labeled as a cut.

### 23.6.3 Experimental Results and Discussion

The method was tested on several newscasts from the TRECVID 2003 reference video test set (see Table 23.3), containing video sequences of more than 6 h duration that has been digitized with a frame rate of 29.97 fps at a resolution of $352 \times 264$ pixels. We used spatially downsampled frames for our experiments, with a resolution of $176 \times 132$ pixels, in order to speed up calculations. The ground truth provided by TRECVID was used to assess the performance of this method.

The experimental tests for abrupt cut detection were performed by setting $N_W = 3$ and $\epsilon_c = 3.1$. The results are summarized in Table 23.4. The recall–precision curve obtained by changing the threshold $\epsilon_c$ is drawn in Figure 23.6. The elapsed time for obtaining results (abrupt cuts and fades) for a video sequence having 51,384 frames was 1,517 sec. Thus, the algorithm can operate in real time. The large majority of the cuts were correctly detected, even in the case of the video sequences that contain fast object and camera movements. Parts of some video sequences where a big object moves in front of the camera are often wrongly characterized as transitions by other methods, whereas this method correctly does not detect a transition in such cases.

The mutual information metric is significantly less sensitive to shot illumination changes (camera flashes), even in the RGB color space, compared to histogram-based methods. This is clear from Equation 23.10 and the properties of conditional entropy. In the case of histogram comparisons, the peaks produced by camera flashes are sometimes more significant than the peaks corresponding to cuts, and this can cause false detections.

**TABLE 23.4**

Shot Cut Detection Results

| Video | Recall | Precision |
|-------|--------|-----------|
| 6 debate videos | 1.00 | 0.99 |
| 4 CNN News | 0.96 | 0.96 |
| 4 ABC News | 0.97 | 0.94 |
| TREC total | 0.97 | 0.95 |

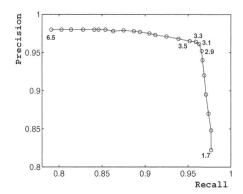

**FIGURE 23.6**

The recall–precision graph obtained for the shot cut detection method by varying threshold $\epsilon_c$ in the range [1.7, 6.5].

False cut detections were caused by artistic camera edits used in the commercials. Missed shot cut detections were caused mainly by shot changes between two images with similar spatial color distribution or in cases where the shot change occurs only in a part of the video frame.

The experimental tests for fade detection were performed using $\epsilon_f = 0.15$ and $T = 3$ for all video sequences. The results are summarized in Table 23.5. The recall–precision curve for fades obtained by changing threshold $\epsilon_f$ is shown in Figure 23.7. Using this setup, the fade boundaries were detected with an accuracy of $\pm 2$ frames. In most cases,

**TABLE 23.5**

Evaluation of Fade Detection by the Proposed Joint Entropy Method

| Video | Fade-ins | | Fade-outs | |
|---|---|---|---|---|
|  | Recall | Precision | Recall | Precision |
| CNN News | 1.00 | 0.84 | 1.00 | 0.84 |
| 4 ABC News | 0.93 | 0.90 | 0.92 | 0.92 |

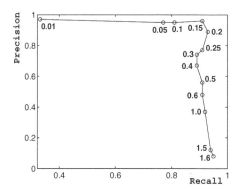

**FIGURE 23.7**

The recall–precision graph obtained for the fade detection method by varying threshold $\epsilon_f$ in the range [0.01, 1.5] and choosing $T = 3$.

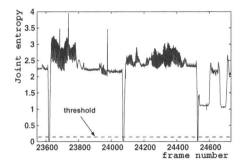

**FIGURE 23.8**
The joint entropy signal from "ABC News" video sequence having three fades.

the boundaries toward black frames were recognized without any error. An example of the joint entropy signal used for fade detection is presented in Figure 23.8. The use of joint entropy for detecting fades is robust (i.e., it does not produce a false detection) when big objects move in front of the camera and when blank frames exist in the video sequence. For the experiments, the threshold was set to a very low value to avoid false detections. Some fades were missed when noise appeared in a black frame or when the fading was not complete and the end frame was just very dark gray instead of black.

## 23.7 Shot Transition Detection Using Singular Value Decomposition

In this section, a method for automated shot boundary detection using singular value decomposition (SVD) will be briefly described. This method can detect all types of gradual transitions. A more detailed description of this method can be found in Reference [41].

The method relies on performing singular value decomposition on the matrix $\mathbf{A}$ created by the 3-D color histograms of single frames. Every video frame $f_i$ is represented by an $M$-dimensional normalized feature vector $\mathbf{a}_i$, with elements that correspond to the bins of the frame's histogram. The $M$-dimensional feature vectors of all the frames are used as columns to create the $M \times N$ matrix $\mathbf{A} = [\mathbf{a}_1 | \mathbf{a}_2 | \ldots | \mathbf{a}_N]$. SVD was used for its capabilities to derive a refined low-dimensional feature space from a high-dimensional raw feature space, where pattern similarity can easily be detected. The original feature vector $\mathbf{a}_i$ is projected from the $M$-dimensional feature space to a $K$-dimensional feature space, which is created by the eigenvectors corresponding to the $K$ largest singular values of matrix $A$ ($K \ll M$). Thus, each column vector $\mathbf{a}_i$ in $\mathbf{A}$ is mapped to a row vector $\widetilde{\mathbf{v}}_i^T$. The frame similarity measure is computed using the the cosine measure $\Phi(f_i, f_j)$ [42], [43] between two frames $f_i$ and $f_j$, that is the cosine of the angle between the vectors $\widetilde{\mathbf{v}}_i$ and $\widetilde{\mathbf{v}}_j$

$$\Phi(f_i, f_j) = \cos(\widetilde{\mathbf{v}}_i, \widetilde{\mathbf{v}}_j) = \frac{(\widetilde{\mathbf{v}}_i^T \cdot \widetilde{\mathbf{v}}_j)}{\|\widetilde{\mathbf{v}}_i\| \|\widetilde{\mathbf{v}}_j\|} \tag{23.16}$$

To detect video shot cuts, a dynamic clustering method is used to create the frame clusters. Frame feature vectors are clustered into $L$ frame clusters, $\{\mathcal{C}_i\}_{i=1}^L$, by comparing the similarity measure (Equation 23.16) between the feature vector of each frame and the average feature vector of the current cluster. The frames are considered in time order, and if the difference is above a threshold $\delta$, a new cluster is started. Each series of consecutive low cardinality clusters (i.e., having few frames) is considered to correspond to a shot transition. Conversely,

**TABLE 23.6**

Shot Detection Results Using the Method Described in Section 23.7

| | Cuts | | Gradual Transitions | | Global | |
|---|---|---|---|---|---|---|
| | Recall | Precision | Recall | Precision | Recall | Precision |
| Basketball | 0.95 | 0.98 | 0.85 | 1.00 | 0.93 | 0.98 |
| News | 0.93 | 0.90 | 1.00 | 1.00 | 0.96 | 0.94 |
| Teste | 1.00 | 1.00 | 1.00 | 1.00 | 1.00 | 1.00 |
| Football | 0.96 | 0.96 | 1.00 | 1.00 | 0.97 | 0.97 |

each large cardinality cluster (i.e., having many frames) is considered to correspond to a shot.

The proposed method was tested on several real TV sequences having many commercials in between, characterized by significant camera effects. In order to evaluate the performance of the method, recall and precision were used. Table 23.6 summarizes the recall and precision measures for cuts, fades, or other gradual transitions (dissolves and wipes) using $\delta = 0.98$ and $K = 10$.

## 23.8　Feature-Level Fusion

Finally, we describe a method for detecting shot boundaries in video sequences by fusing features obtained by singular value decomposition (SVD) and mutual information (MI), as detailed in Reference [44]. According to this method, for every frame $f_i$, a normalized 11-dimensional feature vector $\overline{\mathbf{w}}_i$ is created, by adding to the ten-dimensional feature vector $\widetilde{\mathbf{v}}_i^T$ obtained by applying SVD on frame $f_i$ one additional dimension that corresponds to the mutual information value $I_i$ between consecutive frames $f_i$ and $f_{i+1}$:

$$\overline{\mathbf{w}}_i = [\widetilde{\mathbf{v}}_i \ I_i]^T \quad i = 1, 2, \ldots, N - 1 \tag{23.17}$$

To detect video shot cuts, a two-phase process is used. In the first phase, the same dynamic clustering method as described in Section 23.7 is used to create the frame clusters. After the clustering phase, due to the fixed threshold used in frame feature clustering, it may happen that some shots are split into different clusters. To avoid false shot transition detections, the clusters obtained are tested for a possible merging in a second phase. Merging is performed in two steps applied consecutively. Because the time order of the frames is taken into account in every step, only two consecutive clusters are tested for merging.

The first frame cluster merging step is based on the fact that, if a frame cluster was erroneously split in two clusters (e.g., $\mathcal{C}_k$ and $\mathcal{C}_{k+1}$), the cosine similarity measure between the last frame in cluster $\mathcal{C}_k$ and the first frame in cluster $\mathcal{C}_{k+1}$ is comparable to the average cosine similarity measures of frames assigned to any of these clusters $\mathcal{C}_k$, $\mathcal{C}_{k+1}$.

The second merging step is based on statistical hypothesis testing using the von Mises–Fisher distribution [45], [46], which can be considered as the equivalent of the Gaussian distribution for directional data. The feature vectors in Equation 23.17, if normalized, can be considered as random samples on a $K$-dimensional sphere $S_K$ of unit radius around the origin

$$l_1 = \frac{\overline{\mathbf{w}}_1}{||\overline{\mathbf{w}}_1||}, l_2 = \frac{\overline{\mathbf{w}}_2}{||\overline{\mathbf{w}}_2||}, \ldots, l_n = \frac{\overline{\mathbf{w}}_n}{||\overline{\mathbf{w}}_n||} \in S_K \tag{23.18}$$

One can assume that the normalized feature vectors of frames that have been assigned to a cluster $\mathcal{C}_k$ follow a $K$-variate von Mises–Fisher distribution, with mean direction $\mu$ and

**TABLE 23.7**

The TREC2004 Video Sequences Used in the Experiments

| Video | Frames | Cuts | Fades | Dissolves | Other Transitions |
|---|---|---|---|---|---|
| CNN and ABC News | 307,204 | 1,378 | 117 | 758 | 126 |

concentration parameter $\kappa$ [45], [46]. A cluster merging approach is proposed, where the sample mean direction $\bar{\bar{I}}_k$ and $\bar{\bar{I}}_{k+1}$ of two subsequent shot feature vector clusters $k, k+1$ is compared with the mean direction $\mu_0$ of the cluster after shot merging. These shot clusters are then merged if neither of $\bar{\bar{I}}_k, \bar{\bar{I}}_{k+1}$ is significantly different from $\mu_0$.

The combination of features derived from these methods and subsequent processing through a clustering procedure results in very efficient detection of abrupt cuts and gradual transitions, as demonstrated by experiments on TRECVID 2004 video test set [47] containing different types of shots with significant object and camera motion inside the shots. The ground truth provided by TRECVID was used for evaluating the results. The corresponding data are depicted in Table 23.7.

By adding the mutual information and increasing the dimension of the feature vector, the clusters became better separable. Results verify that the proposed feature-level fusion method outperforms both the decision-level fusion and the SVD method with a recall–precision curve that is also depicted in the same figure (Figure 23.7). Table 23.8 summarizes the recall and precision rates obtained by the proposed method for cuts and gradual transitions, as well as for both of them using a threshold $\delta = 0.98$.

## 23.9  Conclusions

In this chapter, we presented an in-depth discussion of the shot boundary detection problem. We also presented a review of the most important work in the field in the last few years with emphasis on methods utilizing color information, including methods that were submitted to the TREC shot boundary detection task.

In addition, three methods devised by the authors were presented in more detail. The first method detects abrupt cuts and fades using the mutual information measure and the joint entropy measure, respectively, while the second uses SVD on frame color histograms, and the third improves on the other two by using the fusion of their results. These detection techniques were tested on TV video sequences having various types of shots and significant object and camera motion inside the shots, with very good results.

In conclusion, we can say that the video shot boundary detection has matured as a field, being able to perform not only simple cut detection but also the identification of gradual transitions with considerable recall and precision. This maturity is also evidenced by the development of a standard performance evaluation and comparison benchmark in the

**TABLE 23.8**

Shot Detection Results

| CNN and ABC News | Recall | Precision |
|---|---|---|
| Cuts | 0.95 | 0.93 |
| Gradual transitions | 0.86 | 0.85 |
| Overall | 0.91 | 0.89 |

form of the TREC video shot detection task. Available methods have advanced from being simply based on heuristic feature comparison to using rigorous probabilistic methods and complex models of the shot transition formation process. However, there is still room for algorithm improvement. Perhaps the ultimate solution of this problem will first involve an increasingly rigorous inclusion of the *a priori* information about the actual physical process of shot formation, and second, a thorough theoretical analysis of the editing effects, or even better a simulation of it.

## Acknowledgments

The presented work was developed within VISNET, a European Network of Excellence (http://www.visnet-noe.org), funded under the European Commission IST FP6 program.

The C-SPAN video used in this work is provided for research purposes by C-SPAN through the TREC Information-Retrieval Research Collection. C-SPAN video is copyrighted.

## References

[1]  A. Hampapur, R. Jain, and T.E. Weymouth, Production model based digital video segmentation, *Multimedia Tools and Appl.*, 1, 1, 9–46, March 1995.

[2]  R. Lienhart, Reliable transition detection in videos: A survey and practitioner's guide, *Int. J. of Image and Graphics*, 1, 469–486, September 2001.

[3]  R. Lienhart, Comparison of automatic shot boundary detection algorithms, in *Storage and Retrieval for Image and Video Databases VII*, Vol. 3656 of *Proceedings of SPIE*, December 1998, SPIE, Bellingham, WA, pp. 290–301.

[4]  I. Koprinska and S. Carrato, Temporal video segmentation: A survey, *Signal Process.: Image Commun.*, 16, 477–500, January 2001.

[5]  R.M. Ford, C. Robson, D. Temple, and M. Gerlach, Metrics for shot boundary detection in digital video sequences, *ACM Multimedia Syst.*, 8, 37–46, January 2000.

[6]  U. Gargi, R. Kasturi, and S.H. Strayer, Performance characterization of video-shot-change detection methods, *IEEE Trans. on Circuits and Syst. for Video Technol.*, 10, 1–13, February 2000.

[7]  W. Xiong, J.C.-M. Lee, and M. Ip, Net comparison: A fast and effective method for classifying image sequences, in *Storage and Retrieval for Image and Video Databases III*, Vol. 2420 of *Proceedings of SPIE*, February 1995, SPIE, Bellingham, WA, pp. 318–328.

[8]  P. Campisi, A. Neri, and L. Sorgi, Automatic dissolve and fade detection for video sequences, in *Proceedings of the International Conference on Digital Signal Processing*, A.N. Skodras, A.G. Constantinides, Eds., University of Patras, Santorini, Greece, vol. 2, July 2002, pp. 567–570.

[9]  A. Hanjalic, Shot-boundary detection: Unraveled and resolved?, *IEEE Trans. on Circuits and Syst. for Video Technol.*, 12, 90–105, February 2002.

[10]  L. Gu and D.K.K. Tsui, Dissolve detection in MPEG compressed video, in *Proceedings of the 1997 IEEE International Conference on Intelligent Processing Systems*, Vol. 2, October 1997, pp. 1692–1696.

[11]  D. Lelescu and D. Schonfeld, Statistical sequential analysis for real-time video scene change detection on compressed multimedia bitstream, *IEEE Trans. on Multimedia*, 5, 106–117, March 2003.

[12]  H. Zhang and S.S. A. Kankanhalli, Automatic partitioning of full-motion video, *ACM Multimedia Syst.*, 1, 10–28, January 1993.

[13] T. Volkmer and S. Tahaghoghi, RMIT university video shot boundary detection at TRECVID 2005, in *TREC Video Retrieval Evaluation*, NIST, November 2005. http//www-nlpir.nist.gov/projects/tvpubs/tv.pubs.org.html

[14] W. Heng and K. Ngan, An object-based shot boundary detection using edge tracing and tracking, *J. Visual Commun. and Image Representation*, 12, 217–239, September 2001.

[15] R. Zabih, J. Miller, and K. Mai, A feature-based algorithm for detecting and classification production effects, *ACM Multimedia Syst.*, 7, 119–128, January 1999.

[16] H. Yu and G. Bozdagi, Feature-based hierarchical video segmentation, in *Proceedings of the International Conference on Image Processing*, Vol. 2, IEEE, Washington, DC, USA, October 1997, pp. 498–501.

[17] S. Porter, M. Mirmehdi, and B. Thomas, Detection and classification of shot transitions, in *Proceedings of the 12th British Machine Vision Conference*, T. Cootes and C. Taylor, Eds., BMVA Press, Manchester, England, September 2001, pp. 73–82.

[18] J. Sánchez and X. Binefa, Shot segmentation using a coupled Markov chains representation of video contents, in *Proceedings of the Iberian Conference on Pattern Recognition and Image Analysis*, June 2003.

[19] Y. Qi, A. Hauptmann, and T. Liu, Supervised classification for video shot segmentation, in *Proceedings of 2003 IEEE International Conference on Multimedia and Expo*, Baltimore, MD, Vol. II, July 2003, IEEE, pp. 689–692.

[20] A. Miene, T. Hermes, G.T. Ioannidis, and O. Herzog, Automatic shot boundary detection using adaptive thresholds, in *TREC Video Retrieval Evaluation*, November 2003.

[21] R. Lienhart, Reliable dissolve detection, in *Storage and Retrieval for Media Databases 2001*, Vol. 4315 of *Proceedings of SPIE*, SPIE, Bellingham, WA, January 2001, pp. 219–230.

[22] A. Amir, J. Argillander, M. Campbell, A. Haubold, G. Iyengar, S. Ebadollahi, F. Kang, M.R. Naphadez, A.P. Natsev, J.R. Smithz, J. Tesic, and T. Volkmer, IBM research TRECVID-2005 video retrieval system, in *TREC Video Retrieval Evaluation*, November 2005.

[23] A. Nagasaka and Y. Tanaka, Automatic video indexing and full-video search for object appearances, in *Proceedings of the IFIP TC2/WG 2.6 Second Working Conference on Visual Database Systems II*, Stefano Spaccapietra, Ramesh Jain, Eds., Lausanne, Switzerland, January 1995, Chapman & Hall, pp. 113–127.

[24] J.M. Sanchez, X. Binefa, J. Vitria, and P. Radeva, Local color analysis for scene break detection applied to TV commercials recognition, in *Proceedings of the Third International Conference on Visual Information and Information Systems*, Amsterdam, the Netherlands, pp. 237–244, June 1999.

[25] M.J. Swain and D.H. Ballard, Color indexing, *Int. J. Comput. Vision*, 26, 461–470, 1993.

[26] Z.-N. Li, X. Zhong, and M.S. Drew, Spatial temporal joint probability images for video segmentation, *Patt. Recognition*, 35, 1847–1867, September 2002.

[27] W.K. Li and S.H. Lai, Integrated video shot segmentation algorithm, in *Storage and Retrieval for Media Databases*, Vol. 5021 of *Proceedings of SPIE*, Bellingham, WA, January 2003, pp. 264–271.

[28] R. Zhao and W.I. Grosky, Video shot detection using color anglogram and latent semantic indexing: From contents to semantics, in *Handbook of Video Databases: Design and Applications*, B. Furht and O. Marques, CRC Press, Boca Raton, FL, September 2003, pp. 371–392.

[29] X. Liu and T. Chen, Shot boundary detection using temporal statistics modeling, in *Proceedings of the 2002 IEEE International Conference on Acoustics, Speech and Signal Processing*, Vol. 4, May 2002, pp. 3389–3392.

[30] R. Zabih, J. Miller, and K. Mai, A feature-based algorithm for detecting and classifying scene breaks, in *ACM Multimedia*, January 1995, pp. 198–205.

[31] B. Janvier, E. Bruno, S. Marchand-Maillet, and T. Pun, Information-theoretic framework for the joint temporal partitioning and representation of video data, in *Proceedings of the Third International Workshop on Content-Based Multimedia Indexing*, Rennes, France, September 2003.

[32] Z. Cernekova, I. Pitas, and C. Nikou, Information theory-based shot cut/fade detection and video summarization, *IEEE Trans. on Circuits and Syst. for Video Technol.*, 16, 1, 82–91, January 2005.

[33] R. Ruiloba, P. Joly, S. Marchand-Maillet, and G. Quénot, Towards a standard protocol for the evaluation of video-to-shots segmentation algorithms, in *Proceedings of the European Workshop on Content Based Multimedia Indexing*, October 1999, pp. 41–48.

[34] W.J. Heng and K.N. Ngan, Shot boundary refinement for long transition in digital video sequence, *IEEE Trans. on Multimedia*, 4, 434–445, December 2002.

[35] J. Yuan, H. Wang, L. Xiao, D. Wang, D. Ding, Y. Zuo, Z. Tong, X. Liu, S. Xu, W. Zheng, X. Li, Z. Si, J. Li, F. Lin, and B. Zhang, Tsinghua University at TRECVID 2005, in *TREC Video Retrieval Evaluation*, NIST, November 2005. http://www-nlpir.nist.gov/projects/tvpubs/tv.pubs.org.html.

[36] J. Adcock, A. Girgensohn, M. Cooper, T. Liu, L. Wilcox, and E. Rieffel, FXPAL experiments for TRECVID 2004, in *TREC Video Retrieval Evaluation*, NIST, November 2004. http://www-nlpir.nist.gov/projects/tvpubs/tv.pubs.org.html#2004.

[37] G.M. Quenot, D. Moraru, S. Ayache, M. Charhad, M. Guironnet, L. Carminati, P. Mulhem, J. Gensel, D. Pellerin, and L. Besacier, CLIPS-LIS-LSR-LABRI experiments at TRECVID 2005, in *TREC Video Retrieval Evaluation*, NIST, November 2005. http://www-nlpir.nist.gov/projects/tvpubs/tv.pubs.org.html.

[38] T.M. Cover and J.A. Thomas, *Elements of Information Theory*, John Wiley & Sons, New York, 1991.

[39] A. Papoulis, *Probability, Random Variables, and Stochastic Processes*, McGraw-Hill, New York, 1991.

[40] I. Pitas and A. Venetsanopoulos, *Nonlinear Digital Filters: Principles and Applications*, Kluwer, Dordrecht, 1990.

[41] Z. Cernekova, C. Kotropoulos, and I. Pitas, Video shot segmentation using singular value decomposition, in *Proceedings of the 2003 IEEE International Conference on Multimedia and Expo*, Baltimore, MD, Vol. II, July 2003, pp. 301–302.

[42] C. O'Toole, A. Smeaton, N. Murphy, and S. Marlow, Evaluation of automatic shot boundary detection on a large video test suite, *The Challenge of Image Retrieval (CIR99) — Second UK Conference on Image Retrieval*, Newcastle, U.K., Electronic Workshop in Computing, February 25–26, 1999. http://ewic.bcs.org/conferences/1999/imageret/index.htm.

[43] F. Souvannavong, B. Merialdo, and B. Huet, Video content modeling with latent semantic analysis, in *Proceedings of the Third International Workshop on Content-Based Multimedia Indexing*, Rennes, France, September 22–24, 2003.

[44] Z. Cernekova, C. Kotropoulos, N. Nikolaidis, and I. Pitas, Video shot segmentation using fusion of svd and mutual information features, in *Proceedings of IEEE International Symposium on Circuits and Systems (ISCAS 2005)*, Vol. 7, Kobe, Japan, May 2005, pp. 3849–3852.

[45] K.V. Mardia, *Statistics of Directional Data*, Academic Press, London; New York, 1972.

[46] K.V. Mardia, J.T. Kent, and J.M. Bibby, *Multivariate Analysis*, 2nd ed., Academic Press, London, 1980.

[47] TREC Video Retrieval Evaluation, NIST, 2004. http://www-nlpir.nist.gov/projects/tvpubs/tv.pubs. org.html.

# 24

## The Use of Color Features in Automatic Video Surveillance Systems

Stefano Piva, Marcella Spirito, and Carlo S. Regazzoni

**CONTENTS**

## 24.1 Introduction

Today's occidental world is definitely characterized by critical security issues: the international tension and the fast development of information media has led to a present situation where almost no place can actually be considered safe. As a response to this new safety need, applied research has devoted and is devoting strong efforts to finding effective ways to raise security levels where possible. Among many technological solutions, one of the most important and actually applied is the replacement of human guardians with remote visual devices (video cameras) and the replacement of their reasoning capabilities with automatic systems to increase the coverage/personnel ratio and the supervision system effectiveness. With the spread of digital images and video, the core of these systems is automatic (color) image and video processing.

To provide a definition, an automatic video-surveillance (AVS) system can be defined as a computer system that, based on input data and provided by scene understanding capabilities, is oriented either to human operators' attention focusing or to automatic alarm generation. Video-surveillance systems have been developed since the 1960s, and the main technological innovation milestones outline a historical time line in the following four phases:

- *First generation (1960–1990)*: In this kind of system there is no information processing; acquired image sequences are merely transmitted over CCTV networks and displayed through black-and-white (B/W) TV monitors; scene understanding and decision tasks are completely performed by the human operator.

- *Second generation (1990–2000)*: Introduction of digital image conversion, centralized information processing and color images. The system shows acquired scenes and generates alarms helping human operators to face potentially dangerous situations.

- *Third generation (2000–present)*: Distributed digital signal processing. Only the information for signaling and describing a dangerous situation is presented to the human operator in effective symbolic language.

- *Beyond third generation (2004–present)*: Today's research for improved perception and reasoning over monitored events, extended communications, and interaction capabilities: new *Cognitive Surveillance* paradigm. Learning-based smart interactive systems with extended, multimode, and adaptive communications.

In recent systems, sensors acquiring input data from the observed environment can be heterogeneous and arranged in multisensor configurations. Multisensor systems can take advantage of processing either the same type of information acquired from different spatial locations or information acquired by sensors of different types on the same monitored area. Appropriate processing techniques and new sensors providing real-time information related to different scene characteristics can help to both extend the coverage area and to improve performances of danger detection in environments provided with multiple sensors. The highly variable scene conditions an AVS system is subject to imply the necessity of selecting robust scene description and pattern recognition methods that often take advantage of the use of vectorial color information, as will be described later in this chapter.

Automatic learning capabilities are an emerging issue in most advanced new-generation surveillance systems; in particular, unsupervised learning techniques are based on the collection of many heterogeneous input data useful to describe the situations of interest, and color features can often be important discriminating information in many related applications.

In this chapter, we will introduce the use of color in automatic video processing for advanced surveillance applications, pointing out advantages and, where present, drawbacks of the additional information provided by this feature. Going through the logical structure of an AVS system, we will investigate instances belonging to each processing level, to show in detail how color features can improve performances or can actually represent an alternative way to perform classification tasks.

The chapter starts with a brief revision of the state-of-the-art, intended to introduce AVS systems to the possible nonexpert reader. Section 24.2.1 provides the description of the common logical tasks performed by a general-purpose AVS system and follows the line of this architecture to cite the most common approaches developed so far to implement the single architecture modules' functionalities. Section 24.2.2 sketches the motivations to use color features in the introduced serial processing chain. Section 24.3 has the purpose of providing the reader with three examples to show actual solutions to some of many issues related to this kind of system: one algorithmic implementation is presented per each processing level to point out how chromatic features appear to be useful at different data abstraction levels. Section 24.4 draws some general conclusions.

## 24.2 Automatic Vision-Based Monitoring Systems

### 24.2.1 Color AVS Systems Logical Tasks

Usually an AVS system is used to monitor dynamic scenes where interaction activities take place among objects of interest (people or vehicles), and the system reacts to these events

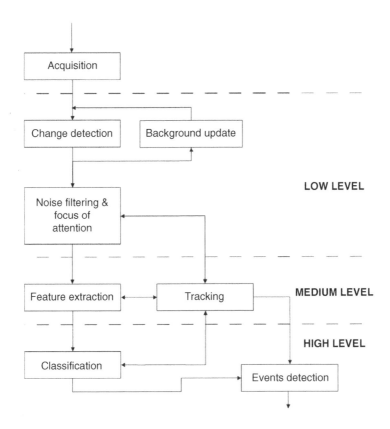

**FIGURE 24.1**
AVS logical architecture.

by rising alarm signals when needed. An AVS system must then be able to detect and track moving objects in order to analyze events. The architecture of an AVS system consists of several logical modules (see Figure 24.1).

A first way to analyze this kind of system is to consider image processing tasks as divided into three hierarchical levels:

- The processed data are pixels.
- Image areas are grouped to be identified as objects.
- An object's behavior is inferred through temporal analysis.

While low-level information deals with the property of the broadcast signal, middle-level information works considering data as objects. Meta-data extracted from the middle level are used in the high level in order to produce semantic information regarding the scene. At a finer resolution level, the AVS activity can be represented as a process performed by means of a modular architecture. If the system is endowed with memory, each module can exploit feedback data coming from following modules to enhance the information. Use of feedbacks presents advantages from an information point of view but has drawbacks from a processing time point of view.

In the following, we explore in detail the architecture modules going through the logical data flow shown in Figure 24.1.

First, an acquisition module directly interacts with sensors. The time employed by the system in order to acquire images places a limit on its performances. If the system uses gray-level images, the information acquired is a scalar value per each pixel of the CCD (charge-coupled device) sensing matrix, while using color cameras the acquired information becomes vectorial, each pixel is described by a vector of three values with different meanings according to color models. Thus, with color cameras, we collect a more complete description of the observed scene at the price of an increased amount of information to be processed.

After having acquired each frame, using static cameras, a robust change detection module is fundamental [1]: because processing image data is an extremely time-consuming and complex operation, it is necessary to reduce the amount of image data before any further processing, detecting the objects of interest. Usually one can assume to possess *a priori* knowledge about the background of the observed scene: in a fixed-camera surveillance system, a reference image (i.e., a frame representing the empty environment) is usually available (background image) to perform a change detection algorithm. This module is able to extract regions of the scene that present color differences with respect to the background image [2]. The output is a binary image with white pixels corresponding to the areas changed with respect to the reference frame.

To compensate for lighting changes or environmental modifications, the reference frame is not static, but a background update module takes care to renew background image when and where needed. A classical background updating algorithm involves a simple weighting operation for generating a new background at time step $k + 1$:

$$B_{k+1}(x, y) = I_k(x, y) + \alpha[B_k(x, y) - I_k(x, y)] \tag{24.1}$$

where $B(x, y)$ is the background image; $I(x, y)$ is the current image; $C(x, y)$ is the change detection output image; and $\alpha$ is the background updating coefficient. It is easy to understand that if $\alpha$ is close to 0, the background updating speed is extremely low, while if $\alpha \approx 1$, the background updating is very fast, with the risk of degrading the image with wrong information. When the guarded environment is rapidly changing (e.g., in outdoor environments), a good choice of these coefficients is very important.

In the filtering and focus of attention module, a morphological filter is applied to the change detection image in order to reduce noise. This operation performs statistical erosion and dilation by using a squared structural element [3], [4]. After, a nonrecursive region growing algorithm is used for finding connected regions in the change detection binary output image. The output of filtering and focus of attention module is a list of regions of interest (ROI) bounded by a set of related minimum bounding rectangles (blob). Each ROI corresponds to one or more moving objects detected in the scene. Usually, algorithms use a set of thresholds to decide whether to merge regions that are partially overlapped or near.

The feature extractor module receives as input the previously obtained list of blobs and outputs their features, such as geometric features (area and perimeter), position, and color-based features (e.g., blob color histogram). Some features are extracted in the image plane domain (e.g., color features and geometric features), others are extracted from the 2-D map plane (e.g., position and speed). Among image level features, a color histogram has the advantage of providing a compact information, rather independent from nonrigid objects' posture and from perspective variations.

At this point of the image elaboration chain, the AVS system has the objects' features data to start the tracking procedure. The goal of this task is to provide a relative association of the objects in a sequence, in terms of a temporally tagged list of attributes of object instances separately detected in successive frames. Different tracking algorithms can be used, as described in Section 24.3.2.

Once the objects in the scene are correctly detected and tracked, for the system, it is sometimes useful to classify them. The main task of a classification algorithm is to define a good decision rule for labeling unknown objects on the basis of information gathered from already classified objects [5], [6]. An *unsupervised* classification algorithm organizes data in structures as partitions or hierarchies by only considering the data. In particular, the self-organizing hierarchical optimal subspace learning and inference framework (SHOSLIF) [7] technique uses the hierarchy that decomposes the problem into manageable pieces to provide approximately an $O(logn)$ time complexity for a retrieval from a database of $n$ objects. The SHOSLIF algorithm has been proven to be a powerful classification and retrieval tool in image retrieval applications; but in the case of a video-surveillance system, one can suppose to classify moving objects, which are mainly pedestrians and vehicles, by inspecting the width-to-height ratio and considering that for a person this ratio is quite low if compared with the same ratio computed for a vehicle [8]. More complex and structured results can be obtained using other classification features (for instance, the objects' corners) bearing shape information [9]. Classification can cover many applications and can be useful as information to be sent as feedback toward the previous modules. A peculiar example of this classification information exploitation will be described in Section 24.3.3.

The last module — events detector — depicted in Figure 24.1, has the aim to provide a list of the events taking place in the scene along with a synthetic description [10], [11]. Abnormal events can be identified by comparing the current scene and a set of allowed situations. For example, this technique is used in traffic monitoring in order to analyze dangerous trajectories or in other applications in order to detect panic disorders analyzing optical flow.

Each of the described modules can be implemented in different ways, and in the literature there are many examples of this diversification. In the following, priority is given to algorithms exploiting color to ascertain the importance of this feature in AVS systems.

### 24.2.2 Color Features in AVS Systems

As stated in the previous section, the use of color in AVS systems increases the amount of information because of its three-dimensional (3-D) nature. In fact, a color model is a specification of a 3-D color coordinate system. Three instances of hardware-oriented color models are RGB (red, green, blue), used with color CRT monitors, YIQ (luminance, inter-modulation, quadrature), the broadcast TV color system, and CMY (cyan, magenta, yellow) for some color printing devices. Considering that none of these models is related directly to the intuitive color notions of hue, saturation, and brightness, the need for other color models has emerged; therefore, a perception-oriented class of models has been developed with ease of use as a goal. Several such models are described in References [12], [13], and [14]. The most used are HSV (hue, saturation, value), HLS (hue, lightness, saturation), and HVC (hue, value, chroma) color spaces.

In some applications, monochrome (black-and-white) processing is enough to assess the alarm condition; the objective of the processing task could be merely to determine the presence of a person or object in the scene. In other applications, the security objective of processing video scenes is to extract more detailed information.

Color cameras usually have lower resolution than black-and-white cameras. However, for some applications, the ability to recognize the color of clothing, the color of vehicles, and so forth is often more important than a more detailed image. For example, in the case of face detection schemes, skin color provides an important cue to achieve the goal [15], [16].

Another example of the important role of color is in shadow detection and removal; both in traffic surveillance systems and more generally in surveillance (airports, car parks, industrial areas), shadow detection is critical. The goal of algorithms for shadows detection is to prevent moving shadows from being misclassified as moving objects or part of them, and all of these algorithms rely on color features. Color is an important feature also widely used to track objects along time and for classification purposes.

We can say that vectorial color information has an important role in all the stages of advanced monitoring-purpose image processing; in the following section, some specific techniques exploiting chromatic properties are described as examples of each of the three listed processing levels of an AVS system.

## 24.3 Color-Based Processing in Video Surveillance Applications

In the following sections, we introduce three more detailed processing technique examples to show how the above-mentioned concepts are actually applied. The guiding choice is to represent an example per each level described in the logical architecture presented above: to represent low-level processing, an example about how color feature can be used to remove the annoying effects of shadows in the definition of the actual objects' boundaries; the representative example of middle-level processing describes the use of color to track objects and keep their relative identity over time; for what concerns high-level processing, the use of skin color detection as an instrument to correctly classify groups of people is presented.

### 24.3.1 Low-Level Algorithms: Filtering and Shadow Removal

In a surveillance system, the output quality of the focus of attention module is very important, because this processing step is devoted to defining number and position of the moving objects detected inside the monitored environment. In the ideal monitored scene, a region of interest should represent only one object; but in common AVS applications, this ideal system behavior is often affected by low-level processing errors due to occlusions, sudden lighting changes, and shadows. The latter problem is due to the fact that while human sight is able to distinguish noticeable objects from their shadows, in computer vision, a specific algorithm is needed to detect and remove shadows from the detected moving areas [17]. Shadows occur when an object partially or totally occludes an illumination source; the shadow projected by the moving object in the opposite direction of the illumination source is called *cast shadow*, while *self-shadow* is the portion of the object that is not directly hit by the illuminating light [18]. Shadows cause serious problems while segmenting and extracting moving objects due to the misclassification of shadow points as foreground. Shadows can cause object merging, object shape distortion, and even object losses (due to the shadow cast over another object). The difficulties associated with shadow detection arise because shadows and objects share two important visual features. First, shadow points are detectable as foreground points, because they typically differ significantly from the background. Second, shadows have the same motion as the objects casting them. For this reason, the shadow identification is critical for both still images and for image sequences (video) and has become an active research area, especially in the recent past [19]. In surveillance systems, the proper algorithms have the duty to locate cast shadows onto background image in order to let the focus of attention module output correct regions of interest. A video-surveillance system without this expedient considers moving shadows as parts of the moving objects, making mistakes in determining the actual bounding boxes. This misunderstanding causes errors in next processing modules: an object's shadow is very close to another object, the focus of attention module can fuse the regions of interest; moreover, the system can be led to misclassify tracking objects because of their wrong size. In other words, the accuracy of low-level modules is extremely important when designing simpler and robust classification modules.

Shadow removal techniques often use color features to distinguish foreground pixels from shadow pixels [20], [21]. A common and effective method is the one to rely on the luminance feature separation achievable through the use of perception-based color models, as described in Section 24.2.2. Most of the proposed approaches take into account the shadow model described in Reference [22].The main distinction among several state-of-the-art systems divides these techniques in deterministic approaches that use an on/off decision process, and statistical approaches using probabilistic functions to describe the class membership. Introducing uncertainty to the class membership assignment can reduce noise sensitivity. In the statistical methods (see References [23] and [24]), the parameter selection is a critical issue. Thus, the statistical approaches can further be divided into parametric and nonparametric methods. Also, the deterministic class [22], [25], [26] can be further subdivided considering whether or not the on/off decision can be supported by model-based knowledge.

Let us describe one of the algorithms present in literature and one of its possible improvements. It is supposed that shadows are projected on a flat surface and no restriction is made on the number and extension of light sources. Better performances are achieved when cast shadows are not interacting with each other. The method uses information detected in each color component in the image in a color space that is invariant with respect to the illumination changes. The method can be divided into two different steps: contour extraction and shadow region extraction. The used invariant color space model is the so-called $c_1c_2c_3$ space [27]. Each component can be computed as follows:

$$c_1 = \arctan\left(\frac{R}{\max(G,B)}\right) \quad c_2 = \arctan\left(\frac{G}{\max(R,B)}\right) \quad c_3 = \arctan\left(\frac{B}{\max(R,G)}\right) \quad (24.2)$$

where $R$, $G$, and $B$ are, respectively, red, green, and blue components in the $RGB$ color space. Contours extraction of the object plus its shadow can be performed by using $RGB$ components of the image. The edge map is obtained through two different steps: first, a Sobel operator per each color channel is applied, then a logical $OR$ is used for combining images obtained through the Sobel operator. The same step is applied in the color invariant space in order to extract an edge map not containing shadow contours. Obtained contours need to be improved and enlarged by using a morphological closing operator. By comparing extracted edges, the shadow removal module is able to classify and remove cast shadows.

Unfortunately, this algorithm [27] cannot work properly for some video-surveillance systems: considered objects can be very small, and this can heavily affect the result.

In order to solve this kind of problem, modified algorithms have been proposed (e.g., the one described in the following). By using the background image, it is possible to extract the binary change detection image representing each object in the scene together with its own shadow (Figure 24.2a). The currently acquired frame is then considered in order to extract contours with the Sobel operator from each color component. The obtained results are combined using a logical OR operator: the generated binary image represents object contours without cast shadow (Figure 24.2b). The application of a pixel-by-pixel logical AND operator leads to the generation of a change detection image without shadow that can be used as a basis for higher processing levels. Figure 24.3 shows a scheme of the proposed algorithm.

The proposed algorithm was tested by using outdoor images acquired during a sunny day. Examining the results shown in Figure 24.4, it can be easily understood how performances of a tracking system are greatly improved using the proposed shadow removal algorithm. A limit of the proposed algorithm is the fact that it is not designed to identify moving objects when shadow is superimposed with shadow zones belonging to the background.

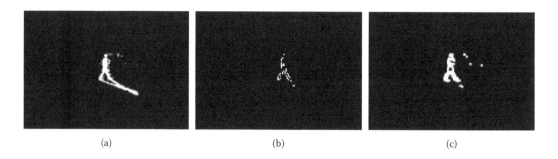

(a)                              (b)                              (c)

**FIGURE 24.2**
(a) Binary change detection output, (b) contours of the object without shadow, and (c) detected object after logical AND operator and a morphological dilatation step.

### 24.3.2  Medium-Level Algorithms: Object Tracking

One of the main problems of the existing video-surveillance systems is the loss of objects' identities in cluttered scenes. If a certain object is occluded by the superimposition of other objects, the tracks and the identities of the objects are lost most of the times.

As one of the main problems in this research field, relative identity objects association along time, is also one of the most studied and explored matter; nevertheless, there are

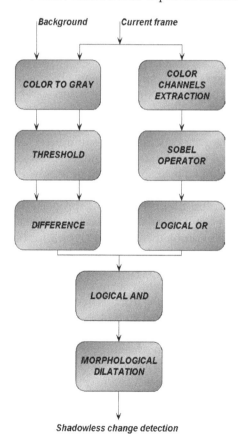

**FIGURE 24.3**
Logical scheme of the proposed algorithm.

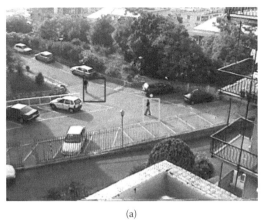 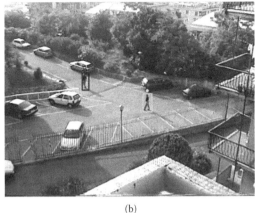

(a) (b)

**FIGURE 24.4**
(a) Object detection without shadow removal module; (b) object detection with shadow removal module.

so many different cases that several are still open issues, and the proposed solutions are countless.

We can classify tracking methods depending on the object attributes (geometric features and color features) to be tracked: they usually involve a phase of search for correspondences, followed by a phase of attribute estimation and regularization. Tracking methods are divided into four major categories: region-based tracking, active-contour-based tracking, feature-based tracking, and model-based tracking (this classification is not absolute in that algorithms from different categories can be integrated [5]). *Region-based tracking* algorithms track objects according to variations of the image regions corresponding to the moving objects [28]. *Active contour-based tracking* algorithms track objects by representing their outlines as bounding contours and updating these contours dynamically in successive frames [29]. *Feature-based tracking* algorithms perform recognition and tracking of objects by extracting elements, clustering them into higher-level features and then matching the features between images. Feature-based tracking algorithms can further be classified into three subcategories according to the nature of selected features: global feature-based algorithms [30], local feature-based algorithms [31], and dependence-graph-based algorithms [32]. *Model-based* tracking algorithms track objects by matching projected object models, produced with prior knowledge, to image data. The models are usually constructed off-line with manual measurement, CAD tools, or computer vision techniques.

According to the outlined classification, the approach described here can be identified as a global feature-based technique. It exploits objects' color histogram extraction and comparison for reassigning correct labels when the objects become visible again after an occlusion phase. If synchronized shots of the same scene from different points of view are available, it is possible to introduce a data fusion module able to refine the scene understanding using the knowledge coming from the processing of the images acquired from different sensors. The object's tracking procedure is based on a long-memory matching algorithm [33] that uses information from blobs extracted by the change detection and focus of attention modules. This operation is based on the features that characterize each blob extracted by the focus of attention module.

The main features of a blob are represented by color-based features (blob color histogram), geometric features (area and proportions of the bounding box), and position on the image plane. The relational link among consecutive instances of each blob along its temporal evolution is expressed by a label that indicates the status of that particular blob. In particular, at each frame, a blob list is filled with the features of the regions that have been found in that frame. Then the current list and the list coming from the previous frame are compared, and the tracking rule is responsible for finding blob correspondences. The comparison is performed considering the degree of overlapping between blobs in subsequent frames. If a blob has no correspondence in the previous frame, it is labeled as "NEW," and a new identifier is given to it. If it is possible to find just one blob that in the previous frame is partially overlapped with the one that is now considered in the current frame, then the blob is labeled as "OLD," and it inherits the identity of the blob that can be considered as its "father." If a certain blob in a certain frame has more than one father (i.e., it is possible to find more than one blob in the previous frame that is partially overlapped with it), the blob is labeled as "MERGED." However, in this case, the identities and the features of the multiple fathers are preserved within the merged blob. Finally, if more than one blob has the same father in the previous frame, two different possibilities can be considered. If the common father is labeled as "OLD" or "NEW," new identities are given to the multiple child of the blob: this basically means that a group of objects entered the scene in one unique group and they split into separated objects or group within the scene guarded by the system. On the other hand, if the father is labeled as "MERGED," it means that a group of previously isolated blobs splits again. In this case, the system is able to give to the splitting blobs the same identifier they had when they were previously detected. This operation is performed on the basis of the color histogram of the objects computed when they were isolated. The measure of the distance between the two histograms is based on the Bhattacharyya coefficient, with the following general form [34]:

$$\beta_{1,2} = \sum_{i=1}^{N_{bin}} H_1(x_i) \cdot H_2(x_i) \tag{24.3}$$

where $H1(\cdot)$ and $H2(\cdot)$ are the color histograms of the areas to be compared, and $N_{bin}$ is the number of color quantization levels used in the histogram computation (bins). A high Bhattacharyya coefficient indicates that the two areas are similar, and they can be identified as the same blob. Thus, if $H_i(k)$ is the color histogram of object $i$ at frame $k$, and $\beta_{i,j}(k)$ is the Bhattacharyya similarity coefficient of objects $i, j$ at frame $k$, the correct associations among objects belonging to subsequent frames $k - 1$ and $k$ is found through the following maximization:

$$max_{i,j}(\beta_{i,j}(k)) = max_{i,j} \left( \sum_{i=1}^{M(k)} \sum_{j=1}^{M(k-1)} H_i(k) \cdot H_j(k-1) \right) \tag{24.4}$$

with $M(k)$ number of objects detected in frame $k$.

An example of tracking and of the correct association obtained through color histograms matching is presented in Figure 24.5a to Figure 24.5c. As can be seen, after the occlusion phase, the two tracked people are identified again by the same object number.

Though not fit to manage heavy and long-time occlusion phases, the presented technique possesses the power of ease and of low computational cost: histograms are very light features to handle, and their comparison is fast. In many applications, the use of color alone or together with other position or shape-based features should be taken into account as a useful and easy instrument to track moving objects.

### 24.3.3 High-Level Algorithms: Classification and Grouped People Splitting

As previously stated in Section 24.2.1, classification in an AVS system is a high-level processing task, operating on symbolic and semantic data. This means that classification can appear in completely different forms in different systems. The following represents an original algorithm in which color model-based face detection is applied to detected moving areas to

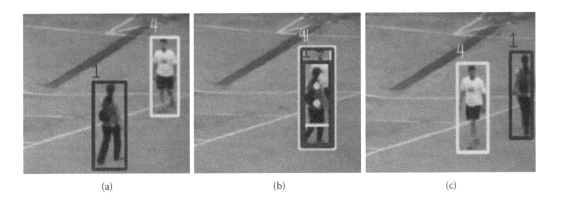

(a)                                    (b)                                    (c)

**FIGURE 24.5**
Color-based tracking example: (a) two people tracked walking one toward the other, (b) occlusion phase, and (c) histogram matching recovers correct relative identity after occlusion phase.

classify the actual number of individuals present in a compact people group. Skin-classified areas of pixels are further classified as faces through the verification of several additional conditions, in order to estimate number and position of people inside the analyzed group.

This application of groups classification represents a possible solution to a classical problem of background subtraction-based video processing algorithms: common techniques are not able to correctly manage the tracking of people entering the monitored scene as a compact group. Many works in literature dealing with groups tracking (e.g., References [35] and [36]) consider only the case of people meeting after having entered the observed environment as individuals and commonly splitting again. The use of skin-color-based classification can be of great help in solving this weakness.

First, we briefly introduce the widely studied topic of face detection techniques. Face detection algorithms can be basically classified in three main categories: template matching techniques [37], [38]; data analysis and representation-based techniques [39]; and neural-networks-based classifiers [40]. Many of these approaches rely at least as a prefiltering step on the hypothesis to locate a face in the processed image where a sufficiently wide area with pixel color that belongs to the common human skin color model is found. Recent years' research in this field demonstrated that the Caucasian human skin color has a clearly bound distribution in the three-dimensional RGB color space. Moreover and surprisingly dealing with color spaces where the luminance component is separated from the chromatic information, it appears that discarding the luminance, also African black human skin has the same chromatic distribution [41]. Then, it is possible to build a model collecting a proper amount of skin-colored image areas and approximate them with a probability density function as in Figure 24.6.

In this example, the distribution is obtained through the collection of about 1,300,000 skin pixels described in the $YCbCr$ color space according to the recommendation Rec601-1, [42]. The final model is the commonly used approximation with a Gaussian distribution. A better function to approximate this distribution should be a bimodal Gaussian function, but the simple Gaussian is often chosen as an easily manageable and sufficient solution.

Processing the target image and comparing each pixel with the model yields a likelihood value, and if the predefined threshold is exceeded, the single pixel is classified as "skin." Local properties can then help the classifier to locate connected skin areas and, to improve the result, obtain segmentation results as that presented in Figure 24.7a and Figure 24.7b.

This color-based technique allows the signal-level classification of skin areas, and further conditions can be applied to infer the actual presence of a face in the processed image.

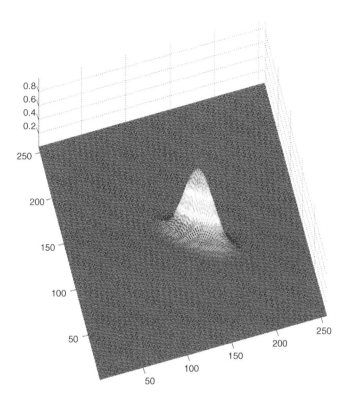

**FIGURE 24.6**
*Cb-Cr* skin color model Gaussian approximation.

To go a step further in the direction of the specific AVS application, we introduce how face detection can be employed to perform higher-level classification. The most moving object detection techniques are based on the change detection paradigm. As previously described in this chapter, connected change areas are then classified and treated as moving objects, and relative interferences, superimpositions, and occlusions are solved along time thanks to features storage of previously detected blobs and tracking. But in the unlucky case that two or more people enter the monitored environment too close to each other, change detection and focus of attention algorithms will classify them as a single blob, afterwards generating

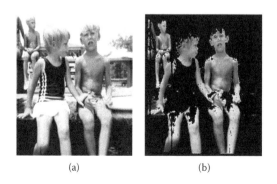

(a)                                    (b)

**FIGURE 24.7  (See color insert.)**
Example of color-based skin detection/segmentation: (a) original image, and (b) image after skin detection.

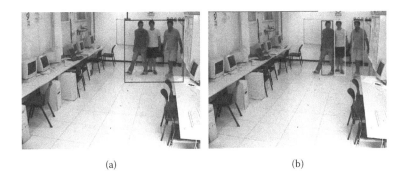

(a)                                    (b)

**FIGURE 24.8**
Object detection: (a) Incorrectly detected group of people; (b) correctly detected group of people.

"new blob" instances when they separate in the video-camera image plane domain (see Figure 24.8a and Figure 24.8b).

A possible idea to solve this problem is to detect faces inside the processed blob and locate the actual number of people contained in it. The first limitation is obviously due to the impossibility of seeing the faces of a group of people: if a person turns with his back toward the camera, it is not possible to detect his skin and an alternative feature must be used to correctly infer the number of people. There are many applications involving, for instance, people walking through a gate, where this approach achieves good performance. With simple conditions, it is possible to obtain, for the group incorrectly classified in Figure 24.8a, the correct classification of Figure 24.8b. This case is relatively simple, because the three people are at the same distance from the camera and appear to be of the same height on the image plane. This allows the system to obtain a correct result through the hypothesis that the candidate skin areas are faces if they are detected in the highest fourth of the change detection blob. For what concerns the bounding boxes, they are drawn with considerations about the distances among the detected skin areas centers of mass. This can solve strongly constrained situations, but it is not general enough for most cases.

Let us consider a more complex situation as the one described by the video shot depicted in Figure 24.9a to Figure 24.9c, where the wrong result of the classical change-detection-based focus of attention techniques is shown. This time the simple "highest bounding box part" constraint and the hypothesis of uniform heights are no longer valid, and their application leads to the result presented in Figure 24.10. Namely, the erroneous hypotheses

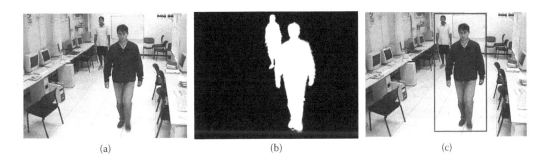

(a)                              (b)                              (c)

**FIGURE 24.9**
Classical change detection system: (a) input image, (b) change detection binary result, and (c) incorrectly classified group.

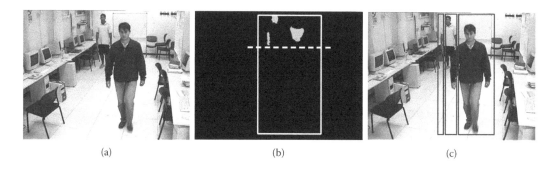

**FIGURE 24.10**
Simple skin color face-detection-based group classification: (a) input image, (b) height-based search area and confirmed face hypotheses, and (c) incorrectly classified group.

on faces positions force the system to classify the blob as a three-people group; the wrong condition on uniform height draws completely wrong bounding boxes.

Solving this kind of situation requires the association of several additional conditions to the skin color classification, including camera calibration-based height estimation and a set of constraints on human body proportions. By preserving the change detection information, we can verify the correctness of all the face hypotheses and achieve the result reported in Figure 24.11a to Figure 24.11c.

More precisely, given a calibrated camera and the model of the mean human height as a function of the position of the detected moving area on the map, the list of check operations to classify multiple people inside a change detection blob is as follows:

1. Detect moving area (change detection image)
2. Segment skin color areas
3. Estimate height and compute search height band
4. Skip out of bounds hypotheses
5. Estimate face area extension threshold versus height
6. Skip hypotheses below threshold
7. Check left hypotheses for body proportions in the binary change detection image

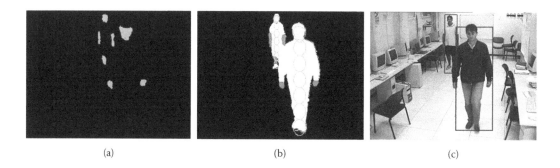

**FIGURE 24.11**
Joint skin color/camera calibration-based height prediction/human body proportions classifier using the input image shown in Figure 24.10a. The results correspond to (a) skin color face hypotheses, (b) face hypotheses verification — a person is seven heads high, and (c) final correct classification result.

**TABLE 24.1**

People Groups Classification Results

| Video Number | Length (Frames) | Actors | Correct Detections Ratio |
|:---:|:---:|:---:|:---:|
| 1 | 87 | 2 | 73.5 |
| 2 | 118 | 2 | 95 |
| 3 | 90 | 3 | 66.7 |
| 4 | 90 | 3 | 84.4 |
| 5 | 88 | 3 | 87.5 |
| 6 | 106 | 3 | 85.4 |
| 7 | 90 | 3 | 86.6 |
| 8 | 26 | 4 | 84.6 |
| 9 | 101 | 4 | 82.1 |
| 10 | 118 | 4 | 77.1 |

8. Estimate bounding boxes of the winning hypotheses

9. Remove confirmed areas from change detection image

10. Remove confirmed face hypotheses

11. If hypotheses $\neq$ {void}, process skipped hypotheses from step 3, else end

Table 24.1 reports some results obtained with this technique on ten different video sequences. Each video contains a group of people entering the scene as a single blob composed of two, three, or four individuals. The environment is an indoor laboratory (see Figure 24.8a and Figure 24.8b) where people are frontally shot by the camera: the face is always visible but several people wear short trousers or T-shirts so that many skin areas can be detected and evaluated by the system. The listed results are computed frame by frame: there is no exploitation of temporal constancy hypotheses, each frame is processed as a stand-alone picture, and the rate results refer to the estimation of the exact number of people. It is easy to understand how temporal regularization could raise these results toward 100 in similar conditions and provide good results in more difficult environments.

To draw some conclusions, the skin-color-based face detection technique can be of great support for blob classification in AVS applications. The easiest way to integrate this capability in a standard system, as the one described in Section 24.2, is to either locate people by using the face detection method or, when the detected face list is empty, go on locating them through the standard change-detection-based technique.

## 24.4 Conclusions

In this chapter, we tried to deliver the message of the actual usefulness of the vectorial color information in many aspects of the video processing chain of a general-purpose automatic video-surveillance system.

When exploring the state-of-the-art literature of this research field, it is not difficult to be convinced of the importance of color in enhancing the results of some processing tasks as well as in providing new solutions to several issues. Because of the limited pages available in a book chapter, it was not possible to describe all the aspects of the use of color features in image and video processing for surveillance application, or to compile an exhaustive list of the known techniques. The choice has then been to provide an overview of the advanced video-surveillance ongoing research, briefly describing a base logical architecture together with the main related known issues and literature solutions. This approach has been used as a guiding line for a deeper investigation of three specific techniques, representative of how color can be used at completely different data abstraction levels, along the serial processing chain: the shadow removal technique of Section 24.3.1 presents the use of color features in low-level processing as an effective improving solution for the filtering and focus of attention module; moving objects relative tracking along subsequent frames is described in Section 24.3.2 as an instance of medium-level processing; a particular use of skin color models to locate faces inside compact people groups for splitting purposes closes the examples inspection, with the aim of representing the high-level classification tasks.

## References

[1] C. Regazzoni, Recognition and tracking of multiple vehicles from complex image sequences, in *Road Vehicle Automation II*, O. Nwagboso, Ed., John Wiley & Sons, New York, 1997, pp. 297–306.

[2] G. Foresti and C. Regazzoni, A change-detection method for multiple object localization in real scenes, in *Proceedings of IECON (International Conference on Industrial Electronics)*, Bologna, Italy, 1994, pp. 984–987.

[3] J. Serra, Ed., *Image Analysis and Mathematical Morphology*, Academic Press, New York, 1982.

[4] A. Yuille, L. Vincent, and D. Geiger, Statistical morphology and Bayesian reconstruction, *J. Math. Imaging and Vision*, 1, 223–238, 1992.

[5] O. Javed and M. Shah, Tracking and object classification for automated surveillance, in *Proceedings of the Seventh European Conference on Computer Vision*, pp. 343–357, May 2002.

[6] Y. Zhai, Z. Rasheed, and M. Shah, A framework for semantic classification of scenes using finite state machines, in *Proceedings of the International Conference on Image and Video Retrieval*, Dublin, Ireland, Springer, 2004, pp. 279–288.

[7] D. Swets and J. Weng, Hierarchical discriminant analysis for image retrieval, *IEEE Trans. on Patt. Anal. and Machine Intelligence*, 21, 386–401, 1999.

[8] Q. Zang and R. Klette, Object classification and tracking in video surveillance, in *Proceedings of CAIP, Computer Analysis of Images and Patterns*, Groningen, the Netherlands, Springer, 2003, pp. 198–205.

[9] L. Marcenaro, M. Gandetto, and C. Regazzoni, Localization and classification of partially overlapped objects using self-organizing trees, in *Proceedings of the IEEE International Conference on Image Processing, 2003 (ICIP 2003)*, Barcelona, Spain, Vol. 3, September 2003, pp. 137–140.

[10] W. Grimson, L. Lee, R. Romano, and C. Stauffer, Using adaptive tracking to classify and monitor activities in a site, in *Proceedings of the International Conference on Computer Vision and Pattern Recognition — CVPR*, Santa Barbara, CA, June 1998, pp. 21–31.

[11] G. Foresti and F. Roli, Learning and classification of suspicious events for advanced visual-based surveillance, in *Multimedia Videobased Surveillance Systems. Requirements, Issues and Solutions*, G.L. Foresti, P. Mhnen, and C.S. Regazzoni, Eds., Kluwer, Norwell, MA, 2000.

[12] G.S.P. Commettee, Ed., *Status Report of the Graphics Standard Planning Committee*, Computer Graphics, 1977.

[13] Jablove and Greenberg, Color spaces for computer graphics, in *SIG-GRAPH*, Proceedings of the 5th annual conference on Computer graphics and interactive techniques, ACM Press, New York, NY, USA, 1978, pp. 20–25.

[14] G. Meyer and D. Greenberg, Perceptual color space for computer graphics, Proceedings of the *7th Annual Conference on Computer Graphics and Interactive Techniques*, Seattle, WA, ACM Press, New York, NY, USA, 1980, pp. 254–261.

[15] D. Maio and D. Maltoni, Real-time face location on gray-scale static images, *Patt. Recognition*, 33, 1525–1539, 2000.

[16] M. Abdel-Mottaleb and A. Elgammal, Face detection in complex environments from color images, in *Proceedings of ICIP (Internatational Conference on Image Processing)*, IEEE Press, 1999, pp. 622–626.

[17] C. Jaynes, S. Webb, and R. Steele, Camera-based detection and removal of shadows from inter-active multiprojector displays, *IEEE Trans. on Visualization and Comput. Graphics*, 10, 290–301, 2004.

[18] M. Kilger, A shadow handler in a video-based real-time traffic monitoring system, in *Proceedings of the IEEE Workshop on Applications of Computer Vision*, Palm Springs, CA, 1992, IEEE Press, pp. 11–18.

[19] A. Prati, I. Mikic, M. Trivedi, and R. Cucchiara, Detecting moving shadows: Algorithms and evaluation, *IEEE Trans. on Patt. Anal. and Machine Intelligence*, 25, 918–923, 2003.

[20] J. Wang, Y. Chung, C. Chang, and S. Chen, Shadow detection and removal for traffic images, in *Proceedings of the IEEE International Conference on Networking, Sensing and Control*, Vol. 1, 2004, IEEE Press, pp. 649–654.

[21] J.-W. Hsieh, S.-H. Yu, Y.-S. Chen, and W.-F. Hu, A shadow elimination method for vehicle analysis, in *Proceedings of the 17th International Conference on Pattern Recognition*, Cambridge, UK, IAPR, Vol. 4, August 2004, pp. 372–375.

[22] J. Stauder, R. Mech, and J. Ostermann, Detection of moving cast shadows for object segmenta-tion, *IEEE Trans. Multimedia*, 1, 65–76, 1999.

[23] I. Mikic, P. Cosman, G. Kogut, and M. Trivedi, Moving shadow and object detection in traffic scenes, in *Proceedings of the International Conference on Pattern Recognition*, IAPR, Barcelona, Spain, September 2000, pp. 321–324.

[24] M. Trivedi, I. Mikic, and G. Kogut, Distributed video networks for incident detection and management, in *Proceedings of the IEEE International Conference Intelligent Transportation Systems*, IEEE Press, Dearborn, MI, 2000, pp. 155–160.

[25] C. Jiang and M. Ward, Shadow identification, in *Proceedings of the IEEE International Conference Computer Vision and Pattern Recognition*, IEEE Press, 1992, pp. 606–612.

[26] D. Koller, K. Daniilidis, and H. Nagel, Model-based object tracking in monocular image sequences of road traffic scenes, *Int. J. on Comput. Vision*, 10, 257–281, 1993.

[27] E. Salvador, A. Cavallaro, and T. Ebrahimi, Shadow identification and classification using invariant color models, in *Proceedings of the IEEE International Conference on Acoustics, Speech, and Signal Processing*, Salt Lake City, UT, 7–11, Vol. 3, May 2001, pp. 1545–1548.

[28] K. Karmann and A. Brandti, Moving object recognition using an adaptive background memory, in *Time-Varying Image Processing and Moving Object Recognition*, Vol. 2, V. Cappellini, Ed., Amsterdam, the Netherlands, Elsevier, Amsterdam; New York, 1990.

[29] A. Mohan, C. Papageorgiou, and T. Poggio, Example-based object detection in images by components, *IEEE Trans. on Patt. Anal. and Machine Intelligence*, 23, 349–361, 2001.

[30] Q. Delamarre and O. Faugeras, 3d articulated models and multi-view tracking with physical forces, *Comput. Vis. Image Understanding*, 81, 328–357, 2001.

[31] B. Coifman, D. Beymer, P. McLauchlan, and J. Malik, A real-time computer vision sys-tem for vehicle tracking and traffic surveillance, *Transportation Res.: Part C*, 6, 271–288, 1998.

[32] W.F. Gardner and D.T. Lawton, Interactive model-based vehicle tracking, *IEEE Trans. on Patt. Anal. and Machine Intelligence*, 18, 1115–1121, 1996.

[33] A. Tesei, A. Teschioni, C. Regazzoni, and G. Vernazza, Long memory matching of interacting complex objects from real image sequences, in *Proceedings of the Conference on Time Varying Image Processing and Moving Objects Recognition*, 1996, pp. 283–286.

[34] T. Kailath, The divergence and Bhattacharyya distance measures in signal detection, *IEEE Trans. on Commun. Technol.*, COM-15, 52–60, 1967.

[35] S. McKenna, S. Jabri, Z. Duric, and A. Rosenfeld, Tracking groups of people, *Comput. Vision Image Understanding*, 80, 42–56, 2000.

[36] F. Cupillard, F. Bremond, and M. Thonnat, Tracking groups of people for video surveillance, in *Video-Based Surveillance Systems*, P. Remagnino, G. Jones, N. Paragios, and C. Regazzoni, Eds., Kluwer, Dordrecht, 2002, pp. 89–100.

[37] J. Cai, A. Goshtasby, and C. Yu, Detecting human faces in color images, in *International Workshop on MultiMedia Database Management Systems*, August 1998, pp. 124–131.

[38] D. Pramadihanto, Y. Iwai, and M. Yachida, A flexible feature matching for automatic face and facial feature points detection, in *Proceedings of the Fourteenth International Conference on Pattern Recognition*, Brisbane, Australia, August 1998, pp. 92–95.

[39]  B. Menser and F. Muller, Face detection in color images using principal components analysis, in *Seventh International Conference on Image Processing and Its Applications*, 1999, pp. 620–624.

[40]  F. Rhee and C. Lee, Region based fuzzy neural networks for face detection, in *Joint 9th IFSA World Congress and 20th NAFIPS International Conference*, 2001, pp. 1156–1160.

[41]  D.J. Kriegman and N. Ahuja, Detecting faces in images: A survey, *IEEE Trans. on Patt. Anal. and Machine Intelligence*, 24, 34–58, 2002.

[42]  S.L. Phung, A. Bouzerdoum, and D. Chai, A novel skin color model in ycbcr color space and its application to human face detection, in *IEEE International Conference on Image Processing (ICIP2002)*, vol. 1, Rochester, NY, USA, 2002, pp. 289–292.

# Index

T - #0044 - 101024 - C26 - 254/178/35 [37] - CB - 9780849397745 - Gloss Lamination